Jonathan Lytton

Handbook of Neurochemistry and Molecular Neurobiology

Neural Membranes and Transport

Abel Lajtha (Ed.)

Handbook of Neurochemistry and Molecular Neurobiology
Neural Membranes and Transport

Volume Editor: Maarten E. A. Reith

With 96 Figures and 22 Tables

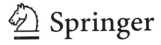 Springer

Editor

Abel Lajtha
Director
Center for Neurochemistry
Nathan S. Kline Institute for Psychiatric Research
140 Old Orangeburg Road
Orangeburg
New York, 10962
USA

Volume Editor

Maarten E. A. Reith, Ph.D.
New York University School of Medicine
Department of Psychiatry
Millhauser Labs, Room MHL-HN–604A
550 First Avenue
New York, N.Y. 10016
USA

Library of Congress Control Number: 2006922553

ISBN: 978-0-387-30347-5

Additionally, the whole set will be available upon completion under ISBN: 978-0-387-35443-9
The electronic version of the whole set will be available under ISBN: 978-0-387-30426-7
The print and electronic bundle of the whole set will be available under ISBN: 978-0-387-35478-1

springer.com

Printed on acid-free paper

SPIN: 11417514 2109 - 5 4 3 2 1 0

Preface

Neural membranes, as plasma membranes of other cells, are composed of lipids, proteins, and carbohydrates. In addition to a structural function for these membrane components, there is a functional role for them as (1) barriers, (2) transporters of ions or other solutes, and (3) receptors or recognition sites. This volume focuses on neural membrane constituents in terms of their functional role. The primary aim of *Neural Membranes and Transport* is to offer a comprehensive picture of the current body of knowledge on neural membranes with an emphasis on their function as barriers and transporters.

The first section of this volume deals with neural membranes and barriers. The main player highlighted here is the blood–brain barrier (BBB), which is covered from many different angles. Tight junctions are discussed, as well as developmental issues, modeling, pathology, astrocytes, and drug transport. There is coverage of P-glycoproteins in the BBB, and of the BBB as an efflux system. The section ends with a discussion of cholesterol, water movement, and endothelial peptide mediators.

The second section covers ion pumps and ion transporters in neural membranes. Sodium/calcium exchange in relation to calcium transport and glutamate excitotoxicity is discussed, as well as copper and zinc transport in the brain.

The final section covers neural membranes and transport of neurotransmitters or other solutes. Various plasma membrane transporters are discussed: GABA and other amino acids, and monoamine transporters. Vesicular transport of GABA, glutamate, acetylcholine, and monoamines is covered, as well as transport of glucose and peptides. Finally, synaptic vesicle recycling and efflux transport are discussed in regard to membrane function.

Each chapter has been put together by experts in the field who have experimentally contributed to advancing knowledge in the area; but coverage goes beyond describing the results of their own research. Rather, these chapters are reviews of the current status of knowledge in each area, aimed at informing the reader about the entire area.

My fascination with neuronal membrane proteins began during undergraduate work as a student in the laboratory of Dr. L.L.M. van Deenen, working on model membrane systems in the form of monolayers and bilayers at Utrecht, the Netherlands. It continued during a predoctoral fellowship at the Center for Neurochemistry in Strasbourg, France with the group of Drs. G. Vincendon, G. Gombos, and I.G. Morgan on purification procedures for plasma membranes from rat brains, during graduate studies on membrane fractionation under the guidance of Drs. D. De Wied, H.S. Jansz, P. Schotman, and W.H. Gispen, and during a postdoctoral fellowship at the Center for Neurochemistry in collaboration with Dr. H. Sershen under the guidance of Dr. A. Lajtha on interactions of nicotine and cocaine with brain membrane components. The latter work laid the foundation for my lasting interest in plasma membrane monoamine transporters. I am honored to be able to contribute to Dr. Lajtha's 3rd edition of the *Handbook of Neurochemistry and Molecular Neurobiology* as editor of this volume. In addition to expressing my gratitude to Dr. Lajtha, I would also like to thank Kristine Immediato for making it possible to edit *Neural Membranes and Transport* while at the same time moving my laboratory from the University of Illinois to New York University. The Internet version of this volume will be updated and will contain future additional chapters to make the subject matter more complete.

Maarten E.A. Reith, PhD
New York, October, 2006

Table of Contents

© Springer-Verlag Berlin Heidelberg 2007

Contributors

M. Adenot
Syntem, Parc Scientifique G.Besse, 30000 Nimes, France

S. Broer
School of Biochemistry & Molecular Biology,
Building 41, The Australian National University,
Canberra ACT 0200, Australia

E. R. Buck
Department of Neurosciences, Division of Neuroscience
Research, Medical University of South Carolina,
Charleston, SC 29425, USA

D. W. Busija
Department of Physiology and Pharmacology,
Wake Forest University Health Sciences,
Winston-Salem, NC, USA

R. P. Clausen
Department of Medicinal Chemistry, Danish University
of Pharmaceutical Sciences, DK-2100 Copenhagen,
Denmark

G. R. de Lores Arnaiz
Instituto de Biología Celular y Neurociencias
"Prof. E. De Robertis", Facultad de Medicina and Cátedra
de Farmacología, Facultad de Farmacia y Bioquímica,
Universidad de Buenos Aires, Buenos Aires, Argentina

M. A. Deli
Laboratory of Molecular Neurobiology, Institute of
Biophysics, Biological Research Centre of the Hungarian
Academy of Sciences, Szeged, Hungary

K. Ebnet
Institute of Cell Biology, ZMBE, University of Münster
Von Esmarch-Straße, D-48149 Münster, Germany

G. P. Eckert
Department of Pharmacology, ZAFES Biocenter
Niederursel, University of Frankfurt, Frankfurt, Germany

E. J. F. Franssen
Department of Pharmacy, Onze Lieve Vrouwe Gasthuis,
Amsterdam, Netherlands

M. Freissmuth
Center for Biomolecular Medicine and
Pharmacology, Institute of Pharmacology,
Medical University Vienna, Währinger Str. 13a, A-1090
Vienna, Austria

B. Frølund
Department of Medicinal Chemistry, Danish University
of Pharmaceutical Sciences, DK-2100 Copenhagen,
Denmark

B. Gasnier
Institut de Biologie Physico-Chimique, Centre National
de la Recherche Scientifique, UPR 1929, Université
Paris 7 Denis Diderot, 13 rue Pierre et Marie Curie,
75005 Paris, France

C. A. Grillo
Department of Pharmacology, Physiology and
Neuroscience, University of South Carolina School
of Medicine, Columbia, SC 29209, USA

M. A. Hediger
Institute for Biochemistry and Molecular Medicine,
University of Bern, Bern, Switzerland

N. H. Hendrikse
Departments of Nuclear Medicine & PET Research and
Clinical Pharmacology & Pharmacy, VU University
Medical Center, Amsterdam, Netherlands

U. Igbavboa
Department of Pharmacology, University of
Minnesota School of Medicine and Geriatric
Research, Education and Clinical Center,
VA Medical Center, Minneapolis,
Minnesota 55414, USA

L. D. Jayanthi
Department of Neurosciences, Division of Neuroscience Research, Medical University of South Carolina, Charleston, SC 29425, USA

A. J. Kastin
Pennington Biomedical Research Center, Baton Rouge, LA, USA

L. Kiedrowski
The Psychiatric Institute, Departments of Psychiatry and Pharmacology, The University of Illinois at Chicago, 1601 West Taylor Street, Room 334W, Chicago, Illinois 60612, USA

B. Kis
Department of Physiology and Pharmacology, Wake Forest University Health Sciences, Winston-Salem, NC, USA and Department of Physiology, University of Occupational and Environmental Health, Kitakyushu, Japan

P. Krogsgaard-Larsen
Department of Medicinal Chemistry, Danish University of Pharmaceutical Sciences, DK-2100 Copenhagen, Denmark

E. M. Lafer
Department of Biochemistry, University of Texas Health Science Center, San Antonio, TX 78229, USA

A. A. Lammertsma
Departments of Nuclear Medicine & PET Research, VU University Medical Center, Amsterdam, Netherlands

C. P. Landowski
Institute for Biochemistry and Molecular Medicine, University of Bern, Bern, Switzerland

O. M. Larsson
Department of Pharmacology and Pharmacotherapy, DK-2100 Copenhagen, Denmark

C. W. Levenson
Program in Neuroscience and Department of Nutrition, Food & Exercise Sciences, Florida State University, Tallahassee, FL 32306-4340, USA

A. Lippoldt
Deptartment Neurology, Schering AG Berlin, Müllerstrasse 178, D-13342 Berlin, Germany

W. Löscher
Department of Pharmacology, Toxicology, and Pharmacy University of Veterinary Medicine, Hannover, Germany; and Center for Systems Neuroscience, Hannover, Germany

G. Luurtsema
Departments of Nuclear Medicine & PET Research, VU University Medical Center, Amsterdam, Netherlands

J. Lytton
Department of Biochemistry & Molecular Biology University of Calgary, Calgary, Alberta, Canada

K. Madsen
Department of Pharmacology and Pharmacotherapy, DK-2100 Copenhagen, Denmark

P. Morin
Institut de Biologie Physico-Chimique, Centre National de la Recherche Scientifique, UPR 1929, Université Paris 7 Denis Diderot, 13 rue Pierre et Marie Curie, 75005 Paris, France

W. E. Müller
Department of Pharmacology, ZAFES Biocenter Niederursel, University of Frankfurt, Frankfurt, Germany

S. Nag
Department of Laboratory Medicine and Pathobiology, University of Toronto, Toronto Western Research Institute, University Health Network, Toronto, Canada

W. Pan
Pennington Biomedical Research Center, Baton Rouge, LA, USA

M. C. Papadopoulos
Departments of Medicine and Physiology, University of California, San Francisco, CA 94143-0521, USA and Academic Neurosurgery Unit and Basic Medical Sciences, St. George's, University of London, SW17 0RE, UK

G. G. Piroli
Department of Pharmacology, Physiology and Neuroscience, University of South Carolina School of Medicine, Columbia, SC 29209, USA and Department of Biochemistry, University of Buenos Aires School of Medicine, Buenos Aires, Argentina

H. Potschka
Department of Pharmacology, Toxicology, and Pharmacy, University of Veterinary Medicine, Hannover, Germany; and Center for Systems Neuroscience, Hannover, Germany

S. Ramamoorthy
Department of Neurosciences, Division of Neuroscience Research, Medical University of South Carolina, Charleston, SC 29425, USA

L. P. Reagan
Department of Pharmacology, Physiology and Neuroscience, University of South Carolina School of Medicine, Columbia, SC 29209, USA

M. E. A. Reith
Department of Psychiatry, New York University School of Medicine, NY 10016, USA

L. R. Reznikov
Department of Pharmacology, Physiology and Neuroscience, University of South Carolina School of Medicine, Columbia, SC 29209, USA

S. Rooker
Department of Neurosurgery, University Hospital Antwerp, B-2650 Antwerp, Belgium

S. Saadoun
Departments of Medicine and Physiology, University of California, San Francisco, CA 94143-0521, USA and Academic Neurosurgery Unit and Basic Medical Sciences, St. George's, University of London, SW17 0RE, UK

C. Sagné
Institut de Biologie Physico-Chimique, Centre National de la Recherche Scientifique, UPR 1929, Université Paris 7 Denis Diderot, 13 rue Pierre et Marie Curie, 75005 Paris, France

D. J. Samuvel
Department of Neurosciences, Division of Neuroscience Research, Medical University of South Carolina, Charleston, SC 29425, USA

B. Schlosshauer
NMI Naturwissenschaftliches und Medizinisches Institut Markwiesenstr. 55, 72770 Reutlingen, Germany

A. Schousboe
Department of Pharmacology and Pharmacotherapy, DK-2100 Copenhagen, Denmark

H. H. Sitte
Center for Biomolecular Medicine and Pharmacology, Institute of Pharmacology, Medical University Vienna, Währinger Str. 13a, A-1090 Vienna, Austria

Y. Suzuki
Institute for Biochemistry and Molecular Medicine, University of Bern, Bern, Switzerland

N. M. Tassabehji
Program in Neuroscience and Department of Nutrition, Food & Exercise Sciences, Florida State University, Tallahassee, FL 32306-4340, USA

Y. Ueta
Department of Physiology, University of Occupational and Environmental Health, Kitakyushu, Japan

B. N. M. van Berckel
Departments of Nuclear Medicine & PET Research, VU University Medical Center, Amsterdam, Netherlands

A. S. Verkman
Departments of Medicine and Physiology, University of California, San Francisco, CA 94143-0521, USA

J. Verlooy
Department of Neurosurgery, University Hospital Antwerp, B-2650 Antwerp, Belgium

H. S. White
Anticonvulsant Drug Development Program, Department of Pharmacology and Toxicology, University of Utah, Salt Lake City, Utah, USA

H. Wolburg
Institute of Pathology, University of Tübingen Liebermeisterstr. 8, D-72076 Tübingen, Germany

W. G. Wood
Department of Pharmacology, University of Minnesota School of Medicine and Geriatric Research, Education and Clinical Center, VA Medical Center, Minneapolis, Minnesota 55414, USA

Part 1

Neural Membranes and Barriers

1 Tight Junctions in the Blood–Brain Barrier

H. Wolburg · A. Lippoldt · K. Ebnet

Abstract: The blood–brain barrier (BBB) protects the neural microenvironment from changes of the blood composition. It is located in the endothelium, which is both seamless and interconnected by tight junctions. The restrictive paracellular diffusion barrier goes along with an extremely low rate of transcytosis and the expression of a high number of channels and transporters for molecules that cannot enter or leave the brain paracellularly.

Many tight junction molecules have been identified and characterized including claudins, occludin, zonula occludens protein-1 (ZO-1), ZO-2, ZO-3, cingulin, 7H6, junctional adhesion molecule (JAM), and endothelial cell-selective adhesion molecule (ESAM). Signaling pathways involved in tight junction regulation include G-proteins; serine, threonine, and tyrosine kinases; extra- and intracellular calcium levels; cAMP levels; proteases; and cytokines. Most of these pathways modulate the connection of the cytoskeletal elements to the tight junction transmembrane molecules. Additionally, cross talk between components of the tight junctions and the adherens junctions suggests a close functional interdependence of the two cell–cell contact systems.

The BBB endothelial cells are situated on top of a basal lamina, which contains various molecules of the extracellular matrix. Pericytes and astrocytes directly contact this basal lamina; however, little is known about the signaling pathways between these cell types and the endothelium, which possibly are mediated by components of the basal lamina. To analyze the interplay between astrocytes, pericytes, the extracellular matrix, and the endothelial cells is a big challenge for understanding the BBB in health and disease.

1   Introduction

The original finding of Ehrlich (1885) that an infused dye did not stain the brain tissue, together with the complementary observation of his pupil Ernst Goldmann that the very same dye if applied into the cerebrospinal fluid did stain the brain tissue, has lead to the concept of a biological barrier between blood and brain. Due to the free access of the dye from brain ventricle to brain tissue, it was concluded that there is no cerebrospinal fluid–brain barrier. However, the staining of circumventricular organs (CVO) and the choroid plexus, when a dye was applied into the general circulation (Goldmann-I-experiment), and the avoidance of staining of these organs, when a dye was applied into the cerebrospinal fluid (Goldmann-II-experiment), suggested the existence of a barrier between the cerebrospinal fluid and the blood. The cellular basis of these barriers was unclear for decades. Today, we know that in most vertebrates the barrier is located within the endothelium (endothelial blood–brain barrier (BBB); only in elasmobranchs, the BBB is located in astrocytes) and in the epithelial choroid plexus cells and the tanycytes of the CVO (glial blood–cerebrospinal fluid barrier (BCSFB) (❷ *Figure 1-1*).

The structure restricting the paracellular permeability is the tight junction, and this structure implies the necessity of transporters for substances that must overcome the barrier for providing the brain with energy-rich substrates. The BBB is only one part of a huge regulatory neurogliovascular machinery, which controls the blood flow and the delivery of oxygen and substrates to the brain according to continuously changing local requirements. The endothelial BBB is regulated by many more factors than all other endothelial cells outside the central nervous system (CNS). The reason for that is the enormous complexity of the consciousness producing brain and the complete dependency from blood perfusion. This situation makes it very difficult to analyze the network of causal relationships between the different components of the neurogliovascular complex. This brief overview tries to follow some lines of evidence that astroglial cells, together with the extracellular matrix between glial endfeet and the endothelium, manage the barrier properties of the BBB, which is primarily established by tight junctions under the control of the brain microenvironment.

2   The Astrocytes Inducers of the Blood–Brain Barrier

It is now generally accepted that the astrocytes play a decisive role in the maintenance if not induction of the BBB (Janzer and Raff, 1987; Raub, 1996; Abbott, 2002; Brillault et al., 2002; Engelhardt, 2003; Wolburg and

□ Figure 1-1

Scheme of the principle of barriers in the brain. The BBB is located within the brain microvessels. The barrier between the blood and the cerebrospinal fluid, the BCSFB, is located within the choroid plexus epithelial cells and the tanycytes of the CVO. The ependymal cells as well as the astrocytic endfeet at the glia limitans do not represent a physiological barrier

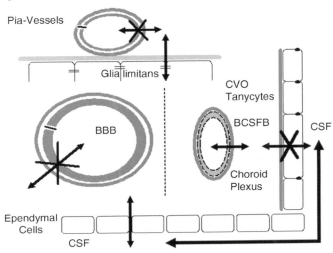

Lippoldt, 2002; Lee et al., 2003; Begley and Brightman, 2003). This concept came up along with experiments showing that astrocytes placed adjacent to endothelial cells in vitro or in vivo supported the development of barrier properties in the endothelial cells. Among the barrier properties tested in these experiments were transendothelial electrical resistance, paracellular permeability of electron-dense tracers, and the expression of barrier-related molecules. Although in vitro models of the BBB have the principal disadvantage of not being able to simulate the whole of the microenvironmental complexity of the brain, they frequently were successful in investigating regulatory mechanisms concerning glio–vascular interactions (Arthur et al., 1987; Méresse et al., 1989; Rubin et al., 1991; Tontsch and Bauer, 1991; Abbott et al., 1992; Wolburg et al., 1994; Stanness et al., 1999; Franke et al., 2000; Gaillard et al., 2001; Cucullo et al., 2002; Nitz et al., 2003; Parkinson et al., 2003). Hamm et al. (2004) demonstrated an increased transendothelial permeability for horseradish peroxidase (HRP) after discontinued coculture with astrocytes, but this change in permeability was not paralleled by a change in tight junction protein expression. The authors concluded that loss of localization of tight junction associated proteins from the BBB tight junctions might be a relatively late event, which is not yet observed in the comparatively short-term in vitro experiments. In vivo, a reversible disruption of tight junctions has been observed after transitory loss of astrocytes as induced by a single dose of 3-chloropropanediol (Willis et al., 2004). Loss of astroglia-derived glial fibrillary acidic protein (GFAP) went along with the fragmentation of occludin immunoreactivity. This observation was in line with experiments performed in GFAP-deficient mice in which an impaired BBB in vivo (Liedtke et al., 1996) or the failure of astrocytes from GFAP-deficient mice to induce BBB properties in aortic endothelial cells in vitro have been described (Pekny et al., 1998). Unfortunately, although close examination of the spatial relationship of glial cells and the expression pattern of GFAP made it tempting to speculate that cellular interactions between neurons, GFAP-expressing glial cells, and endothelial cells supported the establish-ment of barrier properties in endothelial cells (Gerhardt et al., 1999a), the mechanism of how GFAP-expressing glial cells perform this task is still completely unknown.

In an approach to identify factors that are involved in the induction of BBB properties, the glial cell line–derived neurotrophic factor (GDNF) was found to be successful in BBB induction (Igarashi et al., 1999; Utsumi et al., 2000; Yagi et al., 2000). The src-suppressed C-kinase substrate (SSeCKS) in astrocytes has been reported to be responsible for the decreased expression of the angiogenic permeability factor vascular endothelial growth factor (VEGF) and the increased release of the antipermeability factor angiopoietin-1 (Ang-1). SSeCKS overexpression increased the expression of tight junction molecules and decreased the paracellular permeability in endothelial cells (Lee et al., 2003).

An interesting correlation exists between astroglial differentiation and BBB maturation. The astroglial cells form processes to many compartments of the CNS including synapses, Ranvier nodes, and neural–mesenchymal borders at the surface of the CNS and around vessels. They are extremely rich in gap junctions that not only connect processes of different astrocytes, in particular, in the region of superficial and perivascular endfeet (❷ *Figures 1-1* and ❷ *1-2*), but also different domains of the identical cell (Wolff et al., 1998). The network of neurogliovascular interactions (the "neurovascular unit") is involved in manyfold metabolic dependencies between neurons and glial cells on the one hand and glial cells and vascular cells on the other hand (for a comprehensive overview on the neurovascular unit, see Iadecola, 2004). The direct interface between the neuroglial compartment and the vascular compartment is established by the perivascular glial endfeet, forming the glial limiting border (❷ *Figures 1-1,* ❷ *1-2,* and ❷ *1-4a*).

The membranes of astroglial endfeet are characterized by a very special molecular architecture. They not only carry plenty of transporters and ion channels but also the dystrophin–dystroglycan complex (Blake and Kröger, 2000), the water channel protein aquaporin-4 (AQP4) (Amiry-Moghaddam et al., 2004), the so-called orthogonal arrays of particles (OAPs) (❷ *Figures 1-2,* ❷ *1-3b,* and ❷ *1-4*) (Wolburg, 1995a), and a recently identified member of the immunoglobulin superfamily, limitrin (Yonezawa et al., 2003).

One of the most important physiological functions of astrocytes is the maintenance of the extracellular K^+ concentration after neuronal excitation (Orkand et al., 1966). In a series of classical experiments, Newman found in the retinal Müller cell as a model system of astroglial cells that the K^+ conductivity across the surface of the cell is heavily concentrated where the cell contacts the perivascular or the superficial glial limiting membrane (as reviewed in Newman and Reichenbach, 1996; Kofuji and Connors, 2003). The principle of spatial buffering (in the brain) or siphoning (in the retina) means that K^+ efflux takes place spatially apart from the site of K^+ influx effectively stabilizing the extracellular K^+ concentration. Later on, the inwardly rectifying $K^{\pm}$ channel, Kir4.1, was identified as one important member of K^+ channels, which

◼ Figure 1-2
Schematic view of the endothelial BBB. The processes of one endothelial cell (E) are interconnected by tight junctions (TJ). The endothelial cells are underlined by a basal lamina (BL), in which pericytes are embedded and at which astroglial endfeet (A) are attached. These glial endfeet are interconnected by gap junctions (GJ), and their membranes facing the perivascular basal lamina carry numerous OAPs, which were now identified as the water channel protein aquaporin-4

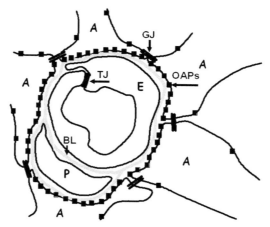

□ Figure 1-3
Schematic view of the distribution of some transporters and receptors at the BBB. A-system of amino acid transport as present in the abluminal membrane (AS), L-system of the amino acid transport (LS) as present in the both the luminal and abluminal endothelial membrane. Receptor-mediated transport (RMT), transferrin receptor (TFR), Insulin receptor (IR), P-glycoprotein (Pgp), orthogonal arrays of particles in the glial endfoot membrane (OAP), representing the site of the water channel protein AQP4, gap junctions (GJ) between astroglial cells (A), endothelial cell (E), pericyte (P), perivascular cell (PC), and microglial cell (M)

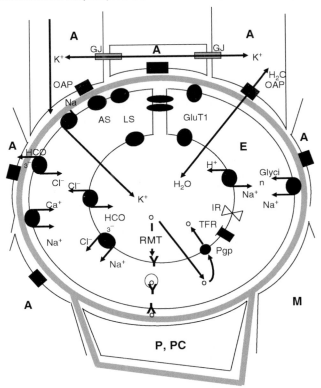

is highly concentrated at glial endfeet membrane domains and responsible for spatial buffering (Kofuji et al., 2002; Kofuji and Newman, 2004). In rodents, the K$^+$ channel is expressed in astrocytes surrounding synapses and perivascular endfeet around blood vessels (Higashi et al., 2001; Li et al., 2001a, b) (❷ *Figure 1-3*).

Interestingly, the distribution of the Kir4.1 channel protein and the K$^+$ conductivity is similar to that of the dystrophin–dystroglycan complex and the water channel protein AQP4 (Blake and Kröger, 2000; Amiry-Moghaddam and Ottersen, 2003; Connors et al., 2004; Nagelhus et al., 2004; Warth et al., 2005). In contrast, within the neuropil the parenchymal astroglial membranes do express these molecules to an essentially less extent. The polarization of astrocytes, which is related to the distribution of OAPs and the K$^+$ conductivity, arises concomitantly with the maturation of the BBB (Wolburg, 1995b; Nico et al., 2001; Brillault et al., 2002; Yonezawa et al., 2003; Nicchia et al., 2004). Regarding the OAPs, it is well-known that they contain at least the water channel protein AQP4 (❷ *Figure 1-4*). Aquaporins mediate water movements between the intracellular, interstitial, vascular, and ventricular compartments, which are under the strict control of osmotic and hydrostatic pressure gradients (Badaut et al., 2002; Papadopoulos et al., 2002). The involvement of AQP4 in the OAP formation was demonstrated by the absence of OAPs in astrocytes of the

☐ Figure 1-4

Electron microscopy of the BBB. (a) Ultrathin section of a mouse brain capillary. The *arrow* points to a tight junction (TJ) interconnecting two processes of an endothelial cell (E). The nucleus of the endothelial cell is at the left-hand side. The points mark the perivascular astroglial membrane, which is shown by means of freeze-fracturing in part b. (b) Freeze-fracture replica of a perivascular astroglial endfoot membrane from the mouse brain, studded with orthogonal arrays of intramembranous particles. (c) Freeze-fracture replica of microvascular endothelial tight junctions from the rat brain. The tight junction particles at the E-face (EF) and the P-face (PF) are roughly equal in density. This BBB-specific high association of tight junctional particles with the P-face is unique among all endothelial cells in the vasculature of the body. (d) Freeze-fracture replica of microvascular endothelial tight junctions from the rat brain cultured in vitro. The density of tight junctional particles at the PF is extremely low such as in non-BBB endothelial cells outside the CNS. Almost all particles of the tight junctions are associated with the E-face (EF)

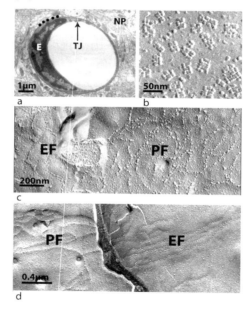

AQP4-deficient mouse (Verbavatz et al., 1997), by formation of OAPs in chinese hamster ovary cells stably transfected with AQP4 cDNA (Yang et al., 1996), and by the immunogold fracture-labeling technique showing that AQP4 is a component of the arrays (Rash et al., 1998, 2004). Moreover, Nielsen et al. (1997) were able to demonstrate by immunogold immunocytochemistry that the distribution of the AQP4-related immunoreactivity was identical to that of the OAPs. It should be stressed that AQP4 is the only member of the aquaporin family, which is associated with a membrane structure demonstrable by electron microscopy (❷ *Figure 1-4b*).

Under brain tumor conditions, the density of OAPs of astroglioma cells has been demonstrated to decrease (Neuhaus, 1990). However, the AQP4 content as detected by immunocytochemistry was increased (Saadoun et al., 2002) and the localization no more restricted at the perivascular endfeet but redistributed across the whole surface of the cell (Warth et al., 2004). These apparently conflicting findings can only be resolved, if one suggests that under glioma conditions AQP4 exists separated from the OAP in the membrane and is no more restricted to the glial membranes contacting the basal membrane. There was a positive correlation between AQP4 restriction at the endfoot membrane (polarization of the astrocyte) and presence of agrin in the vessel basal lamina (Warth et al., 2004). Importantly, the heparan sulfate proteoglycan agrin, an extracellular matrix component, does not bind to AQP4 but to α-dystroglycan

(Gee et al., 1994). AQP4 is connected to the dystrophin–dystroglycan complex via a *postsynaptic density* protein (*PSD*)-*drosophila* disc large-, zonula *occludens* protein (ZO-1) binding protein (PDZ)-binding domain in the C terminus of α-syntrophin (Neely et al., 2001). In human brain tumors, we previously have demonstrated a loss of vessel-associated agrin immunoreactivity, which correlated with loss of different tight junction molecules in the endothelial cells (Rascher et al., 2002). Taken together, we believe that loss of agrin reduces the OAP/AQP4-related polarity of astrocytes leading to a redistribution of "free" AQP4 outside the OAP structure, and this may be one reason for the loss of capability of the glial cell to maintain the BBB properties within the endothelial cell. This is also indirectly supported by the observations of Nico et al. (2003, 2004) and Vajda et al. (2004) who reported the loss of BBB integrity against HRP in a dystrophin-deficient (mdx) mouse. At the molecular level, this increased permeability was accompanied by a faint immunostaining against AQP4 in perivascular glial endfeet compared to controls and a diminished expression of GFAP and zonula occludens protein-1 (ZO-1). Moreover, ZO-1 immunoreactivity was missed at tight junctions; the claudin-1 distribution, AQP4 assembly, and the α-actin cytoskeleton were disturbed; and tight junction openings were observed. Together with our data, these data support our view that the intact α-dystrophin–dystroglycan–α-syntrophin–agrin complex is responsible for clustering AQP4 in polar astrocytes.

3   The Morphology of the Brain Capillary Endothelial Cell

Mature BBB capillaries in the mammalian brain are mainly characterized by the low height of endothelial cells, the interendothelial tight junctions (Brightman and Reese, 1969; for a review, see Wolburg and Lippoldt, 2002) (❷ *Figure 1-2* and ❷ *1-4a*), the small number of caveolae at the luminal surface of the cell (Peters et al., 1991), and the large number of endothelial mitochondria (Coomber and Stewart, 1985). In addition, subendothelial pericytes that are completely surrounded by a basal lamina, phagocytic perivascular cells, and astrocytic processes belong to the set of elements directly adjacent to the cerebral vasculature (Angelov et al., 1998; Balabanov and Dore-Duffy, 1998; Gerhardt and Betsholtz, 2003).

The microvascular endothelial cells are doubtless most important in the restriction of the BBB-related permeability. During brain angiogenesis and differentiation of the BBB, specific molecules have to be expressed in brain endothelial cells. Specific expression of the nonreceptor tyrosine kinase *lyn* (Achen et al., 1995) and gene products encoding P-glycoprotein have been demonstrated early during brain angiogenesis (Qin and Sato, 1995). Whereas the significance of *lyn* expression during brain angiogenesis is not clear so far, expression of P-glycoprotein is required for the differentiation of the BBB (Schinkel et al., 1994) and seems to ensure the rapid removal of toxic metabolites from the neuroectoderm before the BBB has fully differentiated (Begley, 2004). In the developing chicken CNS, it has been shown that angiogenic vessels invading the neuroectoderm express N-cadherin between endothelial cells and pericytes. With the onset of barrier differentiation, N-cadherin labeling decreased suggesting that transient N-cadherin expression in endothelial and perivascular cells may represent an initial signal, which may be involved in the commitment of early blood vessels to express BBB properties (Gerhardt et al., 1999b). The early adhesion between endothelial cells and pericytes might be the result of the release of chemotactic factors by endothelial cells to induce the migration of pericytes toward the endothelial cell wall and subsequent maturation of the vessels by an increased production of extracellular matrix components elicited by the action of activated TGF-β and other proteins (Folkman and D'Amore, 1996). Among these, platelet-derived growth factor (PDGF)-B, a high-affinity ligand for the receptor tyrosine kinase PDGF-Rβ present on pericytes is produced by endothelial cells during development. PDGF-B has been shown to be involved in vascularization of the brain as disruption of the PDGF-B gene leads to pericyte loss, endothelial hyperplasia, and lethal micoraneurysm formation during late embryogenesis (Lindahl et al., 1997). The fine structural investigation of endothelial cells in these PDGF-B-deficient and PDGF-Rβ-deficient mice showed a malformation of brain endothelial cells characterized by the folding of the luminal surface (Hellström et al., 2001). This increase in the luminal surface is also a typical feature of the blood vessels of the pecten oculi that is a convolute of vessels within the vitreous body of the avian eye. In these vessels, the pericytes die by apoptosis during development (Gerhardt et al., 2000). Thus, both the physiological loss of pericytes in the pecten oculi and the pathological loss of pericytes in the PDGF-Rβ-deficient mouse lead to a characteristic alteration of the shape of endothelial cells, suggesting a role for pericytes in the morphogenesis of microvessels.

Establishing the barrier is accompanied by further changes in the phenotype of the brain endothelial cells, such as upregulation of the HT/7-antigen/basigin (Seulberger et al., 1992) or downregulation of the MECA-32 antigen (Hallmann et al., 1995), besides the expression of specific transporters, and metabolic pathways can be observed (Pardridge, 1988, 1991; Mann et al., 2003). As far as the the development of the barrier function of brain capillaries is concerned (Wakai and Hirokawa, 1978; Risau, 1991; Stewart, 2000; Engelhardt, 2003), it has become clear that BBB tightness is not just "switched on" at a specific time point during brain angiogenesis but rather the tightening of the barrier occurs as a gradual process, which is independent from vascular proliferation and begins late during embryogenesis when angiogenes is not complete (Risau et al., 1986). The molecular mechanisms involved in this process are yet poorly understood. From transplantation studies showing that vessels derived from the coelomic cavity gain BBB characteristics when growing into an ectopic brain transplant (Stewart and Wiley, 1981), it is known that the development of BBB characteristics in endothelial cells are not predetermined but rather induced by the neuroectodermal microenvironment.

4　The Structure of Tight Junctions

The notion that tight junctions form an efficient permeability barrier originally came from electron microscopic tracer experiments (Reese and Karnovsky, 1967; Brightman and Reese, 1969). After intravascular perfusion of an electron-dense tracer, such as HRP or lanthanum nitrate, the diffusion of the tracer stopped where tight junctions interconnected endothelial cells or processes. The most important cells responsible for the establishment of the barrier are the capillary endothelial cells in case of the BBB (❷ Figures 1-1, ❷ 1-2, and ❷ 1-4a) and the epithelial (glial) cells in case of the BCSFB (❷ Figure 1-1).

In endothelial cells, these specialized contact zones were already known from ultrathin sections (Muir and Peters, 1962), and in epithelial cells, their morphology was described in detail by Farquhar and Palade (1963). Around the same time when the endothelial nature of the BBB was detected by Reese and Karnovsky (1967) and classically described in the comprehensive study of Brightman and Reese (1969), the freeze-fracturing technique was developed which allowed the cleavage of cytoplasmic membranes. Soon after its introduction, tight junctions were the issue of manyfold freeze-fracture descriptions (as summarized by Staehelin, 1974), including endothelial cell tight junctions of the BBB (Dermietzel, 1975a, b; Tani et al., 1977; Shivers, 1979; Nagy et al., 1984; Mollgard and Saunders, 1986; Wolburg et al., 1994).

If sectioned transversally in ultrathin sections, the tight junction appears as a system of fusion ("kissing") points, each of which represents a sectioned strand. If the tight junctional belt running around the apical circumference of the cell is broad in the apico-basal direction, the number of kissing points in ultrathin sections will be larger as if the belt would be narrow. If cleaved by freeze-fracturing, the tight junctions are visualized directly as a network of strands within the fracture plane of the apical membrane (❷ Figure 1-4c, ❷ 1-4d). Regarding this network, two parameters can be recognized: the complexity of strands and the association of the particles with the inner (P-face) or outer (E-face) lipidic leaflet of the membrane. The complexity of the tight junction network could be described as a logarithmic relationship between the number of tight junction strands and the transcellular electrical resistance (Claude, 1978). Concerning the P-face/E-face association, epithelial tight junctions are mostly associated with the P-face, forming a network of strands, leaving grooves at the E-face, which are occupied by only few particles (Martinez-Palomo et al., 1980; Madara and Dharmsathaphorn, 1985). After adenosine *triphosphate* (ATP) depletion, Madin-Darby canine kidney (MDCK) cells suffer from deterioration of the paracellular barrier ("gate") function, which is accompanied by a reorganization of the actin cytoskeleton (Mandel et al., 1993; Bacallao et al., 1994) and a decreased P-face association of the tight junctions. Taken together, the network complexity as well as the degree of particle association to the P-face seems directly to correlate with the observed transepithelial resistance.

The freeze-fracture structure of the brain capillary endothelial cell tight junctions was investigated by Nagy et al. (1984). The authors found the brain endothelial cell tight junctions most complex in the whole vasculature of the body. In addition, the BBB tight junctions were described to be unique among all endothelial tight junctions in that their P-face association is as high as or even slightly higher than their E-face association (Wolburg et al., 1994) (❯ *Figure 1-4c*). The P-face/E-face ratio of BBB tight junctions continuously increases during development (Kniesel et al., 1996). In cell culture, where the transendothelial resistance is much lower as in vivo, the freeze-fracture morphology of BBB endothelial cells is similar to non-BBB endothelial cells (❯ *Figure 1-4d*) indicating that the association of the strand particles with the membrane leaflets reflects the quality of the barrier and is under the control of the brain microenvironment (Wolburg et al., 1994; Liebnev et al., 2000a).

5 The Molecular Composition of Tight Junctions

In the last 10 years, the knowledge of the molecular composition and regulation of the tight junctions has rapidly extended (Furuse et al., 1993, 1998; Ando-Akatsuka et al., 1996; Morita et al., 1999a; Tsukita et al., 1999, 2001; Heiskala et al., 2001; Huber et al., 2001; D'Atri and Citi, 2002; Gonzalez-Mariscal et al., 2003; Matter and Balda, 2003; Dejana, 2004; Turksen and Troy, 2004) (❯ *Figure 1-5*, ❯ *Table 1-1*). Occludin and the claudin family are the most important membranous components both of which are proteins with four transmembrane domains and two extracellular loops.

5.1 Occludin

Occludin was the first tight junctional transmembrane molecule discovered (Furuse et al., 1993). It was initially isolated from junction-enriched membrane fractions of the chicken liver as a transmembranous tight junction protein of ∼65 kDa, which exists in several isoforms. Occludin shows high interspecies variability between chicken and mammals (Ando-Akatsuka et al., 1996), sharing less than 50% identity in amino acid sequence. In contrast, human, murine, and canine occludins are more closely related, showing ∼90% identity. Besides the high content of tyrosine and glycine in the first extracellular loop (∼60%), the most conserved region of occludin comprises the carboxy terminal ZO-1 binding domain, an α-helical coiled coil structure, putatively linking occludin to the cytoskeleton.

Surprisingly, the tight junctions in occludin-deficient mice (Saitou et al., 2000) were not affected morphologically, and transepithelial resistance as measured in small and large intestine epithelial cells was not altered compared to wild-type mice. However, the mice developed chronic inflammation and

❒ Figure 1-5
Model of the molecular composition of tight junctions (TJ) and adhesion junctions (AJ). PECAM platelet endothelial cell adhesion molecule. The G-protein connected receptor as marked "Rec" is postulated but not found so far. For further explanation, see text and the legend to ❯ Table 1-1

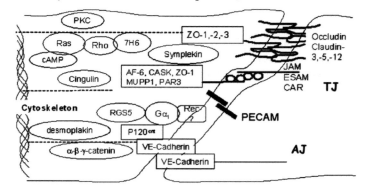

◻ Table 1-1

Molecular composition of tight junctions

Integral membrane proteins	Adaptor proteins first order (direct)	Adaptor proteins second order (indirect)	Signaling proteins	Regulatory proteins
Tight junction strand proteins				
Occludin	ZO-1, -2, -3	AF-6, cingulin	PI3-kinase, CK2, PKC	**Itch**
Claudins	ZO-1	AF-6, cingulin	c-Yes, Gα 12	ZONAB
(Cl-3, -5, -12)	ZO-2	cingulin		c-Jun, c-Fos, C-EBP, SAF-B
	ZO-3	PATJ, cingulin		
	MUPP1			
Ig-superfamily members				
JAM-A	AF-6, ZO-1 PAR-3, MUPP1	PAR-6	aPKC, PP2A Cdc42	
JAM-C	ZO-1, PAR-3	PAR-6	aPKC, PP2A Cdc42	
CAR	?	ZO-1		
ESAM	?			
JAM4	MAGI-1		Rap-GEF	
CLMP	?			
Crumbs homologs				
CRB1	Pals-1	PATJ, PAR-6	aPKC, PP2A Cdc42	
CRB3	Pals-1, PAR-6	PATJ, PAR-6	aPKC, PP2A Cdc42	
Unknown				
?	MAGI-2	JACOP	PTEN	
?	MAGI-3		PTEN, RPTPβ	
–	?		CGEF-H1	
–	?		Rab3B, Rab13	
–	–			huASH1
–	–			symplekin
–	–		Gαs,	
–	–		Gαi2	
–	–		Gα0	
–	–		Gα$_{12}$	
			RGS5	

The molecular components identified at tight junctions are grouped into different classes based on their structures and functions. The first column displays integral membrane proteins. The second column displays adaptor proteins and distinguishes between first- and second-order adaptors based on their direct or indirect association with the integral membrane proteins. The third column contains signaling proteins, which include tyrosine and serine/threonine kinases as well as heterotrimeric G-proteins, small GTP-binding proteins, and guanine-nucleotide exchange factors. Molecules in the fourth column include regulatory proteins such as transcription factors, transcription regulatory proteins, or proteins regulating posttranslational modifications. The inclusion of the molecules listed in the third and fourth column in the table is based on either their association with adaptor proteins or their localization at tight junctions. The mere association with a tight junction associated protein does not necessarily mean that the two proteins are associated at tight junctions. Actin-binding proteins, hyperplasia of the gastric epithelium, calcifications in the brain and around brain vessels, thinning of bones, postnatal growth retardation, testicular atrophy, and abnormalities in sexual behavior (Saitou et al., 2000). The authors concluded that occludin might have a function in tight junction modulation via the induction of intracellular signaling. Moreover, occludin is not required for the formation of tight junction strands. In a number of reports, posttranslational modifications of occludin, such as phosphorylation of its cytoplasmic domains or binding to a ubiquitin-ligase (Traweger et al., 2002), have been described as parts of tight junction regulation (Chen et al., 1997; Sakakibara et al., 1997; Balda et al., 2000; Huber et al., 2000; Hirase et al., 2001). For example, DeMaio et al. (2001) reported on a clear reduction of occludin content in cultured aortic endothelial cells by shear stress (10 dyn/cm^2) but a time-dependent increase of occludin phosphorylation, which could be attenuated by dibutyryl cAMP. An increase of occludin phosphorylation has also been described after treatment with VEGF (Antonetti et al., 1999), suggesting that hormonal and mechanical changes are able to increase the paracellular permeability by an early increase of occludin phosphorylation and a subsequent decrease of the occludin content. Taken together, it seems that mature cells need occludin to regulate rather than establish their barrier properties.

5.2 The Claudin Family

The claudins are the tight junction molecules that seem to fulfill the task of establishing barrier properties (Furuse et al., 1999, 2001; Morita et al., 1999a; Turksen and Troy, 2004) (❷ *Table 1-1*). Claudins share with occludin the overall organization with four transmembrane domains but have no sequence homology to occludin. The first claudins identified were isolated from chicken liver junctional fractions and were called claudin-1 and -2 (Furuse et al., 1998). Since then a number of related proteins have been identified and at present the claudin family contains more than 20 members (Mitic et al., 2000). It is now believed that claudins are responsible for the regulation of paracellular permeability through the formation of homotypic and heterotypic paired strands (for a review, see Tsukita et al., 2001; Turksen and Troy, 2004). In this model, ion selectivity is achieved through the selective expression and combination of distinct claudins in certain tissues (Tsukita and Furuse, 2000). Therefore, it is not surprising that the claudins are not randomly distributed throughout the organs but, at least, in part show a tissue-specific expression pattern. For example, claudin-5 was originally described to be restricted to endothelial cells (Morita et al., 1999b), although it was later found in surface cells of the stomach and of the large and small intestine also (Rahner et al., 2001). In addition, claudin-16 is selectively expressed in the thick ascending limb of Henle in the kidney, where it regulates selectively the permeability for Mg^{2+} ions (Simon et al., 1999).

Functional investigations support the view that the composition of the claudin species directly determines barrier function (Furuse et al., 2001). Tight junction–negative L-fibroblasts when transfected with claudin-1 or -3 form tight junctions, which appeared in freeze-fracture replicas associated with the P-face (Furuse et al., 1999). When transfected with claudin-2 or -5, the cells form tight junctions associated with the E-face (Furuse et al., 1998; Morita et al., 1999b). In contrast, occludin was found to be localized at both fracture faces (Hirase et al., 1997). Whereas occludin induced the formation of short strands, the claudin-induced strands were very long and branched resembling endogenous tight junctions (Tsukita and Furuse, 1999; Furuse et al., 1999).

such as cortactin, synaptopodin, or α-actinin-4, which associate with tight junction proteins and link the tight junctions to actin cytoskeleton are not included in the table. Molecules which are written in **bold** and ***italics*** were described to occur in the BBB AF-6, ALL-1 fusion partner from chromosome 6; *aPKC*, atypical PKC; *ASH1*, absent, small, or homeotic 1; *CAR*, coxsackie- and adenovirus receptor; *C/EBP*, CCAAT/enhancer binding protein; *CK2*, casein kinase 2; *CLMP*, coxsackie- and adenovirus receptor-like membrane protein; *CRB*, Crumbs; *ESAM*, endothelial cell-selective adhesion molecule; *GEF*, guanine nucleotide exchange factor; *JAM*, junctional adhesion molecule; *MAGI*, membrane-associated guanylate kinase inverted; *MUPP1*, multi-PDZ-domain protein; *Pals*, protein associated with Lin-7; *PAR*, partitioning defective; *PATJ*, Pals-1-associated tight junction protein/protein associated with tight junctions; *PI*, phosphatidyl-inositol; *PKC*, protein kinase C; *PP2A*, protein phosphatase 2A; *PTEN*, phosphatase and tensin homolog deleted on chromosome 10; *RGS*, regulator of G-protein signaling; *RPTP*, receptor protein tyrosine phosphatase; *SAF-B*, scaffold attachment factor-B; *ZO*, zonula occludens; *ZONAB*, ZO-1-associated nucleic acid-binding protein; *JACOP*, junction associated coiled-coil protein

Transfection of MDCK cells with claudin-1 increased the transepithelial resistance about fourfold and reduced the paracellular flux (Inai et al., 1999). Transfection with claudin-2 of high-resistant MDCK I cells that normally express claudin-1 and -4, mimicked both the resistance behavior and the tight junction morphology of low-resistant MDCK II cells (Furuse et al., 2001). Claudin-4 was formerly known as the *Clostridium perfringens* enterotoxin receptor (CPE-R). By treatment of MDCK I cells, CPE selectively removed claudin-4 from the tight junctions. Tight junctions were disintegrated to a simple network with only few anastomosing strands, and the transepithelial electrical resistance (TER) was decreased. After CPE removal, barrier properties were reestablished (Sonoda et al., 1999). These results suggested that the combination and stoichiometry of the claudins might be responsible for the outcome of a given resistance or permeability.

The claudins detected in endothelial cells were initially claudin-1 and -5 (Liebner et al., 2000b; Morita et al., 1999b). Later, claudin-3 and -12 were also found to be expressed by BBB endothelial cells (Nitta et al., 2003; Wolburg et al., 2003). Therefore, at least four claudins (claudin-1, -3, -5, and -12) are expressed by BBB endothelial cells.

Concerning claudin-5, the deficiency of this molecule as reported by the Tsukita group (Nitta et al., 2003) could be expected to compromise the quality of the BBB and therefore the viability of the animal. However, astonishingly the newborn knockout animals did not differ from the wild type in terms of macroscopic morphology, and even electron microscopy analysis did not reveal alterations in tight junctions. However, since a low-molecular weight tracer (e.g., Hoechst dye) and not the higher molecular weight tracer microperoxidase extravasated in the claudin-5 knockout mouse out of the brain vessels, it was concluded that the claudin-5 based tight junctions restrict the permeability for small molecules that are less than 800 Da (Nitta et al., 2003). Leaky rat lung endothelial cells transfected with a mutated claudin-5 (substitution of Thr^{207} by Ala) reconstituted a paracellular barrier against inulin (5 kDa) and mannitol. However, phosphorylation of the wild-type claudin-5 at Thr^{207} by cAMP was responsible for a rapid decrease in TER and loosening of the claudin-5–based barrier against mannitol but not inulin (Soma et al., 2004). Also a transfection of MDCK cells with claudin-5 increased TER and reduced the permeability to ions (Wen et al., 2004). These data together with the results reported by Nitta et al. (2003) could also suggest that other tight junction molecules, such as claudin-3 or -12, and their association with claudin-5 are responsible for the establishment of the paracellular barrier against low-molecular weight molecules.

Claudin-12, which was detected as a constituent of the BBB tight junctions, was postulated to be responsible to be selectively restrictive for molecules >800 Da (Nitta et al., 2003). The finding of Willis et al. (2004) that after a 3-chloropropanediol–induced transitory astrocyte loss, the barrier integrity to dextran (10 kDa) and fibrinogen (300 kDa) was reestablished earlier than the return of occludin and claudin-5, was unexpected under the assumption that occludin and claudin-5 would be responsible for the restriction of these proteins. Loss or reappearance of claudin-3 and -12 after the induced transitory astrocyte loss was not tested in this study. We should be aware of the concept of BBB tight junctional components as selectively regulated molecular sieves (Nitta et al., 2003), which may be important for therapeutic procedures in the future.

As mentioned earlier, claudin-3 and -5 if transfected into cultured fibroblasts are associated with the P-face and the E-face, respectively (Furuse et al., 1998; Sonoda et al., 1999). BBB endothelial cells in vivo reveal a P-face/E-face ratio of about 55/45 (Kniesel et al., 1996); as claudin-3 and -5 are well expressed, it can be suggested that the degree of association with the one or the other leaflet roughly reflects the stoichiometry of claudin expression in the tight junctions. In non-BBB endothelial cells, tight junctions are almost completely associated with the E-face, and claudin-3 is rarely or not expressed. BBB endothelial cells cultured in vitro develop tight junctions that are associated with the E-face (Wolburg et al., 1994) and express less claudin-1 (Liebner et al., 2000a, b); however, an antibody was used that is now known to recognize claudin-3 as well. Under pathological conditions, such as malignant glioma or experimental allergic encephalomyelitis (EAE), claudin-1 or -3 was found to be lost and/or the tight junctions were E-face associated (Wolburg et al., 2003).

5.3 Immunoglobulin-like Proteins at Tight Junctions

Almost simultaneously with the identification of claudins, junctional adhesion molecule (JAM) has been reported as the first member of the immunogloblin (Ig) superfamily to be present at tight junctions

(Martin-Padura et al., 1998) (❷ *Figure 1-5*, ❷ *Table 1-1*). JAM, which is now called JAM-A, localizes at homotypic cell–cell contacts of endothelial and epithelial cells and is highly enriched at tight junctions (Martin-Padura et al., 1998; Liu et al., 2000). Two Ig-like proteins closely related to JAM-A, JAM-B, and JAM-C have been identified (Palmeri et al., 2000; Aurrand-Lions et al., 2000). JAM-B and JAM-C are restricted to endothelial cells and are largely absent from epithelial cells. Although ultrastructural analyses for JAM-B and JAM-C in endothelial cell are still missing, the colocalization of JAM-C with occludin and ZO-1 (see later) upon ectopic expression in MDCK epithelial cells suggests its localization at tight junctions (Aurrand-Lions et al., 2001). Additional evidence for a role of JAMs in the formation of tight junctions is based on the observation that anti-JAM-A antibodies as well as soluble JAM-A negatively affect the formation of functional tight junctions after Ca^{2+}-switch–induced cell–cell contact formation (Liang et al., 2000; Liu et al., 2000) and the identification of cytosolic proteins which associate with JAMs and are implicated in the formation/function of tight junctions (see later). In this respect, it is interesting to note that JAM-A and JAM-B are expressed by Sertoli cells in the testis, where they could be involved in the formation and/or maintenance of the blood–testis barrier (Gliki et al., 2004).

Another role of JAMs in endothelial cells might be related to their predicted function in regulating leukocyte–endothelial cell interaction during inflammation through homophilic and heterophilic interactions (for recent reviews, see Johnson-Léger and Imhof, 2003; Muller, 2003; Ebnet et al., 2004). Originally, blocking JAM-A was found to inhibit leukocyte diapedesis in vitro and during inflammation in vivo (Del Maschio et al., 1999). However, there is a considerable body of evidence that leukocyte diapedesis must not follow the paracellular route but the transcellular route via a mechanism called emperipolesis (for overviews of both the classical transmigration studies and the recent literature, see Carman and Springer, 2004; Engelhardt and Wolburg, 2004). The transcellular mechanism as observed in EAE leaves tight junctions intact and implies a complex rearrangement of the luminal and abluminal membranes (Wolburg et al., 2005). This does not exclude that despite leaving tight junctions morphologically intact during transcellular transmigration, these junctions can molecularly be changed. In EAE, we demonstrated a selective loss of anti-claudin-3 immunoreactivity (Wolburg et al., 2003). This molecular alteration is associated with an increase in vascular permeability but not an opening of tight junctions for paracellular leukocyte diapedesis. If we, therefore, assume that transcellular migration of leukocytes delivers a signal to the endothelial junction—probably via the actin cytoskeleton—it is tempting to speculate that functional antibodies that "tickle" junctional molecules, such as VE-cadherin, PECAM-1, the JAM family, or CD99, might trigger these intracellular signaling cascades so that they increase or decrease endothelial mechanisms required for either transcellular or paracellular migration.

Four additional Ig-superfamily members have been identified at tight junctions (❷ *Table 1-1*). These include the coxsackie- and adenovirus receptor (CAR) (Cohen et al., 2001), endothelial cell-selective adhesion molecule (ESAM) (Nasdala et al., 2002), JAM-4 (Hirabayashi et al., 2003), and coxsackie- and adenovirus receptor-like membrane protein (CLMP) (Raschperger et al., 2004). They share with JAM-A, JAM-B, and JAM-C—a similar organization with two Ig-like domains. However, they are more closely related with each other than to the three JAMs and thus form a subfamily within tight junction–associated Ig-superfamily members (Ebnet et al., 2004). CAR, ESAM, and JAM-4 end in a type I PDZ domain-binding motif whereas JAM-A, JAM-B, and JAM-C end in a type II motif, which suggests functional differences between the two subfamilies. The function of these four Ig-superfamily members at tight junctions is not clear. CAR, JAM-4, and CLMP are predominantly expressed by epithelial cells, whereas ESAM is expressed exclusively in endothelial cells including those in brain capillaries (Hirata et al., 2001; Nasdala et al., 2002). Endothelial cells derived from ESAM-deficient mice display defects in endothelial tube formation suggesting a role for ESAM in endothelial cell contact formation (Ishida et al., 2003). How this function relates to its specific localization at tight junctions is not yet clear.

5.4 Peripheral Membrane Components at Tight Junctions

The transmembrane proteins associate in the cytoplasm with peripheral membrane components, which form large protein complexes, the cytoplasmic "plaque" (❷ *Figure 1-5*, ❷ *Table 1-1*). ZO-1, a 220-kDa phosphoprotein, was the first peripheral membrane component identified and characterized at tight junctions (Stevenson et al., 1986). In cellular systems with less elaborate or no tight junctions at all, ZO-1 is found enriched in regions of the adherens junctions (Itoh et al., 1993), where it may interact with components of the cadherin–catenin system (Rajasekaran et al., 1996; Itoh et al., 1997). Since the discovery of ZO-1, many further components of peripheral tight junction proteins have been described. One type of plaque proteins consists of adaptors, proteins with multiple protein–protein interaction domains such as SH-3, guanylate kinase (GUK), and PDZ domains (Vohno, 2001; Harris and Lim, 2001; Pawson and Nash, 2003). The adaptor proteins include members of the membrane-associated guanylate kinase (MAGUK) (Anderson, 1996) and membrane-associated GUK with an inverted orientation of protein–protein interaction domains (MAGI) (Dobrosotskaya et al., 1997) families, such as ZO-1, -2, -3, Pals-1, MAGI-1, -2, and -3, as well as proteins with one or several PDZ domains such as PAR-3, PAR-6, PATJ, and MUPP1 (Ebnet et al., 2001; Ohno, 2001; Hamazaki et al., 2002; Ebnet et al., 2004). The latter two proteins contain 10 and 13 PDZ domains (Ullmer et al., 1998; Roh et al., 2002), respectively, and thus seem to be particularly well suited to assemble large protein complexes. The adaptor proteins serve as scaffolds to organize the close proximity of the second type of plaque proteins, the regulatory and signaling proteins. These include small GTPases like Ras, Rab13, or Cdc42 (Hopkins et al., 2000), and their regulators, e.g., guanine nucleotide exchange factors (Benais-Pont et al., 2003), protein kinases, and phosphatases, such as atypical protein kinase C (aPKC), PP2A, and PTEN (Izumi et al., 1998; Wu et al., 2000; Avila-Flores et al., 2001; Nunbhakdi-Craig et al., 2002), as well as transcriptional regulators like ZO-1-associated nucleic acid-binding protein (ZONAB), huASH1, Jun, Fos, and the CCAAT/enhancer binding protein (C/EBP) (Nakamura et al., 2000; Balda et al., 2003; Betanzos et al., 2004). Furthermore, a new protein called JACOP (junction-associated coiled-coil protein) has been discovered. This protein has been found in the tight junction complex of epithelial and also endothelial cells and is suggested to anchor, especially, the junctional complex to the actin-based cytoskeleton (Ohnishi et al., 2004). JACOP has considerable sequence similarity to cingulin, another previously detected peripheral protein at tight junctions (Citi et al., 1989). In many cases, the role of the regulatory and signaling proteins in tight junction biology is still poorly understood, and it is expected that they are involved in completely different aspects of tight junction biology. The proteins of the PAR-3–aPKC–PAR-6 complex are most likely involved in the regulation of tight junction formation and establishment of cell polarity since overexpression of dominant-negative mutants of these proteins lead to a delayed tight junction formation (Suzuki et al., 2001; Gao et al., 2002; Nagai-Tamai et al., 2002). In addition, when dominant-negative mutants of the PAR-3 ligand JAM-A are overexpressed in epithelial cells, this leads to a delay in tight junction formation and to defects in the establishment of cell polarity (Rehder D and Ebnet K, unpublished results 1918. Both JAM-A and PAR-3 localize to cell–cell contacts of endothelial cells (Ebnet et al., 2003), and therefore it is conceivable that the formation of tight junctions is similarly regulated by JAM-A and the PAR-3–aPKC–PAR-6 complex. Other proteins present at tight junctions might be necessary for signaling to the cell interior, for example, the transcription factors ZONAB and huAsh1. Information on the maturation state of cell–cell contacts is required for many cellular events, which are regulated by cell density (e.g., proliferation), and transcription factors associated with the cytoplasmic plaque at tight junction provide a direct link between tight junctions and the nucleus (Matter and Balda, 2003).

The vast majority of experiments addressing the role of tight junction–associated proteins for tight junction biology were performed with epithelial cells. Our knowledge about their role in tight junction formation in endothelial cells, and in particular those in the BBB, is still limited. However, it is expected that the principal mechanisms underlying tight junction formation operate in both cellular systems in a similar way.

6   Regulatory Mechanisms in the Blood–Brain Barrier

Tight junctions have long been considered as static barriers responsible for both the compartmentalization of the intercellular cleft (gate function) and the polarity of cell (fence function). But in the last years, it came out that the tight junctions are under the control of multiple regulatory systems in which many molecular systems, such as adhesion molecules, extracellular matrix components, and signal transduction pathways, are involved (Matter and Balda, 2003; Sheth et al., 2003). Most data were gathered in epithelial cells. In endothelial cells, in particular in those of the BBB, less data are available, probably due to the fact that the system is considerably more complex as it includes pericytes and astrocytes, a special composition of the extracellular matrix, and not well established in vitro.

6.1 G-Protein Signaling

G-proteins play an essential role in maintaining barrier integrity of epithelial cells (Matter and Balda, 2003). The G-proteins involved are the classical heterotrimeric G-proteins and the small G-proteins/small GTPases (Ras superfamily). Several $G\alpha$ subunits have been localized within the tight junctions of cultured epithelial cells, such as $G\alpha_{i2}$ (Denker et al., 1996), $G\alpha s$ (Dodane and Kachar, 1996), $G\alpha_{12}$ (Dodane and Kachar, 1996), and $G\alpha_O$, when transfected into MDCK cells (Nakamura et al., 2000). Moreover, $G\alpha_O$ (Denker et al., 1996) and $G\alpha_{12}$ (Meyer et al., 2002) could be coprecipitated with ZO-1. The activation of heterotrimeric G-proteins leads to activation of second messengers like cAMP/cGMP or Ca^{2+} and to an increased transepithelial resistance of the cell monolayer. Additionally, $G\alpha_O$ accelerated tight junction biogenesis, whereas $G\alpha_{i2}$ was important for development and maintenance of the tight junctions (Denker and Nigam, 1998; Saha et al., 2001). $G\alpha_{12}$, in contrast, has been demonstrated to be involved in the tight junction maintenance in part through Src tyrosine kinase pathways. A constitutively active $G\alpha_{12}$ disrupted adherens and tight junctions and increased actin stress fibers leading to increased paracellular permeability in MDCK cells (Meyer et al., 2003). The inhibition of the protein kinase A (PKA) has been shown to result in the preservation of tight junctions and low permeability in MDCK cells during removal of calcium (Klingler et al., 2000), suggesting that in epithelial cells the PKA could be involved in the destabilization of tight junctions (Balda et al., 1991). As activated $G\alpha_i$ evokes a decrease in cAMP and thus probably a decrease in the amount of activated PKA, G-protein signaling could influence epithelial permeability via inhibiting the cAMP/PKA-pathway. In contrast, in endothelial cells, elevation of cAMP by forskolin resulted in a stabilization of tight junctions and decrease of permeability (Rubin et al., 1991; Wolburg et al., 1994; Raub, 1996). Accordingly, elevation of cAMP by forskolin or cholera toxin was able to reverse the permeability increasing effect of pertussis toxin (PTX) on cerebral endothelial cells in vitro (Brückener et al., 2003). PTX is known to inhibit G-protein signaling by ADP-ribosylation of $G\alpha_i$ proteins. The pathway by which PTX permeabilized the barrier was shown to include the PKC (Brückener et al., 2003), probably by operating via extracellular signal-regulated kinase (ERK) activation (Garcia et al., 2001).

A family of G-protein signaling regulating proteins has been identified. These so-called RGS proteins (regulators of G-protein signaling) interact with the $G\alpha$ subunit of heterotrimeric G-proteins (❷ Figure 1-5). They inactivate the $G\alpha$ subunit by accelerating GTP hydrolysis (De Vries and Farquahr, 1999). A genomic suppression subtractive hybridization (SSH) approach has been used to identify specific genes expressed at the BBB (Li et al., 2001a, b). Among other genes, RGS5 was found to be expressed at the BBB and also in other tissues. By using the same approach in hypertensive rats, the RGS5 mRNA was identified in isolated brain capillaries and localized in the BBB endothelial cells (Kirsch et al., 2001) (❷ Figure 1-5). Immunocytochemical detection of RGS5 at the light and electron microscope level revealed its occurrence in tight junctions of BBB endothelial cells (Lippoldt et al., in preparation). In an in vitro model of capillary morphogenesis using human umbilical vein endothelial cells (HUVECs), RGS5 was mostly downregulated during the time of extensive branching (Bell et al., 2001) pointing to its importance in endothelial cell differentiation. However, the function of RGS5 in endothelial cells or the signaling pathway RGS5 is acting on is not yet clear. The G-protein connected receptor as marked in ❷ Figure 1-5 as "Rec" is postulated but not found so far.

6.2 Small GTPases

The RhoA and Rac1 small GTPases were shown to play a promoting role in the regulation of tight and adhesion junction structure and function (Adamson et al., 2002; Van Hinsbergh et al., 2002; Matter and Balda, 2003) (❷ Figure 1-5). In MDCK-cells expressing RhoA and Rac1 mutants, the organization of tight junctions is disturbed and the permeability for inulin, anionic or neutral dextran increased and the TER decreased (Jou and Nelson, 1998; Jou et al., 1998). At the molecular level, the GTPases RhoA, Rac1, and Cdc42 promoted the internalization of the tight junction transmembrane molecules occludin, claudin-1 and -2, JAM-1, and ZO-1 depending on their activation status and in a GTPase specific manner (Bruewer et al., 2004). In T84 cells, the inhibition of the Rho pathway by *Clostridium botulinum* toxin C3 transferase resulted in a disorganization of the perijunctional actin ring and ZO-1 distribution, whereas the transient expression of RhoC resulted in actin concentration at intercellular contacts (Nusrat et al., 1995). On the other hand, *Escherichia coli* cytotoxic necrotizing factor-1 (CNF-1) activated the Rho pathway but reduced the gate function of tight junctions in T84 cells and impaired tight junction assembly in the calcium switch assay (Hopkins et al., 2002) by occludin and caveolin-1 internalization in endosomal-caveolar–like structures and ZO-1 and JAM-1 displacement from the tight junctions (Hopkins et al., 2003). In addition, a guanine nucleotide exchange factor (GEF) has been identified, which activated Rho associated with tight junctions and increased the paracellular permeability in MDCK cells (Benais-Pont et al., 2003). Regarding cerebral endothelial cells, the activation of the Rho pathway in vitro by lysophosphatidic acid (LPA) (van Leeuwen et al., 2003) disrupted the paracellular barrier (Schulze et al., 1997). Accordingly, the inhibition of the Rho pathway prevented the LPA-induced increase in permeability (Balda et al., 2000). Inflammation, as caused by bradykinin, thrombin, histamin cytokines, matrix metalloproteinases (Lum and Malik, 1996; Wójciak-Stothard et al., 1998; Johnson-Léger et al., 2000; Mayhan, 2000; Liu et al., 2001; Petty and Lo, 2002), or by bacterial toxins (Essler et al., 1998, 2000; Adamson et al., 1999, 2002) increases the transendothelial permeability by affecting tight and adherens junctions via reorganization of the actin cytoskeleton and formation of intercellular gaps. Also the transendothelial migration of lymphocytes was shown to be dependent on Rho signaling—when activation of Rho as a consequence of leukocyte binding to the adhesion receptor ICAM-1 was blocked by C3-transferase the leukocyte transmigration was compromised (Adamson et al., 1999). Whereas the extracellular domain of endothelial ICAM-1 suffices to mediate T cell adhesion, the cytoplasmic domain is required to mediate transmigration of T cells probably by inducing Rho-signaling within the endothelial cells (Etienne et al., 1998). In HUVECs, affection of the permeability requires the activation of the Cdc42-, rac-, Rho-cascade following stimulation by TNF-α (Lum and Malik, 1996). Furthermore, in vitro studies demonstrated that a Rho/Rho kinase-dependent pathway is a central target for an increase of vascular permeability by inactivating the myosin light chain (MLC) phosphatase, thus enhancing MLC phosphorylation. This leads to endothelial cell contraction and increased permeability (Essler et al., 2000).

7   Conclusions

The neurogliovascular complex is involved in the regulation of blood flow and nutrient supply within the CNS. This regulation includes: (1) control of perfusion parameters differentially realized in specific brain regions according to local requirements, (2) maintenance of energy supply from blood to neuronal and synaptic metabolism via glial cells, and (3) the protection of the nervous parenchyma from alterations of blood composition, in particular, from neurotoxic compounds including reactive oxygen species. Although the cellular partners of the neurogliovascular complex, such as neurons, astrocytes, pericytes, and endothelial cells, are well-known since many years, a functional understanding of what and to which end is signaled between these cells in order to establish the blood–brain interface is far away from being complete. The most important advance in the last years in this field seems to be the recognition of the fact that this interface is not simply an attribute of the brain microvessels but the result of an intense active interaction of all cellular and molecular partners during brain development and barrier maintenance. The formation and continuous maintainance of tight junctions between BBB endothelial cells is only the last step in a long chain of processes characterized now as the common effort of the brain microenvironmental factors to realize energy supply, control of perfusion, and protection from the blood.

Tight junctions have been primarily described as a network of protein particles using freeze-fracture electron microscopy. But, it needed almost 30 years and a great methodological advance in molecular biology to discover protein components of the tight junctional complex and to identify the protein particles within the replicas. Moreover, due to the advances in molecular biological methods, like knockout and GFP-technologies, it is now possible to recognize the tight junctional complex as a very dynamic structure. Using these approaches (Sasaki et al., 2003), it turned out that paired claudin strands are the molecular equivalents of the so-called "kissing points" seen in transmission electron microscopy. In vitro time lapse studies of annealing tight junction strands possessing different types of claudins for the first time demonstrated the high dynamic organization potential of the tight junctional complex. Now, it might be possible to go more into detail to characterize the interplay of these molecules and their regulation by and association with cellular signaling cascades and cytoskeletal components. These data then will allow us to use this knowledge for therapeutic interventions in pathologies influencing BBB integrity.

References

Abbott NJ. 2002. Astrocyte-endothelial interactions and blood-brain barrier permeability. J Anat 200: 629-638.

Abbott NJ, Hughes CCW, Revest PA, Greenwood J. 1992. Development and characterization of a rat capillary endothelial culture. Towards an in vitro BBB. J Cell Sci 103: 23-38.

Achen MG, Clauss M, Schnürch H, Risau W. 1995. The non-receptor tyrosine kinase Lyn is localised in the developing murine blood-brain barrier. Differentiation 59: 15-24.

Adamson P, Etienne S, Couraud PO, Calder V, Greenwood J. 1999. Lymphocyte migration through brain endothelial cell monolayers involves signaling through endothelial ICAM-1 via a rho-dependent pathway. J Immunol 162: 2964-2973.

Adamson RH, Curry FE, Adamson G, Liu B, Jiang Y, et al. 2002. Rho and rho kinase modulation of barrier properties: Cultured endothelial cells and intact microvessels of rats and mice. J Physiol 539: 295-308.

Anderson JM. 1996. Cell signalling: MAGUK magic. Curr Biol 6: 382-384.

Ando-Akatsuka Y, Saitou M, Hirase T, Kishi M, Sakakibara A, et al. 1996. Interspecies diversity of the occludin sequence: cDNA cloning of human, mouse, dog, and rat-kangaroo homologues. J Cell Biol 133: 43-48.

Angelov DN, Walther M, Streppel M, Guntinas-Lichius O, Neiss WF. 1998. The cerebral perivascular cells. Adv Anat Embryol Cell Biol 147: 1-87.

Antonetti DA, Barber AJ, Hollinger LA, Wolpert EB, Gardner TW. 1999. Vascular endothelial growth factor induces rapid phosphorylation of tight junction proteins occludin and zonula occludens 1. A potential mechanism for vascular permeability in diabetic retinopathy and tumors. J Biol Chem 174: 23463-23467.

Amiry-Moghaddam M, Ottersen OP. 2003. The molecular basis of water transport in the Brain. Nature Rev Neurosci 4: 991-1001.

Amiry-Moghaddam M, Frydenlund DS, Ottersen OP. 2003. Anchoring of aquaporin-4 in brain: Molecular mechanisms and implications for the physiology and pathophysiology of water transport. Neuroscience 129: 999-1010.

Arthur FE, Shivers RR, Bowman PD. 1987. Astrocyte-mediated induction of tight junctions in brain capillary endothelium: An efficient in vitro model. Dev Brain Res 36: 155-159.

Aurrand-Lions MA, Duncan L, Du Pasquier L, Imhof BA. 2000. Cloningv of JAM-2 and JAM-3: An emerging junctional adhesion molecular family? Curr Top Microbiol Immunol 251: 91-98.

Avila-Flores A, Rendon-Huerta E, Moreno J, Islas S, Betanzos A, et al. 2001. Tight-junction protein zonula occludens 2 is a target of phophorylation by protein kinase C. Biochem J 360: 295-304.

Bacallao R, Garfinkel A, Monke S, Zampighi G, Mandel LJ. 1994. ATP-depletion: A novel method to study junctional properties in epithelial tissues. I. Rearrangement of the actin cytoskeleton. J Cell Sci 107: 3301-3313.

Badaut J, Lasbennes F, Magistretti PJ, Regli L. 2002. Aquaporins in brain: Distribution, physiology and pathophysiology. J Cereb Blood Flow Metabol 22: 367-378.

Balabanov R, Dore-Duffy P. 1998. Role of the CNS microvascular pericyte in the blood-brain barrier. J Neurosci Res 53: 637-644.

Balda MS, Gonzalez-Mariscal L, Contreras RG, Macias-Silva M, Torres-Marquez ME, et al. 1991. Assembly and sealing of tight junctions: Possible participation of G-proteins, phospholipase C, protein kinase C and calmodulin. J Membr Biol 122: 193-202.

Balda MS, Flores-Maldonado C, Cereijido M, Matter K. 2000. Multiple domains of occludin are involved in the regulation of paracellular permeability. J Cell Biochem 78: 85-96.

Balda MS, Garrett MD, Matter K. 2003. The ZO-1-associated Y-box factor ZONAB regulates epithelial cell proliferation and cell density. J Cell Biol 160: 423-432.

Begley DJ. 2004. ABC transporters and the blood-brain barrier. Curr Pharma Design 10: 1295-1312.

Begley DJ, Brightman MW. 2003. Structural and functional aspects of the blood-brain barrier. Prog Drug Res 61: 39-78.

Bell SE, Mavila A, Salazar R, Bayless KJ, Kanagala S, et al. 2001. Differential gene expression during capillary morphogenesis in 3D collagen matrices: Regulated expression of genes involved in basement membrane matrix assembly, cell cycle progression, cellular differentiation and G-protein signaling. J Cell Sci 114: 2755-2773.

Benais-Pont G, Punn A, Flores-Maldonado C, Eckert J, Raposo G, et al. 2003. Identification of a tight junction-associated guanine nucleotide exchange factor that activates Rho and regulates paracellular permeability. J Cell Biol 160: 729-740.

Betanzos A, Huerta M, Lopez-Bayghen E, Azuara E, Amerena J, et al. 2004. The tight junction protein ZO-2 associates with Jun, Fos and C/EBP transcription factors in epithelial cells. Exp Cell Res 292: 51-66.

Blake DJ, Kröger S. 2000. The neurobiology of Duchenne muscular dystrophy: Learning lessons from muscle? Trends Neurosci 23: 92-99.

Brightman MW, Reese TS. 1969. Junctions between intimately apposed cell membranes in the vertebrate brain. J Cell Biol 40: 648-677.

Brillault J, Berezowski V, Cecchelli R, Dehouck MP. 2002. Intercommunications between brain capillary endothelial cells and glial cells increase the transcellular permeability of the blood-brain barrier during ischemia. J Neurochem 83: 807-817.

Bruewer M, Hopkins AM, Hobert ME, Nusrat A, Madara JL. 2004. RhoA, Rac1, and Cdc42 exert distinct effects on epithelial barrier via selective structural and biochemical modulation of junctional proteins and F-actin. Am J Physiol Cell Physiol 287: C327-C335.

Brückener KE, El Baya A, Galla HJ, Schmidt MA. 2003. Permeabilization in a cerebral endothelial barrier model by pertussis toxin involves the PKC effector pathay and is abolished by elevated levels of cAMP. J Cell Sci 116: 1837-1846.

Carman CV, Springer TA. 2004. A transmigratory cup in leukocyte diapedesis both through individual vascular endothelial cells and between them. J Cell Biol 167: 377-388.

Chen Y, Merzdorf C, Paul DL, Goodenough DA. 1997. COOH terminus of occludin is required for tight junction barrier function in early Xenopus embryos. J Cell Biol 138: 891-899.

Citi S, Sabanay H, Kendrick-Jones J, Geiger B. 1989. Cingulin: Characterization and localization. J Cell Sci 93: 107-122.

Claude P. 1978. Morphologic factors influencing transepithelial permeability. A model for the resistance of the zonula occludens. J Membr Biol 39: 219-232.

Cohen CJ, Shieh JT, Pickles RJ, Okegawa T, Hsieh JT, et al. 2001. The coxsackievirus and adenovirus receptor is a transmembrane component of the tight junction. Proc Natl Acad Sci USA 98: 15191-15196.

Connors NC, Adams ME, Froehner SC, Kofuji P. 2004. The potassium channel Kir4.1 associates with the dystrophin glycoprotein complex via alpha-syntrophin in glia. J Biol Chem 279: 28387-28392.

Coomber BL, Stewart PA. 1985. Morphometric analysis of CNS microvascular endothelium. Microvasc Res 30: 99-115.

Cucullo L, McAllister MS, Kight K, Krizanac-Bengez L, Marroni M, et al. 2002. A new dynamic in vitro model for the multidimensional study of astrocyte-endothelial cell interactions at the blood-brain barrier. Brain Res 951: 243-254.

D'Atri F, Citi S. 2002. Molecular complexity of vertebrate tight junctions. Mol Membr Biol 19: 103-112.

Dejana E. 2004. Endothelial cell-cell junctions: Happy together. Nature Rev Mol Cell Biol 5: 261-270.

Del Maschio A, Luigi AD, Martin-Padura I, Brockhaus M, Bartfai T, et al. 1999. Leukocyte recruitment in the cerebrospinal fluid of mice with experimental meningitis is inhibited by an antibody to junctional adhesion molecule (JAM). J Exp Med 190: 1351-1356.

DeMaio L, Chang YS, Gardner TW, Tarbell JM, Antonetti DA. 2001. Shear stress regulates occludin content and phosphorylation. Am J Physiol Heart Civc Physiol.

Denker BM, Nigam SK. 1998. Molecular structure and assembly of the tight junction. Am J Physiol 274: F1-F9.

Denker BM, Saha C, Khawaja S, Nigam SK. 1996. Involvement of a heterotrimeric G protein alpha subunit in tight junction biogenesis. J Biol Chem 271: 25750-25753.

Dermietzel R. 1975a. Junctions in the central nervous system of the cat. IV. Interendothelial junctions of cerebral blood vessels from selected areas of the brain. Cell Tissue Res 164: 45-62.

Dermietzel R. 1975b. Junctions in the central nervous system of the cat. V. The junctional complex of the pia-arachnoid memvbrane. Cell Tissue Res 164: 309-329.

De Vries L, Farquahr MG. 1999. RGS proteins: More than just GAPs for heterotrimeric G proteins. Trends Cell Biol 9: 138-144.

Dobrosotskaya I, Guy RK, James GL. 1997. MAGI-1, a membrane-associated guanylate kinase with a unique arrangement of protein-protein interaction domains. J Biol Chem 272: 31589-31597.

Dodane V, Kachar B. 1996. Identification of isoforms of G proteins and PKC that colocalize with tight junctions. J Membr Biol 149: 199-209.

Ebnet K, Suzuki A, Horikoshi Y, Hirose T, Meyer Zu Brickwedde MK, et al. 2001. The cell polarity protein ASIP/PAR-3 directly associates with junctional adhesion molecule (JAM). EMBO J 20: 3738–3748.

Ebnet K, Aurrand-Lions M, Kuhn A, Kiefer F, Butz S, et al. 2003. The junctional adhesion molecule (JAM) family members JAM-2 and JAM-3 associate with the cell polarity protein PAR-3: A possible role for JAMs in endothelial cell polarity. J Cell Sci 116: 3879-3891.

Ebnet K, Suzuki A, Ohno S, Vestweber D. 2004. Junctional adhesion molecules (JAMs): More molecules with dual functions? J Cell Sci 117: 19-29.

Ehrlich P. 1885. Das Sauerstoff-Bedürfnis des Organismus. Eine farbenanalytische Studie. PhD thesis Herschwald, Berlin. 69–72.

Engelhardt B. 2003. Development of the blood-brain barrier. Cell Tissue Res 314: 119-129.

Engelhardt B, Wolburg H. 2004. Transendothelial migration of leukocytes: Through the front door or around the side of the house? Eur J Immunol 34: 2955-2963.

Essler M, Amano M, Kruse HJ, Kaibuchi K, Weber PC, et al. 1998. Thrombin inactivates myosin light chain phosphatase via rho and its target rho kinase in human endothelial cells. J Biol Chem 273: 21867-21874.

Essler M, Staddon JM, Weber PC, Aepfelbacher M. 2000. Cyclic AMP blocks bacterial lipopolysaccharide-induced myosin light chain phosphorylation in endothelial cells through inhibition of rho/rho kinase signaling. J Immunol 164: 6543-6549.

Etienne S, Adamson P, Greenwood J, Strosberg AD, Cazaubon S, et al. 1998. ICAM-1 signaling pathways associated with rho activation in microvascular brain endothelial cells. J Immunol 161: 5755-5761.

Farquhar MG, Palade GE. 1963. Junctional complexes in various epithelial. J Cell Biol 17: 375-412.

Folkman J, D'Amore PA. 1996. Blood vessel formation: What is its molecular basis? Cell 87: 1153-1155.

Franke H, Galla H-J, Beuckmann CT. 2000. Primary cultures of brain microvessel endothelial cells: A valid and flexible model to study drug transport through the blood-brain barrier in vitro. Brain Res Protocols 5: 248-256.

Furuse M, Hirase T, Itoh M, Nagafuchi A, Yonemura S, et al. 1993. Occludin: A novel integral membrane protein localizing at tight junctions. J Cell Biol 123: 1777-1788.

Furuse M, Fujita K, Hiiragi T, Fujimoto K, Tsukita S. 1998. Claudin-1 and -2: Novel integral membrane proteins localizing at tight junctions. J Cell Biol 141: 1539-1550.

Furuse M, Sasaki H, Tsukita S. 1999. Manner of interaction of heterogenous claudin species within and between tight junction strands. J Cell Biol 147: 891-903.

Furuse M, Furuse K, Sasaki H, Tsukita S. 2001. Conversion of Zonulae occludentes from tight to leaky strand type by introducing claudin-2 into Madin-Darby canine kidney I cells. J Cell Biol 153: 263-272.

Gaillard PJ, Voorwinden LH, Nielsen JL, Ivanov A, Atsumi R, et al. 2001. Establishment and functional characterization of an in vitro model of the blood-brain barrier, comprising a co-culture of brain capillary endothelial cells and astrocytes. Eur J Pharmac Sci 12: 215-222.

Gao L, Joberty G, Macara I. 2002. Assembly of epithelial tight junctions is negatively regulated by Par6. Curr Biol 12: 221-225.

Garcia JG, Wang P, Liu F, Hershenson MB, Borbiev T, et al. 2001. Pertussis toxin directly activates endothelial cell p42/p44 MAP kinases via a novel signaling pathway. Am J Physiol 280: C1233-C1241.

Gee SH, Montanaro F, Lindenbaum MH, Carbonetto S. 1994. Dystroglycan-α: A dystrophin-associated glyoprotein, is a functional agrin receptor. Cell 77: 675-686.

Gerhardt H, Schuck J, Wolburg H. 1999a. Differentiation of a unique macroglial cell type in the pecten oculi of the chicken. Glia 28: 201-214.

Gerhardt H, Liebner S, Redies C, Wolburg H. 1999b. N-cadherin expression in endothelial cells during early angiogenesis in the eye and brain of the chicken: Relation to blood-retina and blood-brain barrier development. Eur J Neurosci 11: 1191-1201.

Gerhardt H, Rascher G, Schuck J, Weigold U, Redies C, et al. 2000. R- and B-cadherin expression defines subpopulations of glial cells involved in axonal guidance in the optic nerve head of the chicken. Glia 31: 131-143.

Gerhardt H, Betsholtz C. 2003. Endothelial-pericyte interactions in angiogenesis. Cell Tissue Res 314: 15-23.

Gliki G, Ebnet K, Aurrand-Lions M, Imhof BA, Adams RH. 2004. Spermatid differentiation requires the assembly of a cell polarity complex downstream of junctional adhesion molecule-C. Nature 431: 320-324.

Gonzalez-Mariscal L, Betanzos A, Nava P, Jaramillo BE. 2003. Tight junction proteins. Prog Biophys Mol Biol 81: 1-44.

Hallmann R, Mayer DN, Berg EL, Broermann R, Butcher EC. 1995. Novel mouse endothelial cell surface marker is suppressed during differentation of the blood-brain barrier. Dev Dyn 202: 325-332.

Hamazaki Y, Itoh M, Sasaki H, Furuse M, Tsukita S. 2002. Multi-PDZ domain protein 1 (MUPP) is concentrated at tight junctions through its possible interaction with claudin-1 and junctional adhesion molecule. J Biol Chem 277: 455-461.

Hamm S, Dehouck B, Kraus J, Wolburg-Buchholz K, Wolburg H, et al. 2004. Astrocyte mediated modulation of blood-brain barrier permeability does not correlate with a loss of tight junction proteins from the cellular contacts. Cell Tissue Res 315: 157-166.

Harris BZ, Lim WA. 2001. Mechanism and role of PDZ domains in signaling complex assembly. J Cell Sci 114: 3219-3231.

Heiskala M, Peterson PA, Yang Y. 2001. The roles of claudin superfamily proteins in paracellular transport. Traffic 2: 92-98.

Hellström M, Gerhardt H, Kalén M, Li X, Eriksson U, et al. 2001. Lack of pericytes leads to endothelial hyperplasia and abnormal morphogenesis. J Cell Biol 153: 543-553.

Higashi K, Fujita A, Inanobe A, Tanemoto M, Doi K, et al. 2001. An inwardly rectifying K$^+$ channel, Kir4.1, expressed in astrocytes surrounds synapses and blood vessels in brain. Am J Physiol 281: C922-C931.

Hirabayashi S, Tajima M, Yao I, Nishimura W, Mori H, et al. 2003. JAM4, a junctional cell adhesion molecule interacting with a tight junction protein, MAGI-1. Mol Cell Biol 23: 4267-4282.

Hirase T, Staddon JM, Saitou M. 1999. Occludin as a possible determinant of tight junction permeability in ECs. J Cell Sci 11:1603-1613.

Hirase T, Kawashima S, Wong EY, Ueyama T, Rikitake Y, et al. 2001. Regulation of tight junction permeability and occludin phosphorylation by RhoA-p160ROCK-dependent and –independent mechanisms. J Biol Chem 276: 10423-10431.

Hirata K, Ishida T, Penta K, Rezaee M, Yang E, et al. 2001. Cloning of an immunoglobulin family adhesion molecule selectively expressed by endothelial cells. J Biol Chem 276: 16223-16231.

Hopkins AM, Li D, Mrsny RJ, Walsh SV, Nusrat A. 2000. Modulation of tight junction function by G protein-coupled events. Adv Drug Deliv Rev 41: 329-340.

Hopkins AM, Walsh SV, Verkade P, Boquet P, Nusrat A. 2002. Constitutive activation of Rho proteins by CNF-1 influences tight junction structure and epithelial barrier function. J Cell Sci 116: 725-742.

Hopkins AM, Walsh SV, Verkade P, Boquet P, Nusrat A. 2003. Constitutive activation od Rho proteins by CNF-1 influences tight junction structure and epithelial barrier function. J Cell Sci 116: 725-742.

Huber D, Balda MS, Matter K. 2000. Occludin modulates transepithelial migration of neutrophils. J Biol Chem 275: 5773-5778.

Huber JD, Egleton RD, Davis TP. 2001. Molecular physiology and pathophysiology of tight junctions in the blood-brain barrier. Trends Neurosci 24: 719-725.

Iadecola C. 2004. Neurovascular regulation in the normal brain and in Alzheimer's disease. Nature Rev Neurosci 5: 347-360.

Igarashi Y, Utsumi H, Chiba H, Yamada-Sasamori Y, Tobioka H, et al. 1999. Glial cell line-derived neurotrophic factor (GDNF) enhances barrier function of endothelial cells forming the blood-brain barrier. Biochem Biophys Res Commun 261: 108-112.

Inai T, Kobayashi J, Shibata Y. 1999. Claudin-1 contributes to the epithelial barrier function in MDCK cells. Eur J Cell Biol 78: 849-855.

Ishida T, Kundu RK, Yang E, Hirata K, Ho YD, et al. 2003. Targeted disruption of endothelial cell-selective adhesion molecule inhibits angiogenic processes in vitro and in vivo. J Biol Chem 278: 34598-34604.

Itoh M, Nagafuchi A, Yonemura S, Kitaniyasuda T, Tsukita S. 1993. The 220 kD protein colocalizing with cadherins in non-epithelial cells is identical to ZO-1, a tight junction associated protein in epithelial cells - cDNA cloning and immunoelectron microscpy. J Cell Biol 121: 491-502.

Itoh M, Nagafuchi A, Moroi S, Tsukita S. 1997. Involvement of ZO-1 in cadherin-based cell adhesion through its direct binding to a-catenin and actin filaments. J Cell Biol 138: 181-192.

Izumi Y, Hirose T, Tamai Y, Hirai S, Nagashima Y, et al. 1998. An atypical PKC directly associates and colocalizes at the epithelial tight junction with ASIP, a mammalian homologue of Caenorhabditis elegans polarity protein PAR-3. J Cell Biol 143: 95-106.

Janzer RC, Raff MC. 1987. Astrocytes induce blood-brain barrier properties in endothelial cells. Nature 325: 253-257.

Johnson-Léger C, Aurrand-Lions M, Imhof BA. 2000. The parting of the endothelium: Miracle, or simply a junctional affair? J Cell Sci 113: 921-933.

Johnson-Léger C, Imhof BA. 2003. Forgoing the endothelium during inflammation: Pushing at a half-open door? Cell Tissue Res 314: 93-105.

Jou TS, Nelson WJ. 1998. Effects of regulated expression of mutant rhoA and rac1 small GTPases on the development of epithelial (MDCK) cell polarity. J Cell Biol 142: 85-100.

Jou TS, Schneeberger EE, Nelson WJ. 1998. Structural and functional regulation of tight junctions by rhoA and rac1 small GTPases. J Cell Biol 142: 101-115.

Kirsch T, Wellner M, Haller H, Lippoldt A. 2001. Altered gene expression in cerebral capillaries of stroke-prone spontaneously hypertensive rats. Brain Res 910: 106-115.

Klingler C, Kniesel U, Bamforth SD, Wolburg H, Engelhardt B, et al. 2000. Disruption of epithelial tight junctions is prevented by protein kinase A (PKA) inhibitors. Histochem Cell Biol 113: 349-361.

Kniesel U, Risau W, Wolburg H. 1996. Development of blood-brain barrier tight junctions in the rat cortex. Dev Brain Res 96: 229-240.

Kofuji P, Connors NC. 2003. Molecular substrates of potassium spatial buffering in glial cells. Mol Neurobiol 28: 195-208.

Kofuji P, Biedermann B, Siddharthan B, Raap M, Iandiev I, et al. 2002. Kir potassium channel subunit expression in retinal glial cells: Implications for spatial potassium buffering. Glia 39: 292-303.

Kofuji P, Newman EA. 2004. Potassium buffering in the central nervous system. Neuroscience 129: 1045-1056.

Lee S-W, Kim W-J, Choi YK, Song HS, Son MJ, et al. 2003. SSeCKS regulates angiogenesis and tight junction formation in blood-brain barrier. Nature Med 9: 900-906.

Li L, Head V, Timpe LC. 2001a. Identification of an inward rectifier potassium channel gene expressed in mouse cortical astrocytes. Glia 33: 57-71.

Li JY, Boado RJ, Pardridge WM. 2001b. Blood-brain barrier genomics. J Cereb Blood Flow Metab 21: 61-68.

Liang TW, DeMarco RA, Mrsny RJ, Gurney A, Gray A, et al. 2000. Characterization of huJAM: Evidence for involvement in cell-cell contact and tight junction regulation. Am J Physiol Cell Physiol 279: C1733-C1743.

Liebner S, Kniesel U, Kalbacher H, Wolburg H. 2000a. Correlation of tight junction morphology with the expression of tight junction proteins in blood-brain barrier endothelial cells. Eur J Cell Biol 79: 707-717.

Liebner S, Fischmann A, Rascher G, Duffner F, Grote E-H, et al. 2000b. Claudin-1 and claudin-5 expression and tight junction morphology are altered in blood vessels of human glioblastoma multiforme. Acta Neuropathol 100: 323-331.

Liedtke W, Edelmann W, Bieri PL, Chiu F-C, Cowan NJ, et al. 1996. GFAP is necessary for the integrity of CNS white matter architecture and long-term maintenance of myelination. Neuron 17: 607-615.

Lindahl P, Johansson BR, Leveen P, Betsholtz C. 1997. Pericyte loss and microaneurysm formation in PDGF-B-deficient mice. Science 277: 242-245.

Liu F, Verin AD, Borbiev T, Garcia JGN. 2001. Role of cAMP-dependent protein kinase A activity in endothelial cell cytoskeleton rearrangement. Am. J. Physiol. 280: L1309-L1317.

Liu Y, Nusrat A, Schnell FJ, Reaves TA, Walsh S, et al. 2000. Human junction adhesion molecule regulates tight junction resealing in epithelia. J Cell Sci 113: 2363-2374.

Lum H, Malik AB. 1996. Mechanisms of increased endothelial permeability. Can J Physiol Pharmacol 74: 787-800.

Madara JL, Dharmsathaphorn K. 1985. Occluding junction structure-function relationships in a cultured epithelial monolayer. J Cell Biol 101: 2124-2133.

Mandel LJ, Bacallao R, Zampighi G. 1993. Uncoupling of the molecular "fence" and paracellular "gate" functions in epithelial tight junctions. Nature 361: 552-555.

Mann GE, Yudilevich DL, Sobrevia L. 2003. Regulation of amino acid and glucose transporters in endothelial and smooth muscle cells. Physiol Rev 83: 183-252.

Martin-Padura I, Lostaglio S, Schneemann M, Williams L, Romano M, et al. 1998. Junctional adhesion molecule, a novel member of the immunoglobulin superfamily that distributes at intercellular junctions and modulates monocyte transmigration. J Cell Biol 142: 117-127.

Martinez-Palomo A, Meza I, Beaty G, Cereijido M. 1980. Experimental modulation of occluding junctions in a cultured transporting epithelium. J Cell Biol 87: 736-745.

Matter K, Balda MS. 2003. Signalling to and from tight junctions. Nature Rev Mol Biol 4: 225-236.

Mayhan WG. 2000. Leukocyte adherence contriburtes to disruption of the blood-brain barrier during activation of mast cells. Brain Res 869: 112-120.

Méresse S, Dehonk M-P, Delorme P, Bensaid M, Tauber J-P, et al. 1989. Bovine brain ECs express tight junctions and monoamine oxidase activity in long-term culture. J Neurochem 53: 1363-1371.

Meyer T, Schwesinger C, Denker BM. 2002. Zonula occludens-1 is a scaffolding protein for signaling molecules. J Biol Chem 277: 24855-24858.

Meyer T, Hunt J, Schwesinger C, Denker BM. 2003. Gα12 regulates epithelial cell junctions through Src tyrosine kinases. Am. J. Physiol. Cell Physiol 285: C1281-C1293.

Mitic LC, Van Itallie CM, Anderson JM. 2000. Molecular physiology and pathophysiology of tight junctions. I. Tight junction structure and function: Lessons from mutant animals and proteins. Am J Physiol 279: G250-G254.

Mollgard K, Saunders NR. 1986. The development of the human blood-brain and blood-CSF barriers. Neuropathol. Appl Neurobiol 12: 337-358.

Morita K, Furuse M, Fujimoto K, Tsukita S. 1999a. Claudin multigene family encoding four-transmembrane domain protein components of tight junction strands. Proc Natl Acad Sci USA 96: 511-516.

Morita K, Sasaki H, Furuse M, Tsukita S. 1999b. Endothelial claudin: Claudin-5/TMVCF constitutes tight junction strands in endothelial cells. J cell Biol 147: 185-194.

Muir AR, Peters A. 1962. Quintuple-layered membrane junctions at therminal bars between endothelial cells. J Cell Biol 12: 443-448.

Muller WA. 2003. Leukocyte-endothelial-cell interactions in leukocyte transmigration and the inflammatory response. Trends Immunol 24: 327-334.

Nagai-Tamai Y, Mizuno K, Hirose T, Suzuki A, Ohno S. 2002. Regulated protein-protein interaction between aPKC and PAR-3 plays an essential role in the polarization of epithelial cells. Genes Cells 7: 1161-1171.

Nagelhus EA, Mathisen TM, Ottersen OP. 2004. Aquaporin-4 in the central nervous system: Cellular and subcellular distribution and coexpression with Kir4.1. Neuroscience 129: 905-913.

Nagy Z, Peters H, Hüttner I. 1984. Fracture faces of cell junctions in cerebral endothelium during normal and hyperosmotic conditions. Lab Invest 50: 313-322.

Nakamura T, Blechman J, Tada S, Rozovskaia T, Itoyama T, et al. 2000. huASH1 protein, a putative transcription factor encoded by a human homologue of the Drosophila ash1 gene, localizes to both nuclei and cell-cell tight junctions. Proc Natl Acad Sci USA 97: 7284-7289.

Nasdala I, Wolburg-Buchholz K, Wolburg H, Kuhn A, Ebnet K, et al. 2002. A transmembrane tight junction protein selectively expressed on endothelial cells and platelets. J Biol Chem 277: 16294-16303.

Neely JD, Amiry-Moghaddam M, Ottersen OP, Froehner SC, Agre P, et al. 2001. Syntrophin-dependent expression and localization of aquaporin-4 water channel protein. Proc Natl Acad Sci USA 98: 14108-14113.

Neuhaus J. 1990. Orthogonal arrays of particles in astroglial cells: Quantitative analysis of their density, size, and correlation with intramembranous particles. Glia 3: 241-251.

Newman E, Reichenbach A. 1996. The Müller cell: A functional element of the retina. Trends Neurosci 19: 307-312.

Nicchia GP, Nico B, Camassa LMA, Mola MG, Loh N, et al. 2004. The role of aquaporin-4 in the blood-brain barrier development and integrity: Studies in animal and cell culture models. Neuroscience 129: 935-945.

Nico B, Frigeri A, Nicchia GP, Quondamatteo F, Herken R, Errede M, et al. 2001. Role of aquaporin-4 water channel in the development and integrity of the blood-brain barrier. J Cell Sci 114: 1297-1307.

Nico B, Frigeri A, Nicchia GP, Corsi P, Ribatti T, et al. 2003. Severe alterations of endothelial and glial cells in the blood-brain barrier of dystrophic mdx mice. Glia 42: 235-241.

Nico B, Nicchia GP, Frigeri A, Corsi P, Mangieri D, et al. 2004. Altered blood-brain barrier development in dystrophic mdx mice. Neuroscience 125: 921-935.

Nielsen S, Nagelhus EA, Amiry-Moghaddam M, Bourque C, Agre P, et al. 1997. Specialized membrane domains for water transport in glial cells: High-resolution immunogold cytochemistry of aquaporin-4 in rat brain. J Neurosci 17: 171-180.

Nitta T, Hata M, Gotoh S, Seo Y, Sasaki H, et al. 2003. Size-selective loosening of the blood-brain barrier in claudin-5-deficient mice. J Cell Biol 161: 653-660.

Nitz T, Eisenblätter T, Psathaki K, Galla HJ. 2003. Serum-derived weaken the barrier properties of cultured porcine brain capillary endothelial cells in vitro. Brain Res 981: 30-40.

Nunbhakdi-Craig V, Machleidt T, Ogris E, Bellotto D, White CL 3rd, et al. 2002. Protein phosphatase 2A associates with and regulates atypical PKC and the epithelial tight junction complex. J Cell Biol 158: 967-978.

Nusrat A, Giry M, Turner JR, Colgan SP, Parkos D, et al. 1995. Rho protein regulates tight junctions and perijunctional actin organization in polarized epithelia. Proc Natl Acad Sci USA 92: 10629-10633.

Ohnishi H, Nakahara T, Furuse K, Sasaki H, Tsukita S, et al. 2004. JACOP, a novel plaque protein localizing at the apical junctional complex with sequence similarity to cingulin. J Biol Chem 279: 46014-46022.

Ohno S. 2001. Intercellular junctions and cellular polarity: The PAR - aPKC complex, a conserved core cassette playing fundamental roles in cell polarity. Curr Opin Cell Biol 13: 641-648.

Orkand RK, Nicholls JG, Kuffler SW. 1966. Effect of nerve impulses on the membrane potential of glial cells in the central nervous system of amphibia. J Neurophysiol 29: 788-806.

Palmeri D, van Zante A, Huang CC, Hemmerich S, Rosen SD. 2000. Vascular endothelial junction-associated molecule, a novel member of the immunoglobulin superfamily, is localized to intercellular boundaries of endothelial cells. J Biol Chem 275: 19139-19145.

Papadopoulos MC, Krishna S, Verkman AS. 2002. Aquaporin water channels and brain edema. Mount Sinai J Med 69: 242-248.

Pardridge WM. 1988. Recent advances in blood-brain barrier transport. Annu Rev Pharmacol Toxicol 28: 25-39.

Pardridge WM. 1991. Advances in cell biology of blood-brain barrier transport. Semin Cell Biol 2: 419-426.

Parkinson FE, Friesen J, Krizanac-Bengez L, et al. 2003. Use of a three-dimensional in vitro model of the rat blood-brain barrier to assay nucleoside efflux from brain. Brain Res 980: 233-241.

Pawson T, Nash P. 2003. Assembly of cell regulatory systems through protein interaction domains. Science 300: 445-452.

Pekny M, Stanness KA, Eliasson C, Betsholtz C, Janigro D. 1998. Impaired induction of blood-brain barrier properties in aortic endothelial cells by astrocytes from GFAP-deficient mice. Glia 22: 390-400.

Peters A, Palay SL, Webster H. 1991. The fine structure of the nervous system. New York : Oxford University Press.

Peters A, Palay SL, Webster H. 1991. The fine structure of the nervous system. New York : Oxford University Press.

Petty MA, Lo EH. 2002. Junctional complexes of the blood-brain barrier: Permeability changes in neuroinflammation. Prog Neurobiol 68: 311-323.

Qin Y, Sato TN. 1995. Mouse multidrug resistance 1a/3 gene is the earliest known endothelial cell differentiation marker during blood-brain barrier development. Dev Dynamics 202: 172-180.

Rahner C, Mitic LL, Anderson JM. 2001. Heterogeneity in expression and subcellular localization of claudins 2, 3, 4, and 5 in rat liver, pancreas, and gut. Gastroenterology 120: 411-422.

Rajasekaran AK, Hojo M, Huima T, Rodriguez-Boulan E. 1996. Catenins and zonula occludens-1 form a complex during early stages in the assembly of tight junctions. J Cell Biol 132: 451-464.

Rascher G, Fischmann A, Kröger S, Duffner F, Grote E-H, et al. 2002. Extracellular matrix and the blood-brain barrier in glioblastoma multiforme: Spatial segregation of tenascin and agrin. Acta Neuropathol 104: 85-91.

Raschperger E, Engstrom U, Pettersson RF, Fuxe J. 2004. CLMP, a novel member of the CTX family and a new component of epithelial tight junctions. J Biol Chem 279: 796-804.

Rash JE, Yasumura T, Hudson CS, Agre P, Nielsen S. 1998. Direct immunogold labeling of aquaporin-4 in square arrays of astrocyte and ependymocyte plasma membranes in rat brain and spinal cord. Proc Natl Acad Sci USA 95: 11981-11986.

Rash JE, Davidson KGV, Yasumura T, Furman CS. 2004. Freeze-fracture and immunogold analysis of aquaporin-4 (AQP4) square arrays, with models of AQP4 lattice assembly. Neuroscience 129: 915-934.

Raub TJ. 1996. Signal transduction and glial cell modulation of cultured brain microvessel endothelial cell tight junctions. Am J Physiol 271: C495-C503.

Reese TS, Karnovsky MJ. 1967. Fine structural localization of a blood-brain barrier to exogenous peroxidase. J Cell Biol 34: 207-217.

Risau W. 1991. Induction of blood-brain barrier endothelial cell differentiation. Ann N Y Acad Sci 633: 405-419.

Risau W, Hallmann R, Albrecht U. 1986. Differentiation-dependent expression of protein in brain endothelium during development of the blood-brain barrier. Dev Biol 117: 537-545.

Roh MH, Makarova O, Liu CJ, Shin K, Lee S, et al. 2002. The Maguk protein, Pals1, functions as an adapter, linking mammalian homologues of crumbs and discs lost. J Cell Biol 157: 161-172.

Rubin LL, Hall DE, Porter S, Barbu K, Cannon C, et al. 1991. A cell culture model of the blood-brain barrier. J Cell Biol 115: 1725-1736.

Saadoun S, Papadopoulos MC, Davies DC, Krishna S, Bell BA. 2002. Aquaporin-4 expression is increased in oedematous human brain tumours. J Neurol Neurosurg Psychiatry 72: 262-265.

Saha C, Nigam SK, Denker, BM. 2001. Expanding role of G proteins in tight junction regulation: Gαs stimulates tight junction assembly. Biochem Biophys Res Commun 285: 250-256.

Saitou M, Furuse M, Sasaki H, Schulzke J-D, Fromm M, et al. 2000. Complex phenotype of mice lacking occludin, a component of tight junction strands. Mol Biol Cell 11: 4131-4142.

Sakakibara A, Furuse M, Saitou M, Ando-Akatsuka Y, Tsukita S. 1997. Possible involvement of phosphorylation of occludin in tight junction formation. J Cell Biol 137: 1393-1401.

Sasaki H, Matsui C, Furuse K, Mimori-Kiyosue Y, Furuse M, et al. 2003. Dynamic behavior of paired claudin strands

within apposing plasma membranes. Proc Natl Acad Sci USA 100: 3971-3976.

Schinkel AH, Smit JJM, van Tellingen O, Beijnen JH, Wagenaar E, et al. 1994. Disruption of the mouse mdr1a P-glycoprotein gene leads to a deficiency in the blood-brain barrier and to increased sensitivity to drugs. Cell 77: 491-502.

Schulze C, Smales C, Rubin LL, Staddon JM. 1997. Lysophophatidic acid increases tight junctional permeability in cultured brain ECs. J Neurochem 68: 991-1000.

Seulberger H, Unger CM, Risau W. 1992. HT7, Neurothelin, Basigin, gp42 and OX-47--many names for one developmentally regulated immuno-globulin-like surface glycoprotein on blood-brain barrier endothelium, epithelial tissue barriers and neurons. Neurosci Lett 140: 93-97.

Sheth P, Basuroy S, Li C, Naren AP, Rao RK. 2003. Role of phosphatidylinositol 3-kinase in oxidative stress-induced disruption of tight junctions. J Biol Chem 278: 49239-49245.

Shivers RR. 1979. The blood-brain barrier of a reptile, *Anolis carolinensis*. A freeze-fracture study. Brain Res 169: 221-230.

Simon DFB, Lu Y, Choate KA, Velazquez H, Al-Sabban E, et al. 1999. Paracellin-1, a renal tight junction protein required for paracellular Mg^{2+} resorption. Science 285: 103-106.

Soma T, Chiba H, Kato-Mori Y, Wada T, Yamashita T, et al. 2004. Thr(207) of claudin-5 is involved in size-selective loosening of the endothelial barrier by cyclic AMP. Exp Cell Res 300: 202-212.

Sonoda N, Furuse M, Sasaki H, Yonemura S, Katahira J, et al. 1999. Clostridium perfringens enterotoxin fragment removes specific claudins from tight junction strands: Evidence for direct involvement of claudins in tight junction barrier. J Cell Biol 147: 195-204.

Staehelin LA. 1974. Structure and function of intercellular junctions. Int Rev Cytol 39: 191-283.

Stanness KA, Neumaier JF, Sexton TJ, Grant GA, Emmi A, et al. 1999. A new model of the blood-brain barrier: Coculture of neuronal, endothelial and glial cells under dynamic conditions. Neuroreport 10: 3725-3731.

Stevenson BR, Siliciano JD, Mooseker MS, Goodenough DA. 1986. Identification of ZO-1: A high molecular weight polypeptide associated with the tight junction (zonula occludens) in a variety of epithelia. J Cell Biol 103: 755-766.

Stewart PA. 2000. Development of the blood-brain barrier. In Morphogenesis of Endothelium, Risau W, Rubanyi GM, editors. Amsterdam: Harwood Academic Publishers; pp. 109-122.

Stewart PA. 2000. Development of the blood-brain barrier. In Morphogenesis of Endothelium, Risau W, Rubanyi GM, editors. Amsterdam: Harwood Academic Publishers; pp. 109-122.

Stewart PA, Wiley MJ. 1981. Developing nervous tissue induces formation of blood-brain barrier characteristics in invading endothelial cells: A study using quail-chick transplantation chimeras. Dev Biol 84: 183-192.

Suzuki A, Yamanaka T, Hirose T, Manabe N, Mizuno K, et al. 2001. Atypical protein kinase C is involved in the evolutionarily conserved PAR protein complex and plays a critical role in establishing epithelia-specific junctional structures. J Cell Biol 152: 1183-1196.

Tani E, Yamagata S, Ito Y. 1977. Freeze-fracture of capillary endothelium in rat brain. Cell Tissue Res 176: 157-165.

Tontsch U, Bauer HC. 1991. Glial cells and neurons induce blood brain barrier related enzymes in cultured cerebral ECs. Brain Res 539: 247-253.

Traweger A, Fuchs R, Krizbai IA, Weiger TM, Bauer HC, et al. 2002. The tight junction specific protein occludin is a functional target of the E3 ubiquitin-protein ligase Itch. J Biol Chem 277: 10201-10208.

Tsukita S, Furuse M. 1999. Occludin and claudins in tight-junction strands: Leading or supporting players? Trends Cell Biol 9: 268-273.

Tsukita S, Furuse, M. 2000. Pores in the wall: Claudins constitute tight junction strands containing aqueous pores. J Cell Biol 149: 13-16.

Tsukita S, Furuse M, Itoh M. 1999. Structural and signalling molecules come together at tight junctions. Curr Opin Cell Biol 11: 628-633.

Tsukita S, Furuse M, Itoh M. 2001. Multifunctional strands in tight junctions. Nature Rev Mol Cell Biol 2: 285-293.

Turksen K, Troy T-C. 2004. Barriers built on claudins. J Cell Sci 117: 2435-2447.

Ullmer C, Schmuck K, Figge A, Lubbert H. 1998. Cloning and characterization of MUPP1, a novel PDZ domain protein. FEBS Lett 424: 63-68.

Utsumi H, Chiba H, Kamimura Y, Osanai M, Igarashi Y, et al. 2000. Expression of GFRa-1, receptor for GDNF, in rat brain capillary during postnatal development of the BBB. Am J Physiol 279: C361-C368.

Vajda Z, Pedersen M, Doczi T, Sulyok E, Nielsen S. 2004. Sudies of mdx mice. Neuroscience 129: 993-998.

Van Hinsbergh VWM, Van Nieuw Amerongen GP. 2002. Intracellular signalling involved in modulating human endothelial barrier function. J Anat 200: 549-560.

van Leeuwen FN, Giepmans BN, van Meeteren LA, Moolenaar, WH. 2003. Lysophosphatidic acid: Mitogen and motility factor. Biochem Soc Trans 31: 1209-1212.

Verbavatz J-M., Ma T, Gobin R, Verkman AS. 1997. Absence of orthogonal arrays in kidney, brain and muscle from transgenic knockout mice lacking water channel aquaporin-4. J Cell Sci 110: 2855-2860.

Wakai S, Hirokawa N. 1978. Development of the blood-brain barrier to horseradish peroxidase in the chick embryo. Cell Tissue Res 195: 195-203.

Warth A, Kröger S, Wolburg H. 2004. Redistribution of aquaporin-4 in human glioblastoma correlates with loss of agrin immunoreactivity from brain capillary basal laminae. Acta Neuropathol 107: 311-318.

Warth A, Mittelbronn M, Wolburg H. 2005. Redistribution of the water channel protein aquaporin-4 and the K^+ channel protein Kir4.1 differs in low and high grade human brain tumors. Acta Neuropathol, 109: 418-426.

Wen H, Warty DD, Marcondes MC, Fox HS. 2004. Selective decrease in paracellular conductance of tight junctions: Role of the first extracellular domain of claudin-5. Mol Cell Biol 24: 8408-8417.

Willis CL, Nolan CC, Reith SN, Lister T, Prior MJ, et al. 2004. Focal astrocyte loss is followed by microvascular damage, with subsequent repair of the blood-brain barrier in the apparent absence of direct astrocytic contact. Glia. 45: 325-337.

Wójciak-Stothard B, Entwistle A, Garg R, Ridley AJ. 1998. Regulation of TNF-α-induced reorganization of the actin cytoskeleton and cell-cell junctions by rho, rac, and cdc42 in human endothelial cells. J Cell Physiol 176: 150-165.

Wolburg H. 1995a. Orthogonal arrays of intramembranous particles. A review with special reference to astrocytes. J Brain Res 36: 239-258.

Wolburg H. 1995b. Glia-neuronal and glia-vascular interrelations in blood-brain barrier formation and axon regeneration in vertebrates. Neuro-Glial Interactions During Phylogeny. Vernadakis A, Roots B, editors. Totowa, NJ: Humana Press Inc; pp. 479–510.

Wolburg H, Lippoldt A. 2002. Tight junctions of the blood-brain barier: Development, composition and regulation. Vascul Pharmacol 38: 323-337.

Wolburg H, Neuhaus J, Kniesel U, Krauss B, Schmid E-H, et al. 1994. Modulation of tight junction structure in blood-brain barrier ECs. Effects of tissue culture, second messengers and cocultured astrocytes. J Cell Sci 107: 1347-1357.

Wolburg H, Wolburg-Buchholz K, Kraus J, Rascher-Eggstein G, Liebner S, et al. 2003. Localization of claudin-3 in tight junctions of the blood-brain barrier is selectively lost during experimental autoimmune encephalomyelitis and human glioblastoma multiforme. Acta Neuropathol 105: 586-592.

Wolburg H, Wolburg-Buchholz K, Engelhardt B. 2005. Diapedesis of mononuclear cells across cerebral venules during experimental autoimmune encephalomyelitis leaves tight junctions intact. Acta Neuropathol, 109: 181-190.

Wolff JR, Stuke K, Missler M, Tytko H, Schwarz P, et al. 1998. Autocellular coupling by gap junctions in cultured astrocytes: A new view on cellular autoregulation during process formation. Glia 24: 121-140.

Wu Y, Dowbenko D, Spencer S, Laura R, Lee J, et al. 2000. Interaction of the tumor suppressor PTEN/MMAC with a PDZ domain of MAGI3, a novel membrane-associated guanylate kinase. J Biol Chem 275: 21477-21485.

Yagi T, Jikihara I, Fukumura M, Watabe K, Ohashi T, et al. 2000. Rescue of ischemic brain injury by adenoviral gene transfer of glial cell line-derived factor after transient global ischemia in gerbils. Brain Res 885: 273-282.

Yang B, Brown D, Verkman, AS. 1996. The mercurial insensitive water channel (AQP-4) forms orthogonal arrays in stably transfected chinese hamster ovary cells. J Biol Chem 271: 4577-4580.

Yonezawa T, Ohtsuka A, Yoshitaka T, Hirano S, Nomoto H, et al. 2003. Limitrin, a novel immunoglobulin superfamily protein localized to glia limitans formed by astrocyte endfeet. Glia 44: 190-204.

2 Blood–Brain Barrier Models

M. A. Deli

Abstract: In the last 25 years, a great number of cell culture–based blood–brain barrier (BBB) models have been developed. First, primary cultures and passages of cerebral endothelial cells were used as monolayers for experiments. Later, immortalized cell lines have been established and used as BBB models. As brain endothelial cells lose easily their specific characteristics in culture, and the importance of signals from the cells of the neurovascular unit in the induction of BBB properties has been recognized, in the next stage of BBB modeling monocultures were replaced by coculture systems using glial cells, neurons, or pericytes. These models are valuable tools to study cell–cell interaction in the neurovascular unit, modulation of BBB permeability in physiological, pathological, and pharmacological conditions. Some of the BBB models can serve as permeability screens for the pharmaceutical industry.

This chapter will summarize the most frequently used types of in vitro BBB models of bovine, human, porcine, and rodent origin, and their main applications.

List of Abbreviations: 1400W, N-(3-aminomethyl)benzylacetamidine; Ac-LDL, acetylated low-density lipoprotein; ACE, angiotensin converting enzyme; ALP, alkaline phosphatase; ASCT2, sodium-dependent neutral amino acid transporter type 2; ATA2, amino acid transporter A2; BBB, blood-brain barrier; BCRP, brain multidrug resistance protein; CNS, central nervous system; CNT-2, sodium-coupled nucleoside transporter; COMT, catechol-ortho-methyl-transferase; CRT, creatine transporter; cyclic AMP, adenosine $3',5'$-cyclic monophosphate; cyclic GMP, guanosine $3',5'$-cyclic monophosphate; DETA-NONOate, 2,2'-(Hydroxynitrosohydrazino)bis-ethanamine; DPPE, N,N-diethyl-2-[4-(phenylmethyl)-phenoxy]ethanamine; EAAT, excitatory amino acid transporter; ECE-1, endothelin converting enzyme-1; eNOS, endothelial nitric oxide synthase; EVOM, epithelial Volt-Ohm meter; FGF1, acidic fibroblast growth factor; FGF2, basic fibroblast growth factor; GAT2, GABA transporter 2 (same as BGT1); γ-GT, γ-glutamyl-transpeptidase; GDNF, glial cell line-derived neurotrophic factor; GLUT-1, glucose transporter-1; gp120, 120 kDa glycoprotein; HIV-1, human immunodeficiency virus-1; HTLV-1, human T-cell leukemia virus type-1; JAM, junctional adhesion molecule; LAT-1, large neutral amino-acid transporter-1; LDL, low density lipoprotein; L-NAME, N_{ω}-nitro-L-arginine methyl ester; LPS, lipopolysaccharide; LRP, low-density lipoprotein-related receptor; MAO A and B, monoamine oxidase A and B; MCT-1, monocarboxylic acid transporter; MK-801, dizocilpine; MRP, multidrug resistance protein; neuroAIDS, neurological symptoms of acquired immunodeficiency syndrome; NET, norepinephrine transporter; NMDA, N-methyl-D-aspartic acid; NO, nitric oxide; OAT3, organic anion transporter 3; OATP2, organic anion-transporting polypeptide 2; OGD, oxygen-glucose deprivation; P_e, endothelial permeability coefficient; PECAM-1, platelet-endothelial cell adhesion molecule-1; PLA2, phospholipase A2; RAGE, receptor for advanced glycation end-products; SERT, serotonin transporter; SKF 96365, 1-[2-(4-Methoxyphenyl)-2-[3-(4-methoxyphenyl)propoxy]ethyl]-1H-imidazole hydrochloride; TAUT, taurin transporter; TEER, transendothelial electrical resistance; TGF-β, transforming growth factor-β; TJ, tight junctions; U83836E, (-)-2-((4-(2,6-Di-1-pyrrolidinyl-4-pyrimidinyl)-1-piperazinyl)methyl)-3,4-dihydro-2,3,7,8-tetramethyl-2H-1-benzopyran-6-ol, 2HCl; UGT, UDP-glucoronyl-transferase; VCAM-1, vascular cell adhesion molecule-1; VEGF, vascular endothelial cell growth factor; ZO-1, -2, zonula occludens protein 1 and 2

1   Introduction

The blood–brain barrier (BBB) can be defined as a dynamic interaction of cerebral endothelial cells and neighboring perivascular cells, namely astroglia, pericytes, microglia, and neurons. This cross talk between the cells of the neurovascular unit is responsible for the induction and maintenance of the unique BBB phenotype of brain capillary endothelial cells (Abbott et al., 2006). The primary role of the BBB is the regulation of brain microenvironment by restricting ionic, fluid and cell movements between the blood and brain, supply of essential nutrients, and removal of metabolites. In addition to the morphological barrier based on inter-endothelial tight junctions (TJs), the uptake and efflux transport systems as well as enzymic and metabolic barriers participate in the creation and protection of the homeostasis of the nervous system (Abbott, 2005).

There are two tightly controlled pathways for molecules and cells to cross the BBB: the paracellular (junctional) and the transendothelial routes. One of the hallmarks of the BBB phenotype is the restrictive paracellular pathway, regulated by interendothelial TJs. The importance of endothelial TJ in permeability regulation was first observed in the tracer experiments of Reese and Karnovsky (1967) and Brightman and Reese (1969). TJ not only restricts paracellular flux but also maintains polarity of enzymes and receptors on luminal and abluminal membrane domains. The most important integral membrane TJ proteins include occludin, claudin-1, -5, and -12, and junctional adhesion molecules (JAMs) (for review see Wolburg and Lippoldt, 2002; Krizbai and Deli, 2003). Paracellular permeability is regulated by diverse signaling cascades (Rubin and Staddon, 1999; Krizbai and Deli, 2003).

The transendothelial pathways are also restricted at the brain microvasculature. In contrast to peripheral endothelium, the rate of pinocytosis is minimal, and free membrane diffusion applies mainly to small lipophilic molecules, e.g., caffeine, ethanol, or nicotine (Pardridge, 2002). Active or catalyzed transport systems can be divided into three main groups. Carrier-mediated bidirectional transport is responsible for nutrient uptake in the brain, these transporters include glucose transporter GLUT-1, monocarboxylic acid transporter MCT-1, large neutral amino acid transporter LAT-1, or sodium-coupled nucleoside transporter CNT2 (Pardridge, 2002) (❯ *Table 2-1*). Efflux transport is unidirectional and delivers metabolites and

❑ Table 2-1

Endothelial and BBB characteristics present in in vitro models

Selected endothelial markers
• Factor VIII/von Willebrandt factor-related antigen
• Acetylated low-density lipoprotein (Ac-LDL) uptake by scavenger receptors
• Vasoactive mediators produced by their respective enzymes
Nitric oxide (eNOS), endothelins (ECE-1), angiotensins (ACE)
• Cell adhesion molecules
Vascular cell adhesion molecule-1 (VCAM-1), platelet-endothelial cell adhesion molecule-1 (PECAM-1 or CD31)
• Lectin binding
Bandeiraea simplicifolia B4, *Ulex europaeus* A

BBB-specific markers
• Tight junction proteins
Zonula occludens protein 1 and 2 (ZO-1, -2); occludin; claudin-3, -5, and 12; junctional adhesion molecules
• Tight junction functions
Transendothelial electrical resistance (TEER) > 200 Ω cm^2, low endothelial permeability coefficients (P_e) for paracellular markers
• Enzymes
Alkaline phosphatase (ALP), γ-glutamyl-transpeptidase (γ-GT), monoamine oxidase A and B (MAO A and B), UDP-glucoronyl-transferase (UGT), catechol-ortho-methyl-transferase (COMT)
• Influx transporters
Glucose transporter-1 (GLUT-1), neutral amino acid transporters (LAT-1; ATA 2), alanine transporter (ASCT 2), taurin transporter (TAUT), monocarboxylic acid trasporter-1 (MCT-1), creatine transporter (CRT)
• Efflux transporters
ABC transporters (P-glycoprotein; multidrug resistance-associated proteins 4, 5, 6; breast cancer resistance protein), organic anion and cation transporters (Oatp2, OAT3), neurotransmitter transporters (EAAT 1, 2, 3, GAT 2/BGT1), serotonin transporter (SERT), norepinephrine transporter (NET)
• Transport receptors
Insulin receptor, transferrin receptor, LDL receptor, low-density lipoprotein-related receptor LRP, receptor for advanced glycation end-products (RAGE)

ABC transporter adenosine triphosphate-binding cassette transporter, *ACE* angiotensin-converting enzyme, *ATA 2* system A amino acid transporter 2, *BBB* blood–brain barrier, *GAT 2/BGT1* gamma amino butyric acid transporter subtype GAT 2, *EAAT* excitatory amino acid transporters, *ECE-1* endothelin-converting enzyme-1, *eNOS* endothelial nitric oxide synthase, *LAT-1* L-type large neutral amino acid transporter 1, *OAT3* organic anion trasporter 3, *Oatp2* organic anion transport protein 2 xenobiotics from the brain to blood. P-glycoprotein (ABCB1) and MRP-1 multidrug resistance protein-1, -4, -5, -6 (ABCC1, -4, -5, -6), brain multidrug resistance protein (ABCG2/BCRP), or organic anion-transporting polypeptide OATP2 belong to the fast-growing group of efflux transporters at the BBB (Kusuhara and Sugiyama, 2001a, b; de Boer et al., 2003). Receptor-mediated transport by transcytosis is important for the brain supply of peptides and proteins such as low-density lipoproteins (LDL), transferrin, leptin, and insulin (Banks, 1999; Pardridge, 2002).

Specific enzymes expressed by brain endothelial cells (monoamine oxidases, epoxy hydrolase, endo-peptidases, etc.) are important elements of the BBB phenotype constituting the so-called metabolic barrier, and participate in the regulation of brain penetration of drugs (Joó, 1993; Pardridge, 2002).

2   In Vitro Models of the Blood–Brain Barrier

Viable microvessels isolated from the brain can be considered as the first in vitro model of the BBB (Joó and Karnushina, 1973). Experiments on isolated brain microvessels provided important data on cerebral endothelial receptors, transporters, and signaling mechanisms (Joó, 1985, 1992). Laser capture microdis-section of different branches of brain microvasculature combined with gene and protein arrays can be a new and powerful tool to analyze heterogeneity of BBB properties in vessels of different brain regions and in vessels of different location on the vascular tree (Ge et al., 2005).

The first observation on endothelial cells growing out of brain capillaries in culture conditions soon followed the establishment of the brain microvessel isolation technique (Panula et al., 1978). In the following decade, several culture methods have been elaborated resulting in an increasing number of very different BBB models. Despite attempts to standardize some of the frequently used models, the divergence of model systems continues (Reichel et al., 2003). All models should show some elements of general endothelial and specific BBB properties, which are characteristic for the BBB in vivo. Several important BBB features present in vivo and described in in vitro BBB models are summarized in ❷ *Table 2-1*.

The tight paracellular barrier is a fundamental characteristic of BBB. To assess the tightness of a model, measurement of the transendothelial electrical resistance (TEER) is one of the most straightforward methods (Deli et al., 2005). In culture conditions, TEER reflects junctional permeability for sodium ions. Passive flux of small water soluble inert tracers is another way to assess monolayer integrity; therefore, endothelial permeability coefficients (P_e) are important parameters of the quality of BBB models (Deli et al., 2005). All relevant models should show a sufficient tightness (150–200 Ω cm^2) to study permeability or transport of molecules (Gaillard and de Boer, 2000; Reichel et al., 2003; Deli et al., 2005). TEER and P_e values are used to compare different BBB models.

2.1   Types of Cell Culture–Based BBB Models

The first in vitro BBB filter model, adaptation of a technique already used in epithelial cell biology, was introduced in the early 1980s (Bowman et al., 1983). The insert was made by the researchers from nylon mesh and polycarbonate tubing, and bovine brain endothelial cells were seeded on it. The cell layer kept in solo or monoculture was used for studying the effect of calcium-free medium and osmotic shock on sucrose flux (Bowman et al., 1983). Since then a variety of chambers and inserts from different materials and with diverse pore sizes became commercially available. However, the appropriate insert to use in permeability screens should be carefully selected, and permeability of cell-free inserts for each molecule tested has to be determined (Cecchelli et al., 1999).

The cell culture insert/filter setup (❷ *Figure 2-1*) made it possible to use brain endothelial cells for permeability studies in vitro (Joó, 1992). The first studies used monocultures (Panula et al., 1978; Bowman et al., 1981, 1983; Rutten et al., 1987; Abbott et al., 1992), but it turned out very soon that the cultivation of brain endothelial cells alone leads to loss of BBB phenotype, including TJs, transporters, and specific enzymes.

◘ Figure 2-1

(a) In vitro reconstituted blood–brain barrier (BBB) models using culture inserts: monoculture of brain endo-thelial cell layer; coculture of brain endothelial cell layer with a second cell type (e.g., astrocyte) on the other side of the porous filter or at the bottom of the culture well; triple culture with brain endothelial cell layers in the upper side of the inserts with the second cell type at the other side of filter and the third type in the culture well. (b) Measurement of transendothelial electrical resistance (TEER) of brain endothelial cell monolayers grown in cell culture inserts with an electrode pair of custom-made or commercially available (e.g., EVOM, epithelial volt-ohm meter, World Precision Instruments, USA) equipment. (c) Flux of tracers or drugs from the upper (luminal) compartment to the lower (abluminal) compartment through a brain endothelial monolayer can be measured during given time intervals and endothelial permeability coefficients (P_e) can be calculated (Deli et al., 2005)

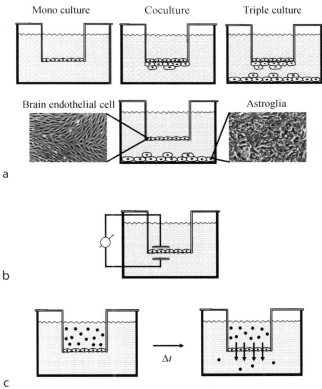

2.1.1 Coculture with Glial Cells

In the first study demonstrating the effect of glia on cultured brain endothelial cells, the activity of a BBB-specific enzyme, γ-glutamyl transpeptidase, could be restored by coculture with glial cells (DeBault and Cancilla, 1980). The results supported the use of brain endothelial cell–astroglia cocultures as in vitro reconstituted BBB models (❷ Figure 2-1). Some systems use cells from different species in coculture, i.e., bovine brain endothelial cells with rat astroglia (Dehouck et al., 1990), others are syngeneic, using for example human cerebral endothelial cells and human astroglia (Kása et al., 1991) or rat brain endothelial cells and rat glia cultures (Kis et al., 2001; Perrière et al., 2005). Both purified type-1 astrocytes and primary mixed glial cultures are efficient in the induction of BBB properties.

The effect of astroglia on endothelial characteristics and functions like permeability has been extensively studied (reviewed by Abbott, 2002; Haseloff et al., 2005; Abbott et al., 2006). It has been demonstrated in the 1980s by electron microscopic techniques that TJ structures are deteriorated in subcultured brain endothelial cells, and coculture with astrocytes or astrocyte-produced factors reenhance endothelial TJ in vitro (Arthur et al., 1987; Tao-Cheng et al., 1987). Resistance and permeability data measured on coculture models with bovine, human, mouse, porcine, and rat brain endothelial cells and immortalized cell lines strongly support these results. In the majority of models using primary rat astroglial cells in a coculture setting, the paracellular barrier properties were increased. Even bovine aortic endothelial cells, which are of non-brain origin, responded to this treatment (Yamagata et al., 1997). Kása et al. (1991) found a similar induction of TEER by fetal human astroglia in human brain endothelial cell monolayers. It has been recently suggested that posthypoxic (Song et al., 2002) or src-suppressed C-kinase substrate overexpressing (Lee et al., 2003) astrocytes induce better TJ integrity than normal cells do; however, the validity of the BBB models used in these experiments was not confirmed by TEER or P_e measurements.

Microglia, present in primary mixed glial cultures, can also influence brain endothelial cells in cocultures. Endothelial monolayer TEER was higher with retinal glial coculture containing microglia (Diaz et al., 1998). Glial cell coculture saved brain endothelial cells from the effects of bacterial lipopolysaccharide (LPS) treatment, and microglial cells or oligodendrocytes, or both, were essential for the protection of the monolayer integrity (Descamps et al., 2003). In a study on feline brain endothelial monolayers, astrocytes had a positive effect on trafficking of peripheral blood mononuclear cells, while microglia had a suppressive effect (Hudson et al., 2005).

Glial cell lines are also used in coculture studies, the rat C6 glioma is the most popular. C6 cells tightened the interendothelial junctions when cocultured with bovine, mouse, and porcine brain endothelial cells or with human ECV304 cell line. In a comparative study, human and rat astroglia and C6 glioma cells were all effective in raising a very low basal TEER of ECV304 monolayers (Tan et al., 2001). However, on a more pertinent BBB model using bovine brain endothelial cells under no condition were C6 cells able to reproduce TEER values as high as in the presence of primary glial cells (Boveri et al., 2005). Furthermore, coculture with C6 cells led to higher sucrose and inulin permeability, less differentiated junction pattern, different morphology, and lower P-glycoprotein expression and activity in brain endothelial cells (Boveri et al., 2005). Elevated levels of vascular endothelial cell growth factor (VEGF) found in the C6 coculture model can be responsible for these effects.

Another cell line, human UC-11 MG astrocytoma, elevated TEER in bovine endothelial cells (Raub et al., 1992), while other malignant glial cells, such as rat gliosarcoma (9L) or human glioblastoma (T98G), had an opposite, permeability increasing effect in rat brain endothelial monolayers (Grabb and Gilbert, 1995). Brain tumors in vivo enhance BBB permeability by secreting angiogenic factors like VEGF. These data indicate that glial cell lines secrete both permeability increasing and decreasing factors, and the final effect will depend on the sum of the opposite actions.

The hypothesis that soluble factors released by glia or glioma cells participate in the induction of BBB phenotype is supported by a large number of studies with glia-conditioned media. In most reports, barrier-enhancing effects were found; however, at least 60-min incubation time was needed (Rubin et al., 1991). The barrier tightening factors secreted by rat C6 glioma cells are unidentified, though a study indicates that nonprotein factors having molecular weight lower than 1,000 Da are responsible for the effect (Ramsohoye and Fritz, 1998). A study trying to clarify the signaling pathways involved in barrier-enhancing effects of C6 cells suggests that the action is not mediated through adenosine 3',5'-cyclic monophosphate (cyclic AMP), but rather by protein kinase C activation via phospholipase D, independently of intracellular calcium increase (Raub, 1996).

All these results are further supported by the finding that removal of astroglia from coculture with brain endothelial cells led to an increase in permeability for sucrose and peroxidase (Hamm et al., 2004). The elevation of junctional permeability was not accompanied by changes in immunostaining of TJ proteins occludin, claudin-3 and -5, and ZO-1 and -2. This clearly indicates that loosening of TJ structure measured by paracellular markers does not mean a complete loss of TJ proteins. Indeed, previous observations on fast and reversible modulation of paracellular permeability in brain endothelial cells by osmotic shock (Bowman et al., 1983; Dehouck et al., 1990; Deli et al., 1995c) and by cyclic AMP (Rubin et al., 1991; Deli et al., 1995a) confirm the importance of TJ protein phosphorylation and dephosphorylation processes in permeability regulation (Rubin and Staddon, 1999).

2.1.2 Coculture with Neurons

Despite their close localization to capillaries, few data are available on the effect of neurons on BBB properties (Bauer and Bauer, 2000). Coculture of RBE4 cells with rat primary neurons decreased transmonolayer dopamine flux (Cestelli et al., 2001). In agreement with these data, organotypic brain slice culture induced differential permeability between L-dopa and dopamine through rat brain endothelial cell monolayers with the reduction of dopamine transport (Duport et al., 1998). No glutamate transport was found in this coculture model compared to monocultures, which indicates the presence of glutamate efflux transporters found in vivo (Duport et al., 1998). In direct contact culture conditions, endothelial cells regulate neural precursor cell differentiation, proliferation, and quiescence showing mutual influence between the two cell types (Shen et al., 2004; Mathieu et al., 2006).

2.1.3 Coculture with Pericytes

Pericytes embedded in brain capillary basement membrane are the nearest neighbors of endothelial cells, and they have a fundamental role in stabilizing brain capillary structure in vivo. The first coculture study gave contradictory results: mouse pericytoma did not change, while bovine retina pericyte-conditioned medium decreased TEER of bovine cerebral endothelial cells (Raub et al., 1992). In the recent years, several papers have been published on the pericytic induction of BBB phenotype. Coculture with rat pericytes in the two sides of the insert (❷ *Figure 2-1*) induced increased tightness of primary rat brain endothelial monolayers measured by higher TEER (Hayashi et al., 2004). Rat pericytes could decrease the paracellular permeability and P-glycoprotein activity in MBEC4 cells, an immortalized mouse brain capillary endothelial cell line (Dohgu et al., 2005). The presence of pericytes also upregulated the endothelial mRNA expression of MRP-6 efflux pump (Berezowski et al., 2004). Human brain pericytes negatively regulated human brain endothelial cell fibrinolysis in a coculture model (Kim et al., 2006).

Soluble factors responsible for the pericytic effect have been identified. The upregulation of BBB properties in MBEC4 cells was mediated by transforming growth factor-β (TGF-β) production in pericytes (Dohgu et al., 2005). Pericyte-derived angiopoietin-1 induced endothelial occludin gene expression through Tie-2 receptor activation, by using conditionally immortalized rat brain endothelial (TR-BBB13) and brain pericyte (TR-PCT1) cell lines (Hori et al., 2004).

2.1.4 Triple Cultures

Cell culture inserts enable the establishment of BBB models using three cell types (❷ *Figure 2-1*). The models published so far use combinations of brain endothelial cells, astrocytes, neurons, and leukocytes.

When RBE4 cells were cultured in the presence of both astrocytes and neurons, a synergistic effect on the induction of occludin expression and junctional localization was observed (Schiera et al., 2003), which is also reflected in the decreased sucrose permeability (Schiera et al., 2005). In the microenvironment of a dynamic in vitro BBB model based on endothelial–glial coculture differentiation of serotonergic neurons was promoted (Stanness et al., 1999). Another variation of the dynamic model includes circulating leukocytes as a third cell type besides endothelial and glial cells (Krizanac-Bengez et al., 2006). This model helped to analyze the role of leukocyte-mediated inflammatory mechanisms in BBB failure induced by loss of flow.

2.1.5 Dynamic Models

Blood vessels are exposed to fluid-induced shear and circumferential stresses. Changes in the hemodynamic forces induce release of endothelial vasoactive mediators and regulation of vascular tone. Pulse pressure and shear stress, relevant physiological forces influencing the endothelium in vivo, are missing from the abovementioned static BBB models.

A dynamic model has been developed by the group of Janigro (Stanness et al., 1999; Krizanac-Bengez et al., 2003, 2006; Parkinson et al., 2003). This BBB model has a three-dimensional tube structure with a continuous flow of culture medium mimicking the physiological shear stress in blood vessels. Insulin and adenosine transport and the contribution of shear stress on BBB integrity were studied on the model.

In a dynamic coculture model of retinal vasculature using bovine retinal microvascular endothelial cells and bovine retinal pericytes, pulsatile flow increased the expression of endothelial nitric oxide synthase (eNOS) prostacyclin and endothelin-1 (Walshe et al., 2005).

2.2 Primary Culture–Based BBB Models

Most in vitro BBB models use bovine, human, porcine, or rodent brain endothelial cell–based systems, and these will be discussed in detail below. Brain microvessel endothelial cells have been isolated from many other species, monkey, dog, gerbil, cat, etc., but well-characterized permeability models using them have not been described.

The common problem of all primary cultures is that besides brain endothelial cell islands they contain contaminating cells, mainly brain pericytes, but also fibroblasts, smooth muscle, or leptomeningeal cells (Abbott et al., 1992). Contaminating cells disturb the development of tight monolayers (Parkinson and Hacking, 2005) and overgrow brain endothelial cells during long-term cultivation. Techniques to purify cultures include the mechanical removal of nonendothelial cells under microscope, cloning of pure colonies of brain capillary endothelial cells, Thy1.1 antibody and complement-mediated immunocytolysis, or separation of cerebral endothelial cells by surface antigens by magnetic beads or fluorescence-activated cell sorting. A new method that proved to be successful to decrease the number of nonendothelial cells is based on the fact that endothelial cells of cerebral capillaries express much higher amounts of efflux pumps, especially P-glycoprotein, than any other cells in the freshly isolated brain microvessel fractions, therefore they can tolerate the otherwise toxic concentrations of P-glycoprotein ligand drugs. Among the P-glycoprotein ligands, puromycin was found to be the best to selectively kill contaminating cells during the first 2 days of the culture (Perrière et al., 2005). This selection can also favor capillary endothelial cells versus those from larger microvessels, and this could lead to tighter monolayers and better BBB models (Ge et al., 2005).

2.2.1 Bovine Models

The first in vitro BBB model with measured permeability characteristics has been established from bovine brain gray matter (Bowman et al., 1983). Bovine systems provide high yield of brain endothelial cells sufficient for pharmacological screening, and they are widely used in basic as well as in applied research. One of the best characterized bovine models developed in the laboratory of Cecchelli (Dehouck et al., 1990, 1992; Cecchelli et al., 1999) is based on coculture of cloned and passaged bovine capillary endothelial cells and rat glia culture showing high TEER ($500–800 \, \Omega \, cm^2$) and low P_e values. The highest TEER values measured on a bovine system exceed $2,000 \, \Omega \, cm^2$, but no P_e values are available on this model (Zenker et al., 2003).

2.2.2 Human Models

Despite the ethical questions and difficulties to have access to the human brain tissue (autopsy material, surgical specimen, and fetal tissue), human BBB models have been established for about 15 years (Reichel et al., 2003). Other problems with human models are the low yield of cells, and whether the tissue, especially from autopsy or surgical material, can be regarded as "healthy." Human models published so far are less robust than bovine or porcine systems, and give lower resistance and permeability values (for review see Deli et al., 2005). The highest published TEER is $500 \, \Omega \, cm^2$ (Zenker et al., 2003), the lowest P_e value for inulin is 3.6×10^{-6} cm/s (Liu et al., 2002).

2.2.3 Mouse Models

Mouse brain yields the least endothelial cells compared to other species. No wonder that few models can be found from mouse primary endothelial cells. The advantages of the murine system, however, include the availability of transgenic and gene-targeted animals, oligoprobes, and wide range of antibodies. In mono-culture conditions, TEER of puromycin-purified mouse brain endothelial monolayers was 200 Ω cm^2 (Weidenfeller et al., 2005). When cultured with C6 cells, mouse cerebral endothelial cell showed higher resistance of 307 Ω cm^2 (Deli et al., 2003). An impressively tight mouse BBB model, using primary brain endothelial and glial cells, could reach 778 Ω cm^2 TEER and 4.5×10^{-6} cm/s P_e for sucrose (Coisne et al., 2005).

2.2.4 Porcine Models

A high-resistance (1800 Ω cm^2) and low-permeability (sucrose P_e is 0.2×10^{-6} to 1.8×10^{-6} cm/s) porcine BBB model has been developed in the laboratory of Galla using serum-free culture condition and hydrocortisone treatment without coculture (Hoheisel et al., 1998; Franke et al., 1999; Nitz et al., 2003). Not all porcine BBB models reach this level of tightness, there is a considerable variation of published TEER (75–800 Ω cm^2) and P_e values for sucrose (3.3×10^{-6} to 33×10^{-6} cm/s) (for review see Deli et al., 2005). The high yield of about 50 million endothelial cells per pig brain and some similarities between porcine and human vascular physiology make the porcine model suitable for drug screening.

2.2.5 Rat Models

Cultures of rat brain endothelial cells are available since the late 1970s; however, models with permeability measurements have been published only since the 1990s. Similarly to the mouse system the yield is low, only 1–2 million endothelial cells per rat brain can be isolated. Barrier properties are similar to mouse models, but they do not reach the level of the best bovine or porcine monolayers (for review see Deli et al., 2005). The advantage of the rat BBB model is that it can be easily compared to in vivo results and measurements, and it is simple to do syngeneic cultures. One such model composed of primary brain endothelial and glial cells was characterized by TEER of 350–500 Ω cm^2 and fluorescein P_e of 4.2×10^{-6} cm/s (Kis et al., 2001). Similar TEER (500 Ω cm^2) and lower P_e (0.75×10^{-6} cm/s) values were measured on another syngeneic model using puromycin treatment (Perrière et al., 2005).

2.3   Cell Line–Based BBB Models

The preparation of primary cultures is expensive, time consuming, and needs expertise. To overcome these difficulties and to establish easy, reproducible and sufficiently tight in vitro BBB models, immortalized brain endothelial cell lines have been generated in growing number in recent years. Until now none of the available (more than 20) cell lines can fulfill all these criteria.

2.3.1 Bovine Cell Lines

Because of the availability of good bovine primary brain endothelial cell models, development of bovine cell lines is not a priority. The only bovine cell line published with comparable permeability data is t-BBEC-117 line, that has a permeability coefficient of 1.8×10^{-6} cm/s for L-glucose (Sobue et al., 1999).

2.3.2 Human Cell Lines

Establishment of good cell line–based human BBB models is a difficult task. Human brain endothelial cell lines are widely used in infectological studies with human pathogens, but the calculated resistance values of the monolayers are rather low, even compared to cell lines from other species (for review see Deli et al., 2005). The first stable, well-characterized human brain endothelial cell line, hCMEC/D3, shows several endothelial and BBB characteristics, including chemokine receptors, TJ proteins, and drug efflux mechanisms (Weksler et al., 2005). D3 cell layers in monoculture give 40 Ω cm^2 TEER value, permeability coefficients of 27.5×10^{-6} cm/s for sucrose, 6×10^{-6} cm/s for inulin, and 5.4×10^{-6} cm/s for 4-kDa FITC-dextran (Weksler et al., 2005). Sucrose permeability of another recently described immortalized human brain capillary endothelial cell line, BB19, was 22.5×10^{-6} cm/s and could not discriminate between passive paracellular flux of sucrose and lipid soluble drug propranolol (Kusch-Poddar et al., 2005).

Although ECV304 proved to be a non-brain and nonendothelial human cell line (Brown et al., 2000), it expresses several endothelial features (Kiessling et al., 1999; Suda et al., 2001) and has been tested in permeability studies by several groups (reviewed in Gumbleton and Audus, 2001; Reichel et al., 2003). There is a large variation in TEER, but values about 200 Ω cm^2 could be reached, and among the cell line models the lowest permeability coefficient for sucrose (0.13×10^{-6} cm/s) was published on ECV304 cells.

2.3.3 Mouse Cell Lines

A spontaneously transformed MB114 mouse brain endothelial monolayer with a low TEER value was the first cell line used for in vitro BBB permeability studies (Hart et al., 1987). Later mouse brain endothelial cell lines became popular models in BBB transporter research (Kusuhara et al., 1998; Tsuji and Tamai, 1999; Kusuhara and Sugiyama, 2001a, b; Reichel et al., 2003). For permeability studies the best characterized mouse lines are TM-BBB4 with a TEER of 105–118 Ω cm^2 (Hosoya et al., 2000; Terasaki et al., 2003), and b.End3 with a basal TEER of 40 Ω cm^2 that can be enhanced to 130 Ω cm^2 by glial factors and treatment elevating intracellular level of cyclic AMP level (Omidi et al., 2003). Sucrose permeability of b.End3 monolayers was 16×10^{-6} cm/s (Omidi et al., 2003).

2.3.4 Rat Cell Lines

Rat brain endothelial cell lines, especially RBE4, have been extensively studied in several areas of BBB research (reviewed by Roux and Couraud, 2005). The main problem with rat cell lines, similarly to all the above-mentioned ones, is that the monolayers are rather leaky. No TEER values are available in the published literature, but sucrose permeability values varying between 11×10^{-6} and 204×10^{-6} cm/s mirror this well. Data on GPNT cells (Romero et al., 2000, 2003), a retransfected and cloned line of the parental GP8 cells (Greenwood et al., 1996), falls in the same range. The resistance of TR-BBB13 cell layers either in solo culture or in coculture with TR-AST4 is 106 Ω cm^2 (Hori et al., 2004).

2.4 Factors Increasing Monolayer Integrity of BBB Models

Besides coculture methods and use of fluid flow (❷ Sect. 2.2.1), several other culture conditions and factors have been tested to induce complex BBB phenotype and tighter paracellular barrier in BBB models. Some of the techniques, like coating culture surfaces with extracellular matrix, defined culture media without serum, or culture additives including growth factors, hormones, and drugs affecting intracellular cyclic AMP levels proved to be effective to improve BBB models (❷ Table 2-2).

■ Table 2-2

Inductive factors used in in vitro BBB models

Basal membrane
Fibronectin, collagen IV, gelled collagen, cornea endothelial matrix
Cocultured cells
Astroglia, pericyte, neuron, microglia
Modulation of intracellular second messenger level
Cyclic AMP analogs, phosphodiesterase inhibitors, adenylate cyclase activators
Hormones
Hydrocortisone, dexamethasone, adrenomedullin
Growth factors
Heparin, basic fibroblast growth factor (FGF2), angiopoietin-1, glia-derived neurotrophic peptide (GDNP), transforming growth factor-β (TGF-β)
Lipids
Eicosapentaenoic acid, γ-linolenic acid, epoxy eicosatrienoic acid
Serum-free conditions
[in the presence of hydrocortisone]

BBB blood–brain barrier, *cyclic AMP* adenosine 3′,5′-cyclic monophosphate

2.4.1 Extracellular Matrix

The fact that extracellular matrix is crucial in the culture of brain endothelial cells and in the local control of TJ biogenesis has long been known (Arthur et al., 1987). Rat tail collagen gel has been found excellent to support monolayer formation of bovine brain endothelial cells, the basis of in vitro modeling, in contrast to laminin, matrigel, or extracellular matrix produced by MDCK cells (Raub et al., 1992). Gelled rat tail collagen is also used in one of the most competent in vitro BBB model systems (Dehouck et al., 1992). Type IV collagen, fibronectin, and laminin either alone or in combination drastically elevated the TEER of low-resistance porcine brain endothelial monolayers (Tilling et al., 1998). A complex biological matrix secreted by corneal endothelial cells improved the growth of cultured brain microvascular endothelial cells (Dömötör et al., 1998) and could support the development of tight monolayers of rat brain endothelial cells.

2.4.2 Serum-Free Conditions

Since the earliest attempts to cultivate living cells, serum and serum components have been used to provide cells with adhesion-promoting molecules, nutrients, trace minerals, transport proteins like transferrin and albumin, growth factors, and hormones. Several in vitro BBB models use serum-containing media. However, few studies examined systematically the effect of serum on permeability (for review see Deli et al., 2005). The ECV304/C6 model shows higher TEER value in the presence of fetal bovine serum, and reduction of serum content or serum deprivation for 24 h led to decreased TEER even in the presence of C6 cells (Hurst and Fritz, 1996). Data from the laboratory of Galla demonstrate an opposite effect of serum on porcine brain endothelial monolayers: bovine serum, ox serum, heat-inactivated ox serum, and human blood plasma all decreased TEER, and disturbed the correct localization of integral TJ proteins on their model (Hoheisel et al., 1998; Franke et al., 1999; Nitz et al., 2003). As fatty acid–free albumin was without effect (Nitz et al., 2003), a variety of known and unidentified serum factors, among them lysophosphatidic acid, can be responsible for the phenomenon.

    The luminal surface of brain endothelial cells is exposed to 6%–8% of plasma protein. Serum deprivation can lead to endothelial cell death by apoptosis and necrosis, a well-known phenomenon, in cerebro-microvascular endothelial cells, too (Ueda et al., 2005). Inclusion of 0.1% serum albumin helps to stabilize TJs in permeability studies (Youdim et al., 2003).

2.4.3 Growth Factors

Basic fibroblast growth factor (bFGF or FGF2) induces not only endothelial cell proliferation and migration, but differentiation too. FGF2 could up-regulate in RBEA cells the activity of alkaline phosphatase and γ-glutamyl transpeptidase, enzymes present at the BBB in vivo (El Hafny et al., 1996). This is the reason why most culture protocols use FGF2 either alone or with heparin to promote the proliferation of brain endothelial cells (Abbott et al., 1992; Dehouck et al., 1992; Kis et al., 2001; Coisne et al., 2005). FGF2, acidic fibroblast growth factor (FGF1), and heparin, which binds and stabilizes them, are devoid of any permeability effect (Raub et al., 1992; Wang et al., 1996). The same applies for epidermal growth factor, platelet-derived growth factor, ciliary neurotrophic factor, and insulin-like growth factor-1 (Rubin et al., 1991; Hoheisel et al., 1998). Similarly to these results, glial cell line–derived neurotrophic factor (GDNF) alone had no effect on monolayer integrity. However, it had a dose-dependent barrier-tightening action in porcine brain capillary endothelial cells, when applied together with cyclic AMP-elevating agents (Igarashi et al., 1999).

Although both GDNF and TGF-β1 belongs to the TGF-β family, the effect of TGF-β1 on monolayer permeability is more controversial. TGF-β1 causes a time-dependent and polarized increase in permeability of bovine brain endothelial monolayers with a basolateral preference through a pertussis toxin-sensitive G protein–coupled pathway (Raub et al., 1992; Raub, 1996). In TR-BBB13 rat brain endothelial cell line, TGF-β1 reduced the occludin mRNA level (Hori et al., 2004). In contrast to these data, the coculture of mouse MBEC4 cells with pericytes decreased fluorescein permeability and rhodamine 123 uptake similarly to TGF-β1 treatment (Dohgu et al., 2005). Both effects in both the coculture and treatment conditions could be inhibited by TGF-β1-specific antibody and TGF-β type I receptor antagonist (Dohgu et al., 2005). The BBB phenotype-inducing and barrier-enhancing effect of astrocytes was also found to be mediated, at least partially, by locally activated TGF-β (Garcia et al., 2004).

2.4.4 Cyclic AMP

Elevated intracellular cyclic AMP levels resulted in barrier tightening in all models tested until now. Increase in intraendothelial cyclic AMP concentration by cell-permeable cyclic AMP analogs activating protein kinase A increases TEER and decreases paracellular flux of sucrose, fluorescein, mannitol, and inulin (reviewed by Deli et al., 2005). Forskolin, a cell-permeable adenylate cyclase activator, has similar effect (Rubin et al., 1991; Brückener et al., 2003; Zenker et al., 2003). Isoproterenol, a selective β-adrenergic agonist that stimulates adenylate cyclase activity and activates mitogen-activated protein kinases, also raised brain endothelial TEER (Rubin et al., 1991). Calcitonin gene-related peptide and adrenomedullin clearly demonstrated a cyclic AMP-like effect (Rubin et al., 1991; Kis et al., 2001).

The permeability decreasing effect of cyclic AMP analogs is more pronounced when phosphodiesterase blockers are used simultaneously to prevent the quick metabolization of cyclic AMP. Both RO 20-1724, a selective inhibitor of cyclic AMP-specific cyclic GMP-independent phosphodiesterase-4, and 3-isobutyl-1-methylxanthine, a nonspecific inhibitor of cyclic AMP and cyclic GMP phosphodiesterases, are widely used for this purpose (Deli et al., 2005). Moreover, treatment of brain endothelial cells with phosphodiesterase inhibitors alone was also able to strengthen monolayer integrity (Raub, 1996; Zenker et al., 2003). Bovine brain endothelial cells reacted better to cyclic AMP increasing treatment in the presence of glial induction by astrocyte-conditioned medium (Rubin et al., 1991).

2.4.5 Glucocorticoids

Physiological concentration of hydrocortisone, a glucocorticoid hormone, considerably improves the barrier properties of porcine cerebral endothelial cells in serum-free culture conditions (Hoheisel et al., 1998; Deli et al., 2005). Similarly to natural steroid hydrocortisone, dexamethasone, an effective synthetic glucocorticoid hormone inhibiting phospholipase A2 (PLA2) activity strengthened specific barrier properties, i.e., increased TEER and decreased P_e for paracellular markers, in the majority of models (Hurst and Clark, 1999; Gaillard et al., 2003; Romero et al., 2003; Cucullo et al., 2004).

2.4.6 Fatty Acids

Fatty acids are major components of the cell membrane and able to regulate junctional permeability. Eicosapentaenoic acids and γ-linolenic acid, two polyunsaturated fatty acids supposed to be mediators in the cross talk between endothelial cells and astroglia, increased TEER of porcine brain endothelial cells after 3 days of serum starvation, whereas linolenic acid had no such effect (Yamagata et al., 2003). The barrier-tightening effect could be blocked by tyrosine kinase inhibitors or protein kinase inhibitors. Cerebral endothelial mitogenesis and morphogenesis were induced by astrocytic epoxy eicosatrieonoic acid (Zhang and Harder, 2002).

3   Use of In Vitro BBB Models

Studies on in vitro reconstituted BBB models have contributed to the present knowledge about the structural and functional organization of the BBB under physiological and pathological conditions. Pharmacology studies on reliable and reproducible in vitro BBB models could accelerate the research and development of new drugs having better brain penetration.

Despite debates that there is no clear correlation between TEER and P_e, the best models with highest TEER give the lowest P_e values. Because of the difficulties in obtaining models with sufficiently tight paracellular barrier from many species and because of the need to develop models for specific applications, a compromise can be made. Models with minimal TEER of 150–200 Ω cm^2 give reasonable solute or drug permeability results (Gaillard and de Boer, 2000; Gumbleton and Audus, 2001; Reichel et al., 2003; Deli et al., 2005).

Many models do not comply with the above-mentioned minimal criteria and results obtained on these systems should be critically evaluated. Cautious interpretation of data and repetition of pivotal experiments in valid and reproducible in vitro BBB models are needed. Even results obtained on the best available models should be compared with in vivo measurements to reach a general conclusion about the effect of a physiological or pathological factor or a drug on the BBB function.

3.1   BBB in Diseases

BBB permeability changes play a crucial role in brain edema formation and central nervous system injuries during human diseases such as stroke, cerebral hypoxia–reoxygenation, head injuries, neurological infections including bacterial and viral meningitis, encephalitis, or HIV-1 infection, and neurodegenerative diseases like Alzheimer's and prion diseases. BBB is not only affected in these pathologies, but BBB damage and dysfunction can lead to secondary neuronal injuries.

In vitro studies on reconstituted BBB models help to reveal the direct effects of pathological conditions on cerebral endothelium, and the contribution of cytokines, reactive oxygen species, nitric oxide (NO), vasoactive mediators, and other pathogenetic factors to the impairment of barrier integrity (❯ *Table 2-3*).

3.1.1   Hypoxia and Reoxygenation

Brain ischemia, a major neuropathological condition in humans, changes BBB permeability in vivo. To better understand the pathomechanism, several studies examined hypoxia and related factors on different in vitro BBB models. Susceptibility of brain endothelial cells to hypoxia differs significantly depending on time, culture and treatment conditions, and validity of the models used (Deli et al., 2005).

❏ Table 2-3
Effects of pathogenetic factors on in vitro BBB models

Hypoxia, ischemia, reoxygenation
- Compromises barrier integrity by time-dependent increase in permeability:
  Hypoxia, hypoxia followed by reoxygenation, hypoxia combined with glucose deprivation
  Cytokines
- Compromises barrier integrity:
  Interferon-γ, interleukin-1, interleukin-6, tumor necrosis factor-α
- Reinforces barrier integrity:
  Interferon-α, interferon-β

Vasoactive mediators and amyloid peptides
- Compromises barrier integrity:
  Amyloid-β peptides, arachidonic acid, atrial natriuretic peptide, bradykinin, endothelin-1, glutamate, histamine, prostaglandin E_2, prostaglandin $F_{2\alpha}$, prion peptide 106–126, serotonin, vascular endothelial growth factor
- Reinforces barrier integrity:
  Adrenomedullin, angiopoietin-1

Infections
- Compromises barrier integrity:
  Living bacteria (*Streptococcus pneumoniae* strain D39), bacterial LPS (*Haemophilus influenzae* type B; *E. coli* O55:B5; *Salmonella typhimurium*), bacterial lipoteichoic acid, HIV-1 gp120 [monoculture], HIV-1 *Nef*, HIV-1 *Tat*, HTLV-1-infected human T-lymphocytes, pertussis toxin
- Neutral effect:
  Living bacteria (*Citrobacter freundii*; *E. coli* strains HB101 or E44 or C5), HIV-1$_{LA1}$ strain, HIV-1 gp120 [coculture], HIV-1$_{ADA-M\ or\ D117III}$-infected human monocytes, fungus *Candida albicans* CAI4 strain
- Reinforces barrier integrity:
  Cholera toxin, schistosomula or excretory/secretory products of parasite *Schistosoma mansoni*

BBB blood–brain barrier, *gp120* 120-kDa glycoprotein, *HIV-1* human immunodeficiency virus-1, *HTLV-1* human T-cell leukemia virus type-1, *LPS* lipopolysaccharide

In monocultures hypoxia (1.5–24 h) induced a drop in TEER, and an increase in sucrose and inulin flux through porcine (Fischer et al., 1995, 1999, 2001) and bovine brain endothelial monolayers (Mark et al., 2004). In coculture systems 2-h hypoxia led to increased fluorescein flux in porcine brain endothelial cell–rat glia model (Giese et al., 1995). In bovine brain endothelial cells cocultured with rat glia 48-h hypoxia was needed to significantly raise sucrose and albumin P_e in endothelial monolayers in the absence of glial cells (Plateel et al., 1995, 1997). The increase in albumin flux was abolished at 4°C, confirming that albumin transport is an active transendothelial process (Plateel et al., 1997). A barrier-weakening effect was demonstrated in rat brain endothelial cell–rat astroglia models, too (Kondo et al., 1996; Utepbergenov et al., 1998). Hypoxia combined with glucose deprivation resulted in a much faster (2–4 h) increase in endothelial permeability for sucrose, inulin, apotransferrin, and albumin than in hypoxia alone (Brillault et al., 2002).

The role of glial factors in mediating the effect of hypoxia is controversial. Bovine brain endothelial permeability was significantly enhanced in hypoxia or oxygen–glucose deprivation (OGD) for sucrose, inulin, and albumin in the presence of glia or conditioned medium of OGD-treated glial cells (Brillault et al., 2002). Other experiments suggest a protective role of glia. Astroglia attenuated the increase in paracellular flux of brain endothelial monolayers following hypoxia and reoxygenation on a rat BBB model (Kondo et al., 1996), in porcine endothelial cells (Fischer et al., 2001), or in bovine cerebral endothelial cells (Brown et al., 2003).

Several pathogenic factors are involved in the regulation of hypoxia-induced changes at the BBB. Among hypoxia-inducible factor 1–regulated genes, endothelin-1, inducible NO synthase, TGF-β, and VEGF contribute to the damage of BBB integrity, whereas adrenomedullin and angiopoietin-1 reinforces the barrier function. VEGF stimulates endothelial cell growth, induces angiogenesis, and increases endothelial permeability. On in vitro BBB models, VEGF increases sucrose and inulin flux, and decreases TEER (Fischer et al., 1999, 2001; Wang et al., 1996). Angiopoietin-1 counteracted the effect of VEGF on a bovine BBB model (Valable et al., 2005). According to a differential protein expression study, brain endothelial cells respond to hypoxia–reoxygenation by adaptive upregulation of proteins involved in the glycolysis, protein synthesis, and stress response (Haseloff et al., 2006).

3.1.2 Infections

The interaction of infectious agents with brain endothelial cells is crucial in the pathogenesis of meningitis, encephalitis, and neurological symptoms of acquired immunodeficiency syndrome (neuroAIDS). Among Gram-negative bacteria causing neonatal meningitis, *Escherichia coli* and *Citrobacter freundii* are able to invade and transcytose human brain endothelial cells without affecting the integrity of the monolayer (Badger et al., 1999; Stins et al., 2001). *Streptococcus pneumoniae*, possessing the cytotoxic virulence factor pneumolysin, dramatically decreases TEER of bovine brain endothelial cells (Zysk et al., 2001).

Bacterial cell wall components and toxins can also cause severe BBB disturbances. LPS is the primary endotoxin involved in inflammatory processes, sepsis, and multiorgan failure caused by Gram-negative bacteria. LPS induced a concentration and time-dependent increase in monolayer permeability in all tested in vitro BBB models (Tunkel et al., 1991; de Vries et al., 1996a; Gaillard and de Boer, 2000; Descamps et al., 2003; Gaillard et al., 2003). Glial cells protected cerebral endothelial cells from LPS-mediated injury in a coculture model (Descamps et al., 2003). Gram-positive bacterial cell wall component lipoteichoic acid disrupted bovine brain endothelial monolayer integrity in a concentration- and time-dependent manner through glia activation (Boveri et al., 2006). Pertussis toxin severely compromises the integrity of brain endothelial monolayers through protein kinase C (Raub, 1996; Brückener et al., 2003). Cholera toxin, an activator of protein kinase A, has a barrier-tightening action similar to forskolin or cyclic AMP treatment (Rubin et al., 1991).

The BBB participates in the penetration of HIV-1 to brain and development of neuroAIDS (Banks, 1999). Infectious HIV-1 penetrates human brain endothelial monolayer by macropinocytosis (Liu et al., 2002) or absorptive endocytosis (Nakaoke et al., 2005) without changing its permeability. In accordance with this result, HIV-1 envelope protein gp120, either in its infectious glycosylated or in nonglycosylated form, did not affect BBB integrity in a coculture model with high TEER (Deli et al., 2005). In a rat brain endothelial cell monolayer with low TEER gp120 was published to increase albumin flux through a substance P-mediated mechanism (Annunziata et al., 1998). HIV-1 infection did not change the barrier-enhancing effect of blood-derived human macrophages in bovine brain endothelial monolayers (Zenker et al., 2003). In contrast, human T-cell leukemia virus type-1 (HTLV-1) infected human lymphocytes showed enhanced adhesion to and migration through rat GPNT cell line monolayers and induced a twofold increase in paracellular permeability (Romero et al., 2000).

The helminth parasite *Schistosoma mansoni*, in its schistosomula stage, developed a special technique to evade from the host immune system. *Schistosoma mansoni* secreted factors elevated cyclic AMP level in bovine brain endothelial cells and enhanced barrier properties (Trottein et al., 1999). *Candida albicans* is the only fungal pathogen tested on BBB permeability in vitro and no specific effect was seen in human brain endothelial monolayers (Jong et al., 2001).

In infectious, inflammatory, or immune-mediated diseases, cytokines interact with the cells of the BBB. Proinflammatory interleukins affected brain endothelial integrity: interleukin-1α increased inulin flux through porcine cerebral endothelial monolayers (Gloor et al., 1997), while interleukin-1β and interleukin-6 decreased TEER of rat brain endothelial cells (de Vries et al., 1996b). On a dynamic BBB model, interleukin-6 production was a crucial component of a BBB protective mechanism triggered by flow cessation and reperfusion (Krizanac-Bengez et al., 2003).

Tumor necrosis factor-α (TNF-α), the most studied proinflammatory cytokine, increases paracellular or transcellular BBB permeability in vitro. TNF-α decreased TEER of endothelial monolayers either in coculture with glia (Hurst and Fritz, 1996; de Vries et al., 1996b; Hurst and Clark, 1997; Dobbie et al., 1999) or in monoculture (Dobbie et al., 1999). TNF-α also increased the flux of sucrose, sodium fluorescein, cisplatin, inulin, FITC-dextran with molecular weight of 3, 4, and 70 kDa, and albumin (for review see Deli et al., 2005). These changes of permeability were accompanied by reorganization of actin filaments into stress fibers (Deli et al., 1995c). TNF-α significantly elevated the transcytosis of transport molecules LDL and lactoferrin (Descamps et al., 1997; Fillebeen et al., 1999) through the MAP kinase pathway (Miller et al., 2005).

Antiviral cytokine interferon-α2a elevated TEER in bovine brain endothelial cell–rat astroglia coculture, and reduced the LPS-induced damage to endothelial monolayer integrity, similarly to interferon-β1b (Gaillard et al., 2003). In contrast, interferon-γ, a proinflammatory cytokine, elevated albumin flux through rat brain endothelial monolayers (Annunziata et al., 2002).

3.1.3 Neurodegenerative Diseases

Amyloid proteins and peptides are involved in the pathogenesis of fatal neurodegenerative conditions like Alzheimer's or prion diseases. Toxic effects of amyloid-β 1–40 and 25–35 peptide treatments were found in RBE4 rat brain endothelial cell line (Preston et al., 1998). Amyloid-β 1–40 peptide increased the paracellular permeability in bovine (Strazielle et al., 2000), and in primary rat brain endothelial cells (Deli et al., 2005). A dose-dependent toxicity by prion peptide 106–126 treatment was described in primary mouse cerebral endothelial cells, which could be attenuated by pentosan polysulfate, a prophylactic agent in scrapie (Deli et al., 2000). Pathogenic factors of neurodegenerative diseases also damage efflux and influx pump mechanisms, metabolic and detoxifying functions in brain endothelial cells in vitro and in vivo (for review see Deli, 2005).

3.2   Drug Targeting to Brain

The BBB is the main regulator of drug transport to the CNS. The problem from clinical point of view is twofold: 98% of potential neuropharmaceuticals do not penetrate the BBB (Pardridge, 2002), while unwanted central nervous system (CNS) side effects develop, if a drug with main peripheral action crosses the BBB (Chishty et al., 2001). Lipid soluble small molecules (molecular weight (400–500 Da), like nicotine, ethanol, caffeine, enter the brain with lipid-mediated free diffusion. In contrast, hydrophilic molecules, substances bigger than 400–500 Da, or ligands of efflux transporters—like majority of medicaments—do not cross the BBB. The strategies can be either the modification of the molecules or the modification of the BBB permeability, or both.

3.2.1 Strategies to Modify Molecules

Several methods exist to enhance brain delivery of molecules by changing their physicochemical properties.

The luminal surface of brain endothelial cells contains glycocalyx residues that establish a negative charge, which contributes to the barrier phenotype. Negatively charged molecules, e.g., FITC-dextrans or nanoparticles, crosses the barrier in significantly lower amount than neutral or cationic ones (Sahagun et al., 1990; Fenart et al., 1999). While nanoparticles did not change basal permeability of brain endothelial cells, their transport was enhanced by lipid coating.

On the other hand, cationization of ferritin (Hart et al., 1987), albumin (Smith and Borchardt, 1989), or anti-tetanus immunoglobulin Fab'2 fragment (Girod et al., 1999) leads to better transcytosis of the above-mentioned macromolecules without changing the barrier integrity. Furthermore, albumin loaded in lipid-coated cationic nanoparticles had a 27-fold-enhanced transport (Fenart et al., 1999). Neutralization of the brain endothelial luminal surface charge by cationic ferritin, as opposed to the treatment with neutral ferritin, resulted in increased transport of Evan's blue dye, a small polar molecule, while TEER and permeability for 20-kDa molecular weight. FITC-dextran was not changed (Hart et al., 1987).

Glycosylation of albumin, similarly to cationization, also resulted in an eightfold elevation of transendothelial transport (Smith and Borchardt, 1989).

Increasing lipid solubility is another successful technique. Monoacylation of ribonuclease A facilitates the transport of the enzyme through the BBB: palmitoylated and stearoylated, but not myristoylated, derivatives show increased BBB transport without degradation of protein or modification of barrier permeability for sucrose or inulin (Chopineau et al., 1998). It is suggested that a minimal length of 16 carbon atoms is required for a translocation of ribonuclease A across monolayers of bovine endothelial cells cocultured with rat astrocytes.

Using antibody phage display technology, single domain antibodies could be selected to effectively cross human in vitro BBB model and in vivo BBB with a potential to use in macromolecule delivery as brain targeting vector (Muruganandam et al., 2002). The transport of FC5, one of the antibodies across human brain endothelial cells, was polarized, charge independent, and temperature dependent, suggesting receptor-mediated process probably involving $\alpha(2,3)$-sialoglycoprotein receptor that triggers clathrin-mediated endocytosis (Abulrob et al., 2005).

Carrier-mediated transporters at the BBB can also be used for drug delivery. The L-glutamate transport system was utilized to facilitate a nonpermeable drug across bovine brain microvessel endothelial monolayers by conjugating the drug with L-glutamate amino acid (Sakaeda et al., 2000).

3.2.2 Strategies to Modify BBB Functions

The efflux pumps and the strictly regulated paracellular barrier are the two major BBB functions in the focus of attempts to enhance drug delivery by modulation of BBB.

P-glycoprotein is the main efflux pump at the BBB to prevent entry of drugs to brain. These drugs include antibiotics, antineoplastic agents, drugs to treat epilepsy and AIDS. BBB models are useful in experiments focused on drug/P-glycoprotein interaction and P-glycoprotein activity modifications.

Rame-β-cyclodextrin and crysme-β-cyclodextrin increased the transport of doxorubicin through a bovine BBB model by a factor of 2 and 3.7, respectively (Tilloy et al., 2006). This increase was attributed to the cholesterol extraction property of these cyclodextrins from brain capillary endothelial cells leading to a modulation of the P-gp activity. Pluronic block copolymer, P85 enhanced BBB transport of digoxin both in vitro and in vivo (Batrakova et al., 2001b). Experiments on bovine brain endothelial cells suggest that both energy depletion (decreasing ATP pool available for P-gp) and membrane fluidization (inhibiting P-gp ATPase activity) are critical factors contributing to the activity of P85 block copolymer at the BBB (Batrakova et al., 2001a).

Selective inhibitors of P-glycoprotein valsprodar and elacridar increase both CNS anticancer drug delivery and therapeutic efficacy in animal models (Doolittle et al., 2005). P-glycoprotein protects the BBB against the disruptive effects of antimicrotubule drugs vinblastine, colchicine, and paclitaxel. When antimicrotubule drugs were used in combination of potent P-glycoprotein modulators, the integrity of bovine brain endothelial cell monolayers was lost (van der Sandt et al., 2001). These data indicate that use of P-glycoprotein blockers with cytostatic drugs should be carefully planned and monitored.

3.3 Modulation of BBB Permeability

Modulation of BBB permeability is another important element of strategies for drug targeting to brain. A safe, rapid, and transient increase of BBB permeability pathways would be optimal for clinical use. Not only the "tight" but also the "leaky" BBB can be a problem. Neurological or other diseases are often associated with BBB dysfunctions and permeability changes. Treatment of BBB dysfunctions could be therapeutic to prevent secondary neuronal damage.

3.3.1 Transient Increase of BBB Permeability

The paracellular or junctional route is modulated by osmotic stress at the BBB. Hyperosmotic concentrations of arabinose or mannitol induces a rapid and reversible decrease in TEER, and increases permeability for sucrose and inulin through brain endothelial cell monolayers (Bowman et al., 1983; Hart et al., 1987; Dehouck et al., 1990; Fischer et al., 1995; Deli et al., 1995c; Hurst and Fritz, 1996; Descamps et al., 1997; Fillebeen et al., 1999; Brillault et al., 2002). *Src* kinase-dependent phosphorylation of the adherens junction protein β-catenin, its subcellular redistribution, and its dissociation from cadherin and α-catenin can be one of the elements of the mode of action of hyperosmotic mannitol treatment (Farkas et al., 2005). The importance of these findings and the usefulness of in vitro models are underlined by the fact that BBB disruption using hyperosmotic mannitol is one of the safest and most effective methods to induce reversible increase of BBB permeability for cytostatic drug delivery to treat brain tumors clinically in the last 20 years (Neuwelt and Rapoport, 1984; Doolittle et al., 2000).

Bradykinin, an established mediator of vasogenic brain edema, decreases TEER in BBB models (Hurst and Clark, 1998; Gaillard and de Boer, 2000; Easton and Abbott, 2002). This effect mediated through B_2 bradykinin receptors has been exploited for reversible and temporal opening of the BBB by receptor agonists RMP-7 or cereport on human brain microvascular endothelial cell monolayers (Mackic et al., 1999) and can be prevented by receptor antagonist HOE-140 (Easton and Abbott, 2002).

Histamine, a mediator of brain edema (Joó, 1993), has a dual action on brain endothelial cells (Abbott, 2000). While low concentrations of this neurotransmitter vasogenic amine increase albumin permeability (Deli et al., 1995b) and decrease TEER value (Hurst and Clark, 1998) via H_2 histamine receptor activation coupled to increased intracellular Ca^{2+} concentration, high concentrations increase TEER (Gaillard and de Boer, 2000) through H_1 receptor and elevation of cyclic AMP level. Intracellular histamine-binding site antagonist N,N-diethyl-2-[4-(phenylmethyl)-phenoxy]ethanamine (DPPE) deteriorated barrier integrity in monolayers of mouse brain endothelial cells cocultured with rat C6 glioma cells (Deli et al., 2003).

The gaseous second messenger NO, involved in brain and BBB pathologies, can exert both damaging and protective effects on the barrier integrity (for review see Deli et al., 2005). NO at concentration lower than 10 μM does not change in vitro permeability (Hurst and Clark, 1997; Utepbergenov et al., 1998). Doses of NO higher than 20 μM induce a rapid drop in TEER and an increase in fluorescein flux (Hurst and Clark, 1997; Hurst et al., 1998; Utepbergenov et al., 1998). This threshold effect can be observed with NO donors, too. SNAP does not change the barrier integrity at 60 μM or below (Raub, 1996; Utepbergenov et al., 1998; Mark et al., 2004), but induces permeability increase at 150 μM (Utepbergenov et al., 1998). For comparison, diethylenetriamine NONOate, a longer acting NO donor, raises sucrose P_e above the dose of 10 μM (Mark et al., 2004). Another NO donor, 3-morpholinosydnonimine is without effect on TEER (Raub, 1996), but sodium nitroprusside enhanced the permeability in all concentrations in all models (Rubin et al., 1991; Raub, 1996; Fischer et al., 1999; Gaillard and de Boer, 2000). Nonselective blocker of NO synthases $N\omega$-nitro-L-arginine methyl ester (L-NAME) N^G-monomethyl-L-arginine (L-NMMA), or 1400W, a selective inhibitor of inducible NO synthase, did not show a permeability-modifying action. On the dynamic in vitro BBB model, exposure to L-NAME during baseline flow with normal shear levels caused a rapid decrease in TEER arguing for protective actions by basal NO production, and that NO can be important in the maintenance of BBB functions (Krizanac-Bengez et al., 2003).

NO activates the soluble guanylate cyclase signal transduction pathway and increases intracellular guanosine $3',5'$-cyclic monophosphate (cyclic GMP) levels. Both exogenous 8-Br-cyclic GMP and atrial natriuretic peptide impair barrier functions (Rubin et al., 1991; Fischer et al., 1999; Deli et al., 2005).

3.3.2 Preventing the Increase of BBB Permeability Induced by Pathological Factors

BBB dysfunction is an early event in many neurological conditions, and damaged BBB became a target for drug action (Abbott et al., 2006). An increasing number of molecules with potential endothelial protective effects are tested on in vitro BBB models mimicking pathological conditions (❷ *Table 2-4*).

■ Table 2-4
Modulation of BBB permeability in vitro

Transient increase of BBB permeability
- Hyperosmotic solutions:
  Arabinose, mannitol, urea
- Receptor-mediated mechanisms:
  Vasogenic amine–related mechanisms
    Bradykinin, cereport (RMP7), histamine, DPPE
  Guanylate cyclase–related mechanisms
    Atrial natriuretic peptide, cyclic GMP analogs, NO donors (sodium nitroprusside, DETA-NONOate),
    Preventing the increase in BBB permeability induced by pathological factors NOS inhibitors (L-NAME)
- Adrenomedullin
- Angiopoietin-1
- Barbiturates
  Methohexital, thiopental
- Calcium channel blockers
  SKF 96365, nifedipine
- Carnosine
- Free radical scavengers
  U83836E
- Glucocorticoids
  Dexamethasone, hydrocortisone
- NMDA antagonists
  Dizocilpine (MK-801)
- NO and NO donors
  Gaseous NO, S-nitroso-N-acetylpenicillamine
- NOS inhibitors
  1400W, L-NAME
- Pentosan polysulfate

1400W N-(3-aminomethyl)benzylacetamidine, *BBB* blood–brain barrier, *DETA-NONOate* 2,2′-(hydroxynitrosohydrazino)*bis*-ethanamine, *DPPE* N,N-diethyl-2-[4-(phenylmethyl)-phenoxy]ethanamine, *L-NAME* Nω-nitro-L-arginine methyl ester, *SKF 96365* 1-[2-(4-methoxyphenyl)-2-[3-(4-methoxyphenyl)propoxy]ethyl-1H-imidazole hydrochloride, *U83836E* (-)-2-((4-(2,6-Di-1-pyrrolidinyl-4-pyrimidinyl)-1-piperazinyl)methyl)-3,4-dihydro-2,3,7,8-tetramethyl-2H-1-benzopyran-6-ol, 2HCl

Hypoxia or OGD-induced brain endothelial hyperpermeability could be effectively blocked by: N-methyl-D-aspartic acid (NMDA) receptor antagonist MK-801 and aminosteroid U83836E (Giese et al., 1995), barbiturates methohexital and thiopental (Fischer et al., 1995), NO and the NO donor S-nitroso-N-acetylpenicillamine (Utepbergenov et al., 1998), nonspecific cation channel blocker SKF 96365 and L-type calcium channel blocker nifedipine (Abbruscato and Davis, 1999), dexamethasone (Fischer et al., 2001), or NO synthase inhibitors L-NAME, and 1400W (Mark et al., 2004). Adrenomedullin, a hypoxia-induced vasodilator peptide, protected rat brain endothelial monolayers from oxidative injury (Chen et al., 2005). On both ischemic in vivo and BBB in vitro models VEGF-enhanced BBB damage and matrix metalloproteinase-9 activity was counteracted by angiopoietin-1 (Valable et al., 2005).

Carnosine, a naturally occurring dipeptide, and pentosan, a clinically used sulfated polysaccharide, inhibited toxic effects of amyloid-β and prion peptides on rat brain endothelial cells (Preston et al., 1998; Deli et al., 2000).

Dexamethasone pretreated bovine brain endothelial cell monolayers were more resistant to LPS-induced TEER decrease and free radical inhibitor N-acetyl-cysteine was also effective (Gaillard et al., 2003). Dexamethasone also provided significant BBB "tightening" effects in the presence of permeability increasing glioma cells (Grabb and Gilbert, 1995). The natural compound glycerophosphoinositol replicated the TEER-increasing effects of dexamethasone on endothelial monolayers and reverted time-dependent TEER decline (Cucullo et al., 2004).

3.4   Permeability Screening

The pharmaceutical industry needs simple, reliable, in vitro BBB models for predicting BBB permeability of CNS drugs. Any in vitro model to serve as a permeability screen should display a restrictive paracellular pathway, a physiologically realistic cell architecture, functional expression of transporter mechanisms, and ease of culture to facilitate drug screening (Gumbleton and Audus, 2001). Though none of the currently available models fits all the criteria, some models can provide reasonable information on drug permeability.

Lundquist et al. (2002) compared bovine brain endothelial cell/rat astroglia coculture, one of the best characterized and tightest BBB models, with Caco-2 cell layers, a popular model for gut permeability screening. There were strong correlations between in vitro and in vivo BBB permeability data, similarly to previous results (Cecchelli et al., 1999). In contrast, a poor correlation was obtained between Caco-2 cell data and in vivo BBB transport (Lundquist et al., 2002).

In a comparative study, several permeability models were tested for a set of test compounds with different properties, transport mechanisms, and degree of permeability (Garberg et al., 2005). Besides primary bovine and human brain endothelial cells cocultured with astrocytes, a rat (SV-ARBEC) and a mouse (MBEC4) immortalized cerebral endothelial cell lines, and non-BBB models ECV/C6, MDCK, and Caco-2 were used. Compounds could be classified into four groups according to their BBB transport: passive diffusion, blood flow–limited passive diffusion, carrier-mediated influx, and active efflux. While several models (primary bovine, MDCK-MDR) could distinguish between passively distributed compounds and efflux substrates, tighter BBB models are needed to identify drugs that are ligands for carrier-mediated or active influx (Garberg et al., 2005). Although studies on passive transport may not require specific BBB models, the presence of specific transporters, metabolic pathways, and receptors make it impossible to replace BBB-derived cell lines with non-BBB-derived cell lines. A long-term goal for drug screening would be a human brain endothelial cell line–based tight BBB model.

4   Conclusions

In the last 30 years, in vitro BBB model systems were successfully used to get information on the physiological functions of the BBB and the complexity of the BBB phenotype. These models were especially valuable for studies on cross talk between cells of the BBB and identifying BBB phenotype-inducing factors. On the basis of results, new double and triple coculture models have been developed, with better BBB properties and tighter paracellular barrier. The best in vitro BBB models are not only suitable for basic research purposes but can be used for testing BBB permeability of drugs and vectors.

New results are expected from gene and protein profiling of brain endothelial cells or isolated brain microvessels under physiological and pathological conditions. A recently published transcriptome catalog of rat brain microvessels revealed gene groups encoding transporters (11%), receptors (5%), proteins involved in vesicle trafficking (4%), structural proteins (10%), and components of signal transduction pathways (17%) emphasizing a unique cellular phenotype (Enerson and Drewes, 2006).

Diseases affecting BBB is another major research area in which in vitro models are used with success in parallel with animal studies. Novel candidate molecules at the level of the BBB could be identified by proteomics and gene array screens in experimental autoimmune encephalomyelitis pathogenesis (Alt et al., 2005), and in TNF-activated human brain endothelial cells (Franzen et al., 2003). BBB models can be useful in the development of targeted therapies for the BBB, an emerging treatment possibility in pathologies involving BBB disorders (Abbott et al., 2006).

An expansion of published papers using cell culture–based BBB models has been seen in the last few years. With the refinement and specialized application of in vitro BBB models this trend will certainly continue.

Acknowledgments

This work was supported by grants from the Hungarian Research Fund (OTKA T37834) and National Office for Research and Technology (RET 08/2004). The help of Dr. Csongor Ábrahám in critical reading of this chapter is gratefully acknowledged.

References

Abbott NJ. 2000. Inflammatory mediators and modulation of blood-brain barrier permeability. Cell Mol Neurobiol 20: 131-147.

Abbott NJ. 2002. Astrocyte-endothelial interactions and the blood-brain barrier permeability. J Anat 200: 629-638.

Abbott NJ. 2005. Dynamics of CNS barriers: Evolution, differentiation and modulation. Cell Mol Neurobiol 25: 5-23.

Abbott NJ, Hughes CCW, Revest PA, Greenwood J. 1992. Development and characterisation of a rat brain capillary endothelial culture: Towards an *in vitro* blood-brain barrier. J Cell Sci 103: 23-37.

Abbott NJ, Rönnbäck L, Hansson E. 2006. Astrocyte-endothelial interactions at the blood-brain barrier. Nat Rev Neurosci 7: 41-53.

Abbruscato TJ, Davis TP. 1999. Combination of hypoxia/aglycemia compromises in vitro blood-brain barrier integrity. J Pharmacol Exp Ther 289: 668-675.

Abulrob A, Sprong H, Van Bergen en Henegouwen P, Stanimirovic D. 2005. The blood-brain barrier transmigrating single domain antibody: Mechanisms of transport and antigenic epitopes in human brain endothelial cells. J Neurochem 95: 1201-1214.

Alt C, Duvefelt K, Franzen B, Yang Y, Engelhardt B. 2005. Gene and protein expression profiling of the microvascular compartment in experimental autoimmune encephalomyelitis in C57Bl/6 and SJL mice. Brain Pathol 15: 1-16.

Annunziata P, Cioni C, Santonini R, Paccagnini E. 2002. Substance P antagonist blocks leakage and reduces activation of cytokine-stimulated rat brain endothelium. J Neuroimmunol 131: 41-49.

Annunziata P, Cioni C, Toneatto S, Paccagnini E. 1998. HIV-1 gp120 increases the permeability of rat brain endothelium cultures by a mechanism involving substance P. AIDS 12: 2377-2385.

Arthur FE, Shivers RR, Bowman PD. 1987. Astrocyte-mediated induction of tight junctions in brain capillary endothelium: An efficient in vitro model. Brain Res 433: 155-159.

Badger JL, Stins MF, Kim KS. 1999. *Citrobacter freundii* invades and replicates in human brain microvascular endothelial cells. Infect Immun 67: 4208-4215.

Banks WA. 1999. Physiology and pathology of the blood-brain barrier: Implications for microbial pathogenesis, drug delivery and neurodegenerative disorders. J Neurovirol 5: 538-555.

Batrakova EV, Li S, Vinogradov SV, Alakhov VY, Miller DW, et al. 2001a. Mechanism of pluronic effect on P-glycoprotein efflux system in blood-brain barrier: Contributions of energy depletion and membrane fluidization. J Pharmacol Exp Ther 299: 483-493.

Batrakova EV, Miller DW, Li S, Alakhov VY, Kabanov AV, et al. 2001b. Pluronic P85 enhances the delivery of digoxin to the brain: In vitro and in vivo studies. J Pharmacol Exp Ther 296: 551-557.

Bauer HC, Bauer H. 2000. Neural induction of the blood-brain barrier: Still an enigma. Cell Mol Neurobiol 20: 13-28.

Berezowski V, Landry C, Dehouck M-P, Cecchelli R, Fenart L. 2004. Contribution of glial cells and pericytes to the mRNA profiles of P-glycoprotein and multidrug resistance-associated proteins in an in vitro model of the blood-brain barrier. Brain Res 1018: 1-9.

Boveri M, Berezowski V, Price A, Slupek S, Lenfant AM, et al. 2005. Induction of blood-brain barrier properties in cultured brain capillary endothelial cells: Comparison between primary glial cells and C6 cell line. Glia 51: 187-198.

Boveri M, Kinsner A, Berezowski V, Lenfant AM, Draing C, et al. 2006. Highly purified lipoteichoic acid from gram-positive bacteria induces in vitro blood-brain barrier disruption through glia activation: Role of pro-inflammatory cytokines and nitric oxide. Neuroscience 137: 1193-1209.

Bowman PD, Betz AL, Wolinsky JS, Penny JB, Shivers RR, et al. 1981. Primary cultures of capillary endothelium from rat brain. In Vitro 17: 353-362.

Bowman PD, Ennis SR, Rarey KE, Betz AL, Goldstein GW. 1983. Brain microvessel endothelial cells in tissue culture: A model for study of blood-brain barrier permeability. Ann Neurol 14: 396-402.

Brightman MW, Reese TS. 1969. Junctions between intimately apposed cell membranes in the vertebrate brain. J Cell Biol 40: 648-677.

Brillault J, Berezowski V, Cecchelli R, Dehouck M-P. 2002. Intercommunications between brain capillary endothelial cells and glial cells increase the transcellular permeability of the blood-brain barrier during ischaemia. J Neurochem 83: 807-817.

Brown J, Reading SJ, Jones S, Fitchett CJ, Howl J, et al. 2000. Critical evaluation of ECV304 as a human endothelial cell model defined by genetic analysis and functional responses: A comparison with the human bladder cancer derived epithelial cell line T24/83. Lab Invest 80: 37-45.

Brown RC, Mark KS, Egleton RD, Huber JD, Burroughs AR, et al. 2003. Protection against hypoxia-induced increase in blood-brain barrier permeability: Role of tight junction proteins and NFκB. J Cell Sci 116: 693-700.

Brückener KE, el Bayâ A, Galla H-J, Schmidt MA. 2003. Permeabilization in a cerebral endothelial barrier model by pertussis toxin involves the PKC effector pathway and is abolished by elevated levels of cAMP. J Cell Sci 116: 1837-1846.

Cecchelli R, Dehouck B, Descamps L, Fenart L, Buée-Scherrer V, et al. 1999. In vitro model for evaluating drug transport across the blood-brain barrier. Adv Drug Deliv Rev 36: 165-178.

Cestelli A, Catania C, D'Agostino S, Di Liegro I, Licata L, et al. 2001. Functional feature of a novel model of blood brain barrier: Studies on permeation of test compounds. J Control Release 76: 139-147.

Chen L, Kis B, Busija DW, Yamashita H, Ueta Y. 2005. Adrenomedullin protects rat cerebral endothelial cells from oxidant damage in vitro. Regul Pept 130: 27-34.

Chishty M, Reichel A, Siva J, Abbott NJ, Begley DJ. 2001. Affinity for the P-glycoprotein efflux pump at the blood-brain barrier may explain the lack of CNS side-effects of modern antihistamines. J Drug Target 9: 223-228.

Chopineau J, Robert S, Fenart L, Cecchelli R, Lagoutte B, et al. 1998. Monoacylation of ribonuclease A enables its transport across an in vitro model of the blood-brain barrier. J Control Release 56: 231-237.

Coisne C, Dehouck L, Faveeuw C, Delplace Y, Miller F, et al. 2005. Mouse syngenic in vitro blood-brain barrier model: A new tool to examine inflammatory events in cerebral endothelium. Lab Invest 85: 734-746.

Cucullo L, Hallene K, Dini G, Dal Toso R, Janigro D. 2004. Glycerophosphoinositol and dexamethasone improve transendothelial electrical resistance in an in vitro study of the blood-brain barrier. Brain Res 997: 147-151.

de Boer AG, van der Sandt ICJ, Gaillard PJ. 2003. The role of drug transporters at the blood-brain barrier. Annu Rev Pharmacol Toxicol 43: 629-656.

de Vries HE, Blom-Roosemalen MC, de Boer AG, van Berkel TJ, Breimer DD, et al. 1996a. Effect of endotoxin on permeability of bovine cerebral endothelial cell layers in vitro. J Pharmacol Exp Ther 277: 1418-1423.

de Vries HE, Blom-Roosemalen MC, van Oosten M, de Boer AG, van Berkel TJ, et al. 1996b. The influence of cytokines on the integrity of the blood-brain barrier in vitro. J Neuroimmunol 64: 37-43.

De Bault LE, Cancilla PA. 1980. Gamma-glutamyl transpeptidase in isolated brain endothelial cells: Induction by glial cells in vitro. Science 207: 653-655.

Dehouck M-P, Méresse S, Delorme P, Fruchart JC, Cecchelli R. 1990. An easier, reproducible, and mass-production method to study the blood-brain barrier in vitro. J Neurochem 54: 1798-1801.

Dehouck M-P, Méresse S, Dehouck B, Fruchart JC, Cecchelli R. 1992. In vitro reconstituted blood-brain barrier. J Control Release 21: 81-92.

Deli MA. 2005. The role of blood-brain barrier in neurodegenerative diseases. Molecular Bases of Neurodegeneration. Di Liegro I, Savettieri G, editors. Kerala, India: Research Signpost; pp. 137-161.

Deli MA, Ábrahám CS, Kataoka Y, Niwa M. 2005. Permeability studies on in vitro blood-brain barrier models: Physiology, pathology, and pharmacology. Cell Mol Neurobiol 25: 59-127.

Deli MA, Ábrahám CS, Niwa M, Falus A. 2003. N,N-diethyl-2-[4-(phenylmethyl)phenoxy]-ethanamide increases the permeability of primary mouse cerebral endothelial cell monolayers. Inflamm Res 52: S39-S40.

Deli MA, Dehouck M-P, Ábrahám CS, Cecchelli R, Joó F. 1995a. Penetration of small molecular weight substances through cultured bovine brain capillary endothelial cells: The early effects of 3′,5′-cyclic adenosine monophosphate. Exp Physiol 80: 675-678.

Deli MA, Dehouck M-P, Cecchelli R, Ábrahám CS, Joó F. 1995b. Histamine induces a selective albumin permeation through the blood-brain barrier in vitro. Inflamm Res 44: S56-S57.

Deli MA, Descamps L, Dehouck M-P, Cecchelli R, Joó F, et al. 1995c. Exposure of tumor necrosis factor α to the luminal membrane induces a delayed increase of permeability and formation of cytoplasmic actin stress fibers in brain capillary endothelial cells cocultured with astrocytes. J Neurosci Res 41: 717-726.

Deli MA, Sakaguchi S, Nakaoke R, Ábrahám CS, Takahata H, et al. 2000. PrP fragment 106–126 is toxic to cerebral endothelial cells expressing PrP(C). Neuroreport 11: 3931-3936.

Descamps L, Cecchelli R, Torpier G. 1997. Effects of tumor necrosis factor on receptor-mediated endocytosis and barrier functions of bovine brain capillary endothelial cell monolayers. J Neuroimmunol 74: 173-184.

Descamps L, Coisne C, Dehouck B, Cecchelli R, Torpier G. 2003. Protective effect of glial cells against lipopolysaccharide-mediated blood-brain barrier injury. Glia 42: 46-58.

Diaz CM, Penfold PL, Provis JM. 1998. Modulation of the resistance of a human endothelial cell line by human retinal glia. Aust N Z J Ophthalmol 26: S62-S64.

Dobbie MS, Hurst RD, Klein NJ, Surtees RAH. 1999. Upregulation of intracellular adhesion molecule-1 expression on human endothelial cells by tumour necrosis factor-α in an in vitro model of the blood-brain barrier. Brain Res 830: 330-336.

Dohgu S, Takata F, Yamauchi A, Nakagawa S, Egawa T, et al. 2005. Brain pericytes contribute to the induction and up-regulation of blood-brain barrier functions through transforming growth factor-beta production. Brain Res 1038: 208-215.

Doolittle ND, Abrey LE, Bleyer WA, Brem S, Davis TP, et al. 2005. New frontiers in translational research in neuro-oncology and the blood-brain barrier: Report of the tenth annual Blood-Brain Barrier Disruption Consortium Meeting. Clin Cancer Res 11: 421-428.

Doolittle ND, Miner ME, Hall WA, Siegal T, Jerome E, et al. 2000. Safety and efficacy of a multicenter study using intraarterial chemotherapy in conjunction with osmotic opening of the blood-brain barrier for the treatment of patients with malignant brain tumors. Cancer 88: 637-647.

Duport S, Robert F, Muller D, Grau G, Parisi L, et al. 1998. An in vitro blood-brain barrier model: Cocultures between endothelial cells and organotypic brain slice cultures. Proc Natl Acad Sci USA 95: 1840-1845.

Dömötör E, Sipos I, Kittel A, Abbott NJ, Ádám-Vízi V. 1998. Improved growth of cultured brain microvascular endothelial cells on glass coated with a biological matrix. Neurochem Int 33: 473-478.

Easton AS, Abbott JN. 2002. Bradykinin increases permeability by calcium and 5-lipoxygenase in the ECV304/C6 cell culture model of the blood-brain barrier. Brain Res 953: 157-169.

El Hafny B, Bourre JM, Roux F. 1996. Synergistic stimulation of gamma-glutamyl transpeptidase and alkaline phosphatase activities by retinoic acid and astroglial factors in immortalized rat brain microvessel endothelial cells. J Cell Physiol 167: 451-460.

Enerson BE, Drewes LR. 2006. The rat blood-brain barrier transcriptome. J Cereb Blood Flow Metab 26: 959-973.

Farkas A, Szatmári E, Orbók A, Wilhelm I, Wejksza K, et al. 2005. Hyperosmotic mannitol induces Src kinase-dependent phosphorylation of beta-catenin in cerebral endothelial cells. J Neurosci Res 80: 855-861.

Fenart L, Casanova A, Dehouck B, Duhem C, Slupek S, et al. 1999. Evaluation of effect of charge and lipid coating on ability of 60-nm nanoparticles to cross an in vitro model of the blood-brain barrier. J Pharmacol Exp Ther 291: 1017-1022.

Fillebeen C, Dehouck B, Benaïssa M, Dhennin-Duthille I, Cecchelli R, et al. 1999. Tumor necrosis factor-α increases lactoferrin transcytosis through the blood-brain barrier. J Neurochem 73: 2491-2500.

Fischer S, Clauss M, Wiesnet M, Renz D, Schaper W, et al. 1999. Hypoxia induces permeability in brain microvessel endothelial cells via VEGF and NO. Am J Physiol Cell Physiol 276: C812-C820.

Fischer S, Renz D, Schaper W, Karliczek GF. 1995. In vitro effects of fentanyl, methohexital, and thiopental brain endothelial permeability. Anesthesiology 82: 451-458.

Fischer S, Renz D, Schaper W, Karliczek GF. 2001. In vitro effects of dexamethasone on hypoxia-induced hyperpermeability and expression of vascular endothelial growth factor. Eur J Pharmacol 411: 231-243.

Franke H, Galla H-J, Beuckmann CT. 1999. An improved low-permeability in vitro-model of the blood-brain barrier: Transport studies on retinoids, sucrose, haloperidol, caffeine and mannitol. Brain Res 818: 65-71.

Franzen B, Duvefelt K, Jonsson C, Engelhardt B, Ottervald J, et al. 2003. Gene and protein expression profiling of human cerebral endothelial cells activated with tumor necrosis factor-alpha. Brain Res Mol Brain Res 115: 130-146.

Gaillard PJ, de Boer AB, Breimer DD. 2003. Pharmacological investigations on lipopolysaccharide-induced permeability changes in the blood-brain barrier in vitro. Microvasc Res 65: 24-31.

Gaillard PJ, de Boer AG. 2000. Relationship between permeability status of the blood-brain barrier and in vitro permeability coefficient of a drug. Eur J Pharm Sci 12: 95-102.

Garberg P, Ball M, Borg N, Cecchelli R, Fenart L, et al. 2005. In vitro models for the blood-brain barrier. Toxicol. In Vitro 19: 299-334.

Garcia CM, Darland DC, Massingham LJ, D'Amore PA. 2004. Endothelial cell-astrocyte interactions and TGF beta are required for induction of blood-neural barrier properties. Brain Res Dev Brain Res 152: 25-38.

Ge S, Song L, Pachter JS. 2005. Where is the blood-brain barrier . . . really? J Neurosci Res 79: 421-427.

Giese H, Mertsch K, Blasig IE. 1995. Effect of MK-801 and U83836E on a porcine brain capillary endothelial cell barrier during hypoxia. Neurosci Lett 191: 169-172.

Girod J, Fenart L, Regina A, Dehouck M-P, Hong G, et al. 1999. Transport of cationized anti-tetanus Fab'2 fragments across an in vitro blood-brain barrier model: Involvement of the transcytosis pathway. J Neurochem 73: 2002-2008.

Gloor SM, Weber A, Adachi N, Frei K. 1997. Interleukin-1 modulates protein tyrosine phosphatase activity and permeability of brain endothelial cells. Biochem Biophys Res Commun 239: 804-809.

Grabb PA, Gilbert MR. 1995. Neoplastic and pharmacological influence on the permeability of an *in vitro* blood-brain barrier. J Neurosurg 82: 1053-1058.

Greenwood J, Pryce G, Devine L, Male DK, dos Santos WL, et al. 1996. SV40 large immortalised cell lines of the rat blood-brain and blood-retinal barriers retain their phenotypic and immunological characteristics. J Neuroimmunol 71: 51-63.

Gumbleton M, Audus KL. 2001. Progress and limitations in the use of in vitro cell cultures to serve as a permeability screen for the blood-brain barrier. J Pharm Sci 90: 1681-1698.

Hamm S, Dehouck B, Kraus J, Wolburg-Buchholz K, Wolburg H, et al. 2004. Astrocyte mediated modulation of blood-brain barrier permeability does not correlate with a loss of tight junction proteins from the cellular contacts. Cell Tissue Res 315: 157-166.

Hart MN, Van Dyk LF, Moore SA, Shasby DM, Cancilla PA. 1987. Differential opening of the brain endothelial barrier following neutralization of the endothelial luminal anionic charge *in vitro*. J Neuropathol Exp Neurol 46: 141-153.

Haseloff RF, Blasig IE, Bauer H-C, Bauer H. 2005. In search of the astrocytic factor(s) modulating blood-brain barrier functions in brain capillary endothelial cells in vitro. Cell Mol Neurobiol 25: 25-39.

Haseloff RF, Krause E, Bigl M, Mikoteit K, Stanimirovic D, et al. 2006. Differential protein expression in brain capillary endothelial cells induced by hypoxia and posthypoxic reoxygenation. Proteomics 6: 1803-1809.

Hayashi K, Nakao S, Nakaoke R, Nakagawa, S., Kitagawa, N., et al. 2004. Effects of hypoxia on endothelial/pericytic co-culture model of the blood-brain barrier. Regul Pept 123: 77-83.

Hoheisel D, Nitz T, Franke H, Wegener J, Hakvoort A, et al. 1998. Hydrocortisone reinforces the blood-brain barrier properties in a serum free cell culture system. Biochem Biophys Res Commun 247: 312-315.

Hori S, Ohtsuki S, Hosoya K, Nakashima E, Terasaki T. 2004. A pericyte-derived angiopoietin-1 multimeric complex induces occludin gene expression in brain capillary endothelial cells through Tie-2 activation in vitro. J Neurochem 89: 503-513.

Hosoya K, Tetsuka K, Nagase K, Tomi M, Saeki S, et al. 2000. Conditionally immortalized brain capillary endothelial cell lines established from a transgenic mouse harboring temperature-sensitive simian virus 40 large T-antigen gene. AAPS Pharmsci 2(3): E27, pp. 1–11. [http://www.pharmsci.org]

Hudson LC, Bragg DC, Tompkins MB, Meeker RB. 2005. Astrocytes and microglia differentially regulate trafficking of lymphocyte subsets across brain endothelial cells. Brain Res 1058: 148-160.

Hurst RD, Clark JB. 1997. Nitric oxide-induced blood-brain barrier dysfunction is not mediated by inhibition of mitochondrial respiratory chain activity and/or energy depletion. Nitric Oxide 1: 121-129.

Hurst RD, Clark JB. 1998. Alterations in transendothelial electrical resistance by vasoactive agonists and cyclic AMP in a blood-brain barrier model system. Neurochem Res 23: 149-154.

Hurst RD, Clark JB. 1999. Butyric acid mediated induction of enhanced transendothelial resistance in an in vitro model blood-brain barrier system. Neurochem Int 35: 261-267.

Hurst RD, Fritz IB. 1996. Properties of an immortalised vascular endothelial/glioma cell co-culture model of the blood-brain barrier. J Cell Physiol 167: 81-88.

Hurst RD, Heales SJR, Dobbie MS, Barker JE, Clark JB. 1998. Decreased endothelial cell glutathione and increased sensitivity to oxidative stress in an in vitro blood-brain barrier model system. Brain Res 802: 232-240.

Igarashi Y, Utsumi H, Chiba H, Yamada-Sasamori Y, Tobioka H, et al. 1999. Glial cell-line-derived neurotrophic factor induces barrier function of endothelial cells forming the blood-brain barrier. Biochem Biophys Res Commun 261: 108-112.

Jong AY, Stins MF, Huang S-H, Chen SHM, Kim KS. 2001. Traversal of *Candida albicans* across human blood-brain barrier in vitro. Infect Immun 69: 4536-4544.

Joó F. 1985. The blood-brain barrier in vitro: Ten years of research on microvessels isolated from the brain. Neurochem Int 7: 1-25.

Joó F. 1992. The cerebral microvessels in culture, an update. J Neurochem 58: 1-17.

Joó F. 1993. The blood-brain barrier *in vitro*: The second decade. Neurochem Int 23: 499-521.

Joó F, Karnushina I. 1973. A procedure for the isolation of capillaries from rat brain. Cytobios 8: 41-48.

Kása P, Pákáski M, Joó F, Lajtha A. 1991. Endothelial cells from human fetal brain microvessels may be cholinoceptive, but do not synthesize acetylcholine. J Neurochem 56: 2143-2146.

Kiessling F, Kartenbeck J, Haller C. 1999. Cell-cell contacts in the human cell line ECV304 exhibit both endothelial and epithelial characteristics. Cell Tissue Res 297: 131-140.

Kim JA, Tran ND, Li Z, Yang F, Zhou W, et al. 2006. Brain endothelial hemostasis regulation by pericytes. J Cereb Blood Flow Metab 26: 209-217.

Kis B, Deli MA, Kobayashi H, Ábrahám CS, Yanagita T, et al. 2001. Adrenomedullin regulates blood-brain barrier functions in vitro. Neuroreport 12: 4139-4142.

Kondo T, Kinouchi H, Kawase M, Yoshimoto T. 1996. Astroglial cells inhibit the increasing permeability of brain endothelial cell monolayer following hypoxia/reoxygenation. Neurosci Lett 208: 101-104.

Krizanac-Bengez L, Kapural M, Parkinson F, Cucullo L, Hossain M, et al. 2003. Effects of transient loss of shear stress on blood-brain barrier endothelium: Role of nitric oxide and IL-6. Brain Res 977: 239-246.

Krizanac-Bengez L, Mayberg MR, Cunningham E, Hossain M, Ponnampalam S, et al. 2006. Loss of shear stress induces leukocyte-mediated cytokine release and blood-brain barrier failure in dynamic in vitro blood-brain barrier model. J Cell Physiol 206: 68-77.

Krizbai IA, Deli MA. 2003. Signalling pathways regulating the tight junction permeability in the blood-brain barrier. Cell Mol Biol (Noisy-le-grand) 49: 23-31.

Kusch-Poddar M, Drewe J, Fux I, Gutmann H. 2005. Evaluation of the immortalized human brain capillary endothelial cell line BB19 as a human cell culture model for the blood-brain barrier. Brain Res 1064: 21-31.

Kusuhara H, Sugiyama Y. 2001a. Efflux transport systems for drugs at the blood-brain barrier and blood-cerebrospinal fluid barrier (Part 1). Drug Discov Today 6: 150-156.

Kusuhara H, Sugiyama Y. 2001b. Efflux transport systems for drugs at the blood-brain barrier and blood-cerebrospinal fluid barrier (Part 2). Drug Discov Today 6: 206-212.

Kusuhara H, Suzuki H, Naito M, Tsuruo T, Sugiyama Y. 1998. Characterization of efflux transport of organic anions in a mouse brain capillary endothelial cell line. J Pharmacol Exp Ther 285: 1260-1265.

Lee S-W, Kim WJ, Choi YK, SongHS, Son M. J., et al. 2003. SSeCKS regulates angiogenesis and tight junction formation in blood-brain barrier. Nat Med 9: 900-906.

Liu NQ, Lossinsky AS, Popik W, Li X, Gujuluva C, et al. 2002. Human immunodeficiency virus type 1 enters brain microvascular endothelia by macropinocytosis dependent on lipid rafts and the mitogen-activated protein kinase signaling pathway. J Virol 76: 6689-6700.

Lundquist S, Renftel M, Brillault J, Fenart L, Cecchelli R, et al. 2002. Prediction of drug transport through the blood-brain barrier in vivo: A comparison between two in vitro cell models. Pharm Res 19: 976-981.

Mackic JB, Stins M, Jovanovic S, Kim KS, Bartus RT, et al. 1999. Cereport (RMP-7) increases the permeability of human brain microvascular endothelial cell monolayers. Pharm Res 16: 1360-1365.

Mark KS, Burroughs AR, Brown RC, Huber JD, Davis TP. 2004. Nitric oxide mediates hypoxia-induced changes in paracellular permeability of cerebral microvasculature. Am J Physiol Heart Circ Physiol 286: H174-H180.

Mathieu C, Fouchet P, Gauthier LR, Lassalle B, Boussin FD, et al. 2006. Coculture with endothelial cells reduces the population of cycling LeX neural precursors but increases that of quiescent cells with a side population phenotype. Exp Cell Res 312: 707-718.

Miller F, Fenart L, Landry V, Coisne C, Cecchelli R, et al. 2005. The MAP kinase pathway mediates transcytosis induced by TNF-alpha in an in vitro blood-brain barrier model. Eur J Neurosci 22: 835-844.

Muruganandam A, Tanha J, Narang S, Stanimirovic D. 2002. Selection of phage-displayed llama single-domain antibodies that transmigrate across human blood-brain barrier endothelium. FASEB J 16: 240-242.

Nakaoke R, Ryerse JS, Niwa M, Banks WA. 2005. Human immunodeficiency virus type 1 transport across the in vitro mouse brain endothelial cell monolayer. Exp Neurol 193: 101-109.

Neuwelt EA, Rapoport SI. 1984. Modification of the blood-brain barrier in the chemotherapy of malignant brain tumors. Fed Proc 43: 214-219.

Nitz T, Eisenblatter T, Psathaki K, Galla H-J. 2003. Serum-derived factors weaken the barrier properties of cultured porcine brain capillary endothelial cells in vitro. Brain Res 981: 30-40.

Omidi Y, Campbell L, Barar J, Connell D, Akhtar S, et al. 2003. Evaluation of the immortalised mouse brain capillary endothelial cell line, b.End3, as an in vitro blood-brain barrier model for drug uptake and transport studies. Brain Res 990: 95-122.

Panula P, Joó F, Rechardt L. 1978. Evidence for the presence of viable endothelial cells in cultures derived from dissociated rat brain. Experientia 34: 95-97.

Pardridge WM. 2002. Drug and gene targeting to brain with molecular Trojan horses. Nat Rev Drug Discov 1: 131-139.

Parkinson FE, Friesen J, Krizanac-Bengez L, Janigro D. 2003. Use of three-dimensional in vitro model of the rat blood-brain barrier to assay nucleoside efflux from brain. Brain Res 980: 233-241.

Parkinson FE, Hacking C. 2005. Pericyte abundance affects sucrose permeability in cultures of rat brain microvascular endothelial cells. Brain Res 1049: 8-14.

Perrière N, Demeuse P, Garcia E, Regina A, Debray M, et al. 2005. Puromycin-based purification of rat brain capillary endothelial cell cultures. Effect on the expression of blood-brain barrier-specific properties. J Neurochem 93: 279-289.

Plateel M, Dehouck M-P, Torpier G, Cecchelli R, Teissier E. 1995. Hypoxia increases the susceptibility to oxidant stress and the permeability of the blood-brain barrier endothelial cell monolayer. J Neurochem 65: 2138-2145.

Plateel M, Teissier E, Cecchelli R. 1997. Hypoxia dramatically increases the nonspecific transport of blood-borne proteins to the brain. J Neurochem 68: 874-877.

Preston JE, Hipkiss AR, Himsworth DT, Romero IA, Abbott JN. 1998. Toxic effects of beta-amyloid(25-35) on immortalised rat brain endothelial cell: Protection by carnosine, homocarnosine and beta-alanine. Neurosci Lett 242: 105-108.

Raub TJ. 1996. Signal transduction and glial cell modulation of cultured brain microvessel endothelial cell tight junctions. Am J Physiol Cell Physiol 271: C495-C503.

Raub TJ, Kuentzel SL, Sawada GA. 1992. Permeability of bovine brain microvessel endothelial cells *in vitro*: Barrier tightening by a factor released from astroglioma cells. Exp Cell Res 199: 330-340.

Ramsohoye PV, Fritz IB. 1998. Preliminary characterization of glial-secreted factors responsible for the induction of high electrical resistances across endothelial monolayers in a blood-brain barrier model. Neurochem Res 23: 1545-1551.

Reese TS, Karnovsky MJ. 1967. Fine structural localization of a blood-brain barrier to exogenous peroxidase. J Cell Biol 34: 207-217.

Reichel A, Begley DJ, Abbott NJ. 2003. An overview of in vitro techniques for blood-brain barrier studies. The Blood-Brain Barrier: Biology and Research Protocols. Nag S, editor. Methods in Molecular Medicine, Vol. 89. Totowa, NJ: Humana Press.

Romero IA, Prevost M-C, Perret E, Adamson P, Greenwood J, et al. 2000. Interactions between brain endothelial cells and human T-cell leukemia virus type 1-infected lymphocytes: Mechanisms of viral entry into the central nervous system. J Virol 74: 6021-6030.

Romero IA, Radewicz K, Jubin E, Michel CC, Greenwood J, et al. 2003. Changes in cytoskeletal and tight junctional proteins correlate with decreased permeability induced by dexamethasone in cultured rat brain endothelial cells. Neurosci Lett 344: 112-116.

Roux F, Couraud P-O. 2005. Rat brain endothelial cell lines for the study of blood-brain barrier permeability and transport functions. Cell Mol Neurobiol 25: 41-58.

Rubin LL, Hall DE, Porter S, Barbu K, Cannon C, et al. 1991. A cell culture model of the blood-brain barrier. J Cell Biol 115: 1725-1735.

Rubin LL, Staddon JM. 1999. The cell biology of the blood-brain barrier. Annu Rev Neurosci 22: 11-28.

Rutten MJ, Hoover RL, Karnovsky MJ. 1987. Electrical resistance and macromolecular permeability of brain endothelial monolayer cultures. Brain Res 425: 301-310.

Sahagun G, Moore SA, Hart MN. 1990. Permeability of neutral vs. anionic dextrans in cultured brain microvascular endothelium. Am J Physiol 259: H162-H166.

Sakaeda T, Siahaan TJ, Audus KL, Stella VJ. 2000. Enhancement of transport of D-melphalan analogue by conjugation with L-glutamate across bovine brain microvessel endothelial cell monolayers. J Drug Target 8: 195-204.

Schiera G, Bono E, Raffa MP, Gallo A, Pitarresi GL, et al. 2003. Synergistic effects of neurons and astrocytes on the differentiation of brain capillary endothelial cells in culture. J Cell Mol Med 7: 165-170.

Schiera G, Sala S, Gallo A, Raffa MP, Pitarresi GL, et al. 2005. Permeability properties of a three-cell type in vitro model of blood-brain barrier. J Cell Mol Med 9: 373-379.

Shen Q, Goderie SK, Jin L, Karanth N, Sun Y, et al. 2004. Endothelial cells stimulate self-renewal and expand neurogenesis of neural stem cells. Science 304: 1338-1340.

Smith KR, Borchardt RT. 1989. Permeability and mechanism of albumin, cationized albumin, and glycosylated albumin transcellular transport across monolayers of cultured bovine brain capillary endothelial cells. Pharm Res 6: 466-473.

Sobue K, Yamamoto N, Yoneda K, Hodgson ME, Yamashiro K, et al. 1999. Induction of blood-brain barrier properties in immortalized bovine brain endothelial cells by astrocytic factors. Neurosci Res 35: 155-164.

Song HS, Son MJ, Lee YM, Kim WJ, Stanness KA, Neumaier JF, Sexton TJ, Grant GA, Emmi A, et al. 1999. A new model of the blood-brain barrier: Co-culture of neuronal, endothelial, and glial cells under dynamic conditions. Neuroreport 10: 3725-3731.

Stins MF, Badger J, Kim KS. 2001. Bacterial invasion and transcytosis in transfected human brain microvascular endothelial cells. Microb Pathog 30: 19-28.

Strazielle N, Ghersi-Egea JF, Ghisoi, Dehouck M-P, Frangione B, et al. 2000. In vitro evidence that beta-amyloid peptide 1-40 diffuses across the blood-brain barrier and affects its permeability. J Neuropathol Exp Neurol 59: 29-38.

Suda K, Rothen-Rutishauser B, Gunthert M, Wunderli-Allenspach H. 2001. Phenotypic characterization of human umbilical vein endothelial (ECV304) and urinary carcinoma (T24) cells: Endothelial versus epithelial features. In Vitro Cell Dev Biol Anim 37: 505-514.

Tan KH, Dobbie MS, Felix RA, Barrand MA, Hurst RD. 2001. A comparison of the induction of immortalized endothelial cell impermeability by astrocytes. Neuroreport 12: 1329-1334.

Tao-Cheng JH, Nagy Z, Brightman MW. 1987. Tight junctions of brain endothelium *in vitro* are enhanced by astroglia. J Neurosci 7: 3293-3299.

Terasaki T, Ohtsuki S, Hori S, Takanaga H, Nakashima E, et al. 2003. New approaches to in vitro models of blood-brain barrier drug transport. Drug Discov Today 8: 944-954.

Tilling T, Korte D, Hoheisel D, Galla H-J. 1998. Basement membrane proteins influence brain capillary endothelial barrier function in vitro. J Neurochem 71: 1151-1157.

Tilloy S, Monnaert V, Fenart L, Bricout H, Cecchelli R, et al. 2006. Methylated beta-cyclodextrin as P-gp modulators for deliverance of doxorubicin across an in vitro model of blood-brain barrier. Bioorg Med Chem Lett 16: 2154-2157.

Trottein F, Descamps L, Nutten S, Dehouck M-P, Angeli V, et al. 1999. *Schistosoma mansoni* activates host microvascular endothelial cells to acquire an anti-inflammatory phenotype. Infect Immun 67: 3403-3409.

Tsuji A, Tamai I. 1999. Carrier-mediated or specialized transport of drugs across the blood-brain barrier. Adv Drug Deliv Rev 36: 277-290.

Tunkel AR, Rosser SW, Hansen EJ, Scheld WM. 1991. Blood-brain barrier alterations in bacterial meningitis: Development of an in vitro model and observations on the effects of lipopolysaccharide. In Vitro Cell Dev Biol 27A:113-120.

Ueda Y, Nakagawa T, Kubota T, Ido K, Sato K. 2005. Glioma cells under hypoxic conditions block the brain microvascular endothelial cell death induced by serum starvation. J Neurochem 95: 99-110.

Utepbergenov DI, Mertsch K, Sporbert A, Tenz K, Paul M, et al. 1998. Nitric oxide protects blood-brain barrier in vitro from hypoxia/reoxygenation-mediated injury. FEBS Lett 424: 197-201.

Valable S, Montaner J, Bellail A, Berezowski V, Brillault J, et al. 2005. VEGF-induced BBB permeability is associated with an MMP-9 activity increase in cerebral ischemia: Both effects decreased by Ang-1. J Cereb Blood Flow Metab 25: 1491-1504.

van der Sandt IC, Gaillard PJ, Voorwinden HH, de Boer AG, Breimer DD. 2001. P-glycoprotein inhibition leads to enhanced disruptive effects by anti-microtubule cytostatics at the in vitro blood-brain barrier. Pharm Res 18: 587-592.

Walshe TE, Ferguson G, Connell P, O'Brien C, Cahill PA. 2005. Pulsatile flow increases the expression of eNOS, ET-1, and prostacyclin in a novel in vitro coculture model of the retinal vasculature. Invest Ophthalmol Vis Sci 46: 375-382.

Wang W, Merrill MJ, Borchardt RT. 1996. Vascular endothelial growth factor affects permeability of brain microvessel endothelial cells in vitro. Am J Physiol Cell Physiol 271: C1973-C1980.

Weidenfeller C, Schrot S, Zozulya A, Galla H-J. 2005. Murine brain capillary endothelial cells exhibit improved barrier properties under the influence of hydrocortisone. Brain Res 1053: 162-174.

Weksler BB, Subileau EA, Perrière N, Charneau P, Holloway K, et al. 2005. Blood-brain barrier-specific properties of a human adult brain endothelial cell line. FASEB J 19: 1872-1874.

Wolburg H, Lippoldt A. 2002. Tight junctions of the blood-brain barrier: Development, composition and regulation. Vascul Pharmacol 38: 323-337.

Yamagata K, Tagami M, Nara Y, Fujino H, Kubota A, et al. 1997. Faulty induction of blood-brain barrier functions by astrocytes isolated from stroke-prone spontaneously hypertensive rats. Clin Exp Pharmacol Physiol 24: 686-691.

Yamagata K, Tagami M, Takenaga F, Yamori Y, Nara Y, et al. 2003. Polyunsaturated fatty acids induce tight junctions to form in brain capillary endothelial cells. Neuroscience 116: 649-656.

Youdim KA, Avdeef A, Abbott NJ. 2003. In vitro trans-monolayer permeability calculations: Often forgotten assumptions. Drug Discov Today 8: 997-1003.

Zenker D, Begley D, Bratzke H, Rübsamen-Waigmann H, von Briesen H. 2003. Human blood-derived macrophages enhance barrier function of cultured brain capillary endothelial cells. J Physiol 551: 1023-1032.

Zhang C, Harder DR. 2002. Cerebral capillary endothelial cell mitogenesis and morphogenesis induced by astrocytic epoxyeicosatrienoic acid. Stroke 33: 2957-2964.

Zysk G, Schneider-Wald BK, Hwang JH, Bejo L, Kim KS, et al. 2001. Pneumolysin in the main inducer of cytotoxicity to brain microvascular endothelial cells caused by *Streptococcus pneumoniae*. Infect Immun 69: 845-852.

3 Structure and Pathology of the Blood–Brain Barrier

S. Nag

Abstract: The presence of a blood-brain barrier to protein (BBB) was recognized as early as 1885. However, it was not until electron microscopy became available that the structural components of the BBB to protein were localized to cerebral endothelium. Fewer endothelial caveolae and the presence of circumferential tight junctions at the interendothelial spaces constitute the anatomic substrate of the BBB to protein. Further technological advances in the last few decades have resulted in the discovery of numerous proteins in cerebral endothelium. This chapter provides information about many of these proteins and what is known about their role during BBB breakdown in brain diseases. The pathogenesis of BBB breakdown has to be understood before therapy can be designed to control BBB breakdown and the subsequent cerebral edema in various diseases.

List of Abbreviations: AD, Alzheimer's disease; ADP, Adenosine diphosphate; AF-6, ALL-1 fusion partner from chromosome 6; Ang, Angiopoietin; ATP, Adenosine triphosphate; BBB, Blood-brain barrier; Ca^{2+}-ATPase, Calcium-activated adenosine triphosphatase; CNS, Central nervous system; CSF, Cerebrospinal fluid; CT, Computed tomography; EAE, Experimental allergic encephalomyelitis; G-protein, Membrane receptor; GBM, Glioblastoma multiforme; GM-CSF, Granulocyte-Macrophage-colony stimulating factor; GTPase, Guanosine 5'-triphosphate; HGF, Hepatocyte growth factor; 7H6, Tight junction-associated antigen; HIV-1, Human immunodeficiency virus-1; HRP, Horseradish peroxidase; Ig, Immunoglobulin; IL, Interleukin; JAM, Junctional adhesion molecule; Mg^{2+}, Magnesium; MMP, Matrix metalloproteinases; MW, Molecular weight; NEF, N-ethyl maleimide; Nm, Nanometers; NSF, NEF-sensitive fusion factor; PECAM-1, Platelet/Endothelial cell adhesion molecules; SF, Scatter factor; SNAP, Soluble NSF attachment protein; v-SNARE, Vesicle-associated SNAP receptor; VAMP-2, Vesicle-associated membrane protein-2; Ser/Thr kinase, Serine/Threonine kinase; Tie2, Tyrosine kinase with Immunoglobulin-like loops and epidermal growth factor homology domains; TGF, Transforming growth factor; TNF, Tumor necrosis factor; UTP, Uridine 5'-triphosphate; VCAM, Vascular cell adhesion molecule; VEGF, Vascular endothelial growth factor; ZO, Zonula occludens

1   Introduction

The classical experiments of Ehrlich (1885) led to the recognition that cerebral endothelium had different permeability properties to plasma proteins than nonneural endothelium, and this feature forms one component of the blood–brain barrier (BBB) which includes numerous physiological and biochemical processes that maintain cerebral homeostasis. The era of electron microcopy provided information about the structural components of the BBB to plasma proteins, namely fewer endothelial caveolae and the presence of circumferential tight junctions at interendothelial spaces. The molecular era has resulted in the discovery of many new proteins in both caveolae and tight junctions, and studies are now underway to determine the function of many of these proteins and to determine which are crucial for maintenance of the normal BBB and their role in BBB breakdown in diseases.

2   Structural and Molecular Components of Normal Cerebral Endothelium

2.1   Caveolae

In the premolecular era, electron microscopists described membrane-bound spherical structures having a mean diameter of ~70 nm free in the endothelial cytoplasm of all body vessels. These structures open to both the luminal and abluminal plasmalemma through a neck of 10–40 nm in diameter (❷ *Figure 3-1*). Known previously as pinocytotic vesicles, these structures are now referred to as plasmalemmal vesicles or caveolae. These noncoated structures are distinct from clathrin-coated vesicles, which have an electron-dense coat and are involved in receptor-mediated endocytosis. Studies of frog mesenteric capillaries suggest that caveolae are part of two racemose systems of invaginations of the luminal and abluminal cell surfaces and not freely moving entities (Frokjaer-Jensen, 1980). There is considerable heterogeneity in endothelium in different parts of a single organ, hence, the findings in frog mesenteric capillaries may not necessarily

◘ Figure 3-1

Segment of cerebral cortical arteriolar endothelium from a control rat injected with HRP intravenously. Tight junctions are present along the interendothelial space (*arrowheads*) and the endothelium contains caveolae, two of which contain HRP reaction product. × 101,400

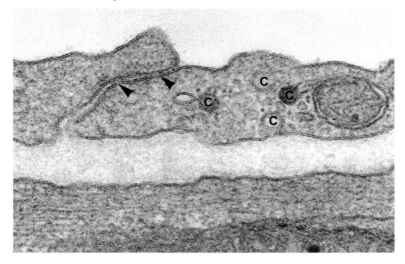

apply to all species or to brain capillaries. Morphometric studies established that normal cerebral endothelium contains a mean of 5 caveolae/μm^2 in arteriolar (Nag, 1998) and capillary endothelium (Nag, 2003a). The numbers of caveolae are 14-fold fewer in cerebral endothelial cells as compared with nonneural endothelial cells, such as myocardial capillaries (Simionescu et al., 1974), suggesting limited transcellular traffic of solutes at the level of cerebral endothelium.

2.1.1 Molecular Structure of Caveolae

The principal proteins in caveolae are the caveolin-1, -2, and -3. Caveolin-1, a major component of caveolae is an integral membrane protein (20–22 kDa) having both amino and carboxyl ends exposed on the cytoplasmic aspect of the membrane (Monier et al., 1995). In brain, caveolin-1 and caveolin-2 are primarily expressed in endothelial cells while caveolin-3 is predominantly expressed in astrocytes (Ikezu et al., 1998). In addition to the full-length proteins (α-isoform), both caveolin-1 and -2 have other smaller sized isoforms. Caveolae have a unique lipid composition, of which cholesterol and sphingolipids (sphingomyelin and glycosphingolipid) are the main components. The sphingolipids are substrates for synthesis of a second intracellular messenger, the ceramides (Liu and Anderson, 1995). Cholesterol may create the frame in which all other caveolar elements are inserted.

Caveolin acts as a multivalent docking site for recruiting and sequestering signaling molecules through the caveolin-scaffolding domain that recognizes a common sequence motif within caveolin-binding signaling molecules (Li et al., 1996). Proteins associated with endothelial caveolae include membrane proteins, G-protein–coupled receptors, G-proteins, nonreceptor tyrosine kinases, nonreceptor Ser/Thr kinases, other enzymes, GTPases, cellular proteins/adaptors, and structural proteins (❯ *Table 3-1*).

2.1.2 Caveolae and Transcytosis

Caveoli contain the molecular machinery that promotes vesicle formation, fission, docking, and fusion with the target membrane. Isolated caveoli from lung capillaries demonstrate *N*-ethyl maleimide (NEF)-sensitive

☐ Table 3-1
Proteins Associated with Endothelial Caveolae (Frank *et al.* 2003)

Protein	Function	References
Membrane Proteins		
PDGF-R	PDGF receptor	(Liu *et al.* 1997).
CD36	Lipoprotein receptor	(Lisanti *et al.* 1994); (Uittenbogaard *et al.* 2000).
RAGE	Advanced glycated end products receptor	(Lisanti *et al.* 1994).
Gp60	Albumin receptor	(Minshall *et al.* 2000).
SR-BI	Lipoprotein receptor	(Uittenbogaard *et al.* 2000); (Yuhanna *et al.* 2001).
Flk-1/KDR	VEGF receptor	(Feng *et al.* 1999).
Tissue factor pathway inhibitor	Down regulates the procoagulant activity of tissue factor	(Lupu *et al.* 1997).
PV-1	Component of stomatal diaphragms of caveolae and transendothelial channels	(Stan *et al.* 1999).
P-glycoprotein	ABC transporter	(Demeule *et al.* 2000).
MMP-1	Matrix metalloproteinase	(Annabi *et al.* 2001)
MMP-2	Matrix metalloproteinase	(Puyraimond *et al.* 2001)
EDG-1 receptor	Endothelial Differentiation gene-1 product	(Igarashi and Michel 2000)
uPAR	Urokinase receptor	(Wei *et al.* 1999)
G protein-coupled receptors		
B2R	Bradykinin receptor	(Ju *et al.* 2000)
ET_A	Endothelin receptor	(Chun *et al.* 1994)
G Proteins		
$G\alpha_S$, $G\alpha_{i1}$, $G\alpha_{i2}$, $G\beta\gamma$, Gq	Regulate G protein-coupled receptor activity	(Lisanti *et al.* 1994) (Lisanti *et al.* 1994); (Oh and Schnitzer 2001)
Nonreceptor tyrosine kinases		
Src, Fyn, Yes, Lck, Lyn	Regulation of growth factor response	(Lisanti *et al.* 1994); (Liu *et al.* 1997)
Tyk2	Regulation of growth factor response	(Ju *et al.* 2000)
STAT3	Signal transduction and activator of transcription	(Ju *et al.* 2000)
Nonreceptor Ser/Thr kinases		
Raf	Signal transduction of mitogenic signals	(Rizzo *et al.* 1998)
MEK	Signal transduction of mitogenic signals	(Lisanti *et al.* 1994)
PI-3 kinase	Phosphorylation of phosphatidyl-inositol	(Lisanti *et al.* 1994); (Liu *et al.* 1997)
PKC α, β	Ser/Thr kinase	(Lisanti *et al.* 1994); (Liu *et al.* 1997)
Other Enzymes		
eNOS	Production of NO	(Shaul *et al.* 1996); (Garcia-Cardena *et al.* 1996)
PLCγ	Phospho-lipase	(Liu *et al.* 1997)
Prostacyclin synthase	Production of prostacyclin (PGI2)	(Spisni *et al.* 2001)

⬛ Table 3-1 (continued)

Protein	Function	References
GTPases		
Ras, Rap1, Rap2	GTPase	(Lisanti *et al.* 1994)
Cellular proteins/ adaptors		
Shc Grb2	Regulates growth factor response Adaptor protein, associates growth factor receptors	(Lisanti *et al.* 1994)
Other Proteins		
ER α and β	Estrogen receptors	(Chambliss *et al.* 2000)
NCX	Na$^+$/Ca$^+$ exchanger	(Teubl *et al.* 1999)
Ca^{2+}-ATPase	Calcium pump	(Fujimoto 1993); (Schnitzer *et al.* 1995b)
IP3 receptor-like protein	Involved in calcium influx	(Schnitzer *et al.* 1995b); (Fujimoto et al. 1992)
Sprouty-1 and -2	Inhibitor of development-associated RTK signaling	(Impagnatiello *et al.* 2001)
Cationic arginine transporter-1	Arginine transporter	(McDonald *et al.* 1997)
Structural Proteins		
Actin	Involved in cell motility	(Lisanti *et al.* 1994)
Annexin II and IV	Promotes membrane fusion and is involved in exocytosis	(Lisanti *et al.* 1994); (Schnitzer *et al.* 1995b)
Dynamin	Involved in vesicular trafficking	(Oh and Schnitzer 2001); (Henley *et al.* 1998)
NSF	Involved in vesicle fusion	(Schnitzer *et al.* 1995b)
SNAP, SNARE	Involved in vesicular transport	(Schnitzer *et al.* 1995b)
VAMP-2	Involved in the targeting/fusion of transported vesicles to their target membranes	(Schnitzer *et al.* 1995b)

fusion factor (NSF) and its attachment protein—soluble NSF attachment protein (SNAP), vesicle-associated SNAP receptor (v-SNARE), vesicle-associated membrane protein-2 (VAMP-2) (McIntosh and Schnitzer, 1999), monomeric and trimeric GTPases, annexins II and IV (Schnitzer et al., 1995a). These molecules interact in the stages of transcytosis as follows: caveoli form at the cell surface through ATP-, GTP-, and Mg^{2+}-polymerization of caveolin-1 and -2, a process stabilized by cholesterol (Monier et al., 1995). Caveolin oligomers may also interact with glycosphingolipids (Fra et al., 1995); these protein–protein and protein–lipid interactions are thought to be the driving force for caveoli formation (Sargiacomo et al., 1995). A component of the caveolar fission machinery is the large GTPase, dynamin, which oligomerises at the neck of caveolae and probably undergoes hydrolysis for fission and release of caveolae, so it becomes free in the cytoplasm (Oh et al., 1998). The transcellular movement of caveolae is facilitated by the association with the actin-cytoskeleton related proteins such as myosin HC, gelsolin, spectrin, and dystrophin (Lisanti et al., 1994). Fusion at the abluminal membrane is aided by NSF, which interacts with SNAPs that can associate with complementary SNAP receptors to form a functional SNARE fusion complex. Prior to fusion of the target and vesicle membrane, v-SNARE (VAMP), the targeting receptor located on the caveolae, recognizes and docks with its cognate t-SNARE (syntaxin) on the target membrane (Rothman, 1994; Hay and Scheller, 1997). Specific docking is aided by endothelial VAMP-2 (McIntosh and Schnitzer, 1999), which is localized in caveolae.

The evidence thus far favors the hypothesis that caveolae are dynamic vesicular carriers budding off from the plasma membrane to form free transport caveolae that fuse with specific target membrane molecules as described previously (Couet et al., 2001; Schnitzer, 2001; Simionescu et al., 2002; Stan, 2002). Caveolae can traffic their cargo across cells (transcytosis) (McIntosh et al., 2002). Transcytosis can be either fluid phase or receptor mediated. The latter requires that the cognate receptor be located within caveolae. Caveolae-mediated transcytosis of albumin (Ghitescu et al., 1986; Schubert et al., 2001), native low-density lipoprotein (Vasile et al., 1983), and hormones, such as insulin (Bendayan and Rasio, 1996), across the endothelial barrier have been clearly demonstrated. Support for the role of caveolae in transcytosis is obtained from caveolin-1 gene knockout mice, which lacks endothelial caveolae and shows defects in the uptake and transport of albumin in vivo (Schubert et al., 2001). Increased vascular permeability in these mice occurs by the paracellular route (Schubert et al., 2002).

Other functions attributed to caveolin-1 are not relevant to this chapter and have been described in further reviews (Razani et al., 2002; Frank et al., 2003; Hnasko and Lisanti, 2003; Minshall et al., 2003).

2.2 Tight Junctions

Transmission electron microscopy (TEM) demonstrated that the junctions between adjacent cerebral endothelial cells are characterized by fusion of the outer leaflets of adjacent plasma membranes at intervals along the interendothelial space, producing a pentalaminar appearance and forming tight or occluding junctions (Muir and Peters, 1962; Brightman and Reese, 1969; Nag et al., 1977) (❷ *Figure 3-1*) that prevent paracellular diffusion of solutes via the intercellular route. These tight junctions form the most apical element of the junctional complex, which includes both tight and adherens junctions. Subsequent studies using horseradish peroxidase (HRP) as a tracer suggested that tight junctions extend circumferentially around cerebral endothelial cells, hence their name zonula occludens (Reese and Karnovsky, 1967; Brightman and Reese, 1969). The physiological correlate of tightness in epithelial membranes is transepithelial resistance. The electrical resistance across the BBB in vivo is estimated to be $\sim$4–8,000 Ω/cm^2 (Crone and Olesen, 1982; Smith and Rapoport, 1986). Freeze-fracture studies show that the tight junctions of cerebral endothelium of mammalian species are characterized by the highest complexity of any other body vessels (Nagy et al., 1984). Around 8 to 12 parallel junctional strands having no discontinuities run in the longitudinal axis of the vessel with numerous lateral anastomotic strands. This pattern extends into the postcapillary venules, although in a less complex fashion (Nagy et al., 1984). Other structural and physiological properties of tight junctions are discussed in Chapter 5.

2.2.1 Molecular Structure of Tight Junctions

Tight junctions are composed of an intricate combination of transmembrane and cytoplasmic proteins linked to an actin-based cytoskeleton that allows these junctions to form a seal while remaining capable of rapid modulation and regulation. Three integral proteins—occludin (Furuse et al., 1993), claudins (Furuse et al., 1998), and junction adhesion molecule (JAM) (Martin-Padura et al., 1998) form the tight junction. High expression of occludin in brain endothelial cells as compared to nonneural endothelial cells provides an explanation for the different properties of both these endothelia (Hirase et al., 1997). Claudins with molecular masses of $\sim$23 kD comprise a multigene family consisting of >20 members (Morita et al., 1999; Tsukita et al., 2001). Claudins may be the major transmembrane proteins of tight junctions as occludin knockout mice are still capable of forming interendothelial connections (Saitou et al., 2000) while claudin knockout mice are nonviable (Gow et al., 1999). Occludin, claudin-1, -3, and -5, and JAM-1 have been localized in cerebral endothelium (Hirase et al., 1997; Sirotkin et al., 1997; Kniesel and Wolburg, 2000; Nag, 2005) (❷ *Figure 3-2*). Brain endothelium also expresses the endothelial cell specific adhesion molecule, which is considered a structural equivalent of JAM (Nasdala et al., 2002).

◻ Figure 3-2
Confocal images of murine brain showing cerebral endothelial tight junction proteins. (a, b) Merged confocal images showing dual labeling for occludin (green) and fibronectin (red). The basement membrane of vessels is immunoreactive with fibronectin, and occludin strands run along the long axis of the vessel, therefore, in cross-sectioned vessels they appear as green dots dispersed along the circumference of the vessel (a). (b) Three-dimensional reconstruction of the Z-series of these vessels shows the longitudinal nature of the occludin strands (*arrowhead*). Claudin-5 immunoreactivity also appears as linear bands, which run along the long axis of vessels connected at intervals by diagonal bands (c). Dual labeling for occludin (green) and claudin 5 (red) show colocalization of both proteins (yellow) in individual strands (d). Claudin-3 strands are present in pial vessels and large intracerebral vessels (e) only and are not visualized in microvessels. Microvessels show endothelial localization of JAM-1 (f) and ZO-1 (g). Magnifications of (a, b, c, d, e, f, and g) are similar. Scale Bars = 25 μm. Figures a–d from Nag (2005) with permission from ISN Neuropath Press

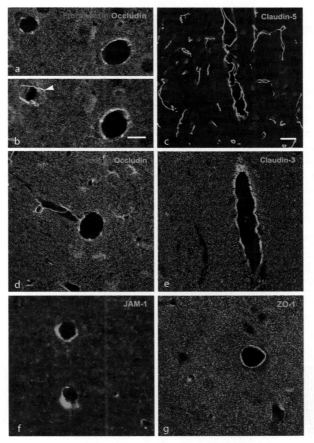

Tight junctions are also made up of several accessory proteins that are necessary for structural support such as zonula occludens (ZO)-1 to -3, AF-6, 7H6, and cingulin. The primary cytoskeletal protein, actin, has known binding sites on all ZO proteins and on claudin and occludin (Itoh et al., 1999). ZO-1 binds to actin filaments and the C terminus of occludin (Itoh et al., 1999), which couples the structural and dynamic properties of perijunctional actin to the paracellular barrier.

Tight junctions are localized at cholesterol-enriched regions along the plasma membrane associated with caveolin-1 (Nusrat et al., 2000). Several cytoplasmic signaling molecules are concentrated at tight junction complexes and are involved in signaling cascades that control assembly and disassembly of tight junctions (Madara et al., 1992). Regulation of tight junctions and further details of the properties of endothelial tight and adherens junctions are discussed in previous reviews (Rubin and Staddon, 1999; Kniesel and Wolburg, 2000; Liebner et al., 2000b; Gloor et al., 2001; Huber et al., 2001; Nag, 2003a; Vorbrodt and Dobrogowska, 2003) and in Chapter 5.

3   Vasogenic Edema

Breakdown of the BBB to plasma proteins leads to vasogenic edema, which occurs in many pathological states such as infection, inflammation, ischemia, seizures, tumors, trauma, and hypertensive encephalopathy (❷ *Figure 3-3a* and *b*). Passage of low-and high-molecular weight (MW) plasma components from blood through intracerebral vessels results in net water influx into the interstitial compartment and a volumetric enlargement of the brain. The compliance of the brain is limited since it is enclosed within the

❑ Figure 3-3
(a) Light microscopy of the brain of a patient who died of hypertensive encephalopathy shows an arteriole with marked BBB breakdown to plasma proteins, which are present in the surrounding neuropil. Plasma proteins stain an intense pink using the Hematoxylin and Eosin stain. (b) Light microscopy of a glioblastoma immunostained for IgG shows BBB breakdown of arterioles to IgG, which is also present in the surrounding neuropil. CT head scans from a patient with ischemic stroke on the day of presentation (c) and at day 3, h prior to death (d). (c) An area of decreased density and loss of grey/white differentiation is present in the right insular region and represents an infarct. (d) A large area of decreased density is present in the right hemisphere involving the entire right middle cerebral artery territory in the area of the infarct and associated edema. There is a shift of midline structures to the opposite side with ipsilateral subfalcial herniation. (a) × 320; (b) × 160; (a) from Nag (2005) with permission from ISN Neuropath Press

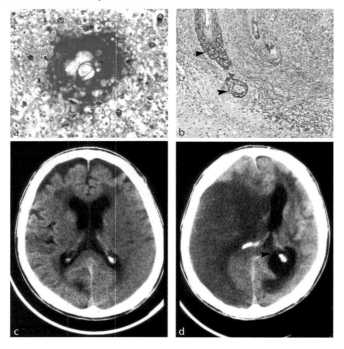

bony calvarium. This volumetric enlargement of brain tissue causes increased intracranial pressure leading to cerebral herniations that are a life-threatening complication (❷ *Figure 3-3c* and *d*).

3.1 Endothelial Protein Permeability Pathways in Vasogenic Edema

Early ultrastructural studies of conditions associated with vasogenic edema, such as acute hypertension (Nag et al., 1977) and septic encephalopathy (Clawson et al., 1966; Papadopoulos et al., 1999), reported increased endothelial caveolae and swelling of astrocytic foot processes. The latter was interpreted as evidence of BBB breakdown and edema formation. The availability of HRP as a marker of BBB permeability led to the demonstration of BBB breakdown in vasogenic edema in diverse experimental models. Transcellular routes for tracer passage are by (1) enhanced transcytosis of caveolae-containing plasma macromolecules, apparently by shuttling their contents adsorbed from blood from the luminal to the antiluminal aspect of endothelium; (2) passage via transendothelial channels, which may form transiently by the fusion of two or more caveolae, providing a direct conduit for the exchange of both small and large plasma molecules; and (3) the interendothelial junctions that constitute a paracellular route for the passive, pressure-driven filtration of water and small solutes.

3.1.1 Enhanced Transcytosis

Multifocal areas of HRP extravasation around cerebral vessels were observed in diverse models, such as hypertension (Nag, 1998); spinal cord injury (Beggs and Waggener, 1976); seizures (Hedley-Whyte et al., 1977; Westergaard, 1980; Nitsch et al., 1986); experimental autoimmune encephalomyelitis (Claudio et al., 1989); excitotoxic brain damage (Nag, 1992); brain trauma (Povlishock et al., 1978), brain tumors (Shivers et al., 1984); and BBB breakdown induced by bradykinin (Raymond et al., 1986; Hashizume and Black, 2002), histamine (Dux and Joo, 1982), and leukotriene C4 (Hashizume and Black, 2002), and other models as reviewed previously (Nag, 2003b; Lossinsky and Shivers, 2004). In these studies, HRP was present in all layers of the vessel wall and extended into the gap junctions between astrocytic foot processes and into the adjacent extracellular spaces. Disruption of vessel walls did not account for the early permeability changes. All these studies reported an increase in endothelial caveolae to account for the permeability change. Quantitative studies in several hypertension models demonstrated a twofold increase in caveolae in arteriolar segments permeable to HRP as compared with the nonpermeable segments and a 16-fold increase when factoring in the caveolae containing HRP (Nag, 1998, 2003b) (❷ *Figure 3-4a*). A similar increment in caveolae numbers occurs in permeable arterioles in BBB breakdown induced by seizures (Petito and Levy, 1980), bradykinin (Raymond et al., 1986), and cytochalasin B (Nag, 1995). In case of capillaries, a fivefold increase in caveole was reported in experimental autoimmune encephalomyelitis (Claudio et al., 1989) and a seven- and fourfold increase in seizures and ischemia, respectively (Petito and Levy, 1980).

Direction of Caveolar Passage in Endothelium Time course studies done in the acute hypertension model established the direction of vesicular passage. Early permeability studies done 90 s after the onset of acute hypertension showed HRP confined to focal segments of penetrating cortical arteriolar walls with very little extravasation into the surrounding neuropil and numerous caveolae many of which contained tracer (Nag et al., 1979). In addition, confluent deposits of HRP were observed in abluminal caveolae and the adjacent endothelial basement membranes, which did not otherwise contain tracer (❷ *Figure 3-4b*), suggesting that caveolae were depositing HRP in the endothelial basement membrane and the direction of caveolar passage was from the vascular lumen to the subendothelium. This finding was observed in all subsequent studies of experimental hypertension (Nag et al., 1980; Nag, 1984a, 1986; Nag and Harik, 1987) and in other models such as spinal cord injury (Beggs and Waggener, 1976), seizures (Hedley-Whyte et al., 1977), bradykinin-induced BBB breakdown (Raymond et al., 1986), and excitotoxic brain damage (Nag, 1992). The active participation of caveolae in transfer of proteins, such as HRP across cerebral endothelium is supported by the absence of such transport in vessels fixed for 45 min before the perfusion of peroxidase (Westergaard and Brightman, 1973).

◘ Figure 3-4

Arteriolar segments of rats with chronic renal hypertension having systolic blood pressures >200 mm Hg prior to death. (a) An arteriolar segment showing BBB breakdown to endogenous plasma proteins, which appear particulate and have expanded the basement membrane. The increased numbers of caveolae are highlighted by their electron-dense deposits of Ca^{2+}-ATPase, which is demonstrated by ultracytochemistry. (b) Segment of arteriolar endothelium permeable to HRP showing tracer in an abluminal caveolae and in the adjacent basement membrane. This was observed within minutes after injection of the tracer, therefore, the direction of tracer passage is from the blood into the basement membrane. (c) A transendothelial channel is highlighted by the Ca^{2+}-ATPase content of the caveolae. (a) × 20,000; (b) × 44,000; (c) × 87,000. From Nag (2005) with permission from ISN Neuropath Press

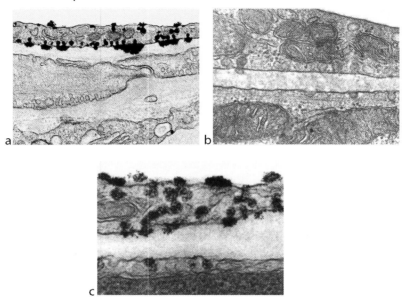

Passage of HRP via interendothelial junctions was not observed in the studies cited earlier. Although tracer was observed focally at the luminal or abluminal end of the interendothelial space, it was never demonstrated along the entire length of the interendothelial space nor was widening of tight junctions seen. These findings support enhanced transcytosis as the principal mechanism resulting in early BBB breakdown to protein.

Drugs and Caveolae Factors reported to decrease caveolae and attenuate BBB breakdown include drugs such as indomethacin, trifluoperazine, or imidazole (Raymond et al., 1986). In the case of imidazole, although the number of vessels showing permeability change was markedly reduced, the magnitude of caveolar increase in the involved vessels was not altered. It is of interest that many of these drugs are used in the treatment of human psychiatric disorders. Dexamethasone, a drug widely used to treat increased intracranial pressure resulting from cerebral edema associated with brain tumors and pseudotumors, is known to decrease the number of endothelial caveolae in normal mouse brain vessels (Hedley-Whyte and Hsu, 1986).

Caveolin-1 and Permeability Our studies of the rat cortical cold-injury model show increased expression of endothelial caveolin-1 in vessels at the injury site as compared with control rats (❷ *Figure 3-5a* and *b*). At 12 h, increased caveolin-1 expression was observed in endothelium of arterioles, particularly, those

◘ Figure 3-5

Cerebral cortex of control rats (a and f) and rats with cortical cold injuries (b–d, e, g, h). (a) Microvessels show endothelial localization of caveolin-1 in cerebral vessels of a control rat. (b) At 12 h, all lesion vessels show increased immunoreactivity for caveolin-1, particularly, arterioles with BBB breakdown to fibronectin, which is demonstrated in the merged confocal image (c). (d) At day 4, following a cortical coldinjury, marked BBB breakdown is present at the lesion site as demonstrated by fibronectin immunostaining. (e) The merged confocal image shows that the endothelium of a vessel with BBB breakdown to fibronectin shows colocalization of VEGF-A (yellow). (f) Merged confocal image from a control rat showing immunoreactivity for VEGF-B (green) in microvessels. The strong VEGF-B signal has masked the weak signal produced by VEGF-A. (g) At day 4, postinjury, a pial vessel shows marked endothelial Ang-2 immunoreactivity, which is also present in the cytoplasm of the macrophages (*arrowheads*). A merged confocal image shows colocalization of Ang-2 and active caspase 3, a marker of apoptosis. Scale bars = 25 μm

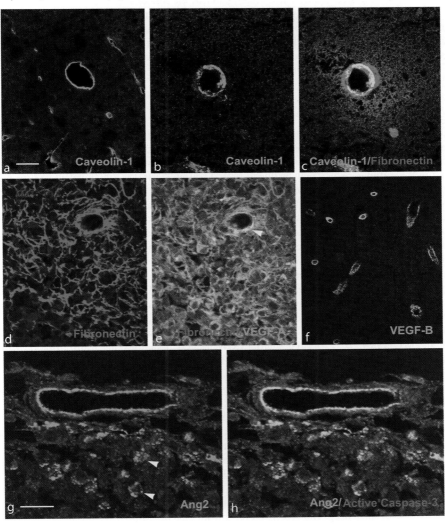

showing BBB breakdown (Nag et al., 2005b) (❷ *Figure 3-5b* and *c*). The latter supports our previous ultrastructural findings of increased endothelial caveolae in vessels with BBB breakdown to HRP.

3.1.2 Transendothelial Channels

Caveolae are known to fuse to form transendothelial channels in normal nonneural vessels. Although such channels have not been demonstrated in normal cerebral endothelium, they do occur following osmotic opening of the BBB (Farrell and Shivers, 1984), hyperglycaemia (Shivers and Harris, 1984), brain trauma (Lossinsky et al., 1989), and acute and chronic hypertension (Nag, 2003b) (❷ *Figure 3-4c*). It must be emphasized that transendothelial channel formation is a transient phenomenon and can only be demonstrated if ultrastructural studies are done within minutes after the onset of the pathological process.

Despite the accumulated evidence from many models, the role of caveolae in the transcytosis of HRP from the circulating blood across the endothelium to the interstitium in pathological states remains a controversial issue, with some opposing this mechanism based on their studies of cerebral endothelial reactivity in steady states (Broadwell, 1989; Stewart, 2000). The major advances made in the molecular biology of endothelial caveolae in the past decade and its role in transcytosis in nonneural vessels should renew interest in this mechanism of BBB breakdown.

3.1.3 Tight Junctions

Structural Changes   Most of the early studies of BBB breakdown in diverse experimental models failed to demonstrate passage of protein tracers, such as HRP via tight junctions, as described under the heading "Direction of Caveolar Passage in Endothelium" Passage of HRP via interendothelial junctions was not observed in these studies, which may be due to several reasons. First, the junctional alterations may be of a minor degree, therefore they are not detectable by HRP, which is a relatively large tracer (MW 40,000). However, BBB breakdown to HRP and larger molecules is relevant to vasogenic edema formation in diseases. Second, it is possible that routine TEM is not the proper technique to detect alterations of tight junctions because only a small segment of the junction is visualized in ultrathin sections. However, tight junction alterations were also not observed by high-voltage electron microscopy, which allows thicker sections and larger areas of the junction to be examined.

Studies of osmotic opening of the BBB by hypertonic solutions, such as mannitol and urea infused via the carotid artery, provided controversial results, with studies for (Brightman et al., 1973) and against this mechanism of tracer passage, with many more studies demonstrating passage of tracer through endothelium by enhanced endothelial caveolae (Hansson and Johansson, 1980; Houthoff et al., 1982; Farrell and Shivers, 1984; Nagy et al., 1984). However, use of molecular markers smaller than HRP, such as ionic lanthanum (MW 138.9 Da) and [^{14}C] sucrose (MW 342 Da), demonstrated BBB breakdown following intracarotid administration of hyperosmotic agents (Rapoport et al., 1980; Dorovini-Zis et al., 1983). These authors estimated that only 0.001% of the endothelial surface need become patent to account for the increased permeability to macromolecules (Dorovini-Zis et al., 1983). These calculations support passage of tracer either through tight junctions or via caveolae.

Acute hypertonic exposure of brain increases cerebral blood volume. The resulting vasodilatation is postulated to stretch cerebrovascular endothelium to mediate tight-junctional opening (Rapoport, 2000). Increased BBB permeability after intracarotid hypertonic infusion is essentially reversed within 10 min in rats (Rapoport et al., 1980) as well as in monkeys (Kessler et al., 1984). Regardless of the mechanism of BBB breakdown, clinical application of osmotic modification of the BBB is used in the treatment of brain tumors to increase the delivery of chemotherapeutic agents in humans up to 100-fold (Neuwelt, 2004). Osmotic BBB disruption is facilitated by hypertonic nonmetabolizable solutes that are injected intra-arterially and can open the BBB to small drugs and proteins reversibly for ~30 min. BBB disruption–enhanced delivery of chemotherapeutic agents has increased survival rates for patients with primary central nervous system (CNS) lymphomas, with outcomes being statistically correlated with the number and degree of BBB disruptions (Kraemer et al., 2001).

Molecular Changes   Decreased immunolocalization of the tight junction proteins—ZO-1 and occludin—has been demonstrated in areas known to have BBB breakdown to HRP following intracerebral injection of interleukin (Bolton et al., 1998) or BBB breakdown to serum proteins in human cerebral malaria (Brown et al., 1999). Dual labeling for occludin and a marker of BBB breakdown demonstrated alterations in tight junction proteins in vessels with BBB breakdown in acute multiple sclerosis lesions (Plumb et al., 2002) and human immunodeficiency virus-1 (HIV-1) encephalitis (Dallasta et al., 1999).

3.1.4 Summary

Early in vivo studies of BBB breakdown using HRP as a tracer in experimental models of diseases demonstrate passage of this tracer via transcytosis and transendothelial channels, suggesting that these are the major routes for early plasma protein passage in diseases associated with vasogenic edema. Demonstration of these processes is dependent on whether an appropriate tracer has been selected to study BBB permeability to protein and when studies are undertaken following the insult. A short insult is associated with transient barrier opening. Persistence of the pathological state results in greater degrees of endothelial damage, resulting in disruption of tight junctions and, eventually, breakdown of the entire endothelial cell occurs. The latter has been observed in brains of patients dying of massive vasogenic edema.

3.2   Factors Affecting BBB Permeability to Protein

Only selected factors affecting BBB permeability to proteins are discussed. Although individual groups study the effect of one or few factors affecting BBB permeability, it should be noted that increased permeability is associated with the concomitant alteration of several factors at a structural and molecular level, and the upregulation of several vasoactive factors that act at different times following injury. As an example, BBB breakdown in the cold-injury model is associated with an increase in several mediators such as bradykinin (Maier-Hauff et al., 1984), polyamines (Trout et al., 1986), oxygen radicals (Murakami et al., 1999), nitric oxide (Nag et al., 2001), vascular endothelial growth factor (VEGF-A) (Nag et al., 1997, 2002), and angiopoietin-2 (Nag et al., 2005a; Nourhaghighi et al., 2003).

3.2.1 Endothelial Surface Properties and BBB Breakdown

The plasma membrane of normal cerebral endothelium has a net negative charge (Nag, 1998), which is greater on the luminal than abluminal plasma membrane (Vorbrodt et al., 1993). In addition, a variety of oligosaccharide residues have been detected on the endothelial plasma membrane by lectin-binding studies. Of the lectins examined, only peanut agglutinin does not bind to the surface of normal cerebral endothelium (Nag, 1985). The net negative charge on endothelium is essential for maintenance of the BBB to protein since its neutralization by intracarotid infusion of positively charged substances, such as polycationic protamine or poly-L-lysine (Nagy et al., 1983; Hardebo and Kahrstrom, 1985), results in BBB breakdown to tracers.

   Following BBB breakdown in acute hypertension (Nag, 1984b) and cold injury (Vorbrodt et al., 1993), vessels with BBB breakdown to HRP show marked reduction or loss of surface charge on endothelium. The loss of charge has been shown to precede BBB breakdown (Nagy et al., 1983). Loss of the terminal sialic acid groups on endothelium in hypertension results in loss of the net negative charge on endothelium and exposes the β-D-gal-(1-3)-D-gal N-acetyl groups, which normally are not accessible to peanut agglutinin, and binding of this lectin occurs (Nag, 1986). The latter is supported by the finding that exposure of cerebral endothelium to neuraminidase, which is known to cleave the terminal sialic acid groups on endothelium, results in loss of the net negative charge on endothelium and allows peanut agglutinin binding (Nag, 1986, 1985; Vorbrodt, 1986). These studies demonstrate that in acute hypertension alterations of the charge and the oligosaccharide residues on the luminal plasma membrane of endothelium allows HRP to be taken up by enhanced transcytosis. These changes are transient and not demonstrable when the BBB is restored.

The surface negative charge on cerebral endothelium is being exploited to introduce chimeric peptides across the BBB. These chimeric peptides are formed when a nontransportable peptide therapeutic is coupled to a BBB drug transport vector, such as cationized albumin, as described previously (Bickel et al., 2001).

3.2.2 The Endothelial Cytoskeleton and BBB Breakdown

Actin Normal cerebral endothelial cells, like most eukaryotic cells, have a cytoskeleton consisting of microfilaments, intermediate filaments, and microtubules (Nag, 1995, 1998). Ultrastructural studies show that microfilament bundles having the dimension of actin are grouped near the cytoplasmic margins and are present in proximity to cell junctions (Nag et al., 1978), and actin has been localized to the endothelial plasma membrane by molecular techniques (Pardridge et al., 1989). Integrity of the endothelial microfilaments is necessary for maintenance of the BBB to protein in steady states since BBB breakdown to HRP occurs in the presence of cytochalasin B, an actin-disrupting agent (Nag, 1995), and is associated with a significant increase in endothelial caveolae in permeable vessels and lack of tracer passage via interendothelial junctions.

Structural organization of actin is necessary for maintenance of tight junction integrity as well since actin-disrupting substances, such as cytochalasin D, cytokines, and phalloidin, disrupt tight junction structure and function (Bentzel et al., 1976; Stevenson and Begg, 1994).

Microtubules Colchicine, an agent, which disrupts microtubules, does not affect BBB permeability in steady states suggesting that the microtubular network has no demonstrable role in normal cerebral homeostasis. However, pretreatment with colchicine attenuates the BBB breakdown that is known to occur in acute hypertension (Nag, 1995). Microtubules are known to form intracellular pathways along which protein-bearing caveolae pass in certain cell types (Allen et al., 1985); (Schnapp et al., 1985). Transport of fluorescein isothiocyanate dextran from the luminal to the abluminal side of bovine aortic endothelial cells was reported to occur by chains of caveolae, and this activity was reduced by colchicine (Liu et al., 1993) supporting the role of microtubules in caveolar passage through endothelium. Hence, a possible explanation for the results observed in acute hypertension is that disruption of microtubules impairs the passage of endothelial caveolae from the luminal to the abluminal plasma membrane, thus attenuating BBB breakdown in acute hypertension.

3.3   Mediators of BBB Breakdown

3.3.1 Vasoactive Agents

Release of vasoactive agents from injured brain tissue appears to play a major role in BBB breakdown and the formation of vasogenic cerebral edema. The criteria used to determine whether agents can mediate cerebral edema include: (1) a permeability-enhancing action under physiological conditions, (2) a vasodilatory action, (3) the ability to induce vasogenic brain edema, (4) an increase of concentration in the tissue or interstitial fluid under pathological conditions, and (5) a decrease of brain edema by specific interference with the release or action of a given autacoid (Schilling and Wahl, 1997). Some of the common vasoactive mediators are shown in ❯ *Table 3-2*, and since their existence has been known for a long time and properties have been reviewed previously (Abbott, 2000; Petty and Lo, 2002), they will not be discussed in this chapter. It should be noted that many of these mediators have only been tested in pial vessels, which differ from intracerebral vessels in structural and permeability properties (Nag, 2003b), therefore, it is uncertain whether the reported effects apply to intracerebral vessels.

□ Table 3-2
Vasoactive substances reported to increase blood–brain barrier permeability

Substance	Reference
Arachidonic acid	Chan et al. (1983); Chan and Fishman (1984); Black and Hoff (1985); Wei et al. (1986); Papadopoulos et al. (1989); Easton and Fraser (1998)
Bradykinin	Raymond et al. (1986); Schilling and Wahl (1999)
Complement-derived polypeptide C3a-desArg	Abbott (2000)
Histamine	Dux and Joo (1982); Joo (1994); Easton et al. (1997)
Interleukins: IL-1α, IL-1β, IL-2	de Vries et al. (1996); Abbott (2000)
Leukotrienes	Black and Hoff (1985)
Macrophage inflammatory proteins: MIP-1, MIP-2	Abbott (2000)
Nitric oxide	Oury et al. (1993)
Oxygen-derived free radicals	Chan et al. (1984); Kontos et al. (1984)
Platelet-activating factor	Abbott (2000)
Prostaglandins	Abbott (2000)
Phospholipase A$_2$	Abbott (2000)
Purine nucleotides: ATP, ADP, AMP	Olesen and Crone (1986); Revest et al. (1991)
Superoxide dismutase	Oury et al. (1993)
Serotonin	Sharma and Dey (1986a); Sharma and Dey (1986b)

3.3.2 Calcium

Calcium is implicated in both transcytosis and the opening of tight junctions.

Calcium and Transcytosis The role of calcium (Ca^{2+}) in BBB breakdown to protein was studied in the acute hypertension model in which enhanced numbers of endothelial caveolae and transcytosis of caveolae led to BBB breakdown to HRP (Nag, 1990, 1998). It was hypothesized that reduced activity of the enzymes responsible for Ca^{2+} homeostasis, such as the endothelial plasma membrane Na^+, K^+-adenosine triphosphatase (ATPase), and Ca^{2+}-ATPase, could result in transient fluxes of increased intra-endothelial calcium that could mediate enhanced permeability by transcytosis in acute hypertension (Nag, 1990). This is supported first by ultracytochemical studies that demonstrate reduced localization of both Ca^{2+}-ATPase and Na^+, K^+-ATPase only in the endothelium of arterioles permeable to HRP in acute hypertension (Nag, 1988, 1990). Subsequent studies demonstrate that reduced activity of the endothelial ATPases precedes BBB breakdown in chronic hypertension (Nag, 1993). Pretreatment of acutely hypertensive rats with the calcium entry blocker, Flunarizine, decreases the number and size of areas of Evans blue extravasation and results in a significant decrease in protein transfer of I^{125}-labeled human serum albumin in total brain as well as in individual brain areas in acute hypertension (Nag, 1991).

Calcium and Tight Junctions Calcium is known to act both extracellularly and intracellularly to regulate tight junction activity. Removal of extracellular Ca^{2+} results in a concurrent decrease in electrical resistance across the membrane and an increase in permeability (Stevenson and Begg, 1994) involving heterotrimeric G-protein and protein kinase C signaling pathways. Intracellular Ca^{2+} plays a role in cell–cell contact (Gumbiner, 1996), increased electrical resistance (Nigam et al., 1992), ZO-1 migration from intracellular sites to the plasma membrane (Stuart et al., 1994), and tight junction assembly (Stuart et al., 1996). Studies of cultured brain endothelial cells demonstrate that vasoactive agents, such as histamine, bradykinin, endothelin, and the nucleotides ATP, ADP, and UTP, which are known to increase BBB permeability, cause activation of phospholipase C and elevation of intracellular Ca^{2+} (Abbott, 1998, 2000). Although it was suggested that the data was consistent with a Ca^{2+}-dependent contractile mechanism for opening of tight junctions, no proof of this was provided. Further data on Ca^{2+} modulation of tight junction function is available in reviews (Denker and Nigam, 1998; Brown and Davis, 2002).

Calcium flux is implicated in structural and functional variations in cultured cerebral endothelial cells during ischemic stress. Bovine brain microvascular endothelial cells exposed to hypoxia and aglycemia for 6 h and hypoxia for 48 h show increased permeability to $[^{14}C]$ sucrose, which is reversed by treatment with the L-type calcium channel blocker nifedipine (Abbruscato and Davis, 1999). Of interest is the finding that 48 h of hypoxia is associated with alteration of the f-actin cytoskeleton of endothelial cells. These authors suggest that endothelial cell calcium flux may be responsible for the observed structural and functional variations.

3.3.3 Endothelial-Specific Growth Factors

The endothelial-specific angiogenic factors, VEGF-A, VEGF-B, and the angiopoietins (Ang), are known to affect BBB permeability (Nag, 2002, 2003b; Zhang and Chopp, 2002).

VEGF-A VEGF-A is one of the best characterized members of the VEGF family. It is known to be a major inducer of endothelial proliferation, migration, sprouting, tube formation, and permeability during embryonic vasculogenesis and in physiological and pathological angiogenesis (Ferrara and Davis-Smyth, 1997; Neufeld et al., 1999). There is low expression of VEGF-A mRNA, and protein in brain in steady states, and expression is increased following brain (Papavassiliou et al., 1997) and spinal cord (Skold et al., 2000) trauma, cerebral ischemia (Lennmyr et al., 1998; Plate et al., 1999), and in multiple sclerosis plaques (Proescholdt et al., 2002). Fewer studies have reported increased VEGF-A expression associated with BBB breakdown following trauma (Nag et al., 1997, 2002; Skold et al., 2005) (❷ *Figure 3-5d, e*), ischemia (Zhang et al., 2000b), and VEGF-A infusion into normal brain (Dobrogowska et al., 1998; Proescholdt et al., 1999).

How VEGF-A produces BBB breakdown has been studied with controversial results. Ultrastructural studies following intracortical injection of VEGF-A shows interendothelial gaps and formation of segmental fenestrae-like narrowings in cortical vessels permeable to endogenous albumin (Dobrogowska et al., 1998). In contrast, VEGF-A-induced hyperpermeability of the blood–retinal barrier is associated predominantly with enhanced numbers of endothelial caveolae while alterations of endothelial tight junctions and fenestrations were not reported (Hofman et al., 2000). VEGF-A is also reported to induce changes in tight junction proteins such as occludin as well as its phosphorylation and that of tyrosine phosphorylation of ZO-1 in retinal endothelial cells both in vivo and in vitro (Antonetti et al., 1999). Exposure of greater than 3 h to VEGF-A reduces occludin expression coinciding with changes in permeability in retinal (Antonetti et al., 1998) or brain (Wang et al., 2001) endothelial cells.

VEGF-A is partly responsible for BBB breakdown and cortical edema formation associated with cerebral infarcts since infarct size is decreased by pretreatment of mice with a soluble VEGF receptor chimeric protein (Flt-(1-3)-IgG), which inactivates endogenous VEGF (vanBruggen et al., 1999). However, administration of VEGF to ischemic rats 1 h after onset of ischemia exacerbates BBB leakage in the ischemic hemisphere but not in the nonischemic hemisphere (Zhang et al., 2000b). These studies suggest that acute inhibition of VEGF-A may have therapeutic potential in control of BBB leakage.

The role of VEGF-A in permeability in brain tumors is discussed in ❷ *Sect. 3.5*.

VEGF-B VEGF-B is expressed constitutively in endothelium of cerebral vessels (Nag et al., 2002) (❷ *Figure 3-5f*). Following injury, loss of endothelial VEGF-B immunoreactivity occurs in endothelium of vessels showing BBB breakdown to fibronectin. This suggests that VEGF-B, unlike VEGF-A, may be an essential factor in maintenance of endothelial homeostasis in steady states (Nag et al., 2002).

Angiopoietins Ang belong to a novel family of endothelial growth factors that function as ligands for the endothelial cell-specific receptor tyrosine kinase, Tie2 (Davis et al., 1996). Angiopoietin1 (Ang-1) and Ang-2 are the best characterized members of this family. Ang-1 induces autophosphorylation of

Tie2 whereas Ang-2 competitively inhibits this effect, suggesting that it may be a naturally occurring inhibitor of Ang-1/Tie2 activity (Maisonpierre et al., 1997). Ang-1 protein is constitutively expressed in endothelium of nonneural and cerebral vessels, consistent with it having a constitutive stabilizing effect by maintaining cell-to-cell and cell-matrix interactions (Maisonpierre et al., 1997) and it also has a strong antileakage effect (Thurston et al., 1999). Normally only weak Ang-2 immunoreactivity is present in occasional vessels.

Time course studies following brain injury demonstrate that early BBB breakdown is associated with loss or decreased endothelial localization of Ang-1 in lesion vessels showing BBB breakdown while there is a concomitant increase in Ang-2 mRNA and protein (Nourhaghighi et al., 2003) (❯ *Figure 3-5g, h*). Ang-2 is known to destabilize vessels to a more plastic state and a recent study demonstrates that Ang-2-like VEGF-A can induce BBB breakdown of intracerebral vessels (Nag et al., 2005a). This study also shows colocalization of Ang-2 and active caspase-3, a marker of apoptosis suggesting that Ang-2 may also be a factor in endothelial cell apoptosis which occurs at days 1 and 2 following the injury. At days 4–6 postinjury, a progressive increase in Ang-1 mRNA and protein results and a decrease in Ang-2 mRNA which coincides with maturation of neovessels and restoration of the BBB (Nourhaghighi et al., 2003).

The leakage-resistant effect of Ang-1 has the potential of being utilized to reduce BBB breakdown in pathological conditions. Recombinant adenoviruses expressing Ang-1 administered to mice before middle cerebral artery occlusion reduces BBB leakage in the ischemic brain and decreases the volume of ischemic tissue (Zhang et al., 2002). A study of nonneural vessels suggests that the leakage-resistant effect of Ang-1 is related to increased expression of junctional proteins such as PECAM-1 and decreased phosphorylation of PECAM-1 and cadherin (Gamble et al., 2000).

Angiopoietin expression in brain tumors is discussed in ❯ *Sect. 3-5*.

4   BBB Breakdown in Infection/Inflammation

4.1   Infections

Studies of cultured brain microvascular endothelial cells have demonstrated microbial proteins, which are the major genetic determinants mediating the penetration of some microorganisms across the BBB (Huang and Jong, 2001). Efficient penetration of *Escherichia coli* across the BBB is mediated by multiple proteins namely ibeA, ibeB, aslA, yijP, and ompA (Hoffman et al., 2000; Huang et al., 2000). A meningococcal protein, PilC, present at the tip of the pilus increases bacterial attachment and invasion of endothelial cells (Pron et al., 1997). Pneumococci bind to the endothelial surface and migrate through the cells via choline-binding protein A (Ring et al., 1998). Invasion of brain endothelial cells by Listeria Monocytogenes is InlB dependent (Greiffenberg et al., 1998). After internalization, the bacterium replicates efficiently over a period of at least 18 h, moves intracellularly by inducing actin tail formation, and spreads from cell to cell. The HIV-1 has an envelop protein, gp120, which can alter the morphology and elevate the permeability of endothelial cells in vitro (Annunziata et al., 1998). The HIV tat protein, known to be secreted extracellularly, has been reported to stimulate interleukin (IL)-8 synthesis by cultured brain endothelial cells—a response that could signal loss of BBB integrity (Hofman et al., 1999). Two surface antigens of *Toxoplasma gondii*, SAG1 and SAG3, have been shown to be important for the invasion process (Dzierszinski et al., 2000).

There is increasing interest in how microorganisms cross the BBB. Microbial pathogens may breach the BBB and enter the CNS through transcellular penetration, paracellular entry, and/or transmigration with infected leukocytes also referred to as the "Trojan horse" mechanism.

The classic transcellular route by which pathogens enter endothelial cells is via clathrin-dependent endocytosis. However, both caveolae and rafts are implicated in the uptake of viruses and bacteria into cells thus avoiding the potentially hazardous environment of lysosomes. A number of viruses, including echovirus, HIV, SV40, polyoma, Ebola, and Marburg viruses, exploit this possibility (Quest et al., 2004). Other organisms, such as *Chlamydia, Brucella, E. coli, Hemophilis influenza, T. gondii*, and *Plasmodium falciparum*, also utilize this route (Huang and Jong, 2001; Quest et al., 2004). Toxins of *Vibrio cholerae* and *Helicobacter pylori* are also internalized in this manner (Shin and Abraham, 2001; Fielding and Fielding, 2003). *T. gondii* and *P. falciparum* remain within the endothelial cells and do not cross the BBB, the effects on the CNS being secondary to sequestration of parasites in the luminal side of the brain microvessels (Gay-Andrieu et al., 1999; Cossart and Lecuit, 2000).

Paracellular penetration through the tight junctions of the BBB has been suggested for the Lyme disease pathogen Borrelia burgdorferi (Szczepanski et al., 1990; Comstock and Thomas, 1991) and Treponema pallidum, which causes syphilis (Haake and Lovett, 1994). A "Trojan horse" mechanism through recruitment of latently infected mononuclear cells from the peripheral circulation has been proposed for the human and simian immunodeficiency viruses (Lawson et al., 1992; Erlander, 1995; Lane et al., 1996). Circulating monocytes, from which perivascular macrophage/microglia are derived, are a possible vehicle for cell-associated transmigration of virus across the BBB. Most HIV enter brain via infected monocytes (Persidsky, 1999), which traverse abnormal tight junctions (Dallasta et al., 1999) and/or penetrate endothelial cells.

The integrity of the BBB varies with the type of infective agent; viruses cause minimal damage making delivery of antiviral agents to the CNS a greater challenge. Pneumococcal meningitis is associated with severe BBB breakdown, which has an advantage as it facilitates the influx of antibiotics such as penicillin across the BBB. The cerebrospinal fluid (CSF) concentrations of penicillin G are usually ∼0.4% of the steady-state serum levels in normal animals, but CSF levels increase approximately tenfold in animals with pneumococcal meningitis (Neuwelt, 2004).

4.2 Inflammation

Inflammation is an essential component in the pathogenesis of brain diseases, such as multiple sclerosis, ischemic stroke, and trauma, and the stages of the inflammatory process are similar in these conditions, although there may be variations in the degree of the stages. During inflammation, the process of leukocyte migration into the brain proceeds via a complex sequence of adhesive and migratory events, beginning with leukocyte rolling along the vascular wall, followed by attachment to the endothelial surface, and concluding with diapedesis of the leukocyte through the endothelial layer. Key regulators in these events are the cytokines which promote interactions between adhesion molecules on the surface of endothelial cells and counterreceptors on the membrane of leukocytes (Mantovani et al., 1997) and cause BBB breakdown (Bolton et al., 1998; Claudio et al., 1989). These processes have been extensively studied using in vitro BBB models as reviewed previously (Pachter et al., 2003).

4.2.1 Cytokines

Upon activation, CNS cells that produce cytokines include macrophages, microglial cells, astrocytes, and cerebral endothelial cells. Thus endothelial cells are not only targets for cytokines but also produce cytokines. Proinflammatory cytokines produced and secreted by cultured brain microvascular endothelial cells include interferon-γ, IL-α and -β, IL-6, and GM-CSF (Fabry et al., 1993; Frigerio et al., 1998; Stanimirovic and Satoh, 2000; Zhang et al., 2000a). Endogenous agents, including many cytokines, such as tumor necrosis factor (TNF)-α, IL-1β, IL-6, interferon-γ, and histamine, show marked permeability increases in cultured cerebral endothelial cells (de Vries et al., 1996; Abbott, 2000; Wong et al., 2004) and in vivo (Ferrari et al., 2004). In multiple sclerosis (Washington et al., 1994; Cannella and Raine, 1995), experimental allergic encephalomyelitis (EAE) (Barten and Ruddle, 1994), and ischemic stroke (Dirnagl et al., 1999; Stanimirovic and Satoh, 2000), cytokines upregulate adhesion molecules on endothelial cells, such as endothelial cell leukocyte adhesion molecule-1 (E-selectin), vascular cell adhesion molecule-1 (VCAM-1), and intercellular adhesion molecule-1 (ICAM-1). E-selectin is responsible for initially capturing the leukocyte from the circulation and setting it rolling on a path toward interactions with VCAM-1 and ICAM-1 (Hogg and Berlin, 1995). VCAM-1 and ICAM-1 utilize the counterreceptors β1 integrin VLA-4 and β2 integrin LFA-1, respectively, present on leukocytes to foster the tight leukocyte/endothelial adhesion required for subsequent leukocyte diapedesis and extravasation. Cerebral endothelial cells also produce factors, which markedly diminish leukocyte migration across CNS endothelial cells and downregulate adhesion molecules such as transforming growth factor (TGF)-β1 and -β2 (Fabry et al., 1995; Prat et al., 2001).

4.2.2 Leukocyte Migration

Leukocyte migration occurs through the endothelium of the venous vascular network (Wisniewski and Lossinsky, 1991; Hirano et al., 1994). The affected endothelial cells of veins and postcapillary venules involved in the immune responses become taller in preparation for leukocyte contact (Raine et al., 1990; Cross and Raine, 1991). Once adhesion molecules establish firm chemical attachment to the upregulated ligand receptors on the leukocyte membranes, pseudopodial projections from the leukocytes penetrate and traverse endothelial cells either through the junctional complexes or directly through the endothelial cell. Ultrastructural studies show lymphocytes and monocytes penetrate the endothelial cell adjacent to the junctional area in autoimmune demyelination (Raine et al., 1990) and in chronic relapsing EAE (Wisniewski and Lossinsky, 1991). It has recently been suggested that inflammatory cells pass through transendothelial channels located in the parajunctional areas (Lossinsky and Shivers, 2004). T lymphocytes can penetrate human brain endothelial cells through tight junctions between these cells without apparent disruption of the integrity or solute permeability of the monolayer (Wong et al., 1999). Polymorphonuclear leukocytes also penetrate the junctional areas between adjacent endothelial cells (Hirano et al., 1994). Increased leukocyte migration is also reported to alter the molecular organization of the tight junction complex, including breakdown of occludin and ZO-1 (Bolton et al., 1998). Abnormalities of ZO-1 and occludin localization associated with BBB breakdown have also been reported in active lesions of multiple sclerosis patients and to a lesser degree in the normal appearing white matter of these patients (Plumb et al., 2002; Vos et al., 2005).

An observation in IL-1-treated human umbilical vein endothelial cells cultured in astrocyte-conditioned medium is that leukocyte migration occurs at tricellular corners where the borders of three endothelial cells meet and where tight and adherens junctions are discontinuous and immunostaining for occludin, ZO-1, cadherin, and β-catenin is not present (Burns et al., 1997). This observation is supported by the finding that neutrophil migration is not associated with widespread proteolytic loss of the tight junction proteins ZO-1, ZO-2, and occludin from endothelial borders and that transendothelial electrical resistance is unaffected (Burns et al., 2000). In this study, the transendothelial electrical resistance of endothelial cells grown in the astrocyte-conditioned medium is reported to be $\sim$12,000 Ω, hence these findings may have relevance to cerebral endothelial cells.

4.2.3 Chemokines

Further passage of leukocytes across the BBB may be promoted by chemokines. Chemokine receptors have been identified on brain microvascular endothelial cells (Andjelkovic and Pachter, 2000). A possible mechanism by which such receptors direct movement of leukocytes into the parenchyma may be through modification of endothelial integrity. In this regard, the chemokine CCL2 (formerly known as MCP-1) has been shown to specifically bind to CCR2, the major cognate receptor for this chemokine (Murphy et al., 2000) on isolated brain microvessels (Andjelkovic and Pachter, 2000). CCL2 has further been reported to diminish expression of the tight junction–associated proteins occludin and ZO-1 in cultured brain microvascular endothelial cells in association with redistribution of these proteins away from their functional association with the detergent-resistant cytoskeleton framework (Song and Pachter, 2004). Chemokine-induced modifications such as these could, hypothetically, allow for facilitated egress of leukocytes through transiently weakened intercellular junctions.

Several chemokines are reported to be synthesized by astrocytes and microglia (Hayashi et al., 1995; Murphy, Jr, et al., 1995), which directly contact the abluminal surface of brain microvessels, and are uniquely positioned to deliver chemokines to the microvascular milieu, thus, affecting mononuclear cell recruitment. The increased chemokine expression reported in EAE (Hulkower et al., 1993; Miyagishi et al., 1997; Ransohoff et al., 1993) supports the concept that release of chemokines by perivascular glia might influence leukocyte interactions at the BBB.

Additional information on the factors influencing leukocyte migration can be obtained from reviews in the literature (Wisniewski and Lossinsky, 1991; de Vries et al., 1996; Pachter et al., 2003; Lossinsky and Shivers, 2004).

4.3   Matrix Metalloproteinases

Matrix metalloproteinases (MMPs) are a family of zinc-containing endopeptidases that target substrates, including collagen IV, fibronectin, and laminin, all of which are critical vascular matrix components. MMP-mediated degradation of these substrates may underlie the development of BBB breakdown and edema. Evidence from both animal models and human studies support a role of MMP-9 in the early BBB disruption in neuroinflammatory diseases. In vitro activation of brain microvascular endothelium with the proinflammatory cytokines TNF-α and IL-β results in selective upregulation of MMP-9 expression (Harkness et al., 2000). MMPs may also contribute to BBB permeability changes after acute cerebral injury (Yong et al., 2001; Lo et al., 2002). Ischemia-reperfusion can trigger the generation of reactive oxygen species, and oxidative stress is a potent signal that upregulates MMP levels in the brain (Gasche et al., 2001). Pharmacologic inhibition of MMPs not only reduces BBB damage but also reduces infarct volume (Rosenberg et al., 1998; Asahi et al., 2001).

MMP's have also been implicated in the neurovascular inflammation accompanying multiple sclerosis (Avolio et al., 2003; Chandler et al., 1997). In the EAE model, clinical symptoms correlate with transcriptional levels of MMP-7 and MMP-9 (Kieseier et al., 1998). In mouse brain, targeted knockout of the MMP-9 gene renders them resistant to EAE (Dubois et al., 1999). Correspondingly, some clinical studies have suggested that MMP-9 is significantly elevated in multiple sclerosis patients (Rosenberg et al., 1996; Trojano et al., 1999), and at least one imaging study has demonstrated a correlation between MMP levels and BBB breakdown detected via contrast-enhanced MRI scans (Lee et al., 1999).

Increases in MMP's may also mediate the inflammation that occurs after meningitis. MMP-8 and MMP-9 are upregulated in CSF of children with bacterial meningitis (Leppert et al., 2000), levels being 10–1,000-fold higher than in viral meningitis (Kolb et al., 1998). The increase of MMP-8 is a specific feature of bacterial meningitis (Leppert et al., 2000). MMP-8 is a typical product of granulocytes and its raised concentration in this neuroinflammatory disease probably reflects the infiltration of CSF with large numbers of neutrophils, a hallmark of the disease. MMP-inhibitors, such as GM6001 and BB1101, have been shown to reduce CSF levels of MMP-9 and TNF-α in experimental bacterial meningitis and lead to significant reduction in mortality and seizure incidence (Leib et al., 2000, 2001).

5   The BBB and Brain Tumors

High-grade gliomas are associated with BBB breakdown due to structural and molecular alterations in endothelial tight junctions. Ultrastructural studies demonstrate lack of fusion of adjacent plasma membranes at tight junctions (Long, 1970), presence of channels through interendothelial junctions, and rare but large breaks in the endothelial wall (Coomber et al., 1987). More recently, BBB breakdown to HRP was studied in an experimental tumor model. Both the number of caveolae and two parameters of tight junction opening, namely the cleft index and the cleft area index, were quantitated in tumor vessels. These authors reported a statistically significant increase of only endothelial caveolae (Hashizume and Black, 2002) in tumor vessels.

Loss of claudin-1 expression has been reported from nearly all microvessels in high-grade astrocytomas while claudin-5 and occludin expression were only downregulated in hyperplastic endothelium, and ZO-1 expression was largely unaffected. (Liebner et al., 2000a). Another study reported that more than two thirds of the microvessels in high-grade astrocytomas and hyperplastic vessels failed to show occludin expression (Papadopoulos et al., 2001). This study also reported a significant inverse correlation between CT enhancement and occludin expression suggesting that loss of junctional proteins is a central event in opening of the BBB. These authors also observed a switch from the 55-kDa form of occludin, which was present only in normal endothelium, to a 60-kDa form in all low-grade and some high-grade gliomas.

Both aquaporin-1 and -4 appear to play important roles in tumor-associated edema. Aquaporin-1 is expressed in microvessel endothelia of astrocytomas and in reactive astrocytes of metastatic carcinoma (Saadoun et al., 2002a) and in glioblastomas (Oshio et al., 2005). Increased expression of aquaporin-4 has been reported in neoplastic astrocytes in high-grade astrocytomas and reactive astrocytes at the margin of the tumor in both high-grade astrocytomas and metastatic carcinomas (Saadoun et al., 2002b). Both tumors showed a significant correlation between aquaporin-4 expression, and the amount of cerebral edema present as indicated by the degree of contrast enhancement on CT scans (Saadoun et al., 2002b). The increased aquaporin-4 expression associated with brain tumors likely functions to enhance edema fluid formation as suggested previously (Davies, 2002).

Factors which initiate BBB breakdown in astrocytomas are still poorly understood. The possibility that neoplastic astrocytes are unable to produce factors necessary to maintain the BBB in the region of the tumor is a possibility, although such a factor is still not defined. A large number of humoral factors are known to modulate BBB permeability (see ❷ *Sect. 3.3.1*) and possibly neoplastic astrocytes release some of these factors.

Increased expression of endothelial-specific growth factors occurs in high-grade gliomas. Molecular studies show an almost 50-fold upregulation of VEGF-A in glioblastomas (Weindel et al., 1994). Increased expression of VEGF-A at the mRNA and protein level has been shown to correlate with edema formation in meningiomas (Goldman et al., 1997; Provias et al., 1997). The structural alterations produced in cerebral endothelial cells by VEGF-A is discussed under the heading "VEGF-A."

In addition, VEGF-A can downregulate occludin expression (Kevil et al., 1998; Wang et al., 2001) leading to increased junctional permeability and cerebral edema in high-grade gliomas. The role of angiopoietins in tumor angiogenesis is well established (Holash et al., 1999; Zagzag et al., 1999). Increased expression of Ang-1 is present in tumor cells (Stratmann et al., 1998) and areas of high-vascular density throughout all stages of GBM progression, which is in keeping with its physiological role of maintaining vascular stability (Maisonpierre et al., 1997). In addition, high expression of endothelial Ang-2 is also reported in high-grade gliomas (Stratmann et al., 1998; Zagzag et al., 1999; Ding et al., 2001; Koga et al., 2001). Ang-2 is known to produce BBB breakdown (Nag et al., 2005a), hence it is another factor contributing to increased permeability in high-grade gliomas. Ang-2 is known to be increased by both hypoxia (Koga et al., 2001) and VEGF-A (Oh et al., 1999).

Scatter factor/hepatocyte growth factor (SF/HGF) is also expressed by astrocytomas, and its expression is upregulated with increasing malignancy (Lamszus et al., 1999). This cytokine also decreases occludin expression and increases endothelial cell permeability (Jiang et al., 1999). Hence both VEGF/SF/HGF expression by neoplastic astrocytes causes the phosphorylation of occludin and its subsequent downregulation, leading to tight junction opening, increased endothelial permeability, and cerebral edema. Current evidence suggests that hypoxia is the driving force for VEGF-A production in high-grade astrocytomas making hypoxia the most important trigger for angiogenesis and edema formation (Plate, 1999).

6   The BBB and Alzheimer's Disease

Alzheimer's disease (AD) is one of the commonest causes of dementia in North America. It is associated with a constellation of brain changes that include neuronal loss, neuritic plaques, neurofibrillary tangles, granulovacuolar degeneration, and Hirano bodies. More than 30% of cases of AD are reported to have cerebrovascular pathology (Kalaria, 1999). About 50% cases of AD show β-amyloid deposition in pial arteries, penetrating arterioles, and capillaries. It is suggested that this vascular deposition compromises BBB function and promotes chronic hypoperfusion (De Jong et al., 1997).

There is evidence that BBB breakdown occurs in AD. Pentraxins, such as P component and C-reactive protein immunoreactivities, have been demonstrated in cerebral lesions in AD, but the lack of their mRNA in brain suggests that these relatively large circulation-derived proteins and possibly others, as yet uncharacterized, originate from liver during the pathogenetic process (Kalaria, 1999). The CSF:serum albumin ratio is a generally accepted method of assessing BBB function in living subjects. Increased CSF: serum ratios have been reported in AD patients, particularly those having peripheral vascular disease (Blennow et al., 1990; Kalaria, 1992; Hampel et al., 1995) but are not apparent in others (Kay et al., 1987; Mecocci et al., 1991). In addition, a population-based study reports that 85-year olds with AD have a higher CSF:serum albumin ratio than nondemented individuals, and there are indications of a disturbed BBB function even before onset of the disease (Skoog et al., 1998).

Alterations in BBB glucose transporter protein (Kalaria and Harik, 1989), decreased mitochondrial content and increased caveolae (Claudio, 1996) and focal necrotic changes in capillary endothelial cells (Claudio, 1996; Kalaria and Hedera, 1995), have also been reported in AD. These endothelial changes could cause BBB breakdown or microvascular insufficiency and promote brain damage in the elderly and deterioration of cognitive function in AD (Andjelkovic and Pachter, 1998; Kalaria, 1999). It has been suggested that the endothelial changes could be produced by β-amyloid (Thomas et al., 1996). A neurovascular hypothesis of AD has also been proposed according to which faulty clearance of amyloid β peptide across the BBB, aberrant angiogenesis, and senescence of the cerebrovascular system could initiate neurovascular uncoupling, vessel regression, brain hypoperfusion, and neurovascular inflammation (Zlokovic, 2005). Ultimately, this would lead to BBB compromise; chemical imbalance in the neuronal environment; and synaptic and neuronal dysfunction, injury, and loss.

7   Concluding Remarks

Research in the past few decades has greatly enhanced our understanding of cerebral endothelial reactivity in disease states. However, much more work is required to determine the function of some of the recently discovered molecules at the BBB in steady states and during BBB breakdown in diseases. Such studies are crucial for designing strategies to modulate the BBB in diseases by opening the BBB for the effective delivery of molecules or to close the BBB during life-threatening vasogenic edema.

Acknowledgements

Grant support from the Heart and Stroke Foundation of Ontario is gratefully acknowledged.

References

Abbott NJ. 1998. Role of intracellular calcium in regulation of brain endothelial permeability. Introduction to the Blood–Brain Barrier. Methodology, Biology and Pathology. Pardridge WM, editor. Cambridge, UK: Cambridge University Press; pp. 345-351.

Abbott NJ. 2000. Inflammatory mediators and modulation of blood–brain barrier permeability. Cell Mol Neurobiol 20: 131-147.

Abbruscato TJ, Davis TP. 1999. Combination of hypoxia/aglycemia compromises in vitro blood–brain barrier integrity. J Pharmacol Exp Ther 289: 668-675.

Allen RD, Weiss DG, Hayden JH, Brown DT, Fujiwake H, et al. 1985. Gliding movement of and bidirectional transport along single native microtubules from squid axoplasm: Evidence for an active role of microtubules in cytoplasmic transport. J Cell Biol 100: 1736-1752.

Andjelkovic AV, Pachter JS. 1998. Central nervous system endothelium in neuroinflammatory, neuroinfectious, and neurodegenerative disease. J Neurosci Res 51: 423-430.

Andjelkovic AV, Pachter JS. 2000. Characterization of binding sites for chemokines MCP-1 and MIP-1alpha on human brain microvessels. J Neurochem 75: 1898-1906.

Annabi B, Lachambre M, Bousquet-Gagnon N, Page M, Gingras D, et al. 2001. Localization of membrane-type 1 matrix metalloproteinase in caveolae membrane domains. Biochem J 353: 547-553.

Annunziata P, Cioni C, Toneatto S, Paccagnini, E. 1998. HIV-1 gp120 increases the permeability of rat brain endothelium cultures by a mechanism involving substance P. AIDS 12: 2377-2385.

Antonetti DA, Barber AJ, Khin S, Lieth E, Tarbell JM, et al. 1998. Vascular permeability in experimental diabetes is associated with reduced endothelial occludin content: Vascular endothelial growth factor decreases occludin in retinal endothelial cells. Diabetes 47: 1953-1959.

Antonetti DA, Barber AJ, Hollinger LA, Wolpert EB, Gardner TW. 1999. Vascular endothelial growth factor induces rapid phosphorylation of tight junction proteins occludin and zonula occluden 1—A potential mechanism for vascular permeability in diabetic retinopathy and tumors. J Biol Chem 274: 23463-23467.

Asahi M, Wang X, Mori T, Sumii T, Jung JC, et al. 2001. Effects of matrix metalloproteinase-9 gene knock-out on the proteolysis of blood–brain barrier and white matter components after cerebral ischemia. J Neurosci 21: 7724-7732.

Avolio C, Giuliani F, Liuzzi GM, Ruggieri M, Paolicelli D, et al. 2003. Adhesion molecules and matrix metalloproteinases in multiple sclerosis: Effects induced by interferon-beta. Brain Res Bull 61: 357-364.

Barten DM, Ruddle NH. 1994. Vascular cell adhesion molecule-1 modulation by tumor necrosis factor in experimental allergic encephalomyelitis. J Neuroimmunol 51: 123-133.

Beggs JL, Waggener JD. 1976. Transendothelial vesicular transport of protein following compression injury to the spinal cord. Lab Invest 34: 428-439.

Bendayan M, Rasio EA. 1996. Transport of insulin and albumin by the microvascular endothelium of the rete mirabile. J Cell Sci 109: 1857-1864.

Bentzel CJ, Hainau B, Edelman A, Anagnostopoulos T, Benedetti EL. 1976. Effect of plant cytokinins on microfilaments and tight junction permeability. Nature 264: 666-668.

Bickel U, Yoshikawa T, Pardridge WM. 2001. Delivery of peptides and proteins through the blood-brain barrier. Adv Drug Deliv Rev 46: 247-279.

Black KL, Hoff JT. 1985. Leukotrienes increase blood-brain barrier permeability following intraparenchymal injections in rats. Ann Neurol 18: 349-351.

Blennow K, Wallin A, Fredman P, Karlsson I, Gottfries CG, et al. 1990. Blood-brain barrier disturbance in patients with Alzheimer's disease is related to vascular factors. Acta Neurol Scand 81: 323-326.

Bolton SJ, Anthony DC, Perry VH. 1998. Loss of the tight junction proteins occludin and zonula occludens-1 from cerebral vascular endothelium during neutrophil-induced blood-brain barrier breakdown in vivo. Neuroscience 86: 1245-1257.

Brightman MW, Reese TS. 1969. Junctions between intimately apposed cell membranes in the vertebrate brain. J Cell Biol 40: 648-677.

Brightman MW, Hori M, Rapoport SI, Reese TS, Westergaard E. 1973. Osmotic opening of tight junctions in cerebral endothelium. J Comp Neurol 152: 317-325.

Broadwell RD. 1989. Transcytosis of macromolecules through the blood-brain barrier: A cell biological perspective and critical appraisal. Acta Neuropathol (Berl) 79: 117-128.

Brown H, Hien TT, Day N, Mai NTH, Chuong LV, et al. 1999. Evidence of blood-brain barrier dysfunction in human cerebral malaria. Neuropathol Appl Neurobiol 25: 331-340.

Brown RC, Davis TP. 2002. Calcium modulation of adherens and tight junction function: A potential mechanism for blood-brain barrier disruption after stroke. Stroke 33: 1706-1711.

Burns AR, Walker DC, Brown ES, Thurmon LT, Bowden RA, et al. 1997. Neutrophil transendothelial migration is independent of tight junctions and occurs preferentially at tricellular corners. J Immunol 159: 2893-2903.

Burns AR, Bowden RA, MacDonell SD, Walker DC, Odebunmi TO, et al. 2000. Analysis of tight junctions during neutrophil transendothelial migration. J Cell Sci 113: 45-57.

Cannella B, Raine CS. 1995. The adhesion molecule and cytokine profile of multiple sclerosis lesions. Ann Neurol 37: 424-435.

Chambliss KL, Yuhanna IS, Mineo C, Liu P, German Z, et al. 2000. Estrogen receptor alpha and endothelial nitric oxide synthase are organized into a functional signaling module in caveolae. Circ Res 87: E44-E52.

Chandler S, Miller KM, Clements JM, Lury J, Corkill D, et al. 1997. Matrix metalloproteinases, tumor necrosis factor and multiple sclerosis: An overview. J Neuroimmunol 72: 155-161.

Chan PH, Fishman RA. 1984. The role of arachidonic acid in vasogenic brain edema. Fed Proc 43: 210-213.

Chan PH, Fishman RA, Caronna J, Schmidley JW, Prioleau G, et al. 1983. Induction of brain edema following intracerebral injection of arachidonic acid. Ann Neurol 13: 625-632.

Chan PH, Schmidley JW, Fishman RA, Longar SM. 1984. Brain injury, edema, and vascular permeability changes induced by oxygen-derived free radicals. Neurology 34: 315-320.

Chun M, Liyanage UK, Lisanti MP, Lodish HF. 1994. Signal transduction of a G protein-coupled receptor in caveolae: Colocalization of endothelin and its receptor with caveolin. Proc Natl Acad Sci USA 91: 11728-11732.

Claudio L. 1996. Ultrastructural features of the blood-brain barrier in biopsy tissue from Alzheimer's disease patients. Acta Neuropathol (Berl) 91: 6-14.

Claudio L, Kress Y, Norton WT, Brosnan CF. 1989. Increased vesicular transport and decreased mitochondrial content in blood-brain barrier endothelial cells during experimental autoimmune encephalomyelitis. Am J Pathol 135: 1157-1168.

Clawson CC, Hartmann JF, Vernier RL. 1966. Electron microscopy of the effect of gram-negative endotoxin on the blood-brain barrier. J Comp Neurol 127: 183-198.

Comstock LE, Thomas DD. 1991. Characterization of Borrelia burgdorferi invasion of cultured endothelial cells. Microb Pathog 10: 137-148.

Coomber BL, Stewart PA, Hayakawa K, Farrell CL, Del Maestro RF. 1987. Quantitative morphology of human glioblastoma multiforme microvessels: Structural basis of blood-brain barrier defect. J Neurooncol 5: 299-307.

Cossart P, Lecuit M. 2000. Microbial pathogens: An overview. Cellular Microbiology. Cossart P, Boquet P, Normark S, Rappuoli R, editors. Washington, DC: American Society for Microbiology Press; pp. 22-25.

Couet J, Belanger MM, Roussel E, Drolet MC. 2001. Cell biology of caveolae and caveolin. Adv Drug Deliv Rev 49: 223-235.

Crone C, Olesen SP. 1982. Electrical resistance of brain microvascular endothelium. Brain Res 241: 49-55.

Cross AH, Raine CS. 1991. Central nervous system endothelial cell-polymorphonuclear cell interactions during autoimmune demyelination. Am J Pathol 139: 1401-1409.

Dallasta LM, Pisarov LA, Esplen JE, Werley JV, Moses AV, et al. 1999. Blood-brain barrier tight junction disruption in human immunodeficiency virus-1 encephalitis. Am J Pathol 155: 1915-1927.

Davies DC. 2002. Blood-brain barrier breakdown in septic encephalopathy and brain tumours. J Anat 200: 639-646.

Davis S, Aldrich TH, Jones PF, Acheson A, Compton DL, et al. 1996. Isolation of angiopoietin-1, a ligand for the TIE2 receptor, by secretion-trap expression cloning. Cell 87: 1161-1169.

De Jong GI, De Vos RA, Steur EN, Luiten PG. 1997. Cerebrovascular hypoperfusion: A risk factor for Alzheimer's disease? Animal model and postmortem human studies. Ann N Y Acad Sci 826: 56-74.

Demeule M, Jodoin J, Gingras D, Beliveau R. 2000. P-glycoprotein is localized in caveolae in resistant cells and in brain capillaries. FEBS Lett 466: 219-224.

de Vries HE, Blom-Roosemalen MC, van OM, De Boer AG, van Berkel TJ, et al. 1996. The influence of cytokines on the integrity of the blood-brain barrier in vitro. J Neuroimmunol 64: 37-43.

Denker BM, Nigam SK. 1998. Molecular structure and assembly of the tight junction. Am J Physiol 274: F1-F9.

Ding H, Roncari L, Wu X, Lau N, Shannon P, et al. 2001. Expression and hypoxic regulation of angiopoietins in human astrocytomas. J Neurooncol 3: 1-10.

Dirnagl U, Iadecola C, Moskowitz MA. 1999. Pathobiology of ischaemic stroke: An integrated view. Trends Neurosci 22: 391-397.

Dobrogowska DH, Lossinsky AS, Tarnawski M, Vorbrodt AW. 1998. Increased blood-brain barrier permeability and endothelial abnormalities induced by vascular endothelial growth factor. J Neurocytol 27: 163-173.

Dorovini-Zis K, Sato M, Goping G, Rapoport S, Brightman M. 1983. Ionic lanthanum passage across cerebral endothelium exposed to hyperosmotic arabinose. Acta Neuropathol (Berl) 60: 49-60.

Dubois B, Masure S, Hurtenbach U, Paemen L, Heremans H, et al. 1999. Resistance of young gelatinase B-deficient mice to experimental autoimmune encephalomyelitis and necrotizing tail lesions. J Clin Invest 104: 1507-1515.

Dux E, Joo F. 1982. Effects of histamine on brain capillaries. Fine structural and immunohistochemical studies after intracarotid infusion. Exp Brain Res 47: 252-258.

Dzierszinski F, Mortuaire M, Cesbron-Delauw MF, Tomavo S. 2000. Targeted disruption of the glycosylphosphatidylinositol-anchored surface antigen SAG3 gene in Toxoplasma gondii decreases host cell adhesion and drastically reduces virulence in mice. Mol Microbiol 37: 574-582.

Easton AS, Fraser PA. 1998. Arachidonic acid increases cerebral microvascular permeability by free radicals in single pial microvessels of the anaesthetized rat. J Physiol 507: 541-547.

Easton AS, Sarker MH, Fraser PA. 1997. Two components of blood-brain barrier disruption in the rat. J Physiol 503: 613-623.

Ehrlich P. 1885. Das Sauerstoff-Bedürfnis des Organismus: Eine farbenanalytische studie. Hirschwald, Berlin.

Erlander SR. 1995. The solution to the seven mysteries of AIDS: The 'Trojan horse'. Med Hypotheses 44: 1-9.

Fabry Z, Fitzsimmons KM, Herlein JA, Moninger TO, Dobbs MB, et al. 1993. Production of the cytokines interleukin 1 and 6 by murine brain microvessel endothelium and smooth muscle pericytes. J Neuroimmunol 47: 23-34.

Fabry Z, Topham DJ, Fee D, Herlein J, Carlino JA, et al. 1995. TGF-beta 2 decreases migration of lymphocytes in vitro and homing of cells into the central nervous system in vivo. J Immunol 155: 325-332.

Farrell CL, Shivers RR. 1984. Capillary junctions of the rat are not affected by osmotic opening of the blood-brain barrier. Acta Neuropathol (Berl) 63: 179-189.

Feng Y, Venema VJ, Venema RC, Tsai N, Behzadian MA, et al. 1999. VEGF-induced permeability increase is mediated by caveolae. Invest Ophthalmol Vis Sci 40: 157-167.

Ferrara N, Davis-Smyth T. 1997. The biology of vascular endothelial growth factor. Endocr Rev 18: 4-25.

Ferrari CC, Depino AM, Prada F, Muraro N, Campbell S, et al. 2004. Reversible demyelination, blood-brain barrier breakdown, and pronounced neutrophil recruitment induced by chronic IL-1 expression in the brain. Am J Pathol 165: 1827-1837.

Fielding CJ, Fielding PE. 2003. Relationship between cholesterol trafficking and signaling in rafts and caveolae. Biochim Biophys Acta 1610: 219-228.

Fra AM, Masserini M, Palestini P, Sonnino S, Simons K. 1995. A photo-reactive derivative of ganglioside GM1 specifically cross-links VIP21-caveolin on the cell surface. FEBS Lett 375: 11-14.

Frank PG, Woodman SE, Park DS, Lisanti MP. 2003. Caveolin, caveolae, and endothelial cell function. Arterioscler Thromb Vasc Biol 23: 1161-1168.

Frigerio S, Gelati M, Ciusani E, Corsini E, Dufour A, et al. 1998. Immunocompetence of human microvascular brain endothelial cells: Cytokine regulation of IL-1beta, MCP-1, IL-10, sICAM-1 and sVCAM-1. J Neurol 245: 727-730.

Frokjaer-Jensen J. 1980. Three-dimensional organization of plasmalemmal vesicles in endothelial cells. An analysis by serial sectioning of frog mesenteric capillaries. J Ultrastruct Res 73: 9-20.

Fujimoto T, Nakade S, Miyawaki A, Mikoshiba K, Ogawa K. 1992. Localization of inositol 1,4,5-trisphosphate receptor-like protein in plasmalemmal caveolae. J Cell Biol 119: 1507-1513.

Fujimoto T. 1993. Calcium pump of the plasma membrane is localized in caveolse. J Cell Biol 120: 1147-1157.

Furuse M, Hirase T, Itoh M, Nagafuch A, Yonemura S, et al. 1993. Occludin: A novel integral membrane protein localizing at tight junctions. J Cell Biol 123: 1777-1788.

Furuse M, Fujita K, Hiiragi T, Fujimoto K, Tsukita S. 1998. Claudin-1 and -2: Novel integral membrane proteins localizing at tight junctions with no sequence similarity to occludin. J Cell Biol 141: 1539-1550.

Gamble JR, Drew J, Trezise L, Underwood A, Parsons M, et al. 2000. Angiopoietin-1 is an antipermeability and anti-inflammatory agent in vitro and targets cell junctions. Circ Res 87: 603-607.

Garcia-Cardena G, Oh P, Liu J, Schnitzer JE, Sessa WC. 1996. Targeting of nitric oxide synthase to endothelial cell caveolae via palmitoylation: Implications for nitric oxide signaling. Proc Natl Acad Sci USA 93: 6448-6453.

Gasche Y, Copin JC, Sugawara T, Fujimura M, Chan PH. 2001. Matrix metalloproteinase inhibition prevents oxidative stress-associated blood-brain barrier disruption after transient focal cerebral ischemia. J Cereb Blood Flow Metab 21: 1393-1400.

Gay-Andrieu F, Cozon GJ, Ferrandiz J, Kahi S, Peyron F. 1999. Flow cytometric quantification of Toxoplasma gondii cellular infection and replication. J Parasitol 85: 545-549.

Ghitescu L, Fixman A, Simionescu M, Simionescu N. 1986. Specific binding sites for albumin restricted to plasmalemmal vesicles of continuous capillary endothelium: Receptor-mediated transcytosis. J Cell Biol 102: 1304-1311.

Gloor SM, Wachtel M, Bolliger MF, Ishihara H, Landmann R, et al. 2001. Molecular and cellular permeability control at the blood-brain barrier. Brain Res Brain Res Rev 36: 258-264.

Goldman CK, Bharara S, Palmer CA, Vitek J, Tsai JC, et al. 1997. Brain edema in meningiomas is associated with increased vascular endothelial growth factor expression. Neurosurgery 40: 1269-1277.

Gow A, Southwood CM, Li JS, Pariali M, Riordan GP, et al. 1999. CNS myelin and sertoli cell tight junction strands are absent in Osp/claudin-11 null mice. Cell 99: 649-659.

Greiffenberg L, Goebel W, Kim KS, Weiglein I, Bubert A, et al. 1998. Interaction of Listeria monocytogenes with human brain microvascular endothelial cells: InlB-dependent invasion, long-term intracellular growth, and spread from macrophages to endothelial cells. Infect Immun 66: 5260-5267.

Gumbiner BM. 1996. Cell adhesion: The molecular basis of tissue architecture and morphogenesis. Cell 84: 345-357.

Haake DA, Lovett MA. 1994. Interjunctional invasion of endothelial cell monolayers. Methods Enzymol 236: 447-463.

Hampel H, Muller-Spahn F, Berger C, Haberl A, Ackenheil M, et al. 1995. Evidence of blood-cerebrospinal fluid-barrier impairment in a subgroup of patients with dementia of the Alzheimer type and major depression: A possible indicator for immunoactivation. Dementia 6: 348-354.

Hansson HA, Johansson BB. 1980. Induction of pinocytosis in cerebral vessels by acute hypertension and by hyperosmolar solutions. J Neurosci Res 5: 183-190.

Hardebo JE, Kahrstrom J. 1985. Endothelial negative surface charge areas and blood-brain barrier function. Acta Physiol Scand 125: 495-499.

Harkness KA, Adamson P, Sussman JD, Davies Jones GAB, Greenwood J, et al. 2000. Dexamethasone regulation of matrix metalloproteinase expression in CNS vascular endothelium. Brain 123: 698-709.

Hashizume K, Black KL. 2002. Increased endothelial vesicular transport correlates with increased blood-tumor barrier permeability induced by bradykinin and leukotriene C4. J Neuropathol Exp Neurol 61: 725-735.

Hayashi M, Luo Y, Laning J, Strieter RM, Dorf ME. 1995. Production and function of monocyte chemoattractant protein-1 and other beta-chemokines in murine glial cells. J Neuroimmunol 60: 143-150.

Hay JC, Scheller RH. 1997. SNAREs and NSF in targeted membrane fusion. Curr Opin Cell Biol 9: 505-512.

Hedley-Whyte ET, Hsu DW. 1986. Effect of dexamethasone on blood-brain barrier in the normal mouse. Ann Neurol 19: 373-377.

Hedley-Whyte ET, Lorenzo AV, Hsu DW. 1977. Protein transport across cerebral vessels during metrazole-induced convulsions. Am J Physiol 233: C74-C85.

Henley JR, Krueger EW, Oswald BJ, McNiven MA. 1998. Dynamin-mediated internalization of caveolae. J Cell Biol 141: 85-99.

Hirano A, Kawanami T, Llena JF. 1994. Electron microscopy of the blood-brain barrier in disease. Microsc Res Tech 27: 543-556.

Hirase T, Staddon JM, Saitou M, Ando-Akatsuka Y, Itoh M, et al. 1997. Occludin as a possible determinant of tight junction permeability in endothelial cells. J Cell Sci 110: 1603-1613.

Hnasko R, Lisanti MP. 2003. The biology of caveolae: Lessons from caveolin knockout mice and implications for human disease. Mol Interv 3: 445-464.

Hoffman JA, Badger JL, Zhang Y, Huang SH, Kim KS. 2000. Escherichia coli K1 aslA contributes to invasion of brain microvascular endothelial cells in vitro and in vivo. Infect Immun 68: 5062-5067.

Hofman FM, Chen P, Incardona F, Zidovetzki R, Hinton DR. 1999. HIV-1 tat protein induces the production of interleukin-8 by human brain-derived endothelial cells. J Neuroimmunol 94: 28-39.

Hofman P, Blaauwgeers HGT, Tolentino MJ, Adamis AP, Cardozo BJN, et al. 2000. VEGF-A induced hyperpermeability of blood-retinal barrier endothelium in vivo is predominantly associated with pinocytotic vesicular transport and not with formation of fenestrations. Curr Eye Res 21: 637-645.

Hogg N, Berlin C. 1995. Structure and function of adhesion receptors in leukocyte trafficking. Immunol Today 16: 327-330.

Holash J, Maisonpierre PC, Compton D, Boland P, Alexander CR, et al. 1999. Vessel cooption, regression, and growth in tumors mediated by angiopoietins and VEGF. Science 284: 1994-1998.

Houthoff HJ, Go KG, Gerrits PO. 1982. The mechanisms of blood-brain barrier impairment by hyperosmolar perfusion. An electron cytochemical study comparing exogenous HRP and endogenous antibody to HRP as tracers. Acta Neuropathol (Berl) 56: 99-112.

Huang SH, Jong AY. 2001. Cellular mechanisms of microbial proteins contributing to invasion of the blood-brain barrier. Cell Microbiol 3: 277-287.

Huang SH, Stins MF, Kim KS. 2000. Bacterial penetration across the blood-brain barrier during the development of neonatal meningitis. Microbes Infect 2: 1237-1244.

Huber JD, Egleton RD, Davis TP. 2001. Molecular physiology and pathophysiology of tight junctions in the blood-brain barrier. Trends Neurosci 24: 719-725.

Hulkower K, Brosnan CF, Aquino DA, Cammer W, Kulshrestha S, et al. 1993. Expression of CSF-1, c-fms, and MCP-1 in the central nervous system of rats with experimental allergic encephalomyelitis. J Immunol 150: 2525-2533.

Igarashi J, Michel T. 2000. Agonist-modulated targeting of the EDG-1 receptor to plasmalemmal caveolae. eNOS activation by sphingosine 1-phosphate and the role of caveolin-1 in sphingolipid signal transduction. J Biol Chem 275: 32363-32370.

Ikezu T, Ueda H, Trapp BD, Nishiyama K, Sha JF, et al. 1998. Affinity-purification and characterization of caveolins from the brain: Differential expression of caveolin-1, -2, and -3 in brain endothelial and astroglial cell types. Brain Res 804: 177-192.

Impagnatiello MA, Weitzer S, Gannon G, Compagni A, Cotton M, et al. 2001. Mammalian sprouty-1 and -2 are membrane-anchored phosphoprotein inhibitors of growth factor signaling in endothelial cells. J Cell Biol 152: 1087-1098.

Itoh M, Furuse M, Morita K, Kubota K, Saitou M, et al. 1999. Direct binding of three tight junction-associated MAGUKs, ZO-1, ZO-2, and ZO-3, with the COOH termini of claudins. J Cell Biol 147: 1351-1363.

Jiang WG, Martin TA, Matsumoto K, Nakamura T, Mansel RE. 1999. Hepatocyte growth factor/scatter factor decreases the expression of occludin and transendothelial resistance TER. and increases paracellular permeability in human vascular endothelial cells. J Cell Physiol 181: 319-329.

Joo F. 1994. Insight into the regulation by second messenger molecules of the permeability of the blood-brain barrier. Microsc Res Tech 27: 507-515.

Ju H, Venema VJ, Liang H, Harris MB, Zou R, et al. 2000. Bradykinin activates the Janus-activated kinase/signal transducers and activators of transcription JAK/STAT. pathway in vascular endothelial cells: Localization of JAK/STAT signalling proteins in plasmalemmal caveolae. Biochem J 351: 257-264.

Kalaria RN. 1992. The blood-brain barrier and cerebral microcirculation in Alzheimer disease. Cerebrovasc Brain Metab Rev 4: 226-260.

Kalaria RN. 1999. The blood-brain barrier and cerebrovascular pathology in Alzheimer's disease. Ann N Y Acad Sci 893: 113-125.

Kalaria RN, Harik SI. 1989. Abnormalities of the glucose transporter at the blood-brain barrier and in brain in Alzheimer's disease. Prog Clin Biol Res 317: 415-421.

Kalaria RN, Hedera P. 1995. Differential degeneration of the cerebral microvasculature in Alzheimer's disease. Neuroreport 6: 477-480.

Kay AD, May C, Papadopoulos NM, Costello R, Atack JR, et al. 1987. CSF and serum concentrations of albumin and IgG in Alzheimer's disease. Neurobiol Aging 8: 21-25.

Kessler RM, Goble JC, Bird JH, Girton ME, Doppman JL, et al. 1984. Measurement of blood-brain barrier permeability with positron emission tomography and [68Ga]EDTA. J Cereb Blood Flow Metab 4: 323-328.

Kevil CG, Payne DK, Mire E, Alexander JS. 1998. Vascular permeability factor/vascular endothelial cell growth factor-mediated permeability occurs through disorganization of endothelial junctional proteins. J Biol Chem 273: 15099-15103.

Kieseier BC, Kiefer R, Clements JM, Miller K, Wells GM, et al. 1998. Matrix metalloproteinase-9 and -7 are regulated in experimental autoimmune encephalomyelitis. Brain 121: 159-166.

Kniesel U, Wolburg H. 2000. Tight junctions of the blood-brain barrier. Cell Mol Neurobiol 20: 57-76.

Koga K, Todaka T, Morioka M, Hamada J, Kai Y, et al. 2001. Expression of angiopoietin-2 in human glioma cells and its role for angiogenesis. Cancer Res 61: 6248-6254.

Kolb SA, Lahrtz F, Paul R, Leppert D, Nadal D, Pfister HW, Fontana A. 1998. Matrix metalloproteinases and tissue inhibitors of metalloproteinases in viral meningitis: Upregulation of MMP-9 and TIMP-1 in cerebrospinal fluid. J Neuroimmunol 84: 143-150.

Kontos HA, Wei EP, Povlishock JT, Christman CW. 1984. Oxygen radicals mediate the cerebral arteriolar dilation from arachidonate and bradykinin in cats. Circ Res 55: 295-303.

Kraemer DF, Fortin D, Doolittle ND, Neuwelt EA. 2001. Association of total dose intensity of chemotherapy in primary central nervous system lymphoma human non-acquired immunodeficiency syndrome and survival. Neurosurgery 48: 1033-1040.

Lamszus K, Laterra J, Westphal M, Rosen EM. 1999. Scatter factor/hepatocyte growth factor SF/HGF. content and function in human gliomas. Int J Neurosci 17: 517-530.

Lane JH, Sasseville VG, Smith MO, Vogel P, Pauley DR, et al. 1996. Neuroinvasion by simian immunodeficiency virus coincides with increased numbers of perivascular macrophages/microglia and intrathecal immune activation. J Neurovirol 2: 423-432.

Lawson LJ, Perry VH, Gordon S. 1992. Turnover of resident microglia in the normal adult mouse brain. Neuroscience 48: 405-415.

Lee MA, Palace J, Stabler G, Ford J, Gearing A, et al. 1999. Serum gelatinase B, TIMP-1 and TIMP-2 levels in multiple sclerosis. A longitudinal clinical and MRI study. Brain 122: 191-197.

Leib SL, Leppert D, Clements J, Tauber MG. 2000. Matrix metalloproteinases contribute to brain damage in experimental pneumococcal meningitis. Infect Immun 68: 615-620.

Leib SL, Clements JM, Lindberg RL, Heimgartner C, Loeffler JM, et al. 2001. Inhibition of matrix metalloproteinases and tumour necrosis factor alpha converting enzyme as adjuvant therapy in pneumococcal meningitis. Brain 124: 1734-1742.

Lennmyr F, Ata KA, Funa K, Olsson Y, Terent A. 1998. Expression of vascular endothelial growth factor VEGF and its receptors Flt-1 and Flk-1 following permanent and transient occlusion of the middle cerebral artery in the rat. J Neuropathol Exp Neurol 57: 874-882.

Leppert D, Leib SL, Grygar C, Miller KM, Schaad UB, et al. 2000. Matrix metalloproteinase MMP-8 and MMP-9 in cerebrospinal fluid during bacterial meningitis: Association with blood-brain barrier damage and neurological sequelae. Clin Infect Dis 31: 80-84.

Liebner S, Fischmann A, Rascher G, Duffner F, Grote EH, et al. 2000a. Claudin-1 and claudin-5 expression and tight junction morphology are altered in blood vessels of human glioblastoma multiforme. Acta Neuropathol (Berl) 100: 323-331.

Liebner S, Kniesel U, Kalbacher H, Wolburg H. 2000b. Correlation of tight junction morphology with the expression of tight junction proteins in blood-brain barrier endothelial cells. Eur J Cell Biol 79: 707-717.

Li S, Couet J, Lisanti MP. 1996. Src tyrosine kinases, Galpha subunits, and H-Ras share a common membrane-anchored scaffolding protein, caveolin. Caveolin binding negatively regulates the auto-activation of Src tyrosine kinases. J Biol Chem 271: 29182-29190.

Lisanti MP, Scherer PE, Vidugiriene J, Tang Z, Hermanowski-Vosatka A, et al. 1994. Characterization of caveolin-rich membrane domains isolated from an endothelial-rich source: Implications for human disease. J Cell Biol 126: 111-126.

Liu J, Oh P, Horner T, Rogers RA, Schnitzer JE. 1997. Organized endothelial cell surface signal transduction in caveolae distinct from glycosylphosphatidylinositol-anchored protein microdomains. J Biol Chem 272: 7211-7222.

Liu P, Anderson RG. 1995. Compartmentalized production of ceramide at the cell surface. J Biol Chem 270: 27179-27185.

Liu SM, Magnusson KE, Sundqvist T. 1993. Microtubules are involved in transport of macromolecules by vesicles in cultured bovine aortic endothelial cells. J Cell Physiol 156: 311-316.

Lo EH, Wang X, Cuzner ML. 2002. Extracellular proteolysis in brain injury and inflammation: Role for plasminogen activators and matrix metalloproteinases. J Neurosci Res 69: 1-9.

Long DM. 1970. Capillary ultrastructure and the blood-brain barrier in human malignant brain tumors. J Neurosurg 32: 127-144.

Lossinsky AS, Shivers RR. 2004. Structural pathways for macromolecular and cellular transport across the blood-brain barrier during inflammatory conditions. Rev Histol Histopathol 19: 535-564.

Lossinsky AS, Song MJ, Wisniewski HM. 1989. High voltage electron microscopic studies of endothelial cell tubular structures in the mouse blood-brain barrier following brain trauma. Acta Neuropathol (Berl) 77: 480-488.

Lupu C, Goodwin CA, Westmuckett AD, Emeis JJ, Scully MF, et al. 1997. Tissue factor pathway inhibitor in endothelial cells colocalizes with glycolipid microdomains/caveolae. Regulatory mechanisms of the anticoagulant properties of the endothelium. Arterioscler Thromb Vasc Biol 17: 2964-2974.

Madara JL, Parkos C, Colgan S, Nusrat A, Atisook K, et al. 1992. The movement of solutes and cells across tight junctions. Ann N Y Acad Sci 664: 47-60.

Maier-Hauff K, Baethmann AJ, Lange M, Schurer L, Unterberg A. 1984. The kallikrein-kinin system as mediator in vasogenic brain edema. Part 2: Studies on kinin formation in focal and perifocal brain tissue. J Neurosurg 61: 97-106.

Maisonpierre PC, Suri C, Jones PF, Bartunkova S, Wiegand SJ, et al. 1997. Angiopoietin-2, a natural antagonist for Tie2 that disrupts in vivo angiogenesis. Science 277: 55-60.

Mantovani A, Bussolino F, Introna M. 1997. Cytokine regulation of endothelial cell function: From molecular level to the bedside. Immunol Today 18: 231-240.

Martin-Padura I, Lostaglio S, Schneemann M, Williams L, Romano M, et al. 1998. Junctional adhesion molecule, a novel member of the immunoglobulin superfamily that distributes at intercellular junctions and modulates monocyte transmigration. J Cell Biol 142: 117-127.

McDonald KK, Zharikov S, Block ER, Kilberg MS. 1997. A caveolar complex between the cationic amino acid transporter 1 and endothelial nitric-oxide synthase may explain the "arginine paradox". J Biol Chem 272: 31213-31216.

McIntosh DP, Schnitzer JE. 1999. Caveolae require intact VAMP for targeted transport in vascular endothelium. Am J Physiol 277: H2222-H2232.

McIntosh DP, Tan XY, Oh P, Schnitzer JE. 2002. Targeting endothelium and its dynamic caveolae for tissue-specific transcytosis in vivo: A pathway to overcome cell barriers to drug and gene delivery. Proc Natl Acad Sci USA 99: 996-2001.

Mecocci P, Parnetti L, Reboldi GP, Santucci C, Gaiti A, et al. 1991. Blood-brain-barrier in a geriatric population: Barrier function in degenerative and vascular dementias. Acta Neurol Scand 84: 210-213.

Minshall RD, Tiruppathi C, Vogel SM, Niles WD, Gilchrist A, et al. 2000. Endothelial cell-surface gp60 activates vesicle formation and trafficking via Gi-coupled Src kinase signaling pathway. J Cell Biol 150: 1057-1070.

Minshall RD, Sessa WC, Stan RV, Anderson RG, Malik AB. 2003. Caveolin regulation of endothelial function. Am J Physiol Lung Cell Mol Physiol 285: L1179-L1183.

Miyagishi R, Kikuchi S, Takayama C, Inoue Y, Tashiro K. 1997. Identification of cell types producing RANTES, MIP-1 alpha and MIP-1 beta in rat experimental autoimmune encephalomyelitis by in situ hybridization. J Neuroimmunol 77: 17-26.

Monier S, Parton RG, Vogel F, Behlke J, Henske A, et al. 1995. VIP21-caveolin, a membrane protein constituent of the caveolar coat, oligomerizes in vivo and in vitro. Mol Biol Cell 6: 911-927.

Morita K, Furuse M, Fujimoto K, Tsukita S. 1999. Claudin multigene family encoding four-transmembrane domain protein components of tight junction strands. Proc Natl Acad Sci USA 96: 511-516.

Muir AR, Peters A. 1962. Quintuple-layered membrane junctions at terminal bars between endothelial cells. J Cell Biol 12: 443-448.

Murakami K, Kondo T, Yang G, Chen SF, Morita-Fujimura Y, et al. 1999. Cold injury in mice: A model to study mechanisms of brain edema and neuronal apoptosis. Prog Neurobiol 57: 289-299.

Murphy GM, Jr, Jia XC, Song Y, Ong E, Shrivastava R, et al. 1995. Macrophage inflammatory protein 1-alpha mRNA expression in an immortalized microglial cell line and cortical astrocyte cultures. J Neurosci Res 40: 755-763.

Murphy PM, Baggiolini M, Charo IF, Hebert CA, Horuk R, et al. 2000. International union of pharmacology. XXII. Nomenclature for chemokine receptors. Pharmacol Rev 52: 145-176.

Nag S. 1984a. Cerebral changes in chronic hypertension: Combined permeability and immunohistochemical studies. Acta Neuropathol (Berl) 62: 178-184.

Nag S. 1984b. Cerebral endothelial surface charge in hypertension. Acta Neuropathol (Berl) 63: 276-281.

Nag S. 1985. Ultrastructural localization of lectin receptors on cerebral endothelium. Acta Neuropathol (Berl) 66: 105-110.

Nag S. 1986. Cerebral endothelial plasma membrane alterations in acute hypertension. Acta Neuropathol (Berl) 70: 38-43.

Nag S. 1988. Localisation of calcium-activated adenosinetriphosphatase Ca^{2+}-ATPase in intracerebral arterioles in acute hypertension. Acta Neuropathol (Berl) 75: 547-553.

Nag S. 1990. Ultracytochemical localisation of Na^+, K^+-ATPase in cerebral endothelium in acute hypertension. Acta Neuropathol (Berl) 80: 7-11.

Nag S. 1991. Protective effect of flunarizine on blood-brain barrier permeability alterations in acutely hypertensive rats. Stroke 22: 1265-1269.

Nag S. 1992. Vascular changes in the spinal cord in N-methyl-D-aspartate-induced excitotoxicity: Morphological and permeability studies. Acta Neuropathol (Berl) 84: 471-477.

Nag S. 1993. Cerebral endothelial mechanisms in increased permeability in chronic hypertension. Adv Exp Med Biol 331: 263-266.

Nag S. 1995. Role of the endothelial cytoskeleton in blood-brain-barrier permeability to protein. Acta Neuropathol (Berl) 90: 454-460.

Nag S. 1998. Blood-brain barrier permeability measured with histochemistry. Introduction to the Blood-Brain Barrier. Methodology, Biology and Pathology. Pardridge WM. editor. Cambridge, UK: Cambridge University Press; pp. 113-121.

Nag S. 2002. The blood-brain barrier and cerebral angiogenesis: Lessons from the cold-injury model. Trends Mol Med 8: 38-44.

Nag S. 2003a. Morphology and molecular properties of cellular components of normal cerebral vessels. Methods Mol Med 89: 3-36.

Nag S. 2003b. Pathophysiology of blood-brain barrier breakdown. Methods Mol Med 89: 97-119.

Nag S. 2005. Anatomy and structure of brain blood vessels. Pathology and Genetics. Cerebrovascular Diseases. Kalimo H, editor. Basel: ISN Neuropath Press; pp. 14-21.

Nag S, Harik SI. 1987. Cerebrovascular permeability to horseradish peroxidase in hypertensive rats: Effects of unilateral locus ceruleus lesion. Acta Neuropathol (Berl) 73: 247-253.

Nag S, Robertson DM, Dinsdale HB. 1977. Cerebral cortical changes in acute experimental hypertension: An ultrastructural study. Lab Invest 36: 150-161.

Nag S, Robertson DM, Dinsdale HB. 1978. Cytoplasmic filaments in intracerebral cortical vessels. Ann Neurol 3: 555-559.

Nag S, Robertson DM, Dinsdale HB. 1979. Quantitative estimate of pinocytosis in experimental acute hypertension. Acta Neuropathol (Berl) 46: 107-116.

Nag S, Robertson DM, Dinsdale HB. 1980. Morphological changes in spontaneously hypertensive rats. Acta Neuropathol (Berl) 52: 27-34.

Nag S, Takahashi JL, Kilty DW. 1997. Role of vascular endothelial growth factor in blood-brain barrier breakdown and angiogenesis in brain trauma. J Neuropathol Exp Neurol 56: 912-921.

Nag S, Picard P, Stewart DJ. 2001. Expression of nitric oxide synthases and nitrotyrosine during blood-brain barrier breakdown and repair after cold injury. Lab Invest 81: 41-49.

Nag S, Eskandarian MR, Davis J, Eubanks JH. 2002. Differential expression of vascular endothelial growth factor-A VEGF-A and VEGF-B after brain injury. J Neuropathol Exp Neurol 61: 778-788.

Nag S, Papneja T, Venugopalan R, Stewart DJ. 2005a. Increased angiopoietin2 expression is associated with endothelial apoptosis and blood-brain barrier breakdown. Lab Invest 85: 1189-1198.

Nag S, Venugopalan R, Stewart DJ. 2005b. Molecular mechanisms in blood-brain barrier breakdown following brain injury. J Neuropathol Exp Neurol 64: 437.

Nagy Z, Peters H, Huttner I. 1983. Charge-related alterations of the cerebral endothelium. Lab Invest 49: 662-671.

Nagy Z, Peters H, Huttner I. 1984. Fracture faces of cell junctions in cerebral endothelium during normal and hyperosmotic conditions. Lab Invest 50: 313-322.

Nasdala I, Wolburg-Buchholz K, Wolburg H, Kuhn A, Ebnet K, et al. 2002. A transmembrane tight junction protein selectively expressed on endothelial cells and platelets. J Biol Chem 277: 16294-16303.

Neufeld G, Cohen T, Gengrinovitch S, Poltorak Z. 1999. Vascular endothelial growth factor VEGF and its receptors. FASEB J 13: 9-22.

Neuwelt EA. 2004. Mechanisms of disease: The blood-brain barrier. Neurosurgery 54: 131-140.

Nigam SK, Rodriguez-Boulan E, Silver RB. 1992. Changes in intracellular calcium during the development of epithelial polarity and junctions. Proc Natl Acad Sci USA 89: 6162-6166.

Nitsch C, Goping G, Laursen H, Klatzo I. 1986. The blood-brain barrier to horseradish peroxidase at the onset of bicuculline-induced seizures in hypothalamus, pallidum, hippocampus, and other selected regions of the rabbit. Acta Neuropathol (Berl) 69: 1-16.

Nourhaghighi N, Teichert-Kuliszewska K, Davis J, Stewart DJ, Nag, S. 2003. Altered expression of angiopoietins during blood-brain barrier breakdown and angiogenesis. Lab Invest 83: 1211-1222.

Nusrat A, Parkos CA, Verkade P, Foley CS, Liang TW, et al. 2000. Tight junctions are membrane microdomains. J Cell Sci 113: 1771-1781.

Oh H, Takagi H, Suzuma K, Otani A, Matsumura M, et al. 1999. Hypoxia and vascular endothelial growth factor selectively up-regulate angiopoietin-2 in bovine microvascular endothelial cells. J Biol Chem 274: 15732-15739.

Oh P, Schnitzer JE. 2001. Segregation of heterotrimeric G proteins in cell surface microdomains. Gq. binds caveolin to concentrate in caveolae, whereas Gi. and Gs. target lipid rafts by default. Mol Biol Cell 12: 685-698.

Oh P, McIntosh DP, Schnitzer JE. 1998. Dynamin at the neck of caveolae mediates their budding to form transport vesicles by GTP-driven fission from the plasma membrane of endothelium. J Cell Biol 141: 101-114.

Olesen SP, Crone C. 1986. Substances that rapidly augment ionic conductance of endothelium in cerebral venules. Acta Physiol Scand 127: 233-241.

Oshio K, Binder DK, Liang Y, Bollen A, Feuerstein B, et al. 2005. Expression of the aquaporin-1 water channel in human glial tumors. Neurosurgery 56: 375-381.

Oury TD, Piantadosi CA, Crapo JD. 1993. Cold-induced brain edema in mice. Involvement of extracellular superoxide dismutase and nitric oxide. J Biol Chem 268: 15394-15398.

Pachter JS, de Vries HE, Fabry Z. 2003. The blood-brain barrier and its role in immune privilege in the central nervous system. J Neuropathol Exp Neurol 62: 593-604.

Papadopoulos MC, Lamb FJ, Moss RF, Davies DC, Tighe D, et al. 1999. Faecal peritonitis causes oedema and neuronal injury in pig cerebral cortex. Clin Sci (Lond) 96: 461-466.

Papadopoulos MC, Saadoun S, Woodrow CJ, Davies DC, Costa-Martins P, et al. 2001. Occludin expression in microvessels of neoplastic and non-neoplastic human brain. Neuropathol Appl Neurobiol 27: 384-395.

Papadopoulos SM, Black KL, Hoff JT. 1989. Cerebral edema induced by arachidonic acid: Role of leukocytes and 5-lipoxygenase products. Neurosurgery 25: 369-372.

Papavassiliou E, Gogate N, Proescholdt M, Heiss JD, Walbridge S, et al. 1997. Vascular endothelial growth factor vascular permeability factor expression in injured rat brain. J Neurosci Res 49: 451-460.

Pardridge WM, Nowlin DM, Choi TB, Yang J, Calaycay J, et al. 1989. Brain capillary 46,000 dalton protein is cytoplasmic actin and is localized to endothelial plasma membrane. J Cereb Blood Flow Metab 9: 675-680.

Persidsky Y. 1999. Model systems for studies of leukocyte migration across the blood-brain barrier. J Neurovirol 5: 579-590.

Petito CK, Levy DE. 1980. The importance of cerebral arterioles in alterations of the blood-brain barrier. Lab Invest 43: 262-268.

Petty MA, Lo EH. 2002. Junctional complexes of the blood-brain barrier: Permeability changes in neuroinflammation. Prog Neurobiol 68: 311-323.

Plate KH. 1999. Mechanisms of angiogenesis in the brain. J Neuropathol Exp Neurol 58: 313-320.

Plate KH, Beck H, Danner S, Allegrini PR, Wiessner C. 1999. Cell type specific upregulation of vascular endothelial growth factor in an MCA-occlusion model of cerebral infarct. J Neuropathol Exp Neurol 58: 654-666.

Plumb J, McQuaid S, Mirakhur M, Kirk J. 2002. Abnormal endothelial tight junctions in active lesions and normal-appearing white matter in multiple sclerosis. Brain Pathol 12: 154-169.

Povlishock JT, Becker DP, Sullivan HG, Miller JD. 1978. Vascular permeability alterations to horseradish peroxidase in experimental brain injury. Brain Res 153: 223-239.

Prat A, Biernacki K, Wosik K, Antel JP. 2001. Glial cell influence on the human blood-brain barrier. Glia 36: 145-155.

Proescholdt MA, Heiss JD, Walbridge S, Muhlhauser J, Capogrossi MC, et al. 1999. Vascular endothelial growth factor VEGF modulates vascular permeability and inflammation in rat brain. J Neuropathol Exp Neurol 58: 613-627.

Proescholdt MA, Jacobson S, Tresser N, Oldfield EH, Merrill MJ. 2002. Vascular endothelial growth factor is expressed in multiple sclerosis plaques and can induce inflammatory lesions in experimental allergic encephalomyelitis rats. J Neuropathol Exp Neurol 61: 914-925.

Pron B, Taha MK, Rambaud C, Fournet JC, Pattey N, et al. 1997. Interaction of Neisseria maningitidis with the components of the blood-brain barrier correlates with an increased expression of PilC. J Infect Dis 176: 1285-1292.

Provias J, Claffey K, deAguila L, Lau N, Feldkamp M, et al. 1997. Meningiomas: Role of vascular endothelial growth factor/vascular permeability factor in angiogenesis and peritumoral edema. Neurosurgery 40: 1016-1026.

Puyraimond A, Fridman R, Lemesle M, Arbeille B, Menashi S. 2001. MMP-2 colocalizes with caveolae on the surface of endothelial cells. Exp Cell Res 262: 28-36.

Quest AF, Leyton L, Parraga M. 2004. Caveolins, caveolae, and lipid rafts in cellular transport, signaling, and disease. Biochem Cell Biol 82: 129-144.

Raine CS, Cannella B, Duijvestijn AM, Cross AH. 1990. Homing to central nervous system vasculature by antigen-specific lymphocytes. II. Lymphocyte/endothelial cell adhesion during the initial stages of autoimmune demyelination. Lab Invest 63: 476-489.

Ransohoff RM, Hamilton TA, Tani M, Stoler MH, Shick HE, et al. 1993. Astrocyte expression of mRNA encoding cytokines IP-10 and JE/MCP-1 in experimental autoimmune encephalomyelitis. FASEB J 7: 592-600.

Rapoport SI. 2000. Osmotic opening of the blood-brain barrier: Principles, mechanism, and therapeutic applications. Cell Mol Neurobiol 20: 217-230.

Rapoport SI, Fredericks WR, Ohno K, Pettigrew KD. 1980. Quantitative aspects of reversible osmotic opening of the blood-brain barrier. Am J Physiol 238: R421-R431.

Raymond JJ, Robertson DM, Dinsdale HB. 1986. Pharmacological modification of bradykinin induced breakdown of the blood-brain barrier. Can J Neurol Sci 13: 214-220.

Razani B, Woodman SE, Lisanti MP. 2002. Caveolae: From cell biology to animal physiology. Pharmacol Rev 54: 431-467.

Reese TS, Karnovsky MJ. 1967. Fine structural localization of a blood-brain barrier to exogenous peroxidase. J Cell Biol 34: 207-217.

Revest PA, Abbott NJ, Gillespie JI. 1991. Receptor-mediated changes in intracellular $[Ca^{2+}]$ in cultured rat brain capillary endothelial cells. Brain Res 549: 159-161.

Ring A, Weiser JN, Tuomanen EI. 1998. Pneumococcal trafficking across the blood-brain barrier. Molecular analysis of a novel bidirectional pathway. J Clin Invest 102: 347-360.

Rizzo V, Sung A, Oh P, Schnitzer JE. 1998. Rapid mechanotransduction in situ at the luminal cell surface of vascular endothelium and its caveolae. J Biol Chem 273: 26323-26329.

Rosenberg GA, Dencoff JE, Correa N, Jr, Reiners CC. Ford M, 1996. Effect of steroids on CSF matrix metalloproteinases in multiple sclerosis: Relation to blood-brain barrier injury. Neurology 46: 1626-1632.

Rosenberg GA, Estrada EY, Dencoff JE. 1998. Matrix metalloproteinases and TIMPs are associated with blood-brain barrier opening after reperfusion in rat brain. Stroke 29: 2189-2195.

Rothman JE. 1994. Intracellular membrane fusion. Adv Second Messenger Phosphoprotein Res 29: 81-96.

Rubin LL, Staddon JM. 1999. The cell biology of the blood-brain barrier. Ann Rev Neurosci 22: 11-28.

Saadoun S, Papadopoulos MC, Davies DC, Bell BA, Krishna S. 2002a. Increased aquaporin 1 water channel expression in human brain tumours. Br J Cancer 87: 621-623.

Saadoun S, Papadopoulos MC, Davies DC, Krishna S, Bell BA. 2002b. Aquaporin-4 expression is increased in oedematous human brain tumours. J Neurol Neurosurg Psychiatry 72: 262-265.

Saitou M, Furuse M, Sasaki H, Schulzke JD, Fromm M, et al. 2000. Complex phenotype of mice lacking occludin, a component of tight junction strands. Mol Biol Cell 11: 4131-4142.

Sargiacomo M, Scherer PE, Tang Z, Kubler E, Song KS, et al. 1995. Oligomeric structure of caveolin: Implications for caveolae membrane organization. Proc Natl Acad Sci USA 92: 9407-9411.

Schilling L, Wahl M. 1997. Brain edema: Pathogenesis and therapy. Kidney Int Suppl 59: S69-S75.

Schilling L, Wahl M. 1999. Mediators of cerebral edema, in Hypoxia. Into the Next Millennium. Roach RC, editor. New York: Kluwer Academic/Plenum Publishing; pp. 123-141.

Schnapp BJ, Vale RD, Sheetz MP, Reese TS. 1985. Single microtubules from squid axoplasm support bidirectional movement of organelles. Cell 40: 455-462.

Schnitzer JE. 2001. Caveolae: From basic trafficking mechanisms to targeting transcytosis for tissue-specific drug and gene delivery in vivo. Adv Drug Deliv Rev 49: 265-280.

Schnitzer JE, Liu J, Oh P. 1995a. Endothelial caveolae have the molecular transport machinery for vesicle budding, docking, and fusion including VAMP, NSF, SNAP, annexins, and GTPases. J Biol Chem 270: 14399-14404.

Schnitzer JE, Oh P, Jacobson BS, Dvorak AM. 1995b. Caveolae from luminal plasmalemma of rat lung endothelium: Microdomains enriched in caveolin, Ca^{2+}.-ATPase, and inositol trisphosphate receptor. Proc Natl Acad Sci USA 92: 1759-1763.

Schubert W, Frank PG, Razani B, Park DS, Chow CW, et al. 2001. Caveolae-deficient endothelial cells show defects in the uptake and transport of albumin in vivo. J Biol Chem 276: 48619-48622.

Schubert W, Frank PG, Woodman SE, Hyogo H, Cohen DE, et al. 2002. Microvascular hyperpermeability in caveolin-1 -/-. knock-out mice. Treatment with a specific nitric-oxide synthase inhibitor, L-name, restores normal microvascular permeability in Cav-1 null mice. J Biol Chem 277: 40091-40098.

Sharma HS, Dey PK. 1986a. Influence of long-term immobilization stress on regional blood-brain barrier permeability, cerebral blood flow and 5-HT level in conscious normotensive young rats. J Neurol Sci 72: 61-76.

Sharma HS, Dey PK. 1986b. Probable involvement of 5-hydroxytryptamine in increased permeability of blood-brain barrier under heat stress in young rats. Neuropharmacology 25: 161-167.

Shaul PW, Smart EJ, Robinson LJ, German Z, Yuhanna IS, et al. 1996. Acylation targets emdothelial nitric-oxide synthase to plasmalemmal caveolae. J Biol Chem 271: 6518-6522.

Shin JS, Abraham SN. 2001. Cell biology. Caveolae—not just craters in the cellular landscape. Science 293: 1447-1448.

Shivers RR, Harris RJ. 1984. Opening of the blood-brain barrier in Anolis carolinensis. A high voltage electron microscope protein tracer study. Neuropathol Appl Neurobiol 10: 343-356.

Shivers RR, Edmonds CL, Del Maestro RF. 1984. Microvascular permeability in induced astrocytomas and peritumor neuropil of rat brain. A high-voltage electron microscope-protein tracer study. Acta Neuropathol (Berl) 64: 192-202.

Simionescu M, Simionescu N, Palade GE. 1974. Morphometric data on the endothelium of blood capillaries. J Cell Biol 60: 128-152.

Simionescu M, Gafencu A, Antohe F. 2002. Transcytosis of plasma macromolecules in endothelial cells: A cell biological survey. Microsc Res Tech 57: 269-288.

Sirotkin H, Morrow B, Saint-Jore B, Puech A, Das GR, et al. 1997. Identification, characterization, and precise mapping of a human gene encoding a novel membrane-spanning protein from the 22q11 region deleted in velo-cardio-facial syndrome. Genomics 42: 245-251.

Skold M, Cullheim S, Hammarberg H, Piehl F, Suneson A, et al. 2000. Induction of VEGF and VEGF receptors in the spinal cord after mechanical spinal injury and prostaglandin administration. Eur J Neurosci 12: 3675-3686.

Skold MK, von GC, Sandberg-Nordqvist AC, Mathiesen T, Holmin S. 2005. VEGF and VEGF receptor expression after experimental brain contusion in rat. J Neurotrauma 22: 353-367.

Skoog I, Wallin A, Fredman P, Hesse C, Aevarsson O, et al. 1998. A population study on blood-brain barrier function in 85-year-olds: Relation to Alzheimer's disease and vascular dementia. Neurology 50: 966-971.

Smith QR, Rapoport SI. 1986. Cerebrovascular permeability coefficients to sodium, potassium, and chloride. J Neurochem 46: 1732-1742.

Song L, Pachter JS. 2004. Monocyte chemoattractant protein-1 alters expression of tight junction-associated proteins in brain microvascular endothelial cells. Microvasc Res 67: 78-89.

Spisni E, Griffoni C, Santi S, Riccio M, Marulli R, et al. 2001. Colocalization prostacyclin PGI2. synthase–caveolin-1 in endothelial cells and new roles for PGI2 in angiogenesis. Exp Cell Res 266: 31-43.

Stanimirovic D, Satoh K. 2000. Inflammatory mediators of cerebral endothelium: A role in ischemic brain inflammation. Brain Pathol 10: 113-126.

Stan RV. 2002. Structure and function of endothelial caveolae. Microsc Res Tech 57: 350-364.

Stan RV, Ghitescu L, Jacobson BS, Palade GE. 1999. Isolation, cloning, and localization of rat PV-1, a novel endothelial caveolar protein. J Cell Biol 145: 1189-1198.

Stevenson BR, Begg DA. 1994. Concentration-dependent effects of cytochalasin D on tight junctions and actin filaments in MDCK epithelial cells. J Cell Sci 107: 367-375.

Stewart PA. 2000. Endothelial vesicles in the blood-brain barrier: Are they related to permeability? Cell Mol Neurobiol 20: 149-163.

Stratmann A, Risau W, Plate KH. 1998. Cell type-specific expression of angiopoietin-1 and angiopoietin-2 suggests a role in glioblastoma angiogenesis. Am J Pathol 153: 1459-1466.

Stuart RO, Sun A, Panichas M, Hebert SC, Brenner BM, et al. 1994. Critical role for intracellular calcium in tight junction biogenesis. J Cell Physiol 159: 423-433.

Stuart RO, Sun A, Bush KT, Nigam SK. 1996. Dependence of epithelial intercellular junction biogenesis on thapsigargin-sensitive intracellular calcium stores. J Biol Chem 271: 13636-13641.

Szczepanski A, Furie MB, Benach JL, Lane BP, Fleit HB. 1990. Interaction between Borrelia burgdorferi and endothelium in vitro. J Clin Invest 85: 1637-1647.

Teubl M, Groschner K, Kohlwein SD, Mayer B, Schmidt K. 1999. Na+/Ca2+ exchange facilitates Ca^{2+}-dependent activation of endothelial nitric-oxide synthase. J Biol Chem 274: 29529-29535.

Thomas T, Thomas G, McLendon C, Sutton T, Mullan M. 1996. Beta-Amyloid-mediated vasoactivity and vascular endothelial damage. Nature 380: 168-171.

Thurston G, Suri C, Smith K, McClain J, Sato TN, et al. 1999. Leakage-resistant blood vessels in mice transgenically overexpressing angiopoietin-1. Science 286: 2511-2514.

Trojano M, Avolio C, Liuzzi GM, Ruggieri M, Defazio G, et al. 1999. Changes of serum sICAM-1 and MMP-9 induced by rIFNbeta-1b treatment in relapsing-remitting MS. Neurology 53: 1402-1408.

Trout JJ, Koenig H, Goldstone AD, Lu CY. 1986. Blood-brain barrier breakdown by cold injury. Polyamine signals mediate acute stimulation of endocytosis, vesicular transport, and microvillus formation in rat cerebral capillaries. Lab Invest 55: 622-631.

Tsukita S, Furuse M, Itoh M. 2001. Multifunctional strands in tight junctions. Nat Rev Mol Cell Biol 2: 285-293.

Uittenbogaard A, Shaul PW, Yuhanna IS, Blair A, Smart EJ. 2000. High density lipoprotein prevents oxidized low density lipoprotein-induced inhibition of endothelial nitric-oxide synthase localization and activation in caveolae. J Biol Chem 275: 11278-11283.

vanBruggen N, Thibodeaux H, Palmer JT, Lee WP, Fu L, et al. 1999. VEGF antagonism reduces edema formation and tissue damage after ischemia/reperfusion injury in the mouse brain. J Clin Invest 104: 1613-1620.

Vasile E, Simionescu M, Simionescu N. 1983. Visualization of the binding, endocytosis, and transcytosis of low-density lipoprotein in the arterial endothelium in situ. J Cell Biol 96: 1677-1689.

Vorbrodt AW. 1986. Changes in the distribution of endothelial surface glycoconjugates associated with altered permeability of brain micro-blood vessels. Acta Neuropathol (Berl) 70: 103-111.

Vorbrodt AW, Dobrogowska DH. 2003. Molecular anatomy of intercellular junctions in brain endothelial and epithelial barriers: Electron microscopist's view. Brain Res Brain Res Rev 42: 221-242.

Vorbrodt AW, Lossinsky AS, Dobrogowska DH, Wisniewski HM. 1993. Cellular mechanisms of the blood-brain barrier BBB opening to albumin-gold complex. Histol Histopathol 8: 51-61.

Vos CM, Geurts JJ, Montagne L, van Haastert ES, Bö L, van der Valk P, Barkhof F, de Vries HE. 2005. Blood–brain barrier alterations in both focal and diffuse abnormalities on postmortem MRI in multiple sclerosis. Neurobiol Dis 20: 953-960.

Wang W, Dentler WL, Borchardt RT. 2001. VEGF increases BMEC monolayer permeability by affecting occludin expression and tight junction assembly. Am J Physiol Heart Circ Physiol 280: H434-H440.

Washington R, Burton J, Todd RF III, Newman W, Dragovic L, et al. 1994. Expression of immunologically relevant endothelial cell activation antigens on isolated central nervous system microvessels from patients with multiple sclerosis. Ann Neurol 35: 89-97.

Wei EP, Ellison MD, Kontos HA, Povlishock JT. 1986. O2 radicals in arachidonate-induced increased blood-brain barrier permeability to proteins. Am J Physiol 251: H693-H699.

Weindel K, Moringlane JR, Marme D, Weich HA. 1994. Detection and quantification of vascular endothelial growth factor/vascular permeability factor in brain tumor tissue and cyst fluid: The key to angiogenesis? Neurosurgery 35: 439-448.

Wei Y, Yang X, Liu Q, Wilkins JA, Chapman HA. 1999. A role for caveolin and the urokinase receptor in integrin-mediated adhesion and signaling. J Cell Biol 144: 1285-1294.

Westergaard E. 1980. Ultrastructural permeability properties of cerebral microvasculature under normal and experimental conditions after application of tracers. Adv Neurol 28: 55-74.

Westergaard E, Brightman MW. 1973. Transport of proteins across normal cerebral arterioles. J Comp Neurol 152: 17-44.

Wisniewski HM, Lossinsky AS. 1991. Structural and functional aspects of the interaction of inflammatory cells with the blood-brain barrier in experimental brain inflammation. Brain Pathol 1: 89-96.

Wong D, Prameya R, Dorovini-Zis K. 1999. In vitro adhesion and migration of T lymphocytes across monolayers of human brain microvessel endothelial cells: Regulation by ICAM-1, VCAM-1, E-selectin and PECAM-1. J Neuropathol Exp Neurol 58: 138-152.

Wong D, Dorovini-Zis K, Vincent SR. 2004. Cytokines, nitric oxide, and cGMP modulate the permeability of an in vitro model of the human blood-brain barrier. Exp Neurol 190: 446-455.

Yong VW, Power C, Forsyth P, Edwards DR. 2001. Metalloproteinases in biology and pathology of the nervous system. Nat Rev Neurosci 2: 502-511.

Yuhanna IS, Zhu Y, Cox BE, Hahner LD, Osborne-Lawrence S, et al. 2001. High-density lipoprotein binding to scavenger receptor-BI activates endothelial nitric oxide synthase. Nat Med 7: 853-857.

Zagzag D, Hooper A, Friedlander DR, Chan W, Holash J, et al. 1999. In situ expression of angiopoietins in astrocytomas identifies angiopoietin-2 as an early marker of tumor angiogenesis. Exp Neurol 159: 391-400.

Zhang W, Smith C, Howlett C, Stanimirovic D. 2000a. Inflammatory activation of human brain endothelial cells by hypoxic astrocytes in vitro is mediated by IL-1beta. J Cereb Blood Flow Metab 20: 967-978.

Zhang Z, Chopp M. 2002. Vascular endothelial growth factor and angiopoietins in focal cerebral ischemia. Trends Cardiovasc Med 12: 62-66.

Zhang ZG, Zhang L, Jiang Q, Zhang RL, Davies K, et al. 2000b. VEGF enhances angiogenesis and promotes blood-brain barrier leakage in the ischemic brain. J Clin Invest 106: 829-838.

Zhang ZG, Zhang L, Croll SD, Chopp M. 2002. Angiopoietin-1 reduces cerebral blood vessel leakage and ischemic lesion volume after focal cerebral embolic ischemia in mice. Neuroscience 113: 683-687.

Zlokovic BV. 2005. Neurovascular mechanisms of Alzheimer's neurodegeneration. Trends Neurosci 28: 202-208.

4 Pathology of the Blood–Brain Barrier

S. Rooker · J. Verlooy

Abstract: It is known that the blood–brain barrier (BBB) plays an important role in the pathophysiology of central nervous system (CNS) disorders. Experimental models of CNS injury based on destabilization of the BBB might therefore be of benefit to understand the pathophysiology of increased intracranial hypertension and allow the exploration of new therapeutic measures. Especially for complex pathologies, such as stroke and neurotrauma, it is highly important that the experimental models as much as possible mimic the pathogenesis and that drugs are delivered at the right time and the right place. Thereby it is not sufficient to counteract solely the endpoint of a traumatic or ischemic process, i.e., irreversible neuronal cell death, but also to interfere with changes in other brain constituents, e.g., the glial and endothelial compartments. Both are structural components of the BBB and play a key role in the development of secondary phenomena as edema formation. The course and structural aspects of edema formation will be discussed based on experience with several animal models of brain ischemia and trauma.

It is concluded that stroke and trauma therapy is not only a matter of neurons and that acute treatment should focus on prevention of brain swelling.

List of Abbreviations: BBB, Blood–brain barrier; CBF, Cerebral blood flow; CHI, Closed head injury; CNS, Central nervous System; ICP, Intra cranial pressure; IL, Interleukine; iNOS, inducible nitric oxide synthase; TNF-α, Tumor necrosis factor-α

1   Introduction

Experimental research in appropriate animal models is required to build knowledge on the complex cascades, which are activated in most disorders of the central nervous system (CNS). Only then can pharmacotherapy be successful to synthesize potent molecular entities to fulfill particular clinical needs. As most clinical disease processes are rather complex, rigorous characterization of pathogenesis, safety, and efficacy in appropriate animal models is also required. For many years now we have been looking into the complex processes, which are activated after traumatic head injury and stroke (Van Reempts et al., 1990, 1994, 2000; Verlooy et al., 1993; Engelborghs et al., 1998, 2000; Rooker et al., 2002, 2003a, b; De Visscher et al., 2005). Although stroke and head injury represent different disease modalities in clinical practice, the specific underlying morphological mechanisms revealed a strong similarity in the neurodegenerative processes, especially with regard to dynamic progression and endpoint parameters. Edema formation is one of the secondary phenomena after trauma and stroke and will lead to neuronal death. Therefore, the treatment strategies should not only focus on protection of neurons but also counteract these secondary phenomena appearing in the subacute phase. Thereby the integrity of the blood–brain barrier (BBB) may play a key role, not only with respect to drug access to critical areas but also in the regulation of uncontrolled swelling of brain tissue.

2   Characterization of Edema

Edema formation leads to worse outcome in clinical practice and has been classified as cytotoxic (or cellular) and vasogenic, depending on whether vascular permeability is increased (Klatzo, 1967). When the BBB is intact, edema will be derived from the blood moving across the BBB without proteins, in a state where the BBB is disrupted these proteins cannot be excluded. Therefore, in fact all edema is vasogenic and the terms "intact barrier" and "open barrier" edema have been proposed (Betz et al., 1989). The multifactorial response of different brain constituents on ischemic or traumatic aggression is rather unpredictable. Although the initial trigger in both diseases is not the same, the progression of destructive cascades leading to neuronal death is in fact the same. As such BBB damage, brain swelling, and ultimate pannecrotic infarction may occur in neurotrauma as well as in stroke (❷ *Figure 4-1*). Edema has to be regarded as a progressively developing secondary symptom originating at the level of the BBB, and not as a disease. Vascular endothelium, the basement membrane, and an almost continuous layer of astrocytic endfeet compose the BBB. Extravasation of plasma proteins may increase in conditions where there is instability of

☐ Figure 4-1
Pathogenesis of cerebral edema and neuronal cell death after traumatic and ischemic challenge

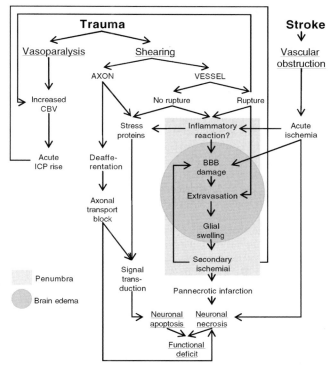

endothelial tight junctions, upregulation of pinocytic vesicles in the endothelial membrane, or destabilization of the basal membrane. Astrocytes play an important role in maintaining the cerebral water balance, probably regulated by aquaporins that are abundantly expressed at the level of the BBB, in particular, the astrocytic endfeet located around blood vessels (Manley et al., 2000). Astrocytes, however, have several additional roles in response to injury, e.g., remodeling the extracellular matrix for wound healing, regulation of immunity, and inflammation by cytokine secretion, promoting neuronal survival by secretion of neurotrophic factors, mobilization of excitotoxic amino acids by secretion of transporter molecules, and protection against neuronal cell death by activation of the antioxidant pathway (Eddleston and Mucke, 1993). Hence, preservation of astrocytic function can be regarded as a prerequisite for ultimate neuronal survival.

3   Edema in Experimental Models

3.1 Edema After Experimental Closed Head Injury

During the past years, a rat model of closed head injury (CHI) has been developed that features several clinically relevant pathological changes, including increased intra cranial pressure (ICP) (Engelborghs et al., 1997, 1998; De Mulder et al., 1999; Rooker et al., 2002), disturbed autoregulation of cerebral blood flow (CBF) (Engelborghs et al., 2000), and increased sensitivity to hypoxia (van Rossem et al., 1999a, b). Recent morphological mapping of injury in different brain areas revealed that the piriform cortex, located remote from the primary impact place at the base of the cranium, is selectively vulnerable in this model of diffuse trauma. Furthermore, there is a rapid upregulation of proinflammatory cytokines and inducible nitric oxide (iNOS) within hours after injury, which extends from the primary injury site to the piriform cortex as a remote site undergoing delayed neurodegeneration. Secondary to trauma, inflammatory processes evolve and are likely to play a major role in the evolution of brain damage. Cytokines are involved in basic neurobiological processes in the injured brain and might provide a target for pharmacological intervention (Gillen et al., 1998; Barone and Feuerstein, 1999). Proinflammatory cytokines, such as tumor necrosis factor-α (TNF-α) and interleukin (IL)-1β, regulate the interaction of immune and inflammatory cells, thereby orchestrating the immune response (Stoll et al., 1998). Moreover, cytokines directly act on neurons and may, therefore, mediate important neurotoxic as well as protective effects (Arai et al., 1990; Hariri et al., 1994; Toulmond and Rothwell, 1995; Merril and Beneviste, 1996; Shohami et al., 1996). iNOS has been implicated as a critical downstream mediator of cytokine-induced neurotoxicity (Hewett et al., 1994). The balance between neurotoxic and protective cytokine effects may be largely determined by the time window, site and dosage of their expression, or exogenous administration both in vitro and in vivo (Jander et al., 2001).

Edema formation after head injury may lead to pannecrotic degeneration. Extreme swelling in the rigid skull can exert mechanical damage due to displacement of brain tissue. In addition, blood flow may become compromised due to increased intracranial pressure (De Visscher et al., 2005), leading to metabolic injury. Edema formation is not necessarily caused by edema alone but may result from acute vasoparalysis and impaired autoregulation (Engelborghs et al., 1998). Thereby the stability of the BBB may be compromised by an increase of transmural pressure and a blockade of venous outflow. Mechanical rupture of the BBB, one of the primary effects of head injury, may induce continuous extravasation or even severe intraparenchymatous hemorrhage (❷ *Figure 4-2*). As in stroke, this induces progressive cellular swelling until flow ultimately ceases and pannecrotic infarction develops. Surrounding this core of necrosis a penumbra develops, this area is not beyond salvation and treatment should focus on rescuing this area (❷ *Figure 4-2d*). The penumbra around the hemorrhagic core shows characteristics of an ischemic penumbra (Van Reempts et al., 2000).

3.2 Edema After Experimental Stroke

In conditions of stroke, tissue swelling is located mainly in the penumbra region, where destabilization of the BBB may lead to extravasation and progressive cellular edema (Welch et al., 1997; Van Reempts et al., 2000). From functional or clinical point of view, the penumbra can be considered as the area at risk for the patient and the area of hope for therapy, since changes detected in this region are largely reversible. Functional deficit and neuronal loss are mainly dependent on duration of ischemia and amount of residual flow (circulatory window) and on the reaction of neurons and their immediate environment (cellular window). Two important cellular aspects deserve attention: selective neuronal necrosis versus pannecrotic infarction and open BBB versus intact BBB.

After a short episode of moderate ischemia (e.g., two-vessel occlusion), the BBB remains intact, edema is absent, and selective neuronal necrosis develops with a considerable delay. After a long episode of severe ischemia, on the other hand (e.g., middle cerebral artery occlusion), the BBB is damaged, leading to extravasation, uncontrolled swelling of astrocytic endfeet, and spongious pannecrotic infarction within a few hours. Another possible model to investigate the role of BBB destabilization in neuronal death is the use of fatty acids. In our laboratory, we injected ultrasound contrast agents which induced lacunar zones of edema formation as soon as 90 min after intracarotid injection in the ipsilateral hemisphere (❷ *Figure 4-3*). These observations could be useful to amplify vasogenic edema in other experimental models (Rooker et al., 2003a, b).

Neurons initially may remain structurally intact, but depending on tissue pH, degree of hyperexcitation, or lack of preconditioning stress, their dendrites can start swelling, thereby sparing the axons. The structural picture in such regions is very typical, i.e., perivascular astrocytes are severely dilated and induce compression of small blood vessels (❷ *Figure 4-3d*). From these pictures, it is evident that microcirculation is considerably hampered. On the one hand, mechanical compression of microvessels should be beneficial

◻ Figure 4-2

(a) Unstained 50-μm vibratome section at the site of impact (*bregma*) showing hemorrhages (*arrow*) surrounded by an extended area of gold tracer extravasation (*asterisk*). (b) Same section as ❷ *Figure 4-1*, viewed by epipolarization to show absence of tracer in the region of mechanically ruptured blood vessels (*arrow*). (c) Vibratome section, adjacent to the one in ❷ *Figure 4-1*, stained with Azure–Eosin to show the morphological aspect of hemorrhages (*arrow*) and the apparently normal surrounding tissue (*asterisk*). (d) Toluidine blue-stained 2-μm epon section to show presence of infarction in areas of extravasation. Compressed blood vessels (*arrow*) and dense stained irreversibly damaged neurons (*arrowhead*) are surrounded by swollen astrocytes (*asterisk*)

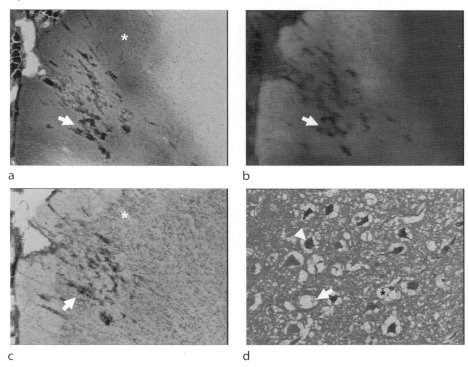

since supply of edema substrate is reduced. Otherwise, in case of preexisting ischemia, oxygen supply will be further reduced resulting in more BBB leaks, increased astrocytic swelling and concomitant dendritic swelling until complete necrosis of all tissue elements takes place.

4 Brain Protection

The majority of pharmacotherapeutic studies focus on neuroprotection. Undoubtedly, prevention of neurodegeneration or restoring of neuronal function must be the main goal of every treatment. However, it is questionable if this can be achieved simply by administering drugs that in vitro have proven to protect neurons from necrotic or apoptotic cell death. In situations of moderate trauma or moderate ischemia of short duration, only neurons will die and this occurs with a certain delay. Neuroprotective agents are the best choice, provided they reach the compromised territory, which is not evident in a situation where the BBB remained intact. Severe trauma with hemorrhage or severe prolonged ischemia, on the other hand, requires another approach. In the acute phase, when the barrier is still open, drugs

■ Figure 4-3

(a) Within 90 min after intracarotid Optison® and i.v. injection of Evans blue tracer unilateral extravasation can be detected macroscopical. (b) Microscopic observation of 50-μm vibratome sections showed that extravasation coincides with multiple lacunar zones of vasogenic edema (*arrows*). (c) In these regions of extravasation (*asterisk*) neurons appear slightly coagulated (*arrowhead*). In the contralateral hemisphere, these effects are absent. (d) Electron micrograph of cerebral microvessel (V) compressed by two swollen astrocytic endfeet (*asterisk*) in the penumbra area 4 h after photochemical ischemic challenge of rat parietal cortex

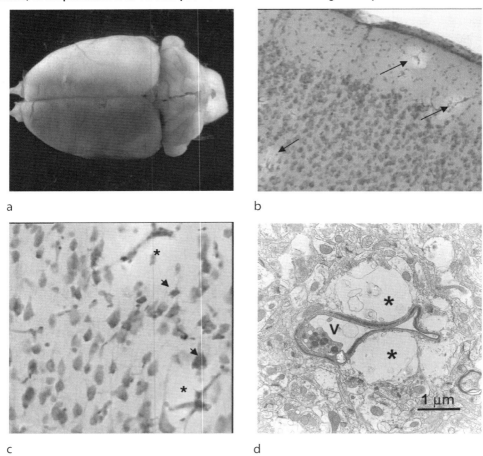

a

b

c

d

have the best chance to arrive at the challenged site. They must primarily counteract extreme cellular swelling by sealing the BBB leaks and/or by regulating astrocytic water transporting systems to finally guarantee sufficient oxygenation. Subsequently, in the subacute phase neuroprotection deserves attention (❯ *Figure 4-4*).

5   Conclusions

The search for cerebroprotective drugs in stroke and neurotrauma till present has not been very successful. So far, there has not been a dramatic improvement of outcome measure such as survival or Glascow outcome scale after trauma. Not only is the pathogenesis extremely complex and far from understanding

◘ Figure 4-4

Dynamic progression and time window for treatment of brain lesions after ischemia or trauma dependent on integrity of the BBB

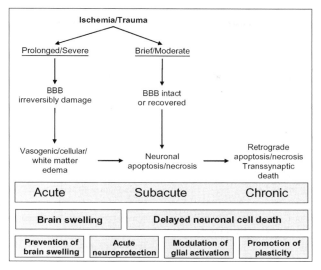

but also pharmacological research has been too much focused exclusively on neuroprotection over the years. A lot of knowledge has been gathered about molecular and cellular processes, and desired action mechanisms for new drugs have been limited to those that play a role in rescue of neurons. However, neurons are not the only actors when the brain is compromised. Their survival also depends on the reactivity of their immediate environment. There is sufficient evidence that a major function of microglial cells and astrocytes, respectively, is modulation of inflammatory response and maintenance of an optimal water balance. Therefore, also the role of microglia and astrocytes in the pathological cascade after stroke and trauma should be investigated. Modulation of these cells could promote neuronal survival without direct action of the pharmacotherapy at the level of neurons. Cellular edema is the very first visible morphological feature after ischemic or traumatic insult. Neurons die with a considerable delay. The BBB, which is situated in between the vascular compartment of fluid supply and the cellular compartment of fluid accumulation, may therefore be considered as a valid target for stroke and trauma therapy. Moreover, temporal destabilization of this barrier can be beneficial because it may allow supply of larger molecular entities in the compromised region. Nowadays, direct actions are undertaken at the site of an accident to prevent brain ischemia using the Advanced Trauma Life Support system. Unraveling the timely progression of pathological events, in the different cellular constituents, is a prerequisite for future pharmacotherapeutic research.

Ideally, there will be one drug or a cocktail of drugs to be given at the site of an accident which influences the pathological cascades, directing them to a situation where neuronal loss will be minimal.

References

Arai K, Lee F, Miyajima A, Arai N, Yokota T. 1990. Cytokines: Coordinators of immune and inflammatory responses. Annu Rev Biochem 59: 783-836.

Barone FC, Feuerstein GZ. 1999. Inflammatory mediators and stroke: New opportunities for novel therapeutics. J Cereb Blood Flow Metab 19: 819-834.

Betz AL, Iannotti F, Hoff JT. 1989. Brain edema: A classification based on blood-brain barrier integrity. Cerebrovasc Brain Metab Rev 1: 133-154.

De Mulder G, van Rossem K, Van Reempts J, Borgers M, Verlooy J. 2000. Validation of a closed head injury model for use in long-term studies. Acta Neurochir Suppl 76: 409-413.

De Visscher G, Rooker S, Jorens PG, Verlooy J, Borgers M, et al. 2005. Pentobarbital fails to reduce cerebral oxygen consumption early after non-hemorrhagic closed head injury in rats. J Neurotrauma 22 (7): 793-806.

Eddleston M, Mucke L. 1993. Molecular profile of reactive astrocytes—implications for their role in neurological disease. Neuroscience 54: 15-36.

Engelborghs K, Haseldonckx M, Van Reempts J, van Rossem K, Wouters L, et al. 2000. Impaired autoregulation of cerebral blood flow in an experimental model of traumatic brain injury. J Neurotrauma 18 (8): 667-677.

Engelborghs K, Verlooy J, Van Deuren B, Van Reempts J, Borgers M. 1997. Intracranial pressure in a modified experimental model of closed head injury. Acta Neurochir Suppl 70: 123-125.

Engelborghs K, Verlooy J, Van Reempts J, Van Deuren B, Van de Ven M, et al. 1998. Temporal changes in intracranial pressure in a modified experimental model of closed head injury. J Neurosurg 89 (5): 796-806.

Gillen C, Jander S, Stoll G. 1998. Sequential expression of mRNA for proinflammatory cytokines and interleukin-10 in the rat peripheral nervous system: Comparison between immune-mediated demyelination and Wallerian degeneration. J Neurosci Res 51: 489-496.

Hariri RJ, Chang VA, Barie PS, Wang RS, Sharif SF, et al. 1994. Traumatic injury induces interleukine-6 production by human astrocyts. Brain Res 636: 139-142.

Hewett SJ, Csernansky CA, Choi DW. 1994. Selection potentiation of NMDA-induced neuronal injury following induction of astrocytic iNOS. Neuron 13: 487-494.

Jander S, Schroeter M, Peters O, Witte OW, Stoll G. 2001. Cortical spreading depression induces proinflammatory cytokine gene expression in the rat brain. J Cerb Blood Flow Metab 21: 218-225.

Klatzo I. 1967. Neuropathological aspects of brain edema. J Neuropathol Exp Neurol 26: 1-14.

Manley JT, Fujimura M, Ma T, Noshita N, Filiz F, et al. 2000. Aquaporin-4 deletion in mice reduces brain edema after acute water intoxication and ischemic stroke. Nat Med 6: 159-163.

Merril JE, Beneviste EN. 1996. Cytokines in inflammatory brain lesions: Helpful and harmful. Trends Neurosci 19: 331-336.

Rooker S, De Visscher G, Van Deuren B, Borgers M, Jorens PG, et al. 2002. Comparison of intracranial pressure measured in the cerebral cortex and the cerebellum of the rat. J Neurosci Methods 119: 83-88.

Rooker S, Jorens PG, Van Reempts J, Borgers M, Verlooy J. 2003b. Continuous measurement of intracranial pressure in awake rats after experimental closed head injury. J Neurosci Methods 131: 75-81.

Rooker S, Van Reempts J, Van Deuren B, Borgers M, Jorens PG, et al. 2003a. Ultrasound agents may open the blood-brain barrier in rats and aggravate pathologic consequences of experimental head trauma. Neuropathology 23 (3): 210-213.

Shohami E, Bass R, Wallach D, Yamin A, Gallily R. 1996. Inhibition of tumor necrosis factor (TNF-α) activity in rat brain is associated with cerebroprotection after closed head injury. J Cereb Blood Flow Metab 16 (3): 378-384.

Stoll G, Jander S, Schroeter M. 1998. Inflammation and glial responses in ischemic brain lesions. Prog Neurobiol 56: 149-171.

Toulmond S, Rothwell NJ. 1995. Interleukin-1 receptor antagonist inhibits neuronal damage caused by fluid percussion injury in the rat. Brain Res 671: 261-266.

Van Reempts J, Borgers M. 1990. Structural damage in experimental cerebral ischemia. Cerebral Ischemia and Resuscitation. Schurr A, Rigor BM, editors. Boca Raton: CRC Press; pp. 235-257.

Van Reempts J, Borgers M. 1994. Histopathological characterization of photochemical damage in nervous tissue. Histol Histopathol 9: 185-195.

Van Reempts J, Borgers M. 2000. Animal models of stroke: Compromise between consistency and clinical relevance? Neurosci Res Commun 26: 161-172.

van Rossem K, Garcia-Martinez S, De Mulder G, Engelborghs K, Van Reempts J, et al. 1999a. Brain oxygenation after experimental closed head injury. Adv Exp Med Biol 471: 209-215.

van Rossem K, Garcia-Martinez S, Wouters L, De Mulder G, Van Deuren B, et al. 1999b. Cytochrome oxidase redox state in brain is more sensitive to hypoxia after closed head injury: A near-infrared spectroscopy (NIRS) study. J Cereb Blood Flow Metab 19 (Suppl. 1): S391.

Verlooy J, Van Reempts J, Peersman G. 1993. Photochemicallyinduced cerebral infarction in the rat: Comparison of NMR imaging and histologic changes. Acta Neurochir (Wien) 122: 250-256.

Welch KMA, Caplan LR, Reis DJ, Siesjö BK, Weir B. 1997. Primer on cerebrovascular diseases. San Diego: Academic Press.

5 Functional Imaging of P-glycoprotein in the Blood–Brain Barrier with PET: State of the Art

N. H. Hendrikse · G. Luurtsema · B. N. M. van Berckel · E. J. F. Franssen · A. A. Lammertsma

Abstract: The blood–brain barrier (BBB) is the main barrier between blood and brain. Its purpose is to maintain homeostasis in and protection of the central nervous system. Therefore, under normal physiological conditions, the BBB is impermeable for endotoxins, but also for exotoxins like drugs.

In the endothelial cells of the BBB, different active influx, but also active drug efflux transporters are presents. An example of drug efflux pumps is P-glycoprotein (P-gp) drug efflux pumps, which are encoded by MDR1 genes in humans.

A different P-gp expression in the blood-brain barrier can play a role in the aetiology of several brain disorders. For this reason, there is a need to develop an assay for the quantification P-gp functionality in the BBB.

We discuss, the relationship of P-gp and brain pathology and the involvement of age in loss of P-gp function.

Furthermore, drugs treatment of brain diseases like Alzheimers's disease and Parkinson's disease are often not effective. Therefore, we discuss the relationship between P-gp and drug availability.

In this chapter, an overview is given in the use of positron emission tomography as a tool for measuring P-gp function in the area of neurology, neurophysiology and pharmacology.

List of Abbreviations: Aβ, beta-amyloid; AD, alzheimer's disease; ATP, adenosine triphospate; BBB, blood–brain barrier; CNS, central nervous system; CsA, cyclosporine A; 4V, fourth ventricle; LV, lateral ventricle; MRI, magnetic resonance image; MRP, multidrug resistance-associated protein; NC, nasal cavity; PET, positron emission tomography; PD, parkinson's disease; P-gp, P-glycoprotein; PIT, pituitary; SUV, standard uptake value; V_d, volume of distribution; WT, wild-type

1   Introduction

1.1 P-glycoprotein and the Blood–Brain Barrier

The blood–brain barrier (BBB) is the main barrier between blood and brain. Its purpose is to maintain homeostasis in the central nervous system (CNS). Furthermore, it protects the CNS from endo- and exogenous toxins that are circulating in blood (Gloor et al., 2001; de Lange and Danhof, 2002).

The BBB consists of a monolayer of brain capillary endothelial cells, joined together by tight junctions. Under normal physiological conditions the BBB is almost impermeable. Only small lipophilic compounds can enter the brain by passive diffusion via the cell membrane. In addition, very small hydrophilic molecules can penetrate the brain via tight junctions between the cells (Pardridge, 1998). All other molecules have to pass the BBB via active transport systems. In the endothelial cells that line the brain capillary, different active influx and efflux transporters have been identified. The most important influx transporters are hexose, amino acid, and monocarboxylic acid transporters (Tsuji and Tamai, 1999). In addition, efflux transporters, such as P-glycoprotein (P-gp) and multidrug resistance-associated proteins (MRP), exist (Taylor, 2002). The estimated total length of brain capillaries in humans is approximately 640 km with a total surface area of 9.3 m². The brain capillaries are separated from each other by a distance of approximately 40 μm (Reese and Karnovsky, 1967) (❷ *Figure 5-1*). In the late 1980s, expression of P-gp in the endothelial cells of the BBB was demonstrated (Cordon-Cardo et al., 1989). Most likely, the physiological role of P-gp in the BBB is to protect the brain from uptake of a variety of harmful and toxic compounds that circulate in the blood (Schinkel, 1999).

P-gp is present at the blood side of the brain capillary endothelial cells. A lipophilic compound is able to penetrate across the lipid bilayer. When the compound is a transport substrate for P-gp, it will immediately be pumped out of the brain into the blood. Because P-gp is an ATP dependent efflux pump, ATP energy is required for substrate transport (Eytan and Kuchel, 1999). For a schematic presentation of P-gp, see ❷ *Figure 5-2*.

1.2 Functional P-gp Measurements with PET

Positron emission tomography (PET), a noninvasive quantitative imaging technique, can provide information about physiological and pharmacokinetic processes in vivo. These processes can be measured

☐ Figure 5-1

A representation of the human brain microvasculature. The estimated total length of brain capillaries in the human head is approximately 640 km with a total surface area of 9.3 m². The brain capillaries are separated from each other by a distance of approximately 40 μm

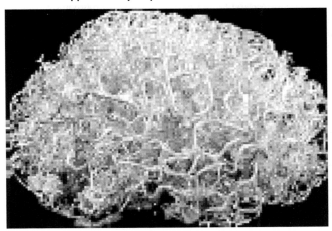

☐ Figure 5-2

A schematic representation of the efflux function of P-gp in endothelial cells

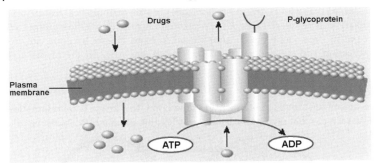

by intravenous injection of a radiotracer labeled with a positron emitter such as ^{15}O ($t_{1/2} = 2$ min), ^{13}N ($t_{1/2} = 10$ min), ^{11}C ($t_{1/2} = 20$ min), and ^{18}F ($t_{1/2} = 110$ min).

PET has proven to be an important tool in the noninvasive diagnosis of human diseases (Lewis et al., 1994; Anderson and Price, 2000). In addition, as it measures function, it can also provide information about effectiveness of therapy (Lammertsma, 2004).

For quantification of functional P-gp in the BBB, the volume of distribution (V_d) of verapamil is a robust parameter. V_d is independent of interindividual differences in tracer bioavailability and cerebral blood flow.

Previously, V_d as determined by Logan graphical analysis (Kortekaas et al., 2005) and the ratio of areas under the tissue and plasma curves (Sasongko et al., 2005) have been used as measures for P-gp mediated transport of verapamil.

Recently, a mathematical model was developed that best describes tracer kinetics for quantification of BBB P-gp (Lubberink et al., 2005).

1.3 P-gp and Brain Pathology

Neurodegenerative brain disorders, such as Alzheimer's disease (AD) and Parkinson's disease (PD), have great impact on patient, family, health care system, and society. The causes of these diseases are largely unknown, although genetic susceptibility and exposure to neurotoxins have been proposed as potential contributors toward brain tissue malfunction and neuronal cell loss (Langston, 2002). Gradual loss of the integrity of the BBB has also been postulated to be a factor in the development of these diseases. Furthermore, it could be hypothesized that the BBB function deteriorates with age and that based on genetic susceptibility individuals may show loss of specific BBB transport functions such as P-gp function. This may allow the entry of neurotoxic substances into the brain. Subsequently, these substances may accumulate to such an extent that they result in neuronal damage.

In a study in a group of PD patients, the entry of neurotoxic compounds was investigated (Drozdzik et al., 2003). Many pesticides from different chemical classes are neurotoxic and can be transported by human P-gp (Bain and LeBlanc, 1996). As not everyone who is exposed to pesticides develops PD, the possible link between environmental and genetic factors was studied. No significant association between patients with PD and polymorphism was found (Furuno et al., 2002). Nevertheless, it was found that the homozygous T3435T genotype, previously associated with a relatively lower P-gp activity, had the highest frequency in the early-onset PD group. Furthermore, in a recent PET study decreased P-gp function in the midbrain in patients with PD was observed. In this study, it was hypothesized that in patients with PD P-gp function in the BBB was reduced. (R,S)-[^{11}C]verapamil which is normally extruded from the brain by P-gp was used to study P-gp function in Parkinson patients and healthy volunteers as a control group. A significant elevated uptake of (R,S)-[^{11}C]verapamil (18%) in the midbrain of PD patients was measured relative to controls (❷ *Figures 5-3* and ❷ *5-4*). This study supports the hypotheses that P-gp dysfunction plays a role in the pathogenesis of PD (Kortekaas et al., 2005).

More evidence for the importance of P-gp in the BBB was found in a study with patients in AD, in whom the deposition of β-amyloid (Aβ) in senile plaques is a key pathological feature (Hardy and Selkoe, 2002; Mattson, 2004). It is of interest that Aβ is a substrate for the P-gp efflux pump (Selkoe, 1999; Lam et al., 2001). In postmortem brain tissue samples, taken from elderly humans, an inverse correlation between P-gp expression and the deposition of both Aβ40 and Aβ42 in the medial temporal lobe was

❏ **Figure 5-3**
Uptake of [^{11}C]verapamil (distribution volume [V_d]) in the brain. This image is representative for all subjects, irrespective of disease. n.c., nasal cavity; L.V., lateral ventricle; pit, pituitary; 4V, fourth ventricle

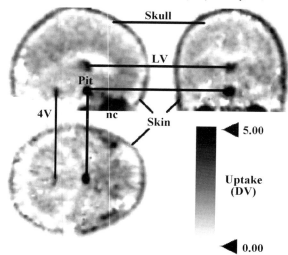

□ Figure 5-4

Individual values of [^{11}C]verapamil uptake in the midbrain. The controls had similar uptake as in the rest of the brain (mean, 102% of the individual brain average), whereas the Parkinson's disease patients showed 18% increase of [^{11}C]verapamil in the midbrain

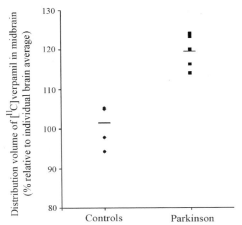

found (Vogelgesang et al., 2002). This indicates a possible protective role of P-gp in the development of amyloid plaques.

Furthermore, in a recent study, labeled ^{125}I-amyloid peptides (Aβ40 and Aβ42) were evaluated in P-gp knockout mice and results were compared with those obtained in wild-type (WT) mice (Cirrito et al., 2005). The investigators showed that, after microinjection of [^{125}I]Aβ40 and [^{125}I]Aβ42 into the CNS, clearance of these amyloid peptides from the brain in P-gp knockout mice was at half the rate as that measured in WT mice. These data establish a direct link between P-gp and Aβ metabolism in vivo and suggest that P-gp activity at the BBB could affect risk for developing AD.

1.4 P-gp, BBB, and Age

The etiology of neurodegenerative diseases like PD is not yet clear. However, it is known that several multifactor events play a role. This may include environmental factors, such as exposure to exogenous toxins like pesticides, genetic factors (Langston, 2002; Di Monte, 2003), and the effect of aging. PD is an age-related neurodegenerative disorder and has a mean age at onset of 55 years. PD affects 2% of the population over the age of 65 years (Corti et al., 2005). It can be hypothesized that due to aging, the BBB loses its protective function and therefore aging could actually be a risk factor for the development of neurological diseases. It is speculated that gradual loss of the integrity of the BBB with age may occur. Consequently, during aging, the human brain may (partly) lose specific transport mechanism in the BBB such as P-gp function. However, in vivo data on age-related changes in P-gp function in the BBB are limited. Therefore, the role of aging on P-gp function in the BBB healthy volunteers was investigated (Toornvliet et al., 2006).

In previous studies, a racemic mixture of (R)- and (S)-[^{11}C]verapamil has been used to assess P-gp function. Due to differences in hepatic metabolism, plasma protein binding and plasma clearance, however, their tissue uptake may be different. Since the difference in plasma and tissue kinetics of a racemic mixture of both enantiomers cannot by separated by radioactivity measurements, use of a selective enantiomer as tracer is a requirement for quantitative measurements. Therefore, enantiomeric pure (R)-[^{11}C]verapamil was developed and it was demonstrated that (R)-[^{11}C]verapamil was superior to (S)-[^{11}C]verapamil for assessing P-gp function (Luurtsema et al., 2003).

The relationship between the volume of distribution of (R)-$[^{11}C]$verapamil in brain and P-gp activity in lymphocytes of healthy volunteers was investigated. The present study is one of the first describing the use of the new radiotracer (R)-$[^{11}C]$verapamil in vivo. Significant differences were found between V_d of young (mean age of 25 ± 2.3 years) and elderly volunteers (mean age of 61 ± 3.6 years). Mean V_d of (R)-$[^{11}C]$ verapamil for young and elderly volunteers was 0.62 ± 0.10 and 0.73 ± 0.07, respectively ($p = 0.03$). Individual results are shown in ❷ *Figure 5-5*.

◻ **Figure 5-5**
V_d of (R)-$[^{11}C]$verapamil in young and elderly volunteers as function of age

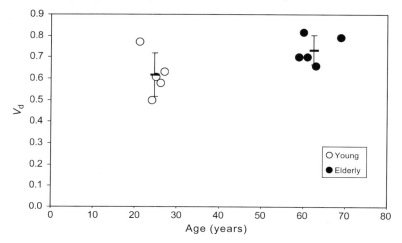

These in vivo results were confirmed with the in vitro data. A significant effect was found in P-gp activity of CD3 positive lymphocytes. The activity index was 2.88 ± 0.77 and 1.76 ± 0.58 in young and elderly volunteers ($p = 0.02$), respectively.

1.5 P-gp and Drug Availability

Often, the administration of drugs for the treatment of diseases of the CNS is not effective. One possible reason for this is that an insufficient amount of drug enters the brain, due to BBB restrictions. Most drugs, however, are lipophilic and can enter the brain by passive diffusion. Despite their lipophilicity, administration of various drugs results in relatively low brain concentrations because they are substrates for efflux transporters such as P-gp. It is clear that this effect leads to ineffective treatment with these drugs (Schinkel et al., 1996; Fellner et al., 2002; Marchi et al., 2004). Some examples of drugs that are subject to P-gp-mediated efflux at the BBB are antidepressants (amitriptyline, nortriptyline) (Roberts et al., 2002; Uhr et al., 2002), chemotherapeutics (paclitaxel, vinblastine) (Schinkel et al., 1994; Rice et al., 2003), and steroids (aldosterone, cortisole, and progesterone) (Uhr et al., 2002). Higher brain uptake of these compounds with affinity for P-gp can be achieved by coadministration of another P-gp substrate or a P-gp inhibitor, so called modulators. For example, in a study in rats pretreated with the P-gp inhibitor cyclosporine A, a higher concentration of nortriptyline in brain tissue was found (Ejsing and Linnet, 2005).

In a recent study in human volunteers, (R,S)-$[^{11}C]$verapamil was administrated after a 1-h infusion of cyclosporine A to investigate the inhibition of P-gp in the BBB (❷ *Figure 5-6*). The brain-to-plasma ratio

□ Figure 5-6

Positron emission tomography images of a normal human brain after [^{11}C]verapamil administration in the absence or presence of cyclosporine (CsA) indicate increased regional uptake (green to red areas) of ^{11}C-radioactivity in the brain in the presence of CsA. Images shown are in standardized uptake value (SUV) summed over a period from 5 to 25 min p.i. SUV is an index of regional radioactivity uptake normalized to the administered dose and weight of the subject. MRI, magnetic resonance image

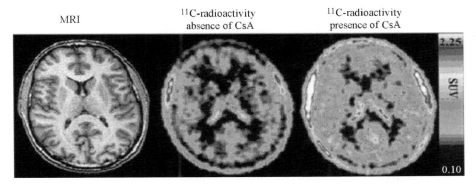

MRI ^{11}C-radioactivity absence of CsA ^{11}C-radioactivity presence of CsA

of the (R,S)-[^{11}C]verapamil activity increased by 88%, demonstrating that inhibition of human functional P-gp by cyclosporine A can be measured with PET (Sasongko et al., 2005).

Furthermore, in a PET study in lung transplant recipients who were treated with cyclosporine A and tacrolimus, both substrates for P-gp, increased brain uptake of (R,S)-[^{11}C]verapamil was shown. This study confirmed that P-gp in the brain plays a role in drug availability in patients. It was concluded that (R,S)-[^{11}C]verapamil and PET could be of value in the improvement of drug delivery to the brain (Bart, 2003).

Moreover, [^{11}C]verapamil has been evaluated in nonhuman primates to study the uptake of [^{11}C] verapamil under control and inhibition conditions. The potent P-gp inhibitor PSC833 caused a significant 4.62-fold increase in brain uptake. These results also confirmed that PET measurement using [^{11}C] verapamil can be used for evaluating P-gp function in the brain (Lee et al., 2005).

2 Conclusion and Perspectives

An overview is given demonstrating that a noninvasive in vivo tool for measuring functional P-gp in the blood–brain barrier can be used in clinical research in the area of neurology, psychiatry, neurophysiology, and pharmacology. PET may be useful in clinical settings to gain more insight in the physiological role of P-gp in various diseases or pathophysiological processes as illustrated in this review. However, more than 48 transporters from the ATP-binding cassette family contribute to transmembrane transport, whereas several of these transporters are expressed in the BBB. Inhibition of only a small number of these transporter types may have only limited effect on drug delivery to the brain. Therefore, further PET studies on the physiological role and clinical relevance of P-gp and other drug transporters in drug delivery to the brain are needed. Insight in the function of these transporters may potentially lead to possibilities for increasing drug delivery to sanctuary sites such as the brain. This, in turn, may result in more optimized drug treatment regimes of brain diseases. In addition, insight in drug transport function in vivo may provide knowledge that could lead to strategies for protecting the brain against toxic side effects of harmful agents.

References

Anderson H, Price P. 2000. What does positron emission tomography offer oncology? Eur J Cancer 36: 2028-2035.

Bain LJ, Le Blanc GA. 1996. Interaction of structurally diverse pesticides with the human MDR1 gene product P-glycoprotein. Toxicol Appl Pharmacol 141: 288-298.

Bart J. 2003. [^{11}C]verapamil PET reveals modulation of P-gp in the BBB by calcineurin blockers in lung transplant recipients. Thesis 2003.

Cirrito JR, Deane R, Fagan AM, Spinner ML, Parsadanian M, et al. 2005. P-glycoprotein deficiency at the blood-brain barrier increases amyloid-beta deposition in an Alzheimer disease mouse model. J Clin Invest 115: 3285-3290.

Cordon-Cardo C, O'Brien JP, Casals D, Rittman-Grauer L, Biedler JL, et al. 1989. Multidrug-resistance gene (P-glycoprotein) is expressed by endothelial cells at blood-brain barrier sites. Proc Natl Acad Sci USA 86: 695-698.

Corti O, Hampe C, Darios F, Ibanez P, Ruberg M, et al. 2005. Parkinson's disease: From causes to mechanisms. C R Biol 328: 131-142.

de Lange EC, Danhof M. 2002. Considerations in the use of cerebrospinal fluid pharmacokinetics to predict brain target concentrations in the clinical setting: Implications of the barriers between blood and brain. Clin Pharmacokin 41: 691-703.

Di Monte DA. 2003. The environment and Parkinson's disease: Is the nigrostriatal system preferentially targeted by neurotoxins? Lancet Neurol 2: 531-538.

Drozdzik M, Bialecka M, Mysliwiec K, Honczarenko K, Stankiewicz J, et al. 2003. Polymorphism in the P-glycoprotein drug transporter MDR1 gene: A possible link between environmental and genetic factors in Parkinson's disease. Pharmacogenetics 13: 259-263.

Ejsing TB, Linnet K. 2005. Influence of P-glycoprotein inhibition on the distribution of the tricyclic antidepressant nortriptyline over the blood-brain barrier. Hum Psychopharmacol 20: 149-153.

Eytan GD, Kuchel PW. 1999. Mechanism of action of P-glycoprotein in relation to passive membrane permeation. Int Rev Cytol 190: 175-250.

Fellner S, Bauer B, Miller DS, Schaffrik M, Fankhanel M, et al. 2002. Transport of paclitaxel (Taxol) across the blood-brain barrier in vitro and in vivo. J Clin Invest 110: 1309-1318.

Furuno T, Landi MT, Ceroni M, Caporaso N, Bernucci I, et al. 2002. Expression polymorphism of the blood-brain barrier component P-glycoprotein (MDR1) in relation to Parkinson's disease. Pharmacogenetics 12: 529-534.

Gloor SM, Wachtel M, Bolliger MF, Ishihara H, Landmann R, et al. 2001. Molecular and cellular permeability control at the blood-brain barrier. Brain Res Brain Res Rev 36: 258-264.

Hardy J, Selkoe DJ. 2002. The amyloid hypothesis of Alzheimer's disease: Progress and problems on the road to therapeutics. Science 297: 353-356.

Kortekaas R, Leenders KL, van Oostrom JC, Vaalburg W, Bart J, et al. 2005. Blood-brain barrier dysfunction in parkinsonian midbrain in vivo. Ann Neurol 57: 176-179.

Lam FC, Liu R, Lu P, Shapiro AB, Renoir JM, et al. 2001. Beta-amyloid efflux mediated by P-glycoprotein. J Neurochem 76: 1121-1128.

Lammertsma AA. 2004. Role of human and animal PET studies in drug development. Int Cong Ser 1265: 3-11.

Langston JW. 2002. Parkinson's disease: Current and future challenges. Neurotoxicology 23: 443-450.

Lee YJ, Maeda J, Kusuhara H, Okauchi T, Inaji M, et al. 2005. In vivo evaluation of P-glycoprotein function at the blood-brain barrier in nonhuman primates using [^{11}C]verapamil. J Pharmacol Exp Ther 316(2): 647-653.

Lewis P, Griffin S, Marsden P, Gee T, Nunan T, et al. 1994. Whole-body ^{18}F-fluorodeoxyglucose positron emission tomography in preoperative evaluation of lung cancer. Lancet 344: 1265-1266.

Lubberink M, Luurtsema G, van Berckel BN, Boellaard R, Toornvliet JR, et al. 2005. Development of a tracer kinetic model for the analysis of (R)-[^{11}C]verapamil PET data. J Cereb Blood Flow Metab 25: S608.

Luurtsema G, Molthoff CFM, Windhorst AD, Smit JW, Keizer H, et al. 2003. (R)- and (S)-[C-11]verapamil as PET-tracers for measuring P-glycoprotein function: In vitro and in vivo evaluation. Nucl Med Biol 30: 747-751.

Marchi N, Hallene KL, Kight KM, Cucullo L, Moddel G, et al. 2004. Significance of MDR1 and multiple drug resistance in refractory human epileptic brain. BMC Med 2: 37.

Mattson MP. 2004. Pathways towards and away from Alzheimer's disease. Nature 430: 631-639.

Pardridge WM. 1998. CNS drug design based on principles of blood-brain barrier transport. J Neurochem 70: 1781-1792.

Reese TS, Karnovsky MJ. 1967. Fine structural localization of a blood-brain barrier to exogenous peroxidase. J Cell Biol 34: 207-217.

Rice A, Michaelis ML, Georg G, Liu Y, Turunen B, et al. 2003. Overcoming the blood-brain barrier to taxane delivery for neurodegenerative diseases and brain tumors. J Mol Neurosci 20: 339-343.

Roberts RL, Joyce PR, Mulder RT, Begg EJ, Kennedy MA. 2002. A common P-glycoprotein polymorphism is associated with nortriptyline-induced postural hypotension in patients treated for major depression. Pharmacogenomics J 2: 191-196.

Sasongko L, Link JM, Muzi M, Mankoff DA, Yang X, et al. 2005. Imaging P-glycoprotein transport activity at the human blood-brain barrier with positron emission tomography. Clin Pharmacol Ther 77: 503-514.

Schinkel AH. 1999. P-Glycoprotein, a gatekeeper in the blood-brain barrier. Adv Drug Deliv Rev 36: 179-194.

Schinkel AH, Smit JJ, van Tellingen O, Beijnen JH, Wagenaar E, et al. 1994. Disruption of the mouse mdr1a P-glycoprotein gene leads to a deficiency in the blood-brain barrier and to increased sensitivity to drugs. Cell 77: 491-502.

Schinkel AH, Wagenaar E, Mol CA, van Deemter L. 1996. P-glycoprotein in the blood-brain barrier of mice influences the brain penetration and pharmacological activity of many drugs. J Clin Invest 97: 2517-2524.

Selkoe DJ. 1999. Translating cell biology into therapeutic advances in Alzheimer's disease. Nature 399: A23-A31.

Taylor EM. 2002. The impact of efflux transporters in the brain on the development of drugs for CNS disorders. Clin Pharmacokinet 41: 81-92.

Toornvliet JR, van Berckel BNM, Luurtsema G, Lubberink M, Geldof AA, et al. 2006. Effect of age on functional P-glycoprotein in the blood brain barrier measured using (R)-[^{11}C]verapamil and positron emission tomography. Clin Pharmacol Ther 79: 540-548.

Tsuji A, Tamai II. 1999. Carrier-mediated or specialized transport of drugs across the blood-brain barrier. Adv Drug Deliv Rev 36: 277-290.

Uhr M, Holsboer F, Muller MB. 2002. Penetration of endogenous steroid hormones corticosterone, cortisol, aldosterone and progesterone into the brain is enhanced in mice deficient for both mdr1a and mdr1b P-glycoproteins. J Neuroendocrinol 14: 753-759.

Vogelgesang S, Cascorbi I, Schroeder E, Pahnke J, Kroemer HK, et al. 2002. Deposition of Alzheimer's beta-amyloid is inversely correlated with P-glycoprotein expression in the brains of elderly non-demented humans. Pharmacogenetics 12: 535-541.

6 A Practical Approach to Computational Models of the Blood–Brain Barrier

M. Adenot

© Springer-Verlag Berlin Heidelberg 2007

Abstract: This article features a practical and critical approach to the development and use of computational blood-brain barrier models; the experimental blood-brain barrier models are also critically examined as the main source of dependant variable that exerts a strong influence on model accuracy and significance. While a very few simple chemical descriptors are generally sufficient to predict the passive diffusion pathway to the brain, we have focused on the inclusion of some other transport components, such as active transport to the brain, transcytosis, internalization and P-glycoprotein active efflux from the brain. These components are fundamental to modeling the behavior of a large panel of drugs, in particular that of complex drugs emerging from biotechnologies that are known to have low passive diffusion.

List of Abbreviations: ADME, Absorption-Distribution-Metabolism-Excretion; AMT, Adsorptive-mediated transcytosis; BBB, Blood-brain barrier; BCSFB, Blood-cerebro-spinal fluid barrier; CNS, Central nervous System; CSF, Cerebro-spinal fluid; CVO, Circumventricular organs; HBA, Hydrogen-bond acceptor; HBD, Hydrogen-bond donor; M6G, Morphine-6-glucuronide; MDR, Multi drug resistance; MFI, Mean fluorescence intensity; MRP, Multidrug resistance protein; MV, Molecular volume; MW, Molecular weight; P-gp, P-glycoprotein; PLS, Partial least squares; PS, Permeability-surface product; PSA, Polar surface area; QSAR, Quantitative structure-activity relationships; RMT, Receptor-mediated transcytosis; RT, Retention time

1   Introduction

For most drugs, the rate of penetration into brain tissues is limited by the diffusion of the drug across the blood–brain barrier (BBB). Existing technologies used to get drugs into the brain are often impractical (invasive neurological delivery) or unsafe (hyperosmotic shock increasing the permeability of the BBB). Knowledge about the ability of a drug to penetrate the brain at a required concentration is of fundamental importance to design central nervous system (CNS) therapeutics or to discard peripheral drugs with unwanted CNS effects. Although new pharmaceutical compounds have the potential for treating specific brain diseases, their development is often impeded by the inability of these drugs to cross the BBB. The field of neurology is growing more and more and BBB remains one of the major limitations for treatments: 95–98% of potential CNS drugs are rejected during research and development (R&D) because of a poor BBB permeability.

The specific issue of BBB permeation has merged in the 1990s with the more general paradigm of absorption–distribution–metabolism–excretion (ADME) as a particular case of biological barrier crossing, drug absorption, and transport. Predicting ADME or druglike properties in large virtual libraries is of major interest for pharmaceutical companies. The empirical rules that are often used in company databases as alerts for poor druglike compounds are extremely simple, neglecting transport phenomenon, formulation improvements, and many aspects of physiological complexity.

The recent increase of published computational BBB/CNS models (3 in 1994 up to 35 at the end of 2003) is an indication of need and interest of the pharmaceutical industry for such a tool and its applications. This article features a practical and critical approach to the development and use of BBB models as well as the experimental data sources they are derived from. While a few very simple descriptors are sufficient to correctly predict the passive diffusion pathway to the brain, we have focused on the necessity to refine BBB models by including all other transport components as a full part of BBB permeation expression. In fact, more or less simple modifications could improve or impair the BBB penetration by passive diffusion for conventional small organic molecules. However, the most promising drugs for the treatment of brain pathologies, such as neurodegenerative diseases, are typically large molecules, peptides, or oligonucleotides that are known for having a very low passive diffusion component as well as vectorized drugs that are especially designed to be transported by alternative pathways. For these reasons, it is of fundamental importance to develop new models aimed at predicting the other transport components, in addition to the more traditional passive diffusion models.

2   From Facts to Models

2.1   How to Conceptualize the BBB?

Modeling as a technique of representing schematically a complex reality, consists in breaking down a system into simplified representations fitting its characteristics as accurately as possible. Such a reductionist method implies to put together different partial complementary views until a global perception of the system is obtained. In this perspective, the BBB like any other biological system can be envisaged from different perspectives.

2.1.1   BBB as a Physiological Function

The BBB is a specialized system of capillary endothelial cells assumed to carry out three main functions:
- Prevention of the entry of undesirable compounds into the brain
- Promotion of the transport of nutrients and metabolites to the brain
- Regulation of the internal environment and the CNS fluid volume by limiting the bulk flow of water across the BBB

The main BBB physiological function (the barrier effect) results from a complex combination of both morphological and biochemical features, but all features are not necessarily correlated to the BBB permeation itself.

BBB Morphological Features   In real conditions, four cellular types are considered as the anatomic basis of the BBB: brain capillary endothelial cells (BCEC), pericytes, astrocytes, and nerve endings. BCEC are distinct from ordinary capillaries: unlike most organs, they are joined by intercellular tight junctions of about 8 nm in diameter (versus 50 nm in other organs) and there is a paucity of cytoplasmic vesicles indicating a poor rate of endocytosis. The tight junctions are responsible for the BBB high-electrical resistance, about 2000 Ω cm^2, across the endothelium. Astrocytes, pericytes, and nerve endings dynamically regulate BBB functions and permeability with still poorly understood mechanisms of interaction with BCEC. Moreover, BCEC population is often heterogeneous. While most in vitro models are based upon only a small surface area, the BBB properties are supposed to be homogenously distributed over all this surface area.

The surface area of the human BBB is estimated around 20 m^2 (Pardridge, 2002). It is noteworthy that some brain areas called the circumventricular organs are BBB-free and the vascular differentiation at the choroid plexus is distinct from the BBB.

BBB Biochemical Features   Different studies have characterized a number of molecular markers and signaling pathways at the BBB and, particularly, at the tight junctions level. Cultured brain endothelial cells, out of their natural environment, lose their physiological properties. Not all markers are correlated to BBB permeation, but experimental in vitro cell models are concerned with maintaining the in vivo metabolic features and biochemical environment of BCEC. Gene expression profiling and protein analysis are used to evaluate the ability of cellular models to reproduce the human BCEC metabolic profile (Marroni et al., 2003).

Some molecular aspects of brain microvessels have been especially evoked such as membrane lipid composition, membrane antigens, endothelial cell secreted factors (NO, endothelines, cytokines, angiopoietines . . .), transporters, channels, or enzymes. At the tight junction level, the morphological integrity is insured by the presence of specific membrane proteins like occludin, cytoplasmic associated proteins, and the cadherin/catenin complex (Rubin et al., 1998; Tsukita et al., 1998).

At physiological pH values, the luminal surface of the brain endothelium presents an overall negative charge mainly due to sialylation. The basolateral side of BCEC contains collagen, fibronectin, laminins, chondroitin, and heparane sulfate forming not only a mechanical supporting structure for the capillary wall but also a negatively charged barrier (Virgintino et al., 1997).

2.1.2 BBB as a Dynamic Regulating Exchange Interface

From a kinetic point of view, the BBB is defined as an interface between the different compartments of a dynamic model (❷ *Figure 6-1*). It is entirely characterized by a set of pharmacokinetic parameters. Unlike

◘ **Figure 6-1**

Model of the blood–brain interfaces and the circulation of a solute between the plasma and the different liquid compartments of the brain. The three major points of entry into the brain are (1) BBB, (2) circumventricular organs (CVO), and (3) CSF uptake. There is no physical barrier between the CSF and the brain parenchyma but the free-diffusion at equilibrium is limited by the CSF bulk flow movement. Practically, drugs do not gain entry to the brain parenchyma via this mechanism and stay in contact with meninges rather than deep subcortical structures

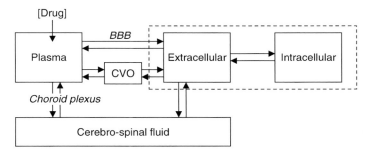

the previous static notion of physical barrier, the BBB should be thought in its real dynamic three-dimensional (3D) environment submitted to physiological constraints like cerebral blood flow, arterial pressure, hormonal stimuli, CSF kinetics . . . . The steady-state concentration of a drug in the brain depends on an equilibrium between various influx/efflux pathways and the available quantity of free drug at the BBB entry. This quantity depends on parameters such as the initial dose, administration route, duration of perfusion, fraction of bound/unbound drug in plasma, metabolic pathway, drug distribution ratio to the brain, and hepatic or pulmonary first-pass effect.

A pharmacokinetic BBB model is aimed at predicting the drug concentration into the brain (or a related variable) as a function of time. A certain number of techniques for acquiring pharmacokinetic data have already been reviewed (de Lange et al., 2000) including quantitative autoradiography, imaging techniques, CSF sampling, or intracerebral microdialysis. Some theoritical models have been based on equations derived from compartment models of the BBB: the free-drug concentration in CNS has been simulated for different rates of transport into and out of the brain in a two-compartment model (Hammarlund-Udenaes et al., 1997); the model has been validated with microdialysis data for five drugs. The rate of equilibration is rapid and mainly determined by the perfusion rate and the distribution ratio. Conversely to the idea that passive diffusion across the BBB is a limiting factor, the above model shows that the time to equilibrium is rapid even for hydrophilic molecules due to the presence of active transporters. The blood concentration profile is a good predictor for concentration profile into the brain even for hydrophilic molecules. More recently, the duration of effects has been simulated as a function of dose, elimination rate constant (k_e), transport parameters (K_m and V_{max}), and EC50 (Mahar Doan and Boje, 2000). This model has been derived in the presence and absence of endogenous transport inhibitors and highlights the influence of transport inhibition on the duration of drug effect.

2.1.3 BBB as a Pathological Function

From a clinical point of view, the BBB can be seen as a physiological function affected by the diseases of the CNS. It is relevant to question the validity of "healthy" BBB models to predict brain permeability to potential CNS drugs while these drugs will be taken by patients with altered BBB. It is admitted that many pathological states like cancers, neurodegenerative diseases, trauma, infections, inflammations, ischemia, hypertension, or epilepsy are associated with a failure of BBB integrity. The local alterations both at the endothelial and the glial level result in the disruption of tight junctions. While BBB breakdown is found in many CNS-associated diseases, the predicted levels of permeation in pathological conditions are different from what is expected. A brain tumor could be seen as one of the most favorable brain area for hydrophilic drug diffusion, but the level and localization of BBB alterations are variable and heterogeneous: the neo-microvasculature is largely abnormal and the increased tissue pressure due to edema leads to unperfused area and limited blood flow to the tumor. As a consequence, the clinical incidence of such alterations are unpredictable and the anticancer drugs or the imagery tracers remain poorly distributed in the brain despite evident BBB alterations.

A model of LPS-mediated BBB alteration has been proposed (Descamps et al., 2003) in which the lipopolysaccharides increases the paracellular permeability of BCEC. This model has been used to demonstrate that glial cells have a protective effect on BCEC. Other models have been used to test the exposure to tumor necrosis factor (TNF-α) (Deli et al., 1995), inflammation, or hypoxia (Plateel et al., 1995; Dehouck et al., 2002).

2.2 Definition of BBB Models Output Variables

In the continuation of this chapter, we consider BBB models as any experimental device or equations able to predict for a given molecule its capacity to cross from bloodstream to brain in human under normal conditions. This implies to define clearly as to which physical quantity could stand for the capacity to cross from bloodstream to brain and how to get access to such an information. Different terminologies have been found to designate the variable of interest: brain penetration, brain uptake, drug transport to the brain, BBB permeability, BBB permeation, transport to the CNS, drug penetration into the CNS ... Even if these terminologies seem to mean more or less the same concept, it is not always clear to which extent they will be of interest in a screening or a drug design process.

2.2.1 Qualitative Variables

A very simple output variable is based on class attribution for each drug. The most used classification is based on the existence of a CNS pharmacological activity, including CNS side effects. It has been used as a means to define the profile of CNS drugs and to design CNS-oriented libraries. But the CNS+/CNS− classification scheme have also been used by many authors as a surrogate for CNS penetration, hence, BBB permeability to a drug, assuming that the existence of a CNS or CNS-mediated activity implies that the drug crosses the BBB. The class attribution is based on claimed pharmacological activities but the belonging to a CNS class is not such a rigid unquestionable concept: the class attribution is a source of discrepancies, as it can be seen by comparing the change of class attribution in Seelig dataset (Fischer et al., 1998) with respect to the previous study (Seelig et al., 1994).

A real BBB+/BBB− classification is based on the ability of a molecule to cross the BBB in vivo in humans. In the absence of such a knowledge, in vivo permeability in animals or in vitro permeability in cell culture are generally used as surrogate variables.

Practically, BBB+/BBB− and CNS+/CNS− concepts are largely confused: many BBB models are in fact CNS+/CNS− models despite the fact that these two concepts do not encode the same level of information. A CNS model includes much more parameters than a BBB model. Upstream from BBB includes:

formulation, route, dose, solubility; metabolism in plasma and at the BBB; sequestration of drugs within the plasma (protein binding) or other organs than the brain; cerebral blood flow, varying between different brain regions both in normal and pathological conditions. Downstream from BBB includes: cerebrospinal fluid distribution; drug metabolism into the brain; diffusion of drugs through brain compartments up to their targets; affinity and intrinsic activity of the compound.

As a consequence, using CNS+/CNS− instead of BBB+/BBB− leads to two classical kind of errors in BBB prediction models as described in the following sections.

BBB+/CNS− Compounds (False BBB−)   CNS activity generally implies BBB permeation (with a few exceptions due to the free-BBB CNS areas), but the converse is not necessarily true: some CNS− drugs may still cross the BBB and show no activity simply because they do not interact with any CNS targets, or they are metabolized, or they do not reach the targeted brain compartment or the required concentration at equilibrium. A molecule classified as CNS-inactive may in fact penetrate the BBB by passive diffusion but is then expelled by an active efflux mechanism. Finally, there is the case of false CNS− compounds, such as undetermined compounds classified CNS− by default or known peripherical drugs, which may also cross the BBB, leads to unwanted CNS side effects and which are in fact CNS+, although they are referenced as non-CNS therapeutics. The case of prodrugs like L-DOPA is another source of confusion as L-DOPA is a BBB+ compound but has no antiparkinsonian activity by itself since it exerts an effect via its metabolite dopamine.

BBB−/CNS+ Compounds (False BBB+)   One additional consideration is that some compounds exert CNS effects without any high-BBB permeation rate:

− A drug can cross the blood–cerebrospinal fluid barrier (BCSFB), mainly located at the choroid plexus.
− A drug can bypass the BBB through the circumventricular organs (BBB-free areas) and exert its action either locally or via neural connection to deeper regions of the brain.
− Some drugs are transported directly from nose to brain via the olfactory pathway (Illum, 2000, 2002; Frey, 2002).

The class attribution is ambiguous for drugs that cannot cross the BBB by themselves but are finally considered as CNS+ despite they are stricto sensu BBB−: naturally occurring CNS molecules like catecholamines are released in situ but (1) they are too polar to enter the CNS from blood by themselves and (2) they are quickly hydrolyzed in the plasma before they can reach the BBB. Prodrugs, like paracetamol or benorilate, are unable to cross the BBB by themselves but finally enter the brain after a metabolic modification.

2.2.2 Quantitative Variables

While the BBB should be seen more like a regulating interface between blood and brain than like a rigid physical barrier, the question is less to know if a molecule crosses the BBB or not than what is the level of drug influx into the brain.

Although customers have a strong natural inclination to believe that the commercial model they bought reflects what it is assumed to, most models are trained to fit surrogate variables rather than target variable. This is a very general limitation of modeling activity due to the fact that, in many cases, an observer has access only to secondary observations.

Apart from a few attempts with NMR or PET imagery, the BBB permeability to a drug in human is not accessible. For this reason, surrogate variables, such as the blood–brain partition coefficient (log BB), the permeability–surface area product (PS), brain uptake index, or brain capillary permeability coefficient, have been used. All these quantities are defined in ❷ *Sect. 10.3.*

BBB models reflect nothing but a partitioning process between blood and lipid material (van de Waterbeemd et al., 2001), and the relevance of blood–brain partition coefficient measurements or predictions to the pharmacological action has not been addressed; moreover, it seems that the free-drug concentration in the cerebral extracellular fluid has a better chance to correlate with CNS pharmacological action (Martin, 2004).

Recently, an interesting discussion arose about the validity of the most popular predictor of BBB permeability (log P) as a surrogate variable of brain penetration (Martin, 2004; Pardridge, 2004). This questions seriously, the interest of most existing models. As a response to Martin, Pardridge explained that if ADME filters are applied (for example, the rejection of compounds with more than 95% plasma-bound fraction), molecules like diazepam will be discarded from the screening (Pardridge, 2004). He suggested that the in vivo BBB PS product replaces the log BB as a standard in the field.

The use of permeability data as a CNS penetration predictor should also be considered with caution while the BBB permeability to a drug is not an intrinsic property for this drug: a lot of external parameters may dynamically modulate the level of BBB permeation such as an increased drug concentration in plasma, or pathological and physiological states.

2.3 Definition of BBB Models Input Data

Within experimental BBB models, a real molecule with convenient formulation (solvent, pH, salt, ionic force, solvent, buffer, presence of serum albumin) is injected in the donor compartment at a certain concentration. Some molecules may be metabolized in a short period of time either in the plasma or as they reached the BBB. Using cellular models, although the reference molecules have a known metabolism, the tested molecules could be structurally modified during the time of experiment.

Within computational models, a virtual molecule defined by its 2D or 3D structure is given as input to an algorithm or an equation. The molecular structure description is the way by which chemical compounds are encoded into a numerical string for mathematical/logical operations and computer-aided processing. In silico, a molecule is considered only as a block of numerical descriptor values. Drug formulation and concentration as well as metabolites are not considered at all, even if these parameters are known to strongly modulate the level of BBB permeation.

A chemical entity will reach the CNS depending on the existence of a transport pathway, its chemical state, and metabolic transformations; predictions for an original molecule cannot be extended to its various metabolites (some metabolites are CNS active, some are not; some do cross the BBB, some do not). Ideally, the BBB permeation should be calculated for the original molecule and its metabolites. This consideration raises two questions:

- What is the exact chemical identity of the molecule, which passes through the BBB?
- To what extent the "calculated" molecule and the real molecule reflect the same entity?

During a screening process, molecular descriptors are computed on the fly over a unique conformation of the molecule and a unique chemical state. Counterions, stereoisomers, ionization, and tautomeric equilibrium are not fully considered albeit often considerable consequences on the descriptor values. The consideration of stereoisomers is largely neglected due to the fact that most descriptors used are 2D descriptors and experimental data on stereoisomers are not available, assuming negligible stereoselectivity in permeation.

All computational models published to date are based on structure–activity relationships: physiological conditions (local cerebral blood flow), concentration level in the donor compartment, and formulation conditions are ignored, although they can dramatically affect the level of permeation.

2.4 Transport Pathways as BBB Functional Components

The BBB, like most physiological functions, acts as a very complex nonisolated system. It can be seen either as a set of embedded transport and regulating systems or as a drug–brain interface. In both cases, drug transport from blood to brain is associated to a continuous variable (the total transflux) that can be thought of as the summation of the individual fluxes through five different routes.

2.4.1 Passive Diffusion

It is the primary process of translocation from the blood stream to the brain for a majority of drugs. For a given biological barrier fully characterized by morphological/biochemical parameters (composition, surface area, water pores, tight junction diameters), the molecular physicochemical properties represent the major rate determinant for passive diffusion. For this reason, they are extensively used as predictors of BBB permeation, which is known to depend on simple parameters that make sense for medicinal chemists (molecular weight [MW], H-bond capacity, rotatable bonds, solvent-accessible surface areas ...) and which are currently used to screen databases.

2.4.2 Paracellular Transport

It is typically used as a transport pathway for small hydrophilic molecules in all organs but the brain. Brain microvessel endothelial cells are characterized by complex tight junctions, the absence of transport pores, a distinct morphological structure, and a low number of pinocytotic vesicles. In these conditions, the entry of small hydrophilic drugs from blood to the brain is very restricted unless specific transporters exist at the cell membranes. Only a provoked disruption of the BBB has been shown to increase the passage of some hydrophilic drugs. While it has a null contribution to the total drug transflux through BBB in normal conditions, the paracellular component could be neglected in first approximation in BBB models. However, it has been demonstrated that the transcellular permeability is locally increased in pathological conditions, mainly under the influence of pro-inflammatory cytokines (Brillault et al., 2002) or viral proteins (Petito, 1998).

2.4.3 Active Transport

It has been seen that hydrophilic compounds cannot cross the BBB in the absence of a specific mechanism. That is the reason why hydrophilic nutrients need specific transporter proteins to deliver them into the brain. They contribute to the molecule influx from blood to brain, but this is limited to a very small number of specific substrates. Active transport concerns essentially known chemical series of endogenous biomolecules. More than 20 transporters have been identified that allow polar molecules to enter the brain: glucose, amines, amino acids and derivatives, small monocarboxylic acids, vitamins, nucleosides, organic anions/cations, and peptides like the opioid peptides, insuline, growth factors, interleukins, thyrotropine-releasing hormone, arginine vasopressine, α-melanocyte stimulating hormone, LHRH, and atrial natriuretic factor (Tsuji and Tamai, 1999, Tamai and Tsuji, 2000).

While transporters are important for CNS penetration, they can also be thought as a gateway to the brain for drugs linked to a specific carrier. This Trojan horse strategy seems to perform better for drugs that mimic the endogenous nutrients rather than for drugs conjugated to the nutrient molecule (Pardridge, 1998, 2002). In fact, the nutrient carriers have generally a very limited capacity of transport. Vectorization by an endogeneous nutrient rarely increases BBB transport. For example, the glucuronidation of morphine does not improve brain delivery by active transport; moreover, it significantly attenuates the brain penetration relative to that of morphine probably due to the presence of the glucuronide moiety of M6G, conferring a higher hydrophilic character (Wu et al., 1997). Recently, kinetic experiments confirmed by in vivo studies indicated that ascorbic acid conjugates of drugs were able to competitively inhibit ascorbate transport in epithelial cells (Manfredini et al., 2002). Most successful applications of the Trojan horse strategy exploit the existence of transport systems for large molecules such as cytokines, transferrine, immunoglobulines, and glycoproteins.

2.4.4 Transcytosis

The drug brain uptake by transcytosis is the result of three mechanisms: (1) endocytosis or internalization at the luminal side of BCEC, (2) diffusion through the cytoplasm without metabolic alterations, and (3) externalization at the basolateral side of BCEC.

Endocytosis as a first step of translocation is an energy-dependent transport process triggered by a nonspecific electrostatic adsorption of polycationic substances (adsorptive-mediated transcytosis) or after receptor binding (receptor-mediated transcytosis [RMT]) (❯ *Figure 6-2*). Despite the fact that endocytosis

☐ **Figure 6-2**
Vector-mediated transport through the BBB. The coupled drug enters the brain by either receptor-mediated endocytosis (1) or adsorptive-mediated endocytosis (2). Once the complex is exocytosed in the brain parenchyma, the linker is cleaved (3), releasing the active drug that may act on its pharmacological receptor. Reproduced from Temsamani et al., 2001 with permission

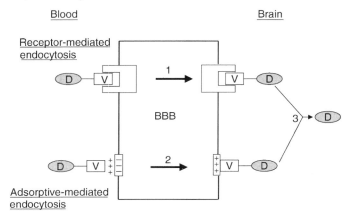

activity in the brain capillaries is rather poor, transcytosis is now considered as an alternative way to active transport for peptide drug brain delivery. Translocated peptides can also be used as a vector strategy: this approach has been successfully used to deliver drugs into live cells (Derossi et al., 1998; Temsamani et al., 2000). The interest of this approach as an effective brain delivery system has been demonstrated for doxorubicin (Rousselle et al., 2000, 2001). The adsorptive-mediated transcytosis (AMT) has been recognized as the main transport mechanism for compounds such as cationized albumin, histone, avidin, dynorphine and dermorphine analogs, ACTH analogs, SynB peptide vectors, or arginine-vasopressine analogs. It is potentially valuable as a drug delivery system for large hydrophobic molecules to the brain. The RMT is implied in the transport of the OX-26 murine monoclonal antibody after binding to the transferrine receptor or the transport of lipid to the brain via the LDL receptors (Dehouck et al., 1997).

2.4.5 Efflux Pumps

An increasing number of transporters have been discovered recently that pump drugs out of cells. The ATP-binding cassette transporter superfamily includes the multidrug resistant gene product 1, also known as P-glycoprotein (P-gp) and multidrug resistance–associated proteins (MRP1 to MRP9). P-gp is a membrane transport protein, very abundant in the luminal membrane of the endothelial cells comprising the BBB. MDR transporters have been proposed to act as "hydrophobic vacuum cleaners" or phospholipids flippases because of their ability to remove drugs and lipids from the inner membrane leaflet. The P-gp efflux transport depends on the drug binding to P-gp, level of expression of P-gp, drug concentration, presence of P-gp inhibitors or modulators, and transport constants at equilibrium. Although they are in vitro P-gp substrates, some compounds like amitriptyline, chlorpromazine, morphine, or disulfiram are also CNS drugs.

The absence of functional P-gp at the BBB level highly increases brain penetration of numerous drugs: MDR-1 knockout mice show an increased sensitivity to CNS toxicity for diverse drugs, suggesting that BBB efficacy is partially or completely abrogated (Schinkel, 1999).

3 Experimental BBB Models

Beyond their intrinsic obvious interest, experimental models are the first step to theoretical models (generally cheaper, quicker, and easy to set up) because they provide the observations needed prior to modeling. The acute comprehension of how experimental data were obtained allows to specify the limits of models, detect internal or interlaboratory variability, and prevent the successive drifts from authors to authors toward useless or far-from-reality computational models.

3.1 Passive Diffusion Models

Classically, the rate of diffusion in solution or through a simple membrane is expressed by the well-known Fick's law that links the amount of solvent diffusing in unit of time to the membrane surface area, diffusion coefficient, and concentration gradient. From Fick's equation, one can derive three interrelated physical quantities quantifying absorption processes.

– The permeability coefficient P_e (cm/s), which designates the ability of a chemical to pass through a material of specified thickness h.
– The influx of substance J (mg/s/cm^2), which is the real quantity of substance passing through the membrane of specified surface area A by unit of time.
– The absorption (or permeation) rate constant k_{obs} (s^{-1}), which is a measure of the rate at which a chemical will pass through the membrane.

$$P_e = \frac{D}{h} \cdot P \qquad J = P_e \cdot (C_1 - C_2) \qquad k_{obs} = P_e \cdot \frac{A}{V_A},$$

where P is the partition coefficient of the chemical between membrane and environment; D, the diffusion coefficient is constant at a given temperature for a given medium, and V_A is the solvent volume in acceptor chamber.

The extension of the simple Fick's membrane model to a biological barrier, such as the BBB, is limited by the nature of the membrane and the anisotropy of the compartments. At least two interfaces should be considered (blood/luminal side and basal side/brain); the fundamental differences between donor and acceptor compartments result in the definition of two partition coefficients. The system is supposed to have reached the steady-state conditions to account for the dynamic conditions in situ.

3.2 In Vitro Models

If in situ observations of BBB are almost difficult to set up, in vitro systems could provide an alternative. Despite a high number of attempts of in vitro BBB modeling, only a few data sets have been publicly provided that are suitable for modeling purposes. The drug diffusion through the in vitro BBB model is currently expressed as the permeability coefficient (P_e in cm/s) or the PS ($\mu L/g/s$).

3.2.1 Measure of In Vitro Partitioning Equilibrium

While BBB permeation depends on physicochemical parameters, such as hydrophobicity/lipophilicity, MW, and hydrogen-bonding potential, some authors attempted to use partition coefficients as determined by chromatography methods in order to predict the BBB permeability coefficient. Partition coefficients have been determined between the aqueous phase and an organic phase (Seelig et al., 1994) or a micelle phase (Kai, 1996) or immobilized artificial membranes (Salminem et al., 1998; Di et al., 2003).

The measure of lipophilicity alone is not sufficient to predict BBB permeation but the addition of surface activity parameters allows a better differentiation between CNS+ and CNS− compounds

(Seelig et al., 1994). A correlation has been found between the enthalpy term of the micelle/partition coefficient and BBB permeability coefficients for a subset of 7 among 14 compounds (Kai, 1996).

More recently, a parallel artificial membrane permeability assay (PAMPA-BBB) has been proposed (Di et al., 2003): the model consists of a modification of the parallel artificial membrane assay (PAMPA) (Kansy et al., 1998) originally developed to predict intestinal absorption. Porcine polar brain lipids composition has been adjusted in order to fit BBB permeation data of 30 commercial drugs. PAMPA-BBB assay directly measures the effective permeability P_e of the compound. The method is fitted to the screening of a high number of drug candidates.

3.2.2 Cell Culture Systems

Cell models must reproduce correctly the main BBB characteristics such as the solute permeability, restrictive paracellular barrier, cell architecture, and functionnal expression of transport mechanism (Gumbleton and Audus, 2001).

Based on the hypothesis that BBB behaves like the intestinal epithelial cells, the human colon cancer cell line Caco-2 has been used to predict BBB permeation. The results emphasize that the BBB and the intestinal mucosa are two fundamentally different biologic barriers and that the in situ BBB characteristics are necessary to accurate predictions (Lundquist et al., 2002). The cell-based BBB models include bovine or porcine brain capillary endothelial cultures, diverse immortalized brain endothelial, or noncerebral cell lines. In primary culture, some BBB characteristics are usually lost. They suffer from a lower transendothelial electrical resistance value, typically around 200 ω cm^2, and higher permeability than in situ BBB. However, these models can express passive and active transports albeit some transport systems are generally underrepresented. A certain number of phenotypic aspects of BBB were correctly reproduced, in particular, when exposing cell cultures to glia factors. The presence of astrocytes has been found to increase the transendothelial resistance in bovine BCEC (Gaillard et al., 2001).

The permeability is determined using a standard method (Siflinger-Birnboim et al., 1987): the average volume cleared during experiment is plotted versus time and the slope is called the PS. The PS is determined across a cell monolayer (PS_e) and across the filter only (PS_f). The in vitro BBB coefficient is:

$$1/PS = 1/PS_e - 1/PS_f$$

The permeability coefficient P_e is simply obtained after dividing PS_e by the surface area of the membrane or calculated as follows:

$$P_e = \left[\frac{V_A}{A \times C_0}\right] \times \frac{dC}{dt},$$

where V_A is the volume of the acceptor compartment, A is the surface area of the cell monolayer, C_0 is the initial concentration in the donor compartment, and dC/dt is the initial slope of the plot of the concentration in the receiver compartment versus time.

The permeability can also be estimated from the luminal fluorescence in confocal imaging using isolated brain capillaries (Miller, 2003).

The standard, commercially available BBB cell models consist in BCEC+astrocytes cocultures, such as the dynamic *DIV-BBB model* (Staness et al., 1996; Janigro et al., 1999) from Flocel (www.flocel.com) or the Cecchelli model (Dehouck et al., 1995; Cecchelli et al., 1999). The former has also been used to study drug efflux from the brain (Parkinson et al., 2003) and the conservation of native cell properties has been validated using gene and protein profiling (Marroni et al., 2003). Cecchelli and coworkers carried out a BBB model where endothelial cells display structural and metabolic characteristics similar to in vivo and developed new models of pathological BBB.

In vitro BBB models are presently developed from BCEC isolated essentially from bovine or porcine species. Since most in vivo BBB permeability studies are performed with rodents, an appropriate in vitro model obtained from rodent cell primary cultures has been codeveloped by INSERM U26 and Synt:em (www.syntem.com): the model has a very low permeability (<0.2 cm/s) for compounds, like sucrose or inulin, which are known to pass through the BBB via a paracellular way. Nevertheless, this model shows a strong correlation with *in vivo* permeability coefficients for many kinds of molecules.

Recently, in vitro BBB models consisting of confluent human brain endothelial cells and human astrocyte cells grown in coculture have been used to study the active transport of drugs (Megard et al., 2002).

Other cell systems have been developed for blood–cerebrospinal fluid barrier (Villalobos et al., 1997; Zheng et al., 1998). A recent review (Terasaki et al., 2003) lists different models of in vitro BBB models, BCSFB models, and some models for studying paracrine interactions between the BBB composing cells.

3.3 In Vivo Models

In vivo methods are distinguished depending on the mode of administration of the drug and the techniques used to measure drug quantity or concentration into the brain.

3.3.1 The Drug Administration Mode

Single Artery Injection Technique   First described in 1970 by Oldendorf, the method consists of measuring the extraction of a radiolabeled drug after a carotid artery single injection in anesthetized rat or rabbit. Tritiated water is added as a diffusible reference isotope. ^{113m}In can be added to the injection mixture, as a nondiffusible reference isotope, in order to evaluate the fraction of the injected test isotope remaining in the intravascular volume. The method is simple but limited in its application while the measure should be made under a very short time (5–15 s after the bolus injection). The very short time period of contact between the test compound and the BBB makes this technique suitable only for drugs with high extraction level. In the case of saturable transport, the Michaelis-Menten transport parameters K_m and V_{max} can be calculated from *PS*. A similar technique has been applied in animal or humans with nonradioactive tracers and is known as the indicator diffusion technique: the bolus is injected into the carotid and blood is sampled from the internal jugular vein. After the extraction coefficient has been measured, the permeability surface area product is calculated knowing the distribution volume and the cerebral blood flow.

In Situ Brain Perfusion   The single bolus injection is replaced by a perfusion. This technique overcomes the short time issue of the Oldendorf's technique and is suited to measure brain penetration for slowly diffusing compounds by allowing an extended exposure of the solute to the BBB. The duration of the experiment (less than 20 min) implies the possible metabolic transformation of the test molecule at the BBB level.

Intravenous Injection   Unlike the Oldendorf's technique, the intravenous injection allows to make measures after multiple passages through the BBB. It provides information about both systemic pharmacokinetics and drug accumulation in the brain. The method is aimed at detecting saturable transport phenomenon (carrier-mediated influx and efflux). The experimental simplicity makes this technique the most widely used approach despite the metabolic transformation both at the BBB level and at the peripheral level during the experiment. Indeed, the brain uptake of metabolites may perturbate the pharmacokinetic evaluation.

3.3.2 The Estimation of Drug Penetration into the Brain

Measure of the Average Free Drug Concentration into the Brain   It can be determined in the whole brain after decapitation and homogenization (one point per animal) or in CSF after sampling (multiple points per animal). If the measure is made on the whole brain, residual drug quantities into the brain vascular compartment could be removed using the brain capillary depletion technique (separation of capillaries from the rest of the brain tissues by density centrifugation). The presence of the drug into the CSF reflects the BCSFB permeability rather than the BBB permeability itself: it indicates the presence of the drug within the ventricles, the spinal canal, and the subarachnoid spaces following the CSF flow circulation but is in no way a marker of the diffusion of the drug into the deeper regions of the brain. Equating drug levels in CSF with drug levels in brain parenchyma may significantly overestimate the real drug penetration into the brain (Groothuis and Levy, 1997). Its interest remains limited to drugs acting at the meninges level.

Quantitative Estimation of Drug Distribution in Brain   It can be determined in the whole brain using noninvasive techniques (imaging) or in brain slices using autoradiography or histochemistry techniques. The brain-imaging techniques, such as positron emission tomography or magnetic resonance imaging, provide quantitative signals that can be related directly to BBB permeability for tracers in human using the amount of tracer in brain tissue (Q_{tracer}^{brain}) and the concentration of tracer in plasma (C_{tracer}^{plasma}):

$$PS = \frac{Q_{tracer}^{brain}}{C_{tracer}^{plasma} \times T}$$

These techniques initially developed for clinical investigations are currently limited to a small number of tracers but could also be extended to labeled drugs (Agon et al., 1991). They remain complex, expensive, and still limited by a low-spatial resolution.

In Situ Measure (Monitoring) of Free Drug Concentration   This measure involves the stereotactic implantation of a probe within localized brain regions. The probe consists of either an electrode (for electrochemically active drugs only) or a microdialysis probe (de Lange et al., 2000). Intracerebral microdialysis provide samples obtained at multiple time points from individual nonanesthetized animals: the dialysate is collected and drug concentrations are directly determined. This is the method of choice for pharmacokinetic studies.

Pharmacological Estimation of the Brain Penetration   A practical way to estimate the penetration of a drug into the brain is simply to detect specific CNS pharmacological activities such as electroencephalogram abnormalities, sleep induction, modification of the mood, psychomotor hyperactivity, seizures, mnesic troubles or anxiety. In some case, the level of brain penetration may be estimated by comparing the pharmacological activity of a compound following administration by subcutaneous and intracerebroventricular routes (Giardina et al., 1995).

3.3.3 Expression of the In Vivo BBB Permeation

The observable target is generally the *PS* product but practically the measured quantities are the extraction coefficient, volume of distribution, or transport coefficient depending on the technique used.

After a Single Capillary Passage Extraction (Single Artery Bolus)   The extraction coefficient (E in %) is the ratio between the amount of substance within the brain (Q^{brain}) and the amount of substance injected in the plasma ($Q^{injected}$) during the same period of time. The brain uptake index (BUI in %) is the ratio between the extraction coefficient of the tested compound and a reference diffusible compound such as water. The tested compound and the reference should be labeled with distinct radionuclei:

$$\mathrm{BUI}(\%) = \frac{[^{14}C]^{brain} \big/ [^3H]^{brain}}{[^{14}C]^{injected} \big/ [^3H]^{injected}} \times 100 = \frac{E^{test}}{E^{reference}} \times 100$$

The extraction coefficient of a nondiffusible reference, generally ^{113m}Indium, is considered as a correction term to estimate the amount of test compound remaining in the vascular space:

$$\text{BUI}(\%) = \frac{[^{14}C]^{\text{brain}} \big/ [^3H]^{\text{brain}} - [^{113m}In]^{\text{brain}} \big/ [^3H]^{\text{brain}}}{[^{14}C]^{\text{injected}} \big/ [^3H]^{\text{injected}} - [^{113m}In]^{\text{injected}} \big/ [^3H]^{\text{injected}}} \times 100 = \frac{E^{\text{test}} - E^{\text{In}}}{E^{\text{reference}}} \times 100$$

The PS product is derived from extraction coefficients using the Renkin-Crone relationship:

$$PS = v \cdot F - \ln(1 - E),$$

where F is the cerebral blood flow and v the fractional volume of blood (without unity) contributing to brain uptake.

After a Multiple Capillary Passage Extraction (Artery or Intravenous Perfusion) The volume of distribution (V_d in µL/g of brain tissue) is another simple expression of brain uptake defined as the ratio of the brain concentration at equilibrium (C^{brain} in mg/mg of tissue) and the perfusate concentration (C^{injected} in mg/mL of perfusate). A nondiffusible reference marker, such as inulin, albumin, or sucrose, can be added in order to evaluate the fraction of the injected drug remaining in the intravascular volume.

$$V_d = \frac{C^{\text{brain}}}{C^{\text{injected}}} \qquad \text{without a nondiffusible reference}$$

$$V_d = \frac{C^{\text{brain}} - [\text{ref}]^{\text{brain}}}{C^{\text{injected}}} \qquad \text{with a nondiffusible reference}$$

Volumes of distribution can be compared only if they have been measured with the same duration of perfusion.

The transport coefficient or unidirectional transfer constant from plasma to brain (K_{in} in µL/g/min) is derived from the measure of V_d in order to take into account the duration of perfusion T in the drug tissue accumulation. The single-time point transport coefficient is calculated as:

$$K_{\text{in}} = \frac{C^{\text{brain}}}{C^{\text{injected}} \cdot T} \qquad \text{without a nondiffusible reference}$$

$$K_{\text{in}} = \frac{C^{\text{brain}} - [\text{ref}]^{\text{brain}}}{C^{\text{injected}} \cdot T} \qquad \text{with a nondiffusible reference}$$

In a multiple-time point analysis, K_{in} is determined with a greater accuracy using the slope of the plot $C^{\text{brain}}/C^{\text{injected}}$ versus time. This analysis requires that animals are sacrificed at various time points after the injection.

The transport coefficient may be converted into the in vivo permeability coefficient knowing the BBB surface area per unit weight of brain S (roughly estimated to 100 cm^2/g, depending on the brain regions):

$$P_e = K_{\text{in}}/S$$

K_{in} may also be expressed as a function of cerebral blood flow and, consequently, of the PS product using the Renkin-Crone relationship:

$$K_{\text{in}} = vF \cdot E = vF\left[1 - \exp\left(\frac{PS}{vF}\right)\right]$$

For low extraction coefficient value ($<10\%$), one can consider that $K_{\text{in}} \cong PS$.

Finally, the blood–brain partition coefficient has been largely used as a surrogate variable for BBB permeation:

$$\log BB = \log\left(C^{\text{brain}}/C^{\text{blood}}\right),$$

where C^{brain} and C^{blood} are respectively the steady-state concentrations of the molecule in brain and blood after a specified time.

4   Computational BBB Models

Experimental data on BBB permeation using experimental in vitro or in vivo models remain difficult to obtain routinely. This explains the need for reliable in silico models to screen virtual libraries of drug compounds. Some qualitative—and often intuitive—rules are currently used by medicinal chemists to predict the BBB permeation of compounds. The computing technology is now used to bypass the need for time- and resource-consuming high-throughput screening of massive compound libraries and reduces the amount of medicinal chemistry required. Most of the computational models have been designed to filter CNS drugs from virtual libraries: clearly, simple diffusion is a well-predicted component of CNS penetration and is generally modeled with a few very simple predictors. It becomes a necessity to improve the accuracy and to extend the validity domain of BBB permeation models: the challenge of BBB computational modeling is to include alternative pathways to the brain as explicit components of the model.

4.1   Empirical Rules

The main objective of theoretical BBB modeling is to identify an accurate computable predictor of the in vivo BBB permeability. Over decades, some molecular properties have appeared as playing a significant role on drug transport properties (and BBB permeation as well) even if the structure–activity relationships have not always been clearly elucidated.

4.1.1 Lipophilicity

Lipophilicity has long been recognized as an essential factor for drug transport across biomembranes. Precisely, this observation is historically related to drug transport into the CNS since Meyer and Overton demonstrated in 1899 that the anesthetic potency of many compounds is nearly linearly related to their oil/water partition coefficients. A well-known medicinal chemistry approach to increase BBB permeation consists in increasing lipophilicity by removing polar groups and/or adding nonpolar groups. In order to give a quantitative rational basis to this empirical approach, log P has been used as a predictor of BBB permeability, as is (Rapoport and Levitan, 1974) or with a correction factor to take into account the role of molecular size (Levin, 1980). Despite a large number of studies, no clear relationship between BBB permeability and lipophilicity has been demonstrated:

1. The simple idea that the higher the lipophilicity, the better the BBB penetration is obviously spurious. The most general relationships between permeability through biomembranes and the lipophilicity have been illustrated by the well-known parabolic (Hansch) or bilinear (Kubinyi) models, but other models have been found linear, hyperbolic, or sigmoid (Camenish et al., 1998), mainly dependent on the used datasets. Interestingly, Lipinski rules, aimed at evaluating drug absorption, indicate an upper limit for log P but no lower limit . . .. An analysis of several classes of CNS-active substances led to the conclusion that BBB crossing is optimal for log P values in the range 1.5–2.7 (Norinder and Haeberlein, 2002).
2. Log P alone (or log D if the pKa for ionizable drugs is taken into account) is not a good predictor of BBB crossing. The existence of such a relationship is strongly related to the composition of the organic phase and its ability to mimic various biological membrane. As an example, there was no relationship between log P and log BB in a set of 20 H2-receptor histamine antagonists (Young et al., 1988). However, a better correlation was found between log BB and log $P_{H/G}$ (heptane/glycol).
3. At the BBB level in vitro, the presence of P-gp decreases the apparent permeability of some lipophilic compounds with respect to a simple phospholipid membrane.

4. At the BBB level in vivo, all other extra-BBB parameters strongly influence the lipophilicity–transport relationships with respect to an isolated membrane system.

Lipophilicity, as determined by the partition coefficient, is a macroscopic observable reflecting the net result of all microscopic contributions involved in the partition process, i.e., the intermolecular and intramolecular forces which govern the solute transfer from one phase to another. These contributions are mainly the hydrophobic interactions, hydrogen-bonds, net charges, polarity, polarizability, aromaticity, and structural factors such as steric effects, tautomerism, and conformation states distribution.

4.1.2 Hydrogen-Bonding Potential

Pardridge suggested that drug uptake into the brain is related to its hydrogen (H)-bonding potential (Pardridge and Mietus, 1979). Indeed, the H-bond potential is inversely correlated to membrane partitioning because of a large energy penalty for breaking the H-bonds between the solute and the aqueous environment.

The influence of H-bond potential has been confirmed in many studies in which a better correlation with BBB permeation was found using $\Delta \log P$ or $\log P_{H/G}$, which reflects H-bond donor capacity (Young et al., 1988).

A very simple estimation of H-bond potential is the count of the number of H-bond donor (HBD) and H-bond acceptor (HBA) atoms. But the definitions of HBD and HBA are not so simple as it appears to vary with the software used. In some cases, it is confused with the count of nitrogen (#N) and oxygen (#O) atoms. Moreover, all H-bonds are not equivalent in terms of energy, geometry, and contribution to the transport process. The solvatochromic parameters $\Sigma \alpha^{H}_{2}$ (solute H-bond acidity) and $\Sigma \beta^{H}_{2}$ (solute H-bond basicity) have been used as a measure or an estimation of the H-bond potential (Abraham et al., 1994). The polar surface area (PSA), i.e., the part of the molecular surface area associated with oxygen, nitrogen, sulfur, and the hydrogens bonded to any of these atoms, is also clearly related to the H-bond potential. PSA has been popularized for the prediction of oral absorption (van de Waterbeemd et al., 1996; Palm et al., 1998) and then applied to BBB permeation models (van de Waterbeemd and Kansy, 1992; Calder and Ganellin, 1994; Clark, 1999; Hou and Xu, 2003). At least, a thermodynamic estimation of H-bonding potential leads to the calculation of the free-energy H-bond donor (C_d) and acceptor (C_a) factors, which was found to correlate better to cell permeability than $\Delta \log P$ (Raevsky and Schaper, 1998).

4.1.3 Number of Heteroatoms

The number of heteroatoms is directly related to the H-bonding potential, polarity, and therefore lipophilicity. Norinder states that molecules with less than five nitrogen and/or oxygen atoms have a high chance of entering the brain (Norinder and Haeberlein, 2002). A large majority of BBB+ compounds have been shown to have no more than nine heteroatoms in their structure. Conversely, most of the BBB− compounds have more than eight heteroatoms (Adenot and Lahana, 2004). The simple consideration of heteroatoms leads to 92% of well-classified compounds (94% for BBB+ and 81% for BBB−) in a large diverse database.

4.1.4 Charge

The molecular net charge depends on molecular pKa and environment pH. It is generally thought that charged species cannot cross a biological membrane. However, different studies have demonstrated that ions contribute to drug influx by various transport mechanisms. The presence of a charge at plasma pH should not be a cause of systematic rejection by a BBB model, and the charged compounds should be examined with caution. A simple decrease of the apical pH in Caco-2 studies leads to a better correlation with in vivo data (Van de Waterbeemd et al., 2001).

4.1.5 Molecular Weight

As with log P, there is no strict relationship between the MW and BBB permeation due to the fact that other favorable factors compensate for too large molecules in the passive diffusion pathway. Levin stated that compounds with significant permeability lies in the range 400–600 Da (Levin, 1980) even if a few exceptions have been noted. The MW only reflects parameters that are important for the diffusion process such as the molecular volume or the molecular size.

4.1.6 Consensus Set of Filters

Globally, a comparative study of CNS versus non-CNS shows that CNS drugs tend to be more lipophilic, more rigid, have fewer H-bond donors, fewer formal charges, and lower polar surface area. While the rules established by Lipinski mainly address the A of absorption (see *infra*), Norinder summarized five rules that specifically address the BBB permeation: $N1[(\#N + \#O) \leq 5]$; $N2[Clog\,P - (\#N + \#O) > 0]$; $N3[PSA < 90\,\text{Å}^2]$; $N4[MW < 450\,\text{Da}]$; and $N5[1 < \log D < 3]$

4.2   Theoritical Studies of the Different Transflux Components

4.2.1 Passive Diffusion Models

Theoritical Transport Models   Camenish (Camenish et al., 1998) demonstrates the equivalence of the two models for homogenous membranes two-step distribution model (van de Waterbeemd and Jansen, 1981) and the diffusional resistance model (De Haan and Jansen, 1985), expressing mathematically the bilinear relationship between permeability and lipophilicity:

$$\log P_e = b_{org} \cdot \log D - \bar{b} \cdot \log[1 + \beta \cdot D] + c,$$

where the two parameters b_{org} and $\bar{b}$ are the determinants for the shape of the curve.
Linear models of permeability–lipophilicity relationships are based on equations of the following type:

$$\log P_e = a_0 + a_1 \cdot \log P$$

$$\text{or,}\quad \log P_e = a_0 + a_1(X_1) + a_2(X_2) + \ldots + a_i(X_i) + \ldots + a_n(X_n),$$

where the X_I's are the different molecular descriptors used in the model. They are not frequently observed.
Nonlinear models of permeability–lipophilicity relationships are based on the description of permeability-related variables as a function of the distribution coefficient using multicompartment models. Depending on the models, the modeled variables may be:
−   The free-drug concentration variations in the monitored compartment (Kubinyi, 1979; Balaz, 2000); the models lead to bilinear equation of the general type:

$$\log C_{aq2} = A \cdot \log P^{\beta} + \Sigma B_i \cdot \log(1 + C_i \cdot P^{\beta}) + D$$

−   The flux through a barrier with thickness h_{ij} separating two phases i and j (Stehle and Higuchi, 1972):

$$J_{ij} = \frac{\overline{D_{ij}} \cdot (C_i - C_j)}{h_{ij}}$$

and the steady-state flux:

$$J = \frac{(C_i - C_j)}{\dfrac{h_{ij} + h_{kl}}{\overline{D}_{ij}} + \dfrac{h_{jk}}{P \cdot \overline{D}_{jk}}}$$

– The permeability coefficient:

$$\frac{1}{P_e} = \sum_i \frac{h_i}{\overline{D}_i \cdot P_i} \quad \text{(Flynn, 1972)}$$

or, $\quad \dfrac{1}{P_e} = \dfrac{\dfrac{\overline{D}_{aq}}{h_{aq}} + \dfrac{\overline{D}_{org}}{h_{org}} \cdot P}{\dfrac{\overline{D}_{org} \cdot \overline{D}_{aq}}{h_{aq}} \cdot P \cdot h_{org}} \quad$ (De Haan and Jansen, 1985)

The choice of the right models depends on the nature of the drug in terms of lipophilicity and amphiphilicity and are determinant for the transport kinetics (Balaz, 2000). The models have also been extended to membrane with pores (Camenish et al., 1998), but this is not of interest in the BBB field. As pointed out by Balaz, such models remain underutilized because the concept is only available as expert knowledge instead of easy-to-use software. However, many other various nonlinear models can help to describe the membrane permeation starting from molecular structure descriptors that differ from the partition coefficient.

$$\log P_e = f(X_1, X_2, \ldots, X_i, X_n)$$

Prediction of Drug Membrane Permeability
Qualitative Predictions   The four Lipinski's filters were aimed at detecting poor solubility and reflecting membrane permeability of drugs (Lipinski et al., 2001): L1 (MW < 500); L2 (Clog $P < 5$); L3 (HBD ≤ 5); and L4 (HBA ≤ 10). Many authors suggest the addition of the polar surface area as an additional determinant for membrane permeability (van de Waterbeemd et al., 1998; Kelder et al., 1999).

Quantitative Prediction by Conversion of N Filters into a Single Continuous Variable   In order to quantify the level of membrane permeability as defined by Lipinski filters, the filters above (L1–L4) have been transformed into a pseudocontinuous variable varying between 0 and 1 (❖ *Figure 6-3*). This variable called C_{diff} score is suitable for ranking structures, performing discriminant analysis, or computing regression models (Adenot and Lahana, 2004). C_{diff} expresses the level of permeation by passive diffusion: a C_{diff} value equal to 0 means that the membrane is totally impermeable to the compound; a C_{diff} value equal to 1 means that the membrane has permeability comparable to a simple porous membrane. The same operation can be applied to the five empirical rules from Norinder, namely N1–N5 (Norinder and Haeberlein, 2002), leading to a score reflecting the level of BBB permeation.

The Particular Case of Passive Diffusion for Peptides
The BBB is a major obstacle to the use of peptides as CNS therapeutic agents. Peptides have long been considered as unable to cross the BBB. The development of more sensitive analytical methods allows to highlight even low rates of penetration for some of them. Various findings have changed the vision of the BBB, and the discovery of peptide transporters leads to a more dynamic vision of the regulating interface between blood and brain. A certain number of physicochemical characteristics naturally prevent the translocation of peptides across BBB (Prokai, 1998): they are unstable, polar, lipid-insoluble compounds with a high-molecular weight. Moreover, they are characterized by a large number of H-bond donors due to the presence of their amide bonds. However, the existence of intramolecular H-bonds improve BBB crossing, and it also appears that some (rare) peptides are able to cross the BBB by a nonsaturable mechanism, i.e., passive diffusion: this is the case for the amphiphilic delta-sleep-inducing peptide (DSIP) and a dermorphin analog (Samii et al., 1994). It has been

□ **Figure 6-3**

The scaling function for each properties may be a plateau or a sigmoid shape function. The plateau function is defined by the slope a_i, the lower threshold t_i, and the upper threshold t_i'

$$f(L) = \begin{cases} 1 & \text{if } L_i > t_i' \\ a_i L + b_i & \text{if } t_i < L_i < t_i' \\ 0 & \text{if } L_i < t_i \end{cases}$$

The sigmoid function is naturally bounded between 0 and 1 and is applied over threshold-centered and scaled data (L'). It is simply defined by the parameter a with ($a > 0$) for a decreasing function of L' and ($a < 0$) for an increasing function of L':

$$f(L') = \frac{1}{1 + \exp(ax)}$$

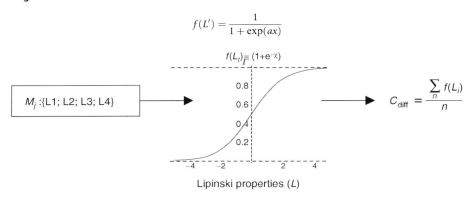

$$f(L_i) = \overline{F}\,(1 + e^{-x})$$

$$M_j : \{L1; L2; L3; L4\} \longrightarrow$$

$$C_{\text{diff}} = \frac{\sum_n f(L_i)}{n}$$

Lipinski properties (L)

suggested that desolvation energy of the polar amide bonds could be a determining factor for intestinal and BBB permeability to peptides (Chikhale et al., 1994).

Like for other drugs, a poor correlation between log P and membrane transport are common for peptides (Conradi et al., 1991, 1992). Some models of membrane permeability to peptides have been established from Caco-2 cells monolayers: it has been found that the permeability correlates with the polar surface area for di- and tripeptides (Stenberg et al., 1999) as well as Δlog P and log P[heptane/ethylene-glycol] (Chikhale et al., 1994). A structure–property model for membrane partitioning with phospholipids as the stationary phase was established for 20 tetrapeptides (Alifranjis et al., 2000). More recently, it has been demonstrated that some dipeptides are passively transported through artificial membranes under influence of H-bond capacity and lipophilicity (Ano et al., 2004). The transfer of acyclic enkephaline analogs from water to membrane has been shown to be an enthalpy driven process, three to seven times more efficient than the entropy-driven transfer of the corresponding cyclic analogs (Boguslavsky et al., 2003).

Explicit or continuum molecular dynamics simulation of bilayer systems allow to develop new theoretical models of peptide–membrane interactions, mainly electrostatic binding of Arg-rich peptides or insertion of amphipathic α-helices. The models are complex, time-consuming, and not routinely available for predictive aims.

4.2.2 Active Transport Models

The active transport pathway was shown to be an important determinant of the brain penetration (Tamai and Tsuji, 2000; Zhang et al., 2002), but the lack of data made this component of BBB transflux largely neglected in BBB models. The transported drugs are characterized by classical transport kinetic studies using parameters such as $V_{\max}$ (mol/min/cm^2), the limiting rate value at substrate saturation, and the Michaelis constant K_m (mM) (concentration of substrate at which the rate of reaction is equal to one half of the maximum rate $V_{\max}$). Imagery techniques can also been used to study the drug transport into the brain (Gruetter, 1996).

Even if some specific structure–transport relationships have been established for intestinal peptide transporters (Schoenmakers et al., 1999; Vabeno et al., 2004), a few systematic studies have been made for the main transporters at the BBB level. Amine drug transport has been investigated for serotonine and nontricyclic antidepressants (Chang, 1993) and later for noradrenaline (Foley, 2002) and dopamine transporter substrates (Vaughan, 1999; Chen, 2000; Appell, 2004). A recent quantitative structure–transport relationship study has been investigated in a series of adenosine A1 receptor agonists (Schaddelee et al., 2003). Pharmacokinetic simulations of drug transport have been established, including the active transport parameters (Mahar Doan and Boje, 2000). The knowledge of the transporter protein structure is not a prerequisite to structure–transport modeling, but structural data can help the interpretation of models. In the absence of structure–transport relationship studies for each homologous series of transported compounds, a simple and economic way to highlight potentially transported compounds in large libraries consists of detecting molecular patterns similar to already known transported molecules.

4.2.3 Transcytosis and Internalization Transport Models

This transport component is fundamental, especially, for the brain uptake of large hydrophilic molecules, such as peptides, proteins, and oligonucleotides, which are of major therapeutic interest.

A quantitative structure–activity relationships (QSAR) model for AMT has been proposed (Tamai et al., 1997; Wakamiya et al., 1998), which established optimal conditions of lipophilicity and cationic charge, independently of peptide length.

We have developed sequence–internalization relationships in order to describe the peptide brain uptake of cationic peptides via a transcytosis pathway. The rational design of optimized sequences is the foundation of the Pep:trans vectors technology to transport drugs across cellular membranes and biological barriers. The SynB peptides family is derived from the antimicrobial protegrin-1, a cell-penetrating peptide (Harwig et al., 1995). SynB3 has shown the ability to bypass the P-gp and transport doxorubicin in resistant K562 cells (Mazel et al., 2001) via an energy-dependent adsorptive-mediated endocytosis mechanism (Rousselle et al., 2001; Drin et al., 2002, 2003). The internalization ability of peptides has been optimized by computer-assisted molecular design. Moreover, the peptide internalization in J774 cell line has been found to correlate ($r = 0.84$) with K_{in} data from brain perfusion study and has been used as a potential predictor for BBB permeation (❯ *Figure 6-4*).

◻ **Figure 6-4**
Relationships between log K_{in} and log (Uptake) in a series of 17 peptide derivatives for K562 (*left*) and J744 (*right*) cell lines

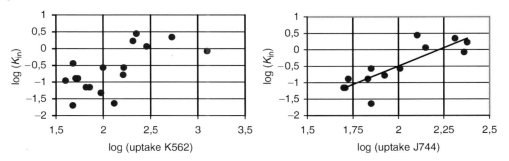

An internalization model has been obtained from 30 peptides, which were D-optimally designed to explore the descriptor space around the reference peptide SynB3. A multiple regression model has been derived using the number of positive charges (CH) and the HPLC retention time (RT), which is related to the hydrophobicity for peptides. The peptide internalization is related to the mean fluorescence intensity

(MFI) into the cell.

$$\log MFI = 1.387 + 0.503 \times \langle CH \rangle + 0.32 \times \langle RT \rangle$$
$$R^2 = 0.82; \quad R^2(\text{cross} - \text{validated}) = 0.79.$$

A PLS model of peptide internalization derived from Z-scales has been successfully used to help the design of a refined peptide vector library under cytotoxicity constraints (❯ *Figure 6-5*): Z-scales are artificial

❏ **Figure 6-5**
Uptake data modeling using the Z-scale

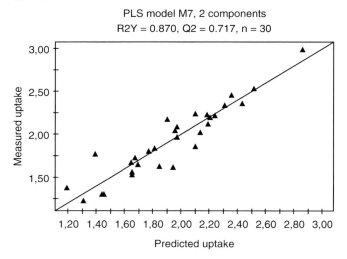

variables, which summarize 29 diverse physicochemical properties for the 20 coded amino acids, reflecting hydrophobicity, size, and electronic properties (Hellberg et al., 1987). They can be easily extended to nonnatural amino acids.

4.2.4 Active Efflux Transport Models

It is highly desirable to predict the P-gp profile of a future drug, either in a CNS-screening perspective or to target P-gp dysfunctions associated with CNS diseases. The therapeutic use of P-gp blockers on a long timescale is debatable because of the major risk of brain toxicity due to the CNS penetration of xenobiotics and impredictible pharmacokinetic variations of cotreatment during P-gp inhibition. The prediction of the P-gp profile of a drug is complicated by the confusion between transported drugs (substrates) and inhibitors, all the more so since substrates may be inhibitors or activators and the P-gp status is in some cases concentration dependent in relation with the passive diffusion ability. The existence of multiple drug-binding sites has been proposed to account for the broad substrate specificities for P-gp (Zhang et al., 2002) implying competitive, noncompetitive, cooperative, and anticooperative allosteric interactions.

In the absence of structural models, it is not well understood how a single protein-like P-gp recognizes and transports so many chemically diverse substrates. The only common structural denominator for substrates seems to be the presence of spatially separated hydrophilic and hydrophobic moieties.

Source of P-gp Efflux Transport Data Each compound can be classified using two classification schemes: the P-gp substrate (P-GP+)/nonsubstrate (P-GP−) classification refers to the affinity of a compound for one of the P-gp-binding site and/or its ability to be effluxed by P-gp; it should be noticed that some nontransported P-gp substrates are also known to be P-gp inducers or P-gp inhibitors (also called MDR reversal agents). Alternatively, the P-gp inhibitor/noninhibitor classification refers to the ability of a compound to inhibit the P-gp efflux transport, independently of any P-gp transport.

Original Quantitative Datasets Twenty-three original datasets from heterogeneous sources, each derived from structurally related compounds, are listed in a review (Stouch and Gudmundsson, 2002).

The P-gp substrate/nonsubstrate classification scheme is based on in vitro measures of P-gp-associated ATPase activity (Litman et al., 1997; Seelig and Landwojtowicz, 2000; Boulton et al., 2002) or the substrate affinity to the verapamil binding site (Doppenschmitt et al., 1999; Neuhoff et al., 2000) or the ratio of efflux to influx apparent permeabilities in monolayer models (Gombar et al., 2004). In vitro efflux studies have also been undertaken on cell suspensions, membrane vesicles, and confluent cell monolayers (Fenart et al., 1998; Parkinson et al., 2003). In vivo, the efflux transport is evaluated by the brain efflux index method (Kakee et al., 1996) or imaging of P-gp kinetics with specific tracers like $[^{11}C]$-verapamil (Luurtsema et al., 2003). The methods can be applied to wild-type, mutant, or transgenic animal models deficient in the expression of drug efflux transporters.

P-gp inhibitors (or MDR reversal agents) have been studied in various structurally related series like phenothiazines (Ford et al., 1989; Ramu and Ramu, 1992), thioxanthenes, propafenone analogs (Chiba et al., 1996; Ecker et al., 1999), and ciclosporin analogs (Loor et al., 2002). The P-gp inhibition is classically measured by IC50 values. In the Ramu standard test system, the MDR reversal activity is estimated by the ratio of ED50 in a cell-growth rate inhibition assay for cells in the presence and absence of adriamycine, respectively. Experimental data on about 20 compounds have been determined for four different types of activity such as inhibition of digoxin transport, inhibition of vinblastine binding to plasma membrane vesicles from multidrug resistant cell line, inhibition of vinblastine, and calcein accumulation into P-gp-expressing cells (Ekins et al., 2002).

Original Qualitative Datasets Ninety-eight compounds have been tested in a monolayer efflux assay and classified as P-gp substrates or nonsubstrates (Polli et al., 2001; Mahar Doan et al., 2002).

Compilations of Qualitative Data One of the major issue, in particular if classification models are used, is the lack of negative data. A hundred of compounds, evaluated for their potential as P-gp substrates, have been compiled from various literature sources and classified into four classes: borderline P-gp substrates, P-gp substrates, P-gp inducers, and no-substrates (Seelig, 1998). A heterogeneous compilation of relative brain level ratios for 22 drugs in P-gp knockout mice and wild-type mice has also been proposed (Ayrton and Morgan, 2001). The first published large library of P-gp agents contained 609 compounds (Klopman, 1997), mostly based upon Ramu's work. A large compilation of 1000 compounds, both substrates and nonsubstrates, has been recently proposed (Didziapetris et al., 2003).

P-gp Substrate Models
P-gp Substrates Pharmacophore Models Early attempts to characterize structural features of P-gp-interacting drugs have been performed on homologous series so that pharmacophores were established only for a limited number of chemical families. It has been noted that P-gp substrates are often lipophilic and possess aromatic ring systems and/or a tertiary nitrogen atom positively charged at physiological pH (Zamora et al., 1988; Pearce et al., 1990; Klopman et al., 1992; Ahkmed et al., 1995). The first attempt to derive a general pharmacophore for P-gp substrate recognition led to a couple of general patterns based on electron-donor groups with a fixed spatial separation based on a hundred of structurally unrelated compounds (Seelig, 1998). Starting from Seelig compounds, a further study based on an extended dataset allowed to derive a multiple pharmacophore model supporting the importance of H-bonding potential, aimed at detecting various chemotypes (Penzotti et al., 2002). Another model, especially derived for compounds related to the verapamil-binding site, led to a six-point-pharmacophore model involving hydrophobic groups and H-bonds donors and acceptors (Pajeva and Wiese, 2002).

P-gp Substrate Classification-Based Models The multiple pharmacophore model has been used as a screening filter to discriminate between substrates (which match at least 20 pharmacophores) and nonsubstrates (Penzotti et al., 2002). More recently, a discriminant analysis has been performed using 254 descriptors, of which 27 were found significant (mainly atom counts and electrotopological states) (Gombar et al., 2004). This analysis based on 95 compounds led to a high rate of well-predicted compounds. The rate of prediction decreased for nonsubstrates in the validation set: in fact, it is common that the P-GP+ prediction performs better than P-GP− using physicochemical parameters as filters, due to the the sparse distribution of P-GP+ compounds within the descriptor space. The classification analysis of P-gp substrate specificity has pointed out the role of molecular size, H-bond capacity, and ionization given by the pKa values (Didziapetris et al., 2003). Authors derived a set of rule for P-gp substrates on the model of the Lipinski filters: P1 $[(N + O) \geq 8]$; P2 (MW > 400); P3 (acid pKa > 4). A $C_{P\text{-}gp}$ score may be derived from P1 to P3 in the same way than the C_{diff} score is derived from Lipinski filters. A recent PLS-DA model allowed a classification based on only one PLS score upon a large compound selection (Adenot and Lahana, 2004): in this model, again, the rate of well-predicted is lower for P-GP+ compounds but the dipole and polarizability components have been shown to increase significantly the prediction for this class (◗ *Table 6-1*).

◼ Table 6-1
P-gp substrates classification models results

Reference	Filters	n	% well-predicted P-GP+	% well-predicted P-GP−
Penzotti et al. (2002)	>20	144 51[a]	64 53	96 79
Gombar et al. (2004)	27	95 58[a]	100 94	99 74
Adenot and Lahana (2004)	1	1.600 88[a]	74 70	96 92

[a]Validation set

P-gp Substrates Regression-Based Models First regression model has been derived using 11 unrelated compounds for which the kinetic parameters of P-gp ATPase have been measured. It highlights the role of the number and strength of H-bonds in V_{max} values. A PLS model based on the 22 compounds from Litman (P-gp ATP-ase activity) pointed out the role of molecular surface area, polarizability, and H-bonding for P-gp activation (Osterberg and Norinder, 2000a, b). Then, a regression model based on the same dataset led to different regression equations aimed for subsets of closely related structures, where molecular size and polarity are key variables (Dearden et al., 2003). The specificity of Dearden study is that, unlike most others, there was little importance given to H-bonding and hydrophobicity. It was also found that dipole moment vectors are significant for P-gp activation, in accordance with previous results from the PLS-DA model (Adenot and Lahana, 2004).

P-gp Inhibitors Models

P-gp Inhibitors Pharmacophore Models The numerous studies establishing the structural features for P-gp inhibitors from various homologous chemical series largely overlap the more general studies for P-gp substrates (vide supra). A large-scale original approach was the application of MULTICASE procedure in order to detect substructural features in a 609 compounds database: this approach led to the identification of 35 biophores (Klopman, 1997). Four pharmacophore models aimed at detecting specific inhibitors of digoxin transport and vinblastin binding have also been proposed (Ekins et al., 2002).

P-gp Inhibitors Classification-Based Models A discriminant analysis based on 220 various descriptors (on which six to nine topological parameters are found significant) was performed using the 609 compounds of the Klopman dataset (Bakken and Jurs, 2000).

P-gp Inhibitors Regression-Based Models   A Free-Wilson analysis (Pajeva and Wiese, 1997) was performed on phenothiazines and thioxanthenes from the Ford dataset and led to optimized substituent sets for these two series. A further ComFA analysis on the same dataset confirmed the role of hydrophobic field to explain the MDR reversal activity (Pajeva and Wiese, 1998). A regression model for 12 propafenone derivatives pointed out the importance of H-bonds acceptor strength (Ecker et al., 1999). QSAR models based on the datasets of Ramu (MDR reversal activity for 157 phenothiazines) and Ayrton (brain level ratio between wild-type and MDR knockout mice for 22 unrelated drugs) led to different regression equations aimed for subsets of closely related structures, where molecular size and polarity are key variables (Dearden et al., 2003). The conclusions are very similar to those found for P-gp substrates.

4.3   In Silico BBB Models

4.3.1   Source of Data

Data sources include large databases, such as MDDR, CMC, WDI, and CISPLINE, where compounds are classified by therapeutic class. No specific information on BBB is generally given, but the CNS penetration is deduced from the pharmacological activity. Conversely, small homogenous series taken from literature provide either qualitative or quantitative data. Experimental data are rare and often questionable but have the merit to exist. A strong emphasis must be placed upon the quality of the data sets, for example, validation sets are not systematically used for external validation of the models. The selection of compounds in the training set delineates a domain of validity of the model. Informative, large, and diverse training sets are a prerequisite for models used for high-throughput screening purposes.

Original Qualitative Datasets   Qualitative data are based on the CNS+/CNS− classification. An initial set of 28 compounds (Seelig et al., 1994) has been extended to 53 compounds (Fischer et al., 1998) and 125 compounds (Van de Waterbeemd et al., 1998) based on their CNS activity. Another dataset of 40 structurally related opioid drugs (Giardina et al., 1995) has been characterized by comparing their antinociceptive potency in the mouse abdominal constriction test after s.c. or i.c.v. administration. This set, completed to 44 compounds, has been used in a QSAR study (Crivori et al., 2000).

   The first large-scale library of CNS-focusing compounds included 15,000 active and 50,000 inactive compounds extracted from CMC and the MDDR databases (Ajay et al., 1999). The claimed objective was not BBB modeling but the design of a CNS-oriented library. Other large datasets extracted from databases have been suggested (Doniger et al., 2002; Engkvist et al., 2003; Adenot and Lahana, 2004).

Original Quantitative Datasets   Little experimental studies have been published, resulting in a poor amount of experimental data suitable for modeling. Large screening studies are mostly funded by private companies and the data remain confidential. However, a few original published datasets, although rather poor in structural diversity, are used from authors to authors.

   Available in vivo permeability data in rats are restricted to the measure of brain capillary permeability coefficients of 20 drugs (Levin, 1980) and the more recent measure of PS products in rats for 18 compounds (Gratton et al., 1997). Log BB in anesthetized rat is more widely used, even if questionable as a predictor of CNS penetration. Experimental values generally lie in the range -2 to $+1$. Molecules with log $BB < (-1)$ are considered as poorly distributed to the brain. The first original data set consisted of 30 log BB values determined by a radioassay method in rats for H2-receptor histamine antagonists (Young et al., 1988). This set was completed up to 65 compounds to increase the structural diversity (Abraham et al., 1994) with in vitro log BB values estimated from air-brain and air-blood partition coefficients. Although heterogeneous by nature and due to the presence of nondrug molecules, the Abraham set has been extensively used by other authors.

   Other in vitro datasets have been based on a measure of cultured cell permeabilities for 9 anti-HIV agents (Glynn and Yazdanian, 1998), 93 drugs (Mahar-Doan, 2002), and on the surface activity data for 37 compounds (Seelig et al., 1994).

Compilation of Quantitative Data   Many papers provide isolated log BB values for particular compounds. This has been the start of literature compilation leading to structurally diverse and heterogeneous datasets (Salminen, 1997; Kaznessis et al., 2001; Keseru and Molnar, 2001; Platts et al., 2001; Ooms et al., 2002; Rose et al., 2002; Lobell et al., 2003). Quantitative models based on a compilation of heterogeneous experimental data should be considered with caution, because of the interlab discrepancies. As an example, imipramine log BB can vary from 0.83 (Young et al., 1998) to 1.30 (Salminem, 1998) and progesterone permeabilities vary from 116×10^6 cm/s (Glynn and Yazdanian, 1998) to 88.5×10^4 cm/s (Shah et al., 1989) depending on the different experimental conditions.

4.3.2 Review of Published Models

A relevant selection of molecular descriptors related to ADME properties and membrane permeation are supposed to give a rational basis to the intuitive and empirical rules governing the passage across biological barriers. It is generally expected that the models become an in-house high-throughput virtual screening tool and, as such, rely upon rapidly calculable molecular descriptors. However, models can also be developed from 3D descriptors derived from conformational analysis. From a practical standpoint, the failure of certain molecular descriptors computation makes the equations impossible to use in virtual-screening applications.

❷ *Tables 6-2* and ❷ *6-3* provide a summary of the main published BBB models up to date with their main characteristics. Equations and algorithms are available in the mentioned references. Most of them are immediately operational, at least, if the molecular description can be computed in the same conditions than the published work in terms of chemical entity definition, software version, and software customization if any.

The modeling techniques used by authors are essentially regression-based techniques (R), partial least square modeling (PLS), discriminant analysis (DA), and neural networks (NN).

Regression-Based Models   These models are based either on simple/multiple regressions or PLS regression. A large number of published equations are now available. Many of these equations are based on more or less complex parameters, sometimes computed from *in-house* software hardly useable by other teams.

Classification-Based Models   Some parameters have been suggested to classify the compounds into the CNS+/CNS− classes with a high rate of prediction (❷ *Table 6-4*). This is the case for the two first PCA components or PLS latent variables derived from 72 3D-descriptors (Crivori et al., 2000), the solvation free-energy (Keseru and Molnar, 2001), 92 atom-types, or a score resulting from substructural analysis (Engkvist et al., 2003).

Discriminant models have been derived, starting from 104 descriptors (on which five to six are found to be significant) and 28 compounds (Basak et al., 1996). A set of discriminant models have been suggested for six different parameter blocks: ADME, geometry, topology, electronic, energy, and surface areas (Adenot and Lahana, 2004). The analysis has been performed on a complete dataset (including P-gp substrates) and a restrained dataset (excluding P-gp substrates). This extensive analysis highlighted the importance of ADME and surface areas parameter blocks with respect to the other blocks for the discrimination between CNS+ and CNS− classes. It is noteworthy that into the ADME block the number of heteroatoms alone led to 92% well-classified compounds.

PLS-DA Based Models   PLS scores derived from 3D parameters in a two-class model have been used as discriminant parameters with a relatively poor level of prediction for CNS− compounds (Crivori et al., 2000). It is a common observation that CNS− are less well-predicted than CNS+ compounds, due to the issue of undetermined status of some drugs included in CNS− by default.

A discriminant equation based on a single parameter like C_{diff} or PLS score has led to high rates of prediction, comparable to those obtained with the ADME and surface areas blocks (Adenot and Lahana, 2004). C_{diff} values are highly correlated to PLS-predicted BBB score values.

Table 6-2
Quantitative models

Year	Reference	Model type	MW, MV	log P	H-bonds	Other parameters	Softwares	Data source	n
1980	Levin	R	✓	Literature				–	22
1988	Young	R	✓	Exp	$\Delta\log P$	PSA**, polarity	SAVOL	–	20
1992	Waterbeemd	R	✓	Exp	$\Delta\log P$	PSA**	MACROMODEL	Y	20
1994	Calder	R	✓	Exp	$\Delta\log P$	$\pi^H_2, V_X, R_2{}^*$		Y+M	25
	Abraham	R			$\Sigma\alpha^H_2, \Sigma\beta^H_2$ $\Sigma\beta^O_2$			Y+M	57
1996	Lombardo	R				Solvation free-energy	AMSOL	A	57
								M	6[a]
1997	Salminen	R	✓	Literature		Nitrogen (0/1) – log K(IAM)		M	26
	Gratton	R		Med Chem	$\Sigma\alpha^H_2, \Sigma\beta^H_2$	$\pi^H_2, V_X, R_2{}^*$		Gratton	18
1998	Norinder	PLS				3D parameters	MOLSURF	A	28
								A	29[a]
1999	Luco	PLS	✓		#HBD #HBA	Topology #Nitrogen Acid (0/1), sulphur (0/1)	MOLCONN-X	A+M	61
								M	39[a]
	Clark	R		Clog P Mlog P		PSA**	Polarsa2	A	57
								A[a]	7[a]
								Lombardo[a]	6[a]
2001	Keserü	R/NN		log P/ACD	#HBD(N + O)		GB/SA	A+M	60
2000	Osterberg	PLS			#HBA(N) #HBA(O)	Solvation free-energy		Clark	70
								Kelder	45
	Feher	R		log P/ACD	#HBA	PSA**	MOE	L	61
								L[a]	39[vs]

◻ **Table 6-2 (continued)**

Year	Reference	Model type	MW, MV	log P	H-bonds	Other parameters	Softwares	Data source	n
2001	Liu	R/NN				E-topology		A	57
	Platts	R			$\Sigma\alpha_2^H, \Sigma\beta_2^H$	π_2^H, V_X, R_2^*		Clark[a]	13[a]
	Jorgensen	R				SA**		M	148
	Kaznessis	R	✓		#HBD	SA**, dipole moment	SAVOL	A+Kelder	105
					#HBA	Solute–solvent interaction energies		A+L+Kelder	85
2002	Rose	R				E-topology	MOLCONN-Z	M	86
								M	20[a]
								Med Chem	2003 9[a]
2003	Ooms	PLS	✓			3D parameters	VOLSURF	M	83
	Hou	R		Slog P	#HBD #HBA	SA**	MSMS	M	78
	Lobell	R	✓	Clog P Alog P98	#HBD #HBA	Molar refractivity PSA**, topology, #Rot pKa	PCMODEL CERIUS2	M M Crivori+Platts	37[a] 48 150
	Hutter	R				Quantum parameters	ACD VAMP	M M	17[a] 90
2004	Subramanian	PLS		Alog P	#HBA	SA**	CERIUS2	M	23[a]
	Sun	PLS				E-topology, #Rot Atom-type classification		L L[a] A	61 39[a] 57
	Fu	NN	✓			Net atomic charges of O and N H-bonds		Clark[a] A Lombardo[a]	13[a] 56 5[a]

The modeled variable is log BB (except Levin, where the variable modeled is log P_e and Gratton, where the variable modeled is log PS). It is examined as a function of molecular weight (MW) or molecular volume (MV), log P, various H-bond parameters, and other parameters. The main data source are Young (Y), Abraham (A), Luco (L), or miscellaneous (M).
[a]Validation set
*Abraham parameters: π_2^H dipolarity/polarizability, V_X volume of MacGowann, R_2 excess molar refraction
**Surface parameters: SA surface areas, PSA polar surface area

■ Table 6-3
Qualitative models based on a binary classification (CNS+/CNS−)

Year	Reference	Model type	MW, MV	log P	H-bonds	Other parameters	Softwares	Data source	n
1996	Basak	DA		Clog P	H-bond (in-house)	Topology	POLLY	S	28
1997	Waterbeemd	Filters	✓	Med Chem	HYBOT	Size, shape Surface activity (exp)	MOLOC	S+M	125
1998	Fischer	Filters				Surface activity (exp)		S+M	53
1999	Luco	PLS-DA	✓		#HBD	Topology	MOLCONN-X	S+M	27[a]
	Ajay	NN			#HBA	#Nitrogen Acid (0/1), Sulphur (0/1) Substructural keys	ISIS	CMC+MDDR MDDR	65000 275[a]
2000	Crivori	PCA PLS-DA				3D parameters	VOLSURF	Giardina M	44 108[a]
2001	Keserü	R/NN		Databases	#HBD	Solvation free-energies	GB/SA	CISPLINE	8.700[vs]
2002	Doniger	NN	✓		#HBA	Hydrophilic-lipophilic Balance PSA** (Literature)		M	324
	Rose	R			$\Sigma\alpha^H_2$, $\Sigma\beta^H_2$	E-topology π^H_2, V_X, R_2*	MOLCONN-Z	Crivori	108[a]
	Mahar-Doan	Filters	✓	Clog P Clog D	#HBD #HBA	SA**, charges			
2003	Engkvist	NN SSA				92 atom-types Substructural keys	SUBSTRUCT	WDI WDI	8678 8678
	Hutter	R				Quantum parameters	VAMP	S	24[a]
	Subramanian	PLS-DA		Alog P	#HBA	SA**, E-topology, #Rot	CERIUS2	M M	61[a] 181[a]
2004	Adenot	DA PLS-DA	✓	Alog P	#HBD #HBA	Geometry, topology Quantum parameters SA**	TSAR VAMP MOLCAD	WDI Crivori[a]	1696 82[a]

The belonging to each class is examined as a function of molecular weight (MW) or molecular volume (MV), log P, various H-bond parameters, and other parameters. The main data source are Seelig (S) or miscellaneous (M)

[a] Validation set

* Abraham parameters: π^H_2 dipolarity/polarizability, V_X volume of MacGowann, R_2 excess molar refraction

** Surface parameters: SA surface areas, PSA polar surface area

◘ Table 6-4
BBB classification-based models results

Reference	Filters	n	% well-predicted CNS+	% well-predicted CNS–
Basak et al. (1996)	5–6	28	100	91
Ajay et al. (1999)	7	>70000	75	65
	174	>70000	83	79
		275[a]	92	71
Crivori et al. (2000)	2	108	90	65
Keser and Molnar (2001)	1	8700	96	n.d.
Doniger et al. (2002)	9	324	83	80
Engkvist et al. (2003)	92	8678	83	77
	1	8678	83	71
Adenot and Lahana (2004)	1	1696	92	78
	(C_{diff})	1605[*]	95	84
		8[a]	90	95
	1	1696	97	73
	(BBB_{pred})	1605[*]	99	89
		82[a]	90	92

[a]Validation set
[*]91 P-gp substrates excluded from models

4.3.3 Composite Models

Although experimental data used to derive models intrinsically encode for active transport components, if any, most BBB models to date rely on passively transported compounds without efflux component, neglecting alternative pathways and excluding drugs with particular mechanisms of transport. We have recently suggested a two-component model for conventional small organic molecules, including P-gp substrates, based on the idea that the predicted BBB permeation is a compromise between the efflux and the influx components (Adenot and Lahana, 2004). The use of composite models accounting for different transport components via their expression onto a continuous scale or a [0–1] range allows to allocate specific weighting coefficients to each transport component (❯ *Figure 6-6*). As an example, $BBB_{pred.}$ or C_{diff} scores reflect passive diffusion (DIF model) while P-gp$_{pred}$ is an estimate of P-gp efflux (P-gp model) (❯ *Figure 6-7*).

For composite classification-based models, the predicted class is the logical result of all transport components classes. Neglecting the fact that some P-gp substrates may also be CNS compounds, it can be written as follows:

$$\text{BBB+} = [(\text{DIF+}) \cap (\text{ACT+}) \cap (\text{TRA+})] \cup (\text{PGP–})$$
$$\text{BBB–} = [(\text{DIF–}) \cup (\text{ACT–}) \cup (\text{TRA–})] \cap (\text{PGP+})$$

CNS-Maps   A CNS-map consists of a plot of two quantitative BBB transport component variables. A CNS-map, including a hundred of P-gp substrates, has been proposed as a powerful tool for CNS drug virtual screening (Adenot and Lahana, 2004): three categories of scores (namely, C_{diff}, BBB_{pred}, and P-gp$_{pred}$) have been suggested to express the level of permeation within a continuous scale, starting from a two-class dataset (BBB+/BBB–). This operation allows the degree to which each compound belongs to an activity class to be given using a membership score. All the compounds are characterized by their passive diffusion component (BBB_{pred} or C_{diff}) and P-gp efflux component (P-gp$_{pred.}$). The application of the composite model to about 1800 CNS+/CNS– compounds have highlighted three distinct regions limited by thresholds $\tau(\text{P-gp})$ and $\tau(C_{diff})$ (❯ *Figure 6-8*):

◘ Figure 6-6
Double optimization of internalization Y (*left*) and cytotoxicity (*right*) in a peptide vector Pep:trans library: the DL50 (in a K562 cell line assay) is plotted as a function of Retention time and cell uptake in logarithmic units. The curve is a representation of the analytical surface, interpolating all the data points. The dark area at the bottom represents the surface related to the peptides with the highest cytotoxicity. The dark area at the top is the surface for the lowest cytotoxicity

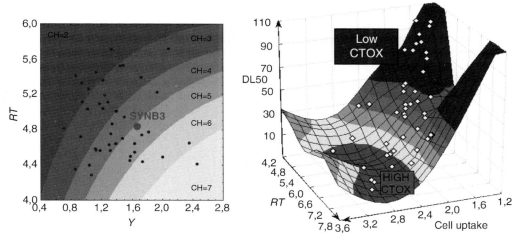

$$\text{P-GP+ drugs: P-gp} > \tau(\text{P-gp}) = 0.14$$

$$\text{BBB+ drugs: P-gp} < \tau(\text{P-gp}) = 0.3 \text{ and } C_{\text{diff}} > \tau(C_{\text{diff}}) = 0.4$$

$$\text{BBB- drugs: P-gp} < \tau(\text{P-gp}) = 0.3 \text{ and } C_{\text{diff}} < \tau(C_{\text{diff}}) = 0.4$$

The CNS profile of individual drugs can be easily compared component by component using the appropriate threshold for detecting good candidates in a database (❯ *Figure 6-9*, ❯ *Figure 6-10*). Molecules, such as morphine, chlorpromazine, disulfiram, or amitryptiline, are in the P-GP+/BBB+ border area, reflecting the clinical fact that some in vitro P-gp substrates may also be CNS drugs anyway. Moreover, the few drugs that are BBB+, although they stand in the low-diffusion score area, are precisely drugs that benefit from active transport with specific transporters, i.e., amino acids like adenosyl methionine or vitamins like folic acid, cobalamine, and thiamine derivatives.

Scaled CNS-Maps A previous standardization of scores S by an appropriate scaling function allows to express the data values into the range $[0–1]$ and to center the discriminant threshold values at 0.5 by translation.

$$\begin{array}{ll} \text{if } S + (0.5 - \tau) > 1 & \\ \text{if } 0 < S + (0.5 - \tau) < 1 & f(S) \begin{cases} = 1 \\ = S + (0.5 - \tau) \\ = 0 \end{cases} \\ \text{if } S + (0.5 - \tau) < 0 & \end{array}$$

While the two components of the model are expressed in a comparable scale, the estimated BBB permeation level (P_e-score) for diffusible compounds may be obtained by orthogonal projections of compounds onto the CNS-map diagonal relatively to the magnitude of the diagonal vector $\overrightarrow{\Delta}$ (i.e., $\sqrt{2}$ for a unity square) (❯ *Figure 6-11*):

☐ **Figure 6-7**

A composite BBB model taking into account the various transport components in BBB permeation. The assumption that P-gp substrates leads to the absence of BBB permeation, hence non-CNS drugs, is supposed to be true as long as the efflux pump is not saturated (i.e., at a normal level of drug concentration). At appropriate plasma concentration level, a P-GP+ drug may pass through the BBB (e.g., morphine, chlorproma-zine, disulfiram, or amitryptiline)

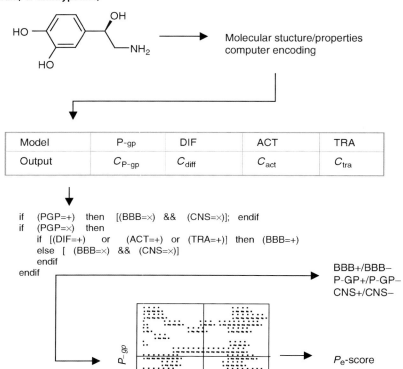

Model	P-gp	DIF	ACT	TRA
Output	C_{P-gp}	C_{diff}	C_{act}	C_{tra}

```
if   (PGP=+)  then  [(BBB=×)  &&  (CNS=×)];  endif
if   (PGP=×)  then
     if [(DIF=+)   or   (ACT=+)  or  (TRA=+)] then  (BBB=+)
     else [ (BBB=×)  &&  (CNS=×)]
     endif
endif
```

BBB+/BBB−
P-GP+/P-GP−
CNS+/CNS−

P_e-score

Passive diffusion

$$P_e\text{-}score = \frac{\text{Proj}_\perp (M_i)}{\left\| \overrightarrow{\Delta} \right\|} = \frac{\left\| \overrightarrow{OM_i} \right\|}{\sqrt{2}} \cos \theta$$

P_e-score values lies below 0.5 each time the efflux component exceeds the diffusion component and are associated with a poor brain penetration. At the opposite, P_e-score values over 0.5 reflects a diffusion/efflux ratio in favor of brain penetration. About 1800 P_e-scores of WDI drugs have been computed within our model showing a good agreement with in vitro and clinical data (❷ *Table 6-5*). The P_e-scores combines both diffusion and efflux terms and significantly increase the number of BBB− compounds with respect to the diffusion term alone (❷ *Table 6-6*). CNS-maps can be easily extended to N-dimensions, including K_m/V_{max} values for active transport or log(MFI) values for transcytosis or any other suitable transport predictor.

◻ **Figure 6-8**
A two-component composite model for conventional small organic molecules, based on the passive diffusion
(DIF model) and the P-gp efflux component (P-gp model)

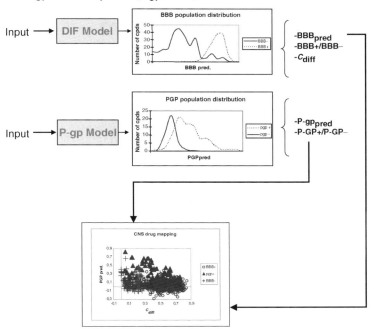

◻ **Figure 6-9**
A CNS-map of 1.691 WDI drugs based on DIF-model and P-gp-model. The compounds are grouped within three
clusters (BBB+, BBB−, and P-GP+). P-GP+ compounds could be either BBB+ or BBB−, showing the practical
interest of CNS-maps for the detection of drugs with CNS clinical incidence

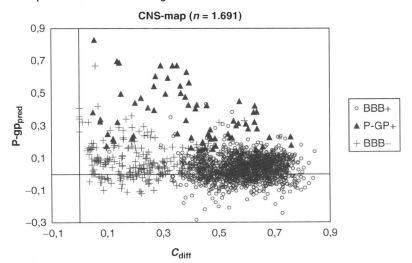

☐ **Figure 6-10**
Comparison of two molecules after prediction with the composite two-components model: a CNS-drug, such as the general anesthetics enflurane, shows low-P-gp efflux and high-passive diffusion (DIF) components. Conversely, a non-CNS drug, such as teniposide, exhibits a high-efflux level and a low-diffusion component

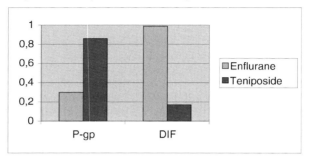

☐ **Figure 6-11**
Projection of compounds onto the CNS-map diagonal. The CNS-map is divided in four domain: (I) High-diffusion/low-efflux in the *lower-right* quarter; (II) High-diffusion/high-efflux in the *upper-right* quarter; (III) Low-diffusion/high-efflux in the *upper-left* quarter; (IV) Low-diffusion/low-efflux in the *lower-left* quarter. The BBB permeation is maximal in area I

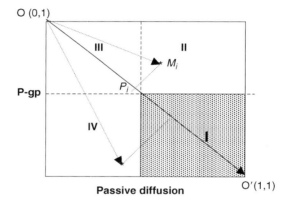

4.4   Commercial Solutions for BBB Predictions

4.4.1   C².ADME/Tox (Accelrys) (www.accelrys.com)

This package of six predictive ADME/Tox models includes a BBB penetration model based on the calculation of properties like log P (Alog $P98$) and FPSA. Two BBB models were developed: a robust regression based on over 120 compounds ($R^2 = 0.889$) or a BBB confidence ellipse derived over 800 CNS+ compounds: molecules outside the BBB confidence ellipse are predicted to have extremely poor log BB. The predicted value is either log BB ratio or a categorical level of BBB penetration scored from 0 to 4.

4.4.2   QikProp (Schrödinger) (www.schrodinger.com)

QikProp includes an automated linear regression package (QikFit) and a similarity program (QikSim) that sorts candidates based on their similarity to a lead molecule (Duffy and Jorgensen, 2000; Jorgensen and

◻ Table 6-5

Some examples of model outputs for known drugs

	DIF substratet	P-gp substrate	P_e-score	CNS domain
Atropine	0.88	0.48	0.70	I
Amphetamine	1.00	0.34	0.83	I
Paracetamol	0.95	0.36	0.80	I
Fluoxetine	1.00	0.48	0.76	I
Modafinil	0.86	0.46	0.70	I
Zolpidem	0.83	0.39	0.72	I
Enflurane	1.00	0.30	0.85	I
Morphine	0.87	0.51	0.68	II
Itraconazole	0.65	0.83	0.41	II
Quinine	0.91	0.71	0.60	II
Levofloxacine	0.67	0.64	0.51	II
Astemizole	0.85	0.63	0.61	II
Nadolol	0.68	0.60	0.54	II
Doxorubicin	0.13	0.61	0.13	III
Teniposide	0.17	0.86	0.17	III
Vinblastine	0.35	0.83	0.35	III
Paclitaxel	0.14	0.92	0.14	III
Digoxine	0.19	0.70	0.19	III
Amphotericin B	0.00	0.61	0.00	III
Ivermectine	0.18	0.57	0.18	III
Teicoplanine	0.00	0.71	0.00	III
Aztreonam	0.15	0.24	0.45	IV
Dibekacine	0.03	0.32	0.35	IV
Gentamicin	0.13	0.36	0.39	IV
Idarubicin	0.29	0.43	0.43	IV

◻ Table 6-6

Composite blood-brain barrier permeation model

Variable entering	Fraction of BBB− well classified	Fraction of P-GP− well classified	Fraction of BBB+ well classified	Fraction of P-GP+ well classified
C_{diff}	0.73		0.97	
P-gp score		0.96		0.74
P_e-score	0.84		0.97	

Discriminant analysis including P-gp substrates (cross-validation method: leaving out each of 3 groups in turn)

Duffy, 2000). BBB predictions are based on the calculation of several 2D and 3D descriptors (number of chemical moieties, MW, surface areas, dipole moment, dipole solvation index, ionization potential, electron affinity ...). QikProp also compare compound properties with those of known drug structures in order to detect non-druglike candidates or to suggest likely metabolic processes. It is suitable to HTS (150,000 structures/h).

4.4.3 VolSurf (Tripos) (www.tripos.com)

VolSurf is described as a computational procedure to compress the information present in 3D molecular interaction maps into a few 2D simple numerical descriptors, which are suitable to predict ADME properties, including BBB (Crivori et al., 2000). Data are analyzed by using multivariate statistics coupled with interactive 2D and 3D plots.

5   Conclusions

Prediction of BBB permeation directly from molecular structures is of great importance in the development of CNS agents, where a high penetration is needed, or in minimizing CNS-related side effects of drugs with a peripherical mechanism of action.

Some very simple models are sufficient to evaluate the passive diffusion component of the BBB permeation in most cases. Lipinski has shown that four simple parameters are good predictors of drug absorption in a large panel of druglike chemical series. We have shown that such a simple descriptor as the number of heteroatoms or the C_{diff} score are sufficient to predict BBB permeation with a high rate of correct classification.

Computational BBB models should ideally consider all the steps of the process flowchart, both upstream and downstream from BBB itself. While this objective is not reachable, three particular points are susceptible to significant improvements in future models: (1) a cautious selection of the datasets, (2) a careful examination of the chemical state of compounds to be predicted, and (3) the consideration of the various pathways into the brain including not only the well-described passive diffusion but also active transport and transcytosis for particular chemical series.

CNS-maps have led to a high rate of discrimination based on a very large number of chemically diverse compounds. The inclusion of P-gp transport as an explicit component of the model allows a clear mapping of drugs in terms of their BBB permeation.

Ackowledgments

We would like to thank Pr JM Scherrmann and Dr. Roger Lahana for their helpful comments.

Annexe Multivariate Data Analysis

Linear Discriminant Analysis. While quantitative BBB permeation data are not abundant, a two-class description (BBB+/BBB−) is certainly a less informative but more reliable way of analyzing such a variable despite its continuous nature. The discriminant technique aims at separating different classes of compounds using a pool of different explanatory variables and may be used to predict class membership. It is commonly used as a direct way to point out the most discriminating variables ("key descriptors") in a descriptor set.

PCA/PLS. Principal components analysis (PCA) and partial least squares (PLS) are now well recognized multivariate methods for reducing large multidimensional data tables in the most informative way. They have been extensively used to predict ADME properties, pharmacological activity, or toxicity. All column data are scaled to unit variance so as to give every variable the same influence in the data analysis. PCA can be used to reduce a large number of variables to a smaller number of components by transformation into an orthogonal set of linear combinations, maximizing the amount of total variance from the original set. PLS is a numerical method aimed at finding the linear relationship between an activity matrix and a numerical descriptors matrix. PLS modeling consists of simultaneous projections of both the pharmacological and chemical spaces onto low-dimensional hyper planes. The model is calculated so as to simultaneously minimize the residuals, and yields latent variables which are optimally correlated. The statistical significance of the PLS model is determined by cross-validation.

PLS-DA. PLS-DA is a practical way to transform a *class*-model into a pseudo *continuous variable*-model. The derivation of a PLS equation from initial X-block and Y-block leads to a new quantitative univariate, Y-variable, varying around two indices of class (0 for BBB− and 1 for BBB+). The predicted variable can be thought of as a predictor of blood–brain barrier (BBB) permeation on a scale from 0 to 1. Discriminant analysis can be used to determine the threshold of PLS-predicted variable that discriminates optimally between the two original classes. The predicted variable value weighs predictions in each class, compounds with a predicted Y around the threshold value being more uncertainly predicted than those with a predicted Y value close to the class indices. With PLS-DA, r^2 and q^2 criteria are meaningless despite the existence of a regression equation. The validation criteria are those of the discriminant analysis (rate of prediction, confidence estimate). The predicted values, e.g., P-gp$_{pred.}$ and BBB$_{pred.}$, allow that the degree to which each compound belongs to an activity class is given using a membership score.

References

Abraham MH, Chadha HS, Mitchell RC. 1994. Hydrogen bonding. 33 factors that influence the distribution of solutes between blood and brain. J Pharm Sci 83: 1257-1268.

Adenot M, Lahana R. 2004. Blood-brain barrier permeation model: Discriminating between CNS and non-CNS potential drugs including P-gp substrates. J Chem Inf Comput Sci 44 (1): 239-248.

Agon P, Goethals P, Van Haver D, Kaufman JM. 1991. Permeability of the blood-brain barrier for atenolol studied by positron emission tomography. J Pharm Pharmacol 43: 597-600.

Ahkmed N, Fojo AT, Bates SE, Scala S. 1995. Pgp substrates diversity among compounds identified by COMPARE analysis in the NCI drug screen. Proc Am Assoc Cancer Res 36: 339.

Ajay, Bemis GW, Murcko MA. 1999. Designing libraries with CNS activity. J Med Chem 42: 4942-4951.

Alifranjis LH, Christensen IT, Berglund A, Sandberg M, Hovgaard L, et al. 2000. Structure-property model for membrane partitioning of oligopeptides. J Med Chem 43: 103-113.

Ano R, Kimura Y, Shima M, Matsuno R, Ueno T, et al. 2004. Relationships between structure and high-throughput screening permeability of peptide derivatives and related compounds with artificial membranes: Application to prediction of Caco-2 cell permeability. Bioorg Med Chem 12: 257-264.

Appell M, Berfield JL, Wang LC, Dunn III WJ, Chen N, Reith MEA. 2004. Structure-activity relationships for substrate recognition by the human dopamine transporter. Biochemical Pharmacology 67: 293-302.

Ayrton A, Morgan P. 2001. Role of transport proteins in drug absorption, distribution and excretion. Xenobiotica 31: 469-497.

Bakken GA, Jurs PC. 2000. Classification of multidrug-resistance reversal agents using structure-based descriptors and linear discriminant analysis. J Med Chem 43: 4534-4541.

Balaz S. 2000. Lipophilicity in trans-bilayer transport and subcellular pharmacokinetics. Perspect Drug Discov Des 19: 157-177.

Basak SC, Gute BD, Drewes LR. 1996. Predicting blood-brain transport of drugs: A computational approach. Pharm Res 13 (5): 775-778.

Boguslavsky V, Hruby VJ, O'Brien DF, Misicka A, Lipkowski AW. 2003. Effect of peptide conformation on membrane permeability. J Pept Res 61 (6): 287-297.

Boulton D, De Vane C, Liston H, Markowitz J. 2002. In vitro P-glycoprotein affinity for atypical and conventional antipsychotics. Life Sci 71: 163-169.

Brillault J, Berezowski V, Ceccheli R, Dehouck MP. 2002. Intercommunications between brain capillary endothelial cells and glial cells increase the transcellular permeability of the blood-brain barrier during ischemia. J Neurochem 83 (4): 807-817.

Calder JAD, Ganellin CR. 1994. Predicting the brain-penetrating capability of histaminergic compounds. Drug Des Discov 11: 259-268.

Camenish G, Folkers G, Waterbeemd van de H. 1998. Shapes of membrane-permeability-lipophilicity curves: Extension of theoritical models with an aqueous pore pathway. Eur J Pharmacol Sci 6: 321-329.

Cecchelli R, Dehouck B, Descamps L, Fenart L, Buee-Scherrer V, et al. 1999. In vitro model for evaluating drug transport across the blood-brain barrier. Adv Drug Deliv Rev 36: 165-178.

Chang AS, Chang SM, Starnes DM. 1993. Structure-activity relationships of serotonin transport : Relevance to non-tricyclic antidepressant interactions. European Journal of Pharmacology 247: 239-248.

Chen N, Jutice Jr JB. 2000. Differential effect of structural modification of human dopamine transporter on the inward and outward transport of dopamine. Molecular Brain Research 75: 208-215.

Chiba P, Ecker G, Schmid D, Drach J, Tell B, et al. 1996. Structural requirements for activity of propafenone-type modulators in P-glycoprotein-mediated multiodrug resistance. Mol Pharmacol 49: 1122-1130.

Chikhale EG, Ng KY, Burton PS, Borchardt RT. 1994. Hydrogen-bonding as a determinant of the in vitro and in situ blood-brain barrier permeability of peptides. Pharm Res 11 (3): 412-419.

Clark DE. 1999. Rapid calculation of polar molecular surface area and its application to the prediction of transport phenomena. 2. Prediction of blood-brain barrier penetration. J Pharm Sci 88 (8): 815-821.

Conradi RA, Hilgers AR, Ho NFH, Burton PS. 1991. The influence of peptide structure on transport across Caco-2 cells. Pharm Res 8: 1453-1460.

Conradi RA, Hilgers AR, Ho NFH, Burton PS. 1992. The influence of peptide structure on transport across Caco-2 cells. II. Peptide modification which results in improved permeability. Pharm Res 9: 435-439.

Crivori P, Cruciani G, Carrupt P-A, Testa B. 2000. Predicting blood-brain permeation from three-dimensional molecular structure. J Med Chem 43: 2204-2216.

Dearden JC, Al-Noobi A, Scott AC, Thomson SA. 2003. QSAR studies on P-glycoprotein-regulated multidrug resistance and on its reversal by phenothiazines. SAR QSAR Environ Res 14: 447-454.

De Haan FHN, Jansen ACA. 1985. Rationally designed model with general applicability for absorption by passive diffusion. QSAR and Strategies in the Design of Bioactive Compounds. Seydel JK, editor. Weinheim: VCH; pp. 198–204.

Dehouck B, Fenart L, Dehouck MP, Pierce A, Torpier G, et al. 1997. A new function for the LDL receptor: Transcytosis of LDL across the blood-brain barrier. J Cell Biol 138 (4): 877-889.

Dehouck MP, Dehouck B, Schluep C, Lemaire M, Cecchelli R. 1995. Drug transport to the brain: Comparison between in vitro and in vivo models of the blood-brain barrier. Eur J Pharm Sci 3: 357-365.

Dehouck MP, Cecchelli R, Green AR, Renftel M, Lundquist S. 2002. In vitro blood-brain barrier permeability and cerebral endothelial cell uptake of the neuroprotective nitrone compound NXY-059 in normoxic, hypoxic and ischemic conditions. Brain Res 955: 229-235.

de Lange EC, de Boer AG, Breimer DD. 2000. Methodological issues in microdialysis sampling for pharmacokinetic studies. Adv Drug Deliv Rev 45: 125-148.

Deli MA, Descamps L, Dehouck MP, Cecchelli R, Joo F, et al. 1995. Exposure of tumor-necrosis factor-alpha to luminal membrane of bovine brain capillary endothelial cells cocultured with astrocytes induced a delayed increase of permeability and cytoplasmic stress fiber formation of actin. J Neurosci Res 41 (6): 717-726.

Derossi D, Chassaing G, Prochiantz A. 1998. Trojan peptides: The penetratin system for intracellular delivery. Trends Cell Biol 8: 84-87.

Descamps L, Coisne C, Dehouck B, Cecchelli R, Torpier G. 2003. Protective effect of glial cells against lipopolysaccharide-mediated blood-brain barrier injury. Glia 42 (1): 46-58.

Didziapetris R, Japertas P, Avdeef A, Petrauskas A. 2003. Classification Analysis of P-glycoprotein substrate specificity. J Drug Target 11 (7): 391-406.

Di L, Kerns EH, Fan K, McConnell OJ, Carter GT. 2003. High throughput artificial membrane permeability assay for blood-brain barrier. Eur J Med Chem 38: 223-232.

Doniger S, Hofmann T, Yeh J. 2002. Predicting CNS permeability of drug molecules: Comparison of neural network and support vector machine algorithms. J Comput Biol 9 (6): 849-864.

Doppenschmitt S, Spahn- Langguth H, Regardh CG, Langguth P. 1999. Role of P-glycoprotein-mediated secretion in absorptive drug permeability: An approach using passive membrane permeability and affinity to P-glycoprotein. J Pharm Sci 88 (10): 1067-1072.

Drin G, Rousselle C, Schermann JM, Rees AR, Temsamani J. 2002. Peptide delivery to the brain via adsorptive-mediated endocytosis: Advances with SynB vectors. AAPS Pharm Sci 4 (4): 1-7.

Drin G, Cottin S, Blanc E, Rees AR, Temsamani J. 2003. Studies on the internalization mechanism of cationic cell-penetrating peptides. J Biol Chem 278 (33): 31192-31201.

Duffy EM, Jorgensen, WL. 2000. Prediction of properties from simulations: Free energies of solvation in hexadecane, octanol, and water. J Am Chem Soc 122: 2878-2888.

Ecker G, Huber M, Schmid D, Chiba P. 1999. The importance of a nitrogen atom in modulators of multidrug resistance. Mol Pharmacol 56: 791-796.

Ekins S, Kim RB, Leake BF, Dantzig AH, Schuetz EG, et al. 2002. Application of three-dimensional quantitative structure-activity relationships of P-glycoprotein inhibitors and substrates. Mol Pharmacol 61: 974-981.

Engkvist O, Wrede P, Rester U. 2003. Prediction of CNS activity of compound libraries using substructure analysis. J Chem Inf Comput Sci 43: 155-160.

Fenart L, Buee-Scherrer V, Descamps L, Duhem C, Poullain MG, et al. 1998. Inhibition of P-glycoprotein: Rapid assessment of its implication in blood-brain barrier integrity and drug transport to the brain by an in vitro model of the blood-brain barrier. Pharm Res 15 (7): 993-1000.

Fischer H, Gottschlich R, Seelig A. 1998. Blood-brain barrier permeation: Molecular parameters governing passive diffusion. J Membr Biol 165: 201-211.

Foley KF, Van Dort ME, Sievert MK, Ruoho AE, Cozzi NV. 2002. Stereospecific inhibition of monoamine uptake transporters by meta-hydroxyephedrine isomers. J Neural Transm 109(10): 1229-40.

Ford JM, Prozialeck WC, Hait WN. 1989. Structural features determining activity of phenothiazines and related drugs for inhibition of cell-growth and reversal of multidrug resistance. Mol Pharmacol 35: 105-115.

Frey WH, 2002. Bypassing the blood-brain barrier to deliver therapeutic agents to the brain and spinal cord. Drug Deliv Technol 2: 5.

Fu XC, Wang GP, Liang WQ, Yu QS. 2004. Predicting blood-brain barrier penetration of drugs using an artificial neural network. Farmazie 59: 126-130.

Gaillard PJ, Voordwinden LH, Nielsen JL, Ivanov A, Atsumi R, et al. 2001. Establishment and functional characterization of an in vitro model of the blood-brain barrier, comprising a co-culture of brain capillary endothelial cells and astrocytes. Eur J Pharm Sci 12: 215-222.

Giardina G, Clarke GD, Grugni M, Sbacchi M, Vecchietti V. 1995. Central and peripheral analgesic agents: Chemical strategies for limiting brain penetration in Kappa-Opioid agonists belonging to different chemical classes. Il Farmaco 50 (6): 405-418.

Glynn SL, Yazdanian M. 1998. In vitro blood-brain barrier permeability of nevirapine compared to other HIV antiretroviral agents. J Pharm Sci 87 (3): 306-310.

Gombar VK, Polli JW, Humphreys JE, Wring SA, Serabjit-Singh CS. 2004. Predicting P-glycoprotein substrates by a quantitative structure-activity relationship model. J Pharm Sci 93 (4): 957-968.

Gratton JA, Abraham MH, Bradbury MW, Chadh S. 1997. Molecular factors influencing drug transfer across the blood-brain barrier. J Pharm Pharmacol 49: 1211-1216.

Groothuis DR, Levy RM. 1997. The entry of antiviral and antiretroviral drugs into the central nervous system. J Neurovirol 3 (6): 387-400.

Gruetter R, Novotny EJ, Boulware SD, Rothman DL, Shulman RG. 1996. 1H NMR studies of glucose transport in the human brain. J Cereb Blood Flow Metab 16(3): 427-38.

Gumbleton M, Audus KL. 2001. Progress and limitations in the use of in vitro cell cultures to serve as permeability screen for the blood-brain barrier. J Pharm Sci 90 (11): 1681-1698.

Hammarlund-Udenaes M, Paalzow LK, De Lange ECM. 1997. Drug equilibration across the blood-brain barrier—pharmacokinetic considerations based on the microdialysis method. Pharm Res 14 (2): 128-134.

Harwig SS, Swiderek KM, Lee TD, Lehrer RI. 1995. Determination of disulphide bridges in PG-2, an antimicrobial peptide from porcine leukocytes. J Pept Sci 1: 207-215.

Hellberg S, Sjöström M, Skagerberg B, Wold S. 1987. Peptide quantitative structure-activity relationships, a multivariate approach. J Med Chem 30 (7): 1126-1135.

Hou TJ, Xu XJ. 2003. ADME evaluation in drug discovery. 3. Modeling blood-brain barrier partitioning using simple molecular descriptors. J Chem Inf Comput Sci 43 (6): 2137-2152.

Hutter MC. 2003. Prediction of blood-brain barrier permeation using quantum chemically derived information. J Comput Aided Mol Des 17: 415-433.

Illum L. 2000. Transport of drugs from the nasal cavity to the central nervous system. Eur J Pharm Sci 11: 1-18.

Illum L. 2002. Nasal drug developments and strategies. Drug Des Today 7: 1184-1189.

Janigro D, Leaman S, Stanness KA, 1999. Dynamic in vitro modelling of the blood-brain barrier: A novel tool for studies of drug delivery to the brain. Pharmacol Sci Technol Today 2 (1): 7-12.

Jorgensen FS, Jensen LH, Capion D, Christensen IT 2001. Prediction of blood-brain barrier penetration. Rational Approaches to Drug Design. Höltje H-D, Sippl W, editors. Prous Science SA, Barcelona pp. 281–285.

Jorgensen WL, Duffy EM. 2000. Prediction of drug solubility from Monte Carlo simulations. Bioorg Med Chem Lett 10 (11): 1155-1158.

Kai J. 1996. Thermodynamic aspects of hydrophobicity and the blood-brain barrier permeability studied with a gel filtration chromatography. J Med Chem 39: 2621-2624.

Kakee A, Terasaki T, Sugiyama Y. 1996. Brain efflux index as a novel method of analyzing efflux transport at the blood-brain barrier. J Pharmacol Exp Ther 277: 1550-1559.

Kansy M, Senner F, Gubernator K. 1998. Physicochemical high throughput screening: Parallel artificial membrane permeation assay in the description of passive absorption processes. J Med Chem 41 (7): 1007-1010.

Kaznessis YN, Snow ME, Blankley CJ. 2001. Prediction of blood-brain partitioning using Monte-Carlo simulations of molecules in water. J Comput Aided Mol Des 15: 697-708.

Kelder J, Grootenhuis PDJ, Bayada DM, Delbressine LPC, Ploemen JP. 1999. Polar Molecular surface as a dominating determinant for oral absorption and brain penetration of drugs. Pharm Res 16: 1514-1519.

Keserü GM, Molnar L. 2001. High-througput prediction of blood-brain partitioning: A thermodynamic approach. J Chem Inf Comput Sci 41: 120-128.

Klopman G, Srivastava S, Kolossvary I, Epoand RF, Ahmed N, et al. 1992. Structure-activity study and design of multidrug-resistant reversal compounds by a computer automated structure evaluation methodology. Cancer Res 52: 4121-4129.

Klopman G, Shi LM, Ramu A. 1997. Quantitative structure-activity relationship of multidrug resistance reversal agents. Molecular Pharmacology 52: 323-334.

Kubinyi H. 1979. Lipophilicity and drug activity. Prog Drug Res 23: 97-198.

Levin VA. 1980. Relationship of octanol/water partition coefficient and molecular weight to rat brain capillary permeability. J Med Chem 23: 682-684.

Lipinski CA, Lombardo F, Dominy BW, Feeney PJ. 2001. Experimental and computational approaches to estimate solubility and permeability in drug discovery and development settings, Adv Drug Deliv Rev 46: 3-25.

Litman T, Zuthen T, Skovsgaard T, Stein W. 1997. Structure-activity relationships of P-glycoprotein interacting drugs: Kinetic characterization of their effects on ATP-ase activity. Biochim Biophys Acta 1361: 159-168.

Liu R, Sun H, So S. 2001. Development of quantitative structure-property relationship models for early ADME evaluation in drug discovery. 2. Blood-brain barrier penetration. J Chem Inf Comput Sci 41: 1623-1632.

Lobell M, Molnar L, Keserü GM. 2003. Recent advances in the prediction of blood-brain partitioning from molecular structure. J Pharm Sci 92 (2): 360-370.

Lombardo F, Blake JF, Curatolo W. 1996. Computation of brain-blood partitioning of organic solutes via free-energy calculations. J Med Chem 39: 4750-4755.

Loor F, Tiberghien F, Wenandy T, Didier A, Traber R. 2002. Cyclosporins: Structure-activity relationships for the inhibition of the human MDR1 P-glycoprotein ABC transporter. 45 (21): 4598–4612.

Luco JM. 1999. Prediction of the brain-blood distribution of a large set of drugs from structurally derived descriptors using partial least-squares (PLS) modeling. J Chem Inf Comput Sci 39: 396-404.

Lundquist S, Renftel M, Brillault J, Fenart L, Cecchelli R, et al. 2002. Prediction of drug transport through the blood-brain barrier in vivo: A comparison between two in vitro cell models. Pharm Res 19 (7): 976-981.

Luurtsema G, Molthoff CFM, Windhorst AD, Smit JW, Keizer H, et al. 2003. (R)- and (S)-[11C]Verapamil as PET-tracers for measuring P-glycoprotein function: In vitro and in vivo evaluation. Nucl Med Biol 30: 747-751.

Mahar Doan KM, Boje KMK. 2000. Theoritical pharmacokinetic and pharmacodynamic simulations of drug delivery mediated by blood-brain barrier transporters. Biopharm Drug Dispos 21: 261-278.

Mahar Doan KM, Humphreys JE, Webster LO, Wring SA, Shampine LJ, et al. 2002. Passive permeability and P-glycoprotein mediated efflux differentiate CNS and non-CNS marketed drugs. J Pharmacol Exp Ther 303: 1029-1037.

Manfredini S, Pavan B, Vertuani S, Scaglianti M, Compagnone D, et al. 2002. Design, synthesis and activity of ascorbic acid prodrugs of nipecotic, kynurenic and diclophenamic acids, liable to increase neurotropic activity. J Med Chem 45 (3): 559-562.

Marroni M, Kight KM, Hossain M, Cucullo L, Desai SY, et al. 2003. Dynamic in vitro model of the blood-brain barrier. Gene profiling using cDNA microarray analysis. Methods Mol Med 89: 419-434.

Martin I. 2004. Prediction of blood-brain barrier penetration: Are we missing the point? Drug Discov Today 9: 161-162.

Mazel M, Clair P, Rousselle C, Vidal P, Scherrmann JM, et al. 2001. Doxorubicin-peptide conjugates overcome multidrug resistance. Anti-Cancer Drugs 12: 107-116.

Megard I, Garrigues A, Orlowski S, Jorajuria S, Clayette, Ezan E, Mabondzo A. 2002. A co-culture-based model of human blood-brain barrier: Application to active transport of indinavir and in vivo-in vitro correlation. Brain Res 927: 153-167.

Miller DS. 2003. Confocal imaging of xenobiotic transport across the blood-brain barrier. J Exp Zoolog A 300: 84-90.

Neuhoff S, Langguth P, Dressler C, Andersson TB, Regardh CG, et al. 2000. Affinities at the verapamil binding site of MDR-1-encoded P-glycoprotein: Drugs and analogs, stereoisomers and metabolites. Int J Clin Pharmacol Ther 293: 376-382.

Norinder U, Haeberlein M. 2002. Computational approaches to the prediction of blood-brain distribution. Adv Drug Deliv Rev 54 (3): 291-313.

Norinder U, Sjöberg P, Osterberg T. 1998. Theoritical calculations and prediction of brain-blood partitionning of organic solutes using mol surf parametrization and PLS statistics. J Pharm Sci 88: 815-821.

Ooms F, Weber P, Carrupt PA, Testa B. 2002. A simple model to predict blood-brain barrier permeation from 3D molecular fields. Biochim Biophys Acta 1587: 118-125.

Osterberg T, Norinder U. 2000a. Theoritical calculation and prediction of p-glycoprotein-interacting drugs using mol surf parametrization and PLS Statistics. Eur J Pharm Sci 10: 295-303.

Osterberg T, Norinder U. 2000b. Prediction of polar surface area and drug transport processes using simple parameters and PLS statistics. J Chem Inf Comput Sci 40: 1408-1411.

Pajeva I, Wiese M. 1997. QSAR and molecular modelling of cataphiphilic drugs able to modulate multidrug resistance in tumors. Quant Struct-Act Relat 16: 1-10.

Pajeva I, Wiese M. 1998. Molecular modelling of phenothiazines and related drugs as multidrug resistance modifiers: A comparative molecular fields analysis study. J Med Chem 41: 1815-1826.

Pajeva I, Wiese M. 2002. Pharmacophore model of drugs incloved in P-glycoprotein multidrug resistance: Explanation of structural variety (Hypothesis). J Med Chem 45: 5671-5686.

Palm K, Luthman K, Ungell AL, Strandlund G, Beigi F, et al. 1998. Evaluation of dynamic polar molecular surface area as predictor of drug absorption: Comparison with other computational and experimental predictors. J Med Chem 41 (27): 5382-5392.

Pardridge WM. 1998. CNS drug design based on principles of blood-brain barrier transport. J Neurochem 70 (5): 1781-1792.

Pardridge WM. 2002. Drug and gene targeting to the brain with molecular Trojan horses. Nat Rev Drug Discov 1: 131-139.

Pardridge WM. 2004. Log (BB), PS products and in silico models of drug brain penetration. Drug Discov Today 9: 392-393.

Pardridge WM, Mietus LJ. 1979. Transport of steroid hormones through the rat blood-brain barrier. Primary role of albumin-bound hormone. J Clin Invest 64: 145-154.

Parkinson FE, Friesen J, Krizanac- Bengez L, Janigro D. 2003. Use of a three-dimensional in vitro model of teh rat blood-brain barrier to assay nucleoside efflux from brain. Brain Res 980: 233-241.

Pearce HL, Winter MA, Beck WT. 1990. Structural characteristics of compounds that modulates P-glycoprotein-associated multidrug resistance. Adv Enzyme Regul 30: 357-373.

Penzotti JE, Lamb ML, Evensen E, Grootenhuis PDJ. 2002. A computational ensemble P harmacophore model for identifying substrates of P-glycoprotein. J Med Chem 45 (9): 1737-1740.

Petito CK, 1998. HIV infection and the blood-brain barrier. Pardridge WM, Introduction to the Blood-Brain Barrier. Pardridge WM, editor. UK: Cambridge University Press.

Plateel M, Dehouck MP, Torpier G, Cecchelli R, Teissier E. 1995. Hypoxia increases the susceptibility to oxidant stress and the permeability of the blood-brain barrier endothelial cell monolayer. J Neurochem 65 (5): 2138-2145.

Platts JA, Abraham MH, Zhao YH, Hersey A, Ijaz L, et al. 2001. Correlation and prediction of a large blood-brain distribution data set—an LFER study. Eur J Med Chem 36: 719-730.

Polli JW, Wring SA, Humphreys JE, Huang L, Morgan JB, et al. 2001. Rational use of in vitro P-glycoprotein assays in drug discovery. J Pharmacol Exp Ther 299: 620-628.

Prokai L. 1998. Peptide drug delivery into the central nervous system. Prog Drug Res 51: 95-131.

Raevsky OA, Schaper KJ. 1998. Quantitative estimation of hydrogen bond contribution to permeability and absorption processes of some chemicals and drugs. Eur J Med Chem 33: 799-807.

Ramu A, Ramu N. 1992. Reversal of multidrug resistance by phenothiazines and structurally related compounds. Cancer Chemother Pharmacol 30: 165-173.

Rapoport SI, Levitan H. 1974. Neurotoxicity of X-ray contrast media. Relation to lipid solubility and blood-brain barrier permeability. Am J Roentgenol Radium Ther Nucl Med 122 (1): 186-193.

Rose K, Hall LH, Kier LB. 2002. Modeling blood-brain barrier partitioning using the electrotopological state. J Chem Inf Comput Sci 42: 651-666.

Rousselle C, Clair P, Lefauconnier JM, Kaczoreck M, Scherrmann JM, et al. 2000. New advances in the transport of doxorubicin through the blood-brain barrier by a peptide vector-mediated strategy. Mol Pharmacol 57: 679-686.

Rousselle C, Smirnova M, Clair P, Lefauconnier JM, Chavanieu A, et al. 2001. Enhanced delivery of doxorubicin into the brain via a peptide-vector-mediated strategy: Saturation kinetics and specificity. J Pharmacol Exp Ther 296 (1): 124-131.

Rubin L, Morgan L, Staddon JM. 1998. Regulation of brain endothelial cell tight junction permeability. Introduction to the Blood-Brain Barrier. Pardridge WM, editor. Cambridge: Cambridge University Press; pp. 293–300.

Salminen T, Pulli A, Taskinen J. 1997. Relationship between immobilised artificial membrane chromatographic retention and the brain penetration of structurally diverse drugs. J Pharm Biomed Anal 15: 469-477.

Samii A, Bickel U, Stroth U, Pardridge WM. 1994. Blood-brain barrier transport of neuropeptides: Analysis with a metabolically stable dermorphin analogue. Am J Physiol 267: E124-E131.

Schaddelee MP, Voorwinden HL, Groenendaal D, Hersey A, Ijzerman AP, et al. 2003. Blood-brain barrier transport of synthetic adenosine A1 receptor agonists in vitro: Structure transport relationships. Eur J Pharm Sci 20 (3): 347-356.

Schinkel AH. 1999. P-glycoprotein, a gatekeeper in the blood-brain barrier. Adv Drug Deliv 36: 179-194.

Schoenmakers RG, Stehouwer MC, Tukker JJ. 1999. Structure-transport relationship for the intestinal small-peptides carrier: Is the carbonyl group of the peptide bond relevant for transport? Pharm Res 16 (1): 62-68.

Seelig A. 1998. A general pattern for substrate recognition by P-glycoprotein. Eur J Biochem 251: 252-261.

Seelig A, Landwojtowicz E. 2000. Structure-activity relationship of P-glycoprotein substrate and modifiers. Eur J Pharm Sci 12: 31-40.

Seelig A, Gottschlich R, Devant RM. 1994. A method to determine the ability of drugs to diffuse through the blood-brain barrier. Proc Natl Acad Sci USA 91, 68-72.

Shah MV, Audus KL, Borchardt RT. 1989. The application of bovine brain microvessel endothelial-cell monolayers grown onto polycarbonate membranes in vitro to estimate the potential permeability of solutes through the blood-brain barrier. Pharm Res 6 (7): 624-627.

Siflinger-Birnboim A, Del Becchio PJ, Cooper JA, Blumenstock FA, Shepard JN, et al. 1987. Molecular sieving characteristics of the cultures endothelial monolayer. J Cell Physiol 132: 111-117.

Staness KA, Guatteo E, Janigro D. 1996. A dynamic model of the blood-brain barrier in vitro. Neurotoxicology 17 (2): 481-496.

Stehle RG, Higuchi WI. 1972. In vitro model for transport of solutes in three-phase system. I. Theoretical principles. J Pharm Sci 61 (12): 1922-1930.

Stenberg P, Luthman K, Artursson P. 1999. Prediction of membrane permeability to peptides from calculated dynamic molecular surface properties. Pharm Res 16 (2): 205-212.

Stouch TR, Gudmundsson O. 2002. Progress in understanding the structure-activity relationships of P-glycoprotein. Adv Drug Deliv Rev 54 (3): 315-328.

Subramanian G, Kitchen DB. 2003. Computational models to predict blood-brain barrier permeation and CNS activity. J Comput Aided Mol Des 17: 643-664.

Sun H. 2004. A universal molecular descriptor system for prediction of LogP, LogS, LogBB and absorption. J Chem Inf Comput Sci 44: 748-757.

Tamai I, Tsuji A. 2000. Transporter-mediated permeation of drugs across the blood-brain barrier. J Pharm Sci 89 (11): 1371-1388.

Tamai I, Sai Y, Kobayashi H, Kamata M, Wakamiya T, et al. 1997. Structure-internalization relationship for adorptive-mediated endocytosis of basic peptides at the blood-brain barrier. J Pharmacol Exp Ther 280: 410-415.

Temsamani J, Scherrmann JM, Rees AR, Kaczoreck M. 2000. Brain drug delivery technologies: Novel approaches for transporting therapeutics. Pharmacol Sci Technol Today 3 (5): 155-162.

Temsamani J, Rousselle C, Rees AR, Scherrmann JM. 2001. Vector-mediated drug delivery to the brain. Expert Opin Biol Ther 1 (5): 1-10.

Terasaki T, Ohtsuki S, Hori S, Takanaga H, Nakashima E, et al. 2003. New approaches to in vitro models of blood-brain barrier drug transport. Drug Discov Today 8 (20): 944-954.

Tsuji A, Tamai I. 1999. Carrier-mediated or specialized transport of drugs across the blood-brain barrier. Adv Drug Deliv Rev 36: 277-290.

Tsukita S, Furuse M, Itoh M. 1998. Molecular dissection of tight junctions: Occludin and ZO-1. Introduction to the Blood-Brain Barrier. Pardridge WM, editor. Cambridge: Cambridge University Press; pp. 322–329.

Vabeno J, Lejon T, Nielsen CU, Steffansen B, Chen W, et al. 2004. Phe-Gly dipeptidomimetics designed for the di-/tripeptide transporters PEPT1 and PEPT2: Synthesis and biological investigations. J Med Chem 47 (4): 1060-1069.

Van de Waterbeemd H, Jansen A. 1981. Transport in QSAR. V: Application of the interfacial drug transfer model. Pharm Weekbl Sci Ed 3: 587-594.

Van de Waterbeemd H, Kansy M. 1992. Hydrogen-bonding capacity and brain penetration. Chimia 46: 299-303.

Van de Waterbeemd H, Camenish G, Folkers G, Raevsky OA. 1996. Estimation of Caco-2 cell permeability using calculated molecular descriptors. Quant Struct-Activity Relat 15: 480-490.

Van de Waterbeemd H, Camenish G, Folkers G, Chretien JR, Raevsky OA. 1998. Estimation of blood-brain barrier crossing of drugs using molecular size and shape, and H-bonding descriptors. J Drug Target 6 (2): 151-165.

Van de Waterbeemd H, Smith DA, Beaumont K, Walker DK. 2001. Property-based design: Optimization of drug absorption and pharmacokinetics. J Med Chem 44 (9): 1313-1333.

Vaughan RA, Agoston GE, Lever JR, Newman AH. 1999. Differential binding of tropane-based photoaffinity ligands on the dopamine transporter. The Journal of Neuroscience 19(2): 630-636.

Villalobos AR, Parmelee JT, Pritchard JB, 1997. Functional characterization of choiroid plexus epithelial cells in primary culture. J Pharmacol Exp Ther 282: 1109-1116.

Virgintino D, Monaghan P, Robertson D. 1997. An immuno-histochemical and morphometric study on asrtocytes and microbasculature in the human cerebral cortex. Histochem J 29: 655-660.

Wakamiya T, Kamata M, Kusumoto S, Kobayashi H, Sai Y, et al. 1998. Design and synthesis of peptides passing through the blood-brain barrier. Bull Chem Soc Jpn 78: 699-709.

Wu D, Kang YS, Bickel U, Pardridge WM. 1997. Blood-brain barrier permeability to morphine-6-glucuronide is markedly reduced compared with morphine. Drug Metab Dispos 25 (6): 768-71.

Young RC, Mitchell RC, Brown TH, Ganellin CR, Griffiths R, et al. 1998. Development of a new physicochemical model for brain penetration and its application to the design of centrally acting H2 receptor histamine antagonists. J Med Chem 31: 656-671.

Zamora JM, Pearce HL, Beck WT. 1988. Physico-chemical properties shared by compounds that modulate multidrug resistance un human leukemic cells. Mol Pharmacol 33: 454-462.

Zhang EY, Phelps MA, Chen C, Ekins S, Swaan PW. 2002. Modeling of active transport systems. Adv Drug Deliv Rev 54: 329-354.

Zheng W, Zhao Q, Graziano JH. 1998. Primary culture of choroidal epithelial cells: Characterization of an in vitro model of blood-CSF barrier. In Vitro Cell Dev Biol Anim 34(1): 40-45.

7 Cholesterol—A Janus-Faced Molecule in the Central Nervous System

W. G. Wood · U. Igbavboa · G. P. Eckert · W. E Müller

Abstract: Understanding the role of cholesterol in normal brain function and its involvement in specific neurodegenerative diseases has attracted considerable attention. One general observation is that there are notable differences in the brain cholesterol properties and dynamics as compared with cholesterol outside of the brain. In addition, much of what is known of brain cholesterol is based on studies focusing on the total or bulk amount of cholesterol; however, it is becoming increasingly recognized that cholesterol domains may provide greater insight into the cellular function of cholesterol. This chapter, therefore, examines the role of cholesterol in brain, compares the properties and dynamics of brain and peripheral cholesterol, and describes cholesterol domains and the contribution of cholesterol to brain pathophysiology, with an emphasis on Alzheimer's disease (AD). Attention is also directed at the participation of other compounds in the brain cholesterol biosynthetic pathway, namely isoprenoids and the cholesterol metabolites, oxysterols.

List of Abbreviations: AD, Alzheimer's disease; APP, amyloid precursor protein; Aβ, amyloid β-protein; BBB, blood–brain barrier; CSF, cerebrospinal fluid; CYP46A1, cholesterol 24-hydroxylase; DHCR7, 3β-hydroxysterol Δ^7-reductase; FPP, farnesyl pyrophosphate; GGPP, geranylgeranyl pyrophosphate; GPI, Glycosylphosphatidylinositol; HD, Huntington's disease; NPC, Niemann–Pick type C; P-gp, P-glycoprotein; LDL, low-density lipoproteins; LRP, low-density lipoprotein receptor-related protein; SLOS, Smith–Lemli–Opitz syndrome

1 Introduction

Poulletier de la Salle is credited with discovering cholesterol in bile and gallstones in 1769 (Dam, 1958), later identified by M. E. Chevreul in 1815 in experiments examining compounds of human gallstones (Vance and Van den Bosch, 2001). Chevreul named it cholesterine (Greek: khole for bile and stereos for solid). Since that time, and particularly in the past 100 years, tremendous advancements have been made in understanding cholesterol regulation and its role in cell function. When Michael Brown and Joseph Goldstein were awarded the Nobel Prize in physiology or medicine in 1985 for their work on cholesterol regulation, in their acceptance speech they described the fascination that cholesterol has had for scientists and labeled cholesterol as a "Janus faced molecule," having both positive and negative consequences. While those comments at the time pertained to cholesterol outside of brain, their elegant comments equally apply to brain cholesterol.

In most species, the total cholesterol concentration (mg/g wet weight) is highest in brain when compared with other organs (Dietschy and Turley, 2004). Cholesterol is an integral part of the brain and like any sterol outside of brain provides structural stability to membranes, involvement in protein function, and is the precursor of steroids. There are, however, key differences in cholesterol dynamics in the brain versus the peripheral system (e.g., ratio of unesterified cholesterol to esterified cholesterol, apolipoprotein and lipoprotein distribution, and abundance of the oxysterol 24S-hydroxycholesterol) distinguishing its action, and these differences will be considered. Much of our knowledge on brain cholesterol has been based on total or bulk cholesterol amounts. It is becoming increasingly recognized that different cholesterol domains in contrast to bulk levels may play an important role in cell function, and these domains will be examined from the perspective of their structure and function in brain. As with cholesterol outside of brain, regulation of this Janus-faced molecule in brain can go awry as demonstrated most pointedly in human malformation syndromes of inborn errors of cholesterol synthesis and Niemann–Pick type C disease (Porter, 2002; Vance et al., 2005). Furthermore, there is evidence suggestive of cholesterol being a factor in neurodegenerative diseases such as Huntington's disease, Alzheimer's disease (AD), and pathophysiology occurring with increasing age (Burns and Duff, 2002; Wood et al., 2002; Valenza et al., 2005). This chapter, therefore, examines the role of cholesterol in the brain, compares the dynamics of brain and peripheral cholesterol, and describes cholesterol domains and the contribution of cholesterol to brain pathophysiology, with an emphasis on AD. Attention is also given to the participation in brain of other compounds in the cholesterol biosynthetic pathway, namely isoprenoids and the cholesterol metabolites, oxysterols.

2 Brain Cholesterol Synthesis and Dynamics

2.1 Cholesterol Synthesis

In the brain and in the peripheral organs, cholesterol synthesis results from the action of HMG-CoA reductase catalyzing the NADPH-dependent reduction of HMG-CoA to mevalonate, as shown in ❯ *Figure 7-1*, which is an abbreviated depiction of the biosynthetic pathway for cholesterol. Early studies on synthesis of brain cholesterol concluded that synthesis occurred in immature organisms but not in

◻ Figure 7-1

Cholesterol synthesis pathway. Acetyl-CoA and acetoacetyl-CoA are converted to 3-hydroxy-3-methylglutaryl-CoA (HMG-CoA), which is then converted to mevalonate through the action of HMG-CoA reductase and the cofactor NADPH. This reaction is the rate-limiting step for cholesterol synthesis and statins are a substrate for HMG-CoA reductase. Through a series of reactions, mevalonate is converted to isopentyl pyrophosphate, which is the precursor for isoprenoid compounds and cholesterol. Geranylgeranyl-pyrophosphate (GGPP) and farnesyl-pyrophosphate (FPP) serve an important role by prenylation of GTP-binding proteins such as Rho, Rac, and Ras, enabling those proteins to be inserted in membranes. FPP is also the precursor for ubiquinone, dolichol, and squalene. Conversion of squalene to cholesterol requires over 19 reactions. Cholesterol can be subsequently converted to neurosteroids beginning with cytochrome P450scc-induced production of pregnenolone and cholesterol converted to oxysterols such as 24S-hydroxycholesterol by cholesterol-24-hydroxylase

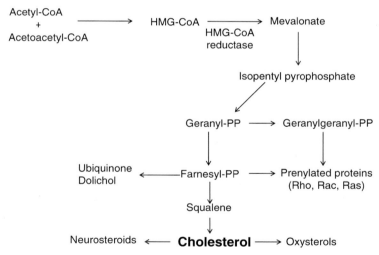

adults (Waelsch et al., 1940; Srere et al., 1950). Studies by Kabara and others in the 1960s and 1970s established the fact that cholesterol was synthesized in the brain in both young and mature organisms, and readers are referred to a review of this early and instructive work on brain cholesterol metabolism (Kabara, 1973). Subsequent studies have shown that the rate of brain cholesterol synthesis is high in the fetus and the newborn animal and that as the animal matures brain cholesterol synthesis decreases but does occur (Dietschy, 1997; Turley and Dietschy, 1997). Cholesterol turnover is quite different between the brain and the whole-body. In mice, the turnover is approximately 0.4% per day in the brain when compared with 8% in the whole body (Dietschy and Turley, 2004). Human cholesterol turnover is lower in both the brain and the whole body, 0.03% and 0.7%, respectively, as compared with mice (Dietschy and Turley, 2004).

2.2 Asymmetry Between Brain and Plasma Cholesterol Levels

A fundamental issue pertaining to brain cholesterol is whether there is equilibrium between brain and plasma cholesterol levels. In a recent review, it was suggested that cholesterol may cross the blood–brain barrier (BBB) (Vance et al., 2005) and this conclusion was based on the following evidence. Administration of cholesterol for 8 weeks to mice expressing amyloid precursor protein (APP) holoprotein and human amyloid β-protein (Aβ) produced a reduction in the amounts of brain APP metabolites including $A\beta_{1-40}$ and $A\beta_{1-42}$ (Howlands et al., 1998). In this study, it was concluded that changes in cholesterol levels can affect APP metabolism although changes in cholesterol levels were minimal. There were no significant differences in the total amounts of brain cholesterol between the control diet mice (cholesterol 6.1 mg/g) and the high-cholesterol diet mice (7.7 mg/g). Serum cholesterol levels were strikingly elevated in the high-cholesterol diet mice (332. 5 mg/dl) versus the control mice (109.9 mg/dl). It was found in the same study that the frontal cortex of the cholesterol group contained 16 mg of cholesterol and the frontal cortex of the control group contained 13.3 mg of cholesterol and this difference of 2.7 mg was statistically significant. A second study presented as support for plasma cholesterol crossing the BBB found that administration of cholesterol diets for 9 months to apoE-null mice, which have been shown to have elevated plasma cholesterol levels and wild-type mice, induced glial activation and that levels of the antioxidant enzyme NADPH/quinone oxidoreductase were higher in the cholesterol apoE-null mice (Crisby et al., 2004). Brain cholesterol levels of the wild type and apoE-null mice were not reported in this study. Most interestingly, the high-cholesterol diets clearly induced changes in brain chemistry but attributing such changes to brain cholesterol is not warranted. Arguing against the idea that cholesterol from the plasma can cross the BBB has been recently reviewed (Dietschy and Turley, 2004). Furthermore, data on plasma and brain cholesterol levels in apoE-null mice and wild-type mice support lack of equilibrium between plasma cholesterol and brain cholesterol. Plasma cholesterol levels of apoE-null mice were sixfold higher than those of wild-type mice (Eckert et al., 2001). However, bulk brain cholesterol levels did not differ between those two groups, which is in agreement with an earlier study (Igbavboa et al., 1997). A study in guinea pigs reported that dietary administration of a high-cholesterol diet (1500 mg/day) had no effect on brain cholesterol levels but increased serum cholesterol twofold in the high-cholesterol diet group when compared with control animals (Lütjohann et al., 2004). Elevated cholesterol in plasma whether from diet or absence of apoE does not appreciably increase brain cholesterol abundance. What is unresolved is the mechanism(s) whereby cholesterol diets induce changes in brain chemistry without increasing brain cholesterol levels.

2.2.1 Properties of Brain Cholesterol Compared with Plasma Cholesterol

There are major differences in characteristics of cholesterol in brain versus outside of brain. Notable differences are levels of unesterified cholesterol compared with esterified cholesterol (i.e., cholesteryl ester), apolipoprotein and lipoprotein distribution, and production of the oxysterol 24S-hydroxycholesterol. In plasma, approximately 70% of cholesterol in low-density lipoproteins (LDL) is esterified. A general consensus is that the mature brain contains little if any esterified cholesterol (Ramsey and Nicholas, 1972; Kabara, 1973; Agranoff, 1989). Exceptions where cholesterol esters are increased in brain are during early development, certain demyelinating diseases, and gliomas (Kabara, 1973; Quarles et al., 1989; Tosi et al., 2003). An explanation for the increase in brain cholesterol ester levels among the different conditions is not well understood. BBB permeability has been noted in patients with astrocytic tumors (Arismendi-Morillo and Castellano, 2005), which might allow passage of LDL- and HDL-containing cholesterol esters to be delivered to the brain, but in the case of developing organisms data indicate that all of the cholesterol results from synthesis within the brain (Dietschy and Turley, 2004).

Apolipoproteins such as apoA-I, apoA-II, apoB, and apoE complex with cholesterol, esterified cholesterol, phospholipids, and triglycerides forming lipoproteins, and these lipid carriers are the primary means by which cholesterol is transported systemically. In the brain, the composition of apolipoproteins and lipoproteins is different as compared with those structures outside of the brain. Apolipoproteins in human brain have been identified and include apoA-I, apoA-IV, apoD, apoE, and apoJ (Harr et al., 1996). Apo B, apo A-II, and apo C-II were not detected in the brain. ApoB has also not been detected in cerebrospinal fluid (CSF) (Roheim et al., 1979; Pitas et al., 1987b). The absence of apoB in brain is of particular interest because of the fact that apoB is the primary protein in LDL suggesting that LDL-containing apoB may not be present in brain. Lipid composition of lipoprotein fractions from CSF have been reported to differ compared with lipoprotein fractions of plasma in normal humans with substantially less total cholesterol, and phospholipids in CSF fractions than in plasma fractions (Koch et al., 2001). It was also noted that CSF cholesterol was concentrated in the HDL fraction whereas plasma cholesterol was observed in the VLDL and LDL fractions.

ApoE and apoJ are the primary apolipoproteins in brain (Boyles et al., 1985; Oda et al., 1994). In the case of apoE, there has been considerable interest in the role of apoE in brain, especially its involvement in AD, and several excellent reviews have addressed these topics (Holtzman, 2004; Huang et al., 2004; Rebeck, 2004; Poirier, 2005). ApoE is a 34-kDa protein that binds to members of the LDL receptor family (Mahley, 1988; Fagan and Holtzman, 2000). ApoE is primarily synthesized by astrocytes (Boyles et al., 1985; Pitas et al., 1987a; Xu et al., 2000). It has been shown that astrocytes are an important source of cholesterol for neurons and that apoE is the transport protein (Mauch et al., 2001). This astrocyte-derived cholesterol is necessary for synapse development. Another study reported that particles containing apoE and cholesterol from astrocytes induced axonal growth in retinal ganglion cells (Hayashi et al., 2004). The target of the apoE particles was distal axons and not the cell body. Astrocytes are also a source of polyunsaturated fatty acids for neurons (Moore et al., 1991), and it has been shown that neuronal membranes of apoE-null mice differed in their polyunsaturated phospholipid molecular species compared with wild-type mice (Igbavboa et al., 2002). ApoE has been proposed to be an important factor in maintaining the stability of the neuron during aging and brain injury (Poirier, 1994; Holtzman et al., 1995; Masliah et al., 1995, 1996). In support of this hypothesis was the finding that there was a loss of brain nerve terminals in apoE-null mice and that aged apoE-null mice displayed the greatest loss of neuronal structure compared with younger apoE-null mice and wild-type mice (Masliah et al., 1995). Lesioning of the hippocampus increased apoE expression and increased binding of fluorescent-labeled LDL to hippocampal brain slices (Poirier et al., 1993a). It was concluded in this study that apoE and the LDL receptor were necessary to recycle neuronal cholesterol for membrane biogenesis.

ApoE in humans has three main isoforms, E2, E3, and E4, differing in amino acids at positions 112 and 158 (Weisgraber et al., 1981; Rall et al., 1982). ApoE2 has cysteines at both positions, apoE3 has a cysteine and arginine, and apoE4 has two arginines. Expression of these isoforms confers specific differences in amounts of lipid released from astrocytes, effects on neurite growth of neurons, plasticity, oxidative insult, membrane cholesterol asymmetry, and their interaction with Aβ, a protein thought to be involved in pathophysiology of AD (Fagan and Holtzman, 2000; Wood et al., 2003). ApoE4 inhibited and apoE3 increased neurite growth in mouse neurons (Nathan et al., 2002). Similar findings were observed in hippocampal slices from mice expressing apoE4 and mice expressing apoE3 (Teter et al., 2002). ApoE isoforms differ in their neuronal distribution as soon as they are taken up by the low-density lipoprotein receptor-related protein (LRP) (Dekroon and Armati, 2003). ApoE3 showed little localization in late endosomes whereas apoE4 showed a high concentration, and such differences might alter cholesterol distribution in neurons. Mouse astrocytes expressing human apoE3 released more cholesterol in apoE3 particles as compared with astrocytes expressing human apoE4 (Gong et al., 2002). However, another study reported that lipoproteins secreted from astrocytes of apoE3- and apoE4-mice were similar in apoE abundance and lipid composition (Fagan et al., 1999). Astrocytes cultured from mice expressing human apoE3 were found to induce greater neurite growth as compared with astrocytes expressing human apoE4 or apoE-null mice (Sun et al., 1998). Mice expressing human apoE4 showed lower immunostaining for synaptophysin than apoE3 mice following entorhinal cortex lesion and was indicative of extent of degeneration and regeneration (White et al., 2001). Cholesterol binds to synaptophysin (Thiele et al., 2000) and it was reported that the interaction of the synaptophysin/synaptobrevin complex was dependent on cholesterol and that such cholesterol may be derived from astrocytes (Mauch et al., 2001; Mitter et al., 2003). The transbilayer distribution of cholesterol is significantly different in synaptic plasma membranes (SPM) of mice expressing human apoE4 as compared with SPM of mice expressing human apoE3 (Hayashi et al., 2002). There is almost a twofold increase in exofacial leaflet cholesterol of apoE4 mice. This increase is similar to what has been reported in aged versus young mice and apoE-null mice (Igbavboa et al., 1996, 1997).

Modification of the transbilayer distribution of cholesterol can alter protein activity, cholesterol transport, and leaflet fluidity leading to cell dysfunction and is discussed later in this chapter. Presence of the apoE4 allele is a risk factor for AD (Saunders et al., 1993). There are data showing that cytotoxicity induced by Aβ was diminished in an isoform-specific manner with apoE2 > apoE3 > apoE4 (Ma et al., 1996; Miyata and Smith, 1996; Titov, 1997). ApoE3 protected cells from Aβ toxicity but apoE4 had no effect and Aβ was toxic (Jordán et al., 1998). ApoE 4 stimulated Aβ production in rat neuroblastoma B103 cells transfected with human APP695 (Ye et al., 2005). In mice expressing human APP and apoE3 or apoE4, synaptic deficits were delayed by apoE3 as compared with apoE4 (Buttini et al., 2002).

2.3 Isoprenoids and Oxysterols

As seen in ❷ *Figure 7-1*, the pathway of cholesterol synthesis includes a family of several other important molecules upstream of cholesterol. These molecules include ubiquinone (coenzyme Q), vitamin D, dolichol, geranylgeranyl pyrophosphate (GGPP), and farnesyl pyrophosphate (FPP). In this section, we focus on GGPP, FPP, dolichol, and oxysterols. There is growing recognition of the important contributions of the isoprenoids in cell function. Mevalonate-derived isoprenoid compounds, FPP and GGPP, are necessary for the prenylation of GTP-binding proteins such as Ras, Rac, and Rho (Holstein and Hohl, 2004). Much of the interest in these isoprenoids is due in part to the mechanisms of action of HMG-CoA reductase inhibitors (statins). These drugs in addition to lowering cholesterol levels concomitantly lower isoprenoid levels. There is increasing evidence that the protective effects of statins in vascular disease may involve cholesterol-independent actions of statins, namely reduction of isoprenoid levels (Mcfarlane et al., 2002). The prenylated protein Rac1 is noteworthy because it has been shown that inhibition of geranylger-anylation of Rac1 by atorvastatin was antiapoptotic in vascular smooth muscle cells (Wassmann et al., 2001). Triggering of apoptosis involving membrane-bound Rac1 is thought to be mediated by a NADPH oxidase-dependent pathway (Chung et al., 2003). Inhibition of geranylgeranylation by atorvastatin reduced angiotensin II free-radical production because of inhibition of isoprenylation of Rac1 leading to a decreased insertion of Rac1 into the membrane of vascular smooth muscle cells (Wassmann et al., 2001). Isoprenoids may play an important role in cell function but a basic issue which has not been addressed in brain pertains to isoprenoid levels both under normal and under different treatment conditions. In mice, it has been reported for example that statins reduce brain cholesterol levels (Johnson-Anuna et al., 2005). Would such an in vivo treatment also reduce isoprenoid levels, and if so, what would be the magnitude of such a reduction? The need for isoprenoid determination also applies to in vitro studies where cells are incubated with statins. Quantifying isoprenoid levels is needed due to the fact that in cell culture studies amounts of isoprenoids added to examine cholesterol-independent effects of statins may far exceed in vivo levels. It was reported in fibroblasts (Tong et al., 2005) that isoprenoid levels were in picomole amounts but in vitro studies including work of our laboratory often use amounts in the micromolar range.

An isoprenoid compound whose levels have been quantified in brain is dolichol (Pullarkat and Reha, 1982; Andersson et al., 1987; Wood et al., 1989b). Dolichols are long-chain polyisoprenols derived from FPP. They are ubiquitous among body organs with the highest levels observed in testis, kidney, brain, and various exocrine glands (Rip et al., 1985). Dolichol can be in free forms or phosphorylated. Dolichol phosphates are intermediates in the synthesis of oligosaccharide groups of glycoproteins. The cellular function of free dolichols is not known. Dolichol increased fluidity of SPM, and it has been detected in membranes where it might function to regulate membrane fluidity (Wood et al., 1986). There is a marked increase of this compound in human brain tissue with aging (Pullarkat and Reha, 1982; Andersson et al., 1987). SPM of 18- and 28-month-old C57BL/6 mice had a 5-fold and 11-fold increase, respectively, in dolichol levels when compared with 6-month-old mice (Wood et al., 1989b). In the same study, it was found that dolichol had a greater fluidizing effect on SPM of young mice than aged mice. Increased dolichol content has been observed in brain tissue from individuals with AD and neuronal lipofuscinosis (Ng Ying Kin et al., 1983; Wolfe et al., 1985). Whether the elevated dolichol levels observed with increasing age and certain neurodegenerative diseases is injurious to cell function has not been established.

Oxysterols are oxygenated derivatives of cholesterol and these sterols have been suggested to be involved in processes such as cholesterol metabolism, apoptosis, and inflammation (Björkhem and Diczfalusy, 2002). A metabolite of cholesterol enriched in brain is the oxysterol 24S-hydroxycholesterol (Lutjohann et al., 1996). This oxysterol is thought to be the primary mechanism for removal of cholesterol from brain because of its polarity. Cholesterol is converted to 24S-hydroxycholesterol by cholesterol 24-hydroxylase (CYP46A1) (Lund et al., 1999). It has been suggested that CYP46A1 may be a risk factor for AD (Papassotiropoulos et al., 2005) but other data do not support this hypothesis (Ingelsson et al., 2004). The importance of CYP46A1 in brain is unclear in that its transcriptional regulation is largely unaffected by changes in cholesterol homeostasis (Ohyama et al., 2005).

3   Cholesterol Domains

3.1 Transbilayer Cholesterol Distribution

Cholesterol is not evenly distributed throughout the membrane but is located in different cholesterol domains as depicted in ❷ *Figure 7-2*, panel a. Two major cholesterol domains are the exofacial and cytofacial leaflets of membranes. These two leaflets differ in their fluidity, lipid distribution, electrical charge, and active sites of certain proteins (Op den Kamp, 1979; Schroeder et al., 1996; Wood et al., 2002, 2003). The cytofacial leaflet contains almost seven times as much cholesterol as the exofacial leaflet and is markedly less fluid as compared with the exofacial leaflet (Wood et al., 2002). The two leaflets differ in their

◻ Figure 7-2

Plasma membrane lipid domains. Panel a illustrates the two leaflets of the plasma membranes, showing the asymmetric distribution of cholesterol and phospholipids. Large globular structures represent proteins. Cholesterol (C), phosphatidylinositol (PI), phosphatidylethanolamine (PE), and phosphatidylserine (PS) are enriched in the cytofacial leaflet. Phosphatidylcholine (PC) and sphingomyelin (SM) are in abundance in the exofacial leaflet, and there is some PC in the cytofacial leaflet. A lipid raft is denoted in the exofacial leaflet (panel a) containing a glycosylphosphatidylinositol-anchored protein (GPI). Panel b is a model of caveolae enriched in cholesterol, sphingolipids, and caveolin

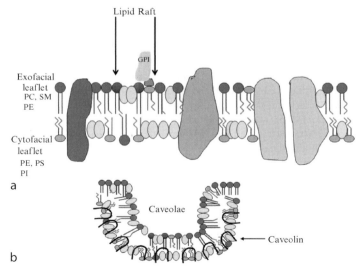

susceptibility to perturbation. Whereas 25 mM ethanol significantly fluidized the exofacial leaflet, ethanol at a concentration as high as 400 mM had no effect on the fluidity of the cytofacial leaflet (Schroeder et al., 1988; Wood et al., 1989a).

SPM transbilayer cholesterol distribution (TCD) is not static but can be modified by in vivo and in vitro treatment conditions. For example, 25-month-old C57BL/6NNIA mice had approximately 30% of cholesterol in the SPM exofacial leaflet in contrast to mice 14–15 months and 3–4 months of age which had approximately 23% and 14% of cholesterol in the exofacial leaflets, respectively (Igbavboa et al., 1996). The total amount of SPM cholesterol among the three different age groups did not significantly differ. HMG-CoA reductase inhibitors (statins) altered SPM TCD of mice when administered for 21 days (Kirsch et al., 2003). An approximately twofold increase in the exofacial leaflet cholesterol was observed in chronic ethanol-treated mice as compared with the pair-fed control group (Wood et al., 1990). Total amounts of SPM cholesterol did not differ between the ethanol-treated and control groups.

Either increasing or decreasing membrane cholesterol has consequences on membrane proteins. For example, it was shown in neuronal tissue that cholesterol reduction in membranes produced a loss in GABA uptake and uptake was restored by the addition of cholesterol (North and Fleischer, 1983). Choline uptake was not affected by changes in cholesterol content in this study. Removing or adding cholesterol to the membrane not only modifies the total amount of cholesterol but such procedures would also alter TCD, which may be important in regulating the activity of certain membrane-bound proteins. Cholesterol enrichment of the erythrocyte exofacial leaflet increased protein sulfhydryl group exposure and antigen exposure (Schachter et al., 1983). Oxidation of cholesterol in the exofacial leaflet of brain synaptosomes significantly reduced Ca^{2+}/Mg^{2+}-ATPase activity (Wood et al., 1995). Na^+/K^+-ATPase activity was not affected. TCD and protein function has received very little attention and certainly warrants further study. Mechanisms regulating TCD are poorly understood in contrast to membrane phospholipid distribution where specific proteins have been identified (Connor and Schroit, 1990; Zachowski, 1993; Diaz and Schroit, 1996). Intracellular protein candidates for TCD regulation have been proposed including fatty acid-binding proteins FABP and sterol carrier protein-2 (Wood et al., 1999). Other potential regulatory proteins are apoE, LDLR, and P-glycoprotein. The SPM exofacial leaflets of apoE-null mice and LDL-receptor-null mice had twice the amount of cholesterol when compared with the exofacial leaflet of control mice (Igbavboa et al., 1997). Differences in TCD were not explainable by differences in the total SPM cholesterol levels. ApoE either may add cholesterol by coupling with the LDLR and other receptors or may remove cholesterol from the membrane which in turn could alter TCD. Even though there was a doubling of cholesterol in the exofacial leaflets of "knockout" mice, cholesterol remained asymmetrically distributed between the two leaflets of the bilayer. While apoE and the LDLR may be involved in regulating TCD, there must be other proteins or possibly lipids that contribute to maintaining membrane cholesterol asymmetry. An additional protein candidate is P-glycoprotein (P-gp), which is an ATP-binding cassette transporter (Schinkel, 1997). On the basis of accessibility of cholesterol in the cell membrane to cholesterol oxidase, it was concluded that overexpression of P-gp induced movement of cholesterol from the cytofacial leaflet to the exofacial leaflet, which was ATPase-dependent (Garrigues et al., 2002). The actual mechanism of how P-gp may induce cholesterol redistribution is not understood and could be an indirect effect or cholesterol complexing with P-gp (Garrigues et al., 2002). Data not supporting cholesterol complexing with P-gp comes from results discussed earlier that reported that statins increased cholesterol distribution in the exofacial leaflet (Kirsch et al., 2003; Burns et al., 2004). Statins are a substrate for P-gp and it would seem that statins would compete with cholesterol for binding to the protein (Bogman et al., 2001).

There is evidence that sphingomyelin may contribute to regulation of TCD (Slotte and Bierman, 1988; Porn et al., 1991). Hydrolysis of sphingomyelin in Leydig tumor cells and fibroblasts resulted in movement of cholesterol from the cell surface to the cell interior where cholesterol was esterified. Sphingomyelin may be involved in regulating cellular cholesterol distribution, but this regulation may involve exofacial leaflet cholesterol and not cytofacial leaflet cholesterol. Sphingomyelin is primarily if not exclusively located in the exofacial leaflet of erythrocytes and SPM (Roelofsen, 1982; Rao et al., 1993; Wood et al., 1993). Sphingomyelin accounts for approximately between 2% and 4% of the total SPM phospholipid (Wood et al., 1989a, 1993; Rao et al., 1993) and that sphingomyelin is not present in the SPM cytofacial leaflet (Rao et al., 1993). In erythrocytes, sphingomyelin content is approximately 25% of total phospholipid (Dougherty et al., 1987) content and the amount in the exofacial leaflet was reported to be between 82% and 100%, depending on species (Roelofsen, 1982). The percent of cholesterol in SPM exofacial leaflet is around 13%–15% of total SPM cholesterol. Cholesterol content in the erythrocyte exofacial leaflet is approximately 25% of the total membrane cholesterol (Schroeder et al., 1991). Thus, increasing sphingomyelin content in the exofacial leaflet is positively associated with increasing cholesterol content in that leaflet. Not supporting the regulation of TCD by sphingomyelin is the fact that the cytofacial leaflet contains the highest amount of cholesterol and the lowest level of sphingomyelin compared with the exofacial leaflet. TCD is altered by several different conditions. Whether a singular mechanism regulates TCD has yet to be determined. It is possible that multiple mechanisms contribute to membrane TCD. It is worth noting that while TCD is modified by apparently unrelated factors, in most instances the cytofacial leaflet maintains the highest level of cholesterol compared with the exofacial leaflet.

3.2 Lipid Rafts and Caveolae

For purposes of this discussion, lipid rafts will refer to structures enriched in cholesterol, glycosphingolipids, and glycosylphosphatidylinositol (GPI)-anchored proteins and not containing the caveolae protein caveolin, as shown in ❷ Figure 7-2, panel A. Other names for lipid rafts have been detergent-insoluble glycolipid-enriched membranes and detergent-resistant membranes (Quest et al., 2004). Caveolae are defined as membrane invaginations containing caveolin enriched in cholesterol and glycosphingolipids (Yamada, 1955) and are discussed later. There have been several recent reviews of lipid rafts (Edidin, 2003; Fielding and Fielding, 2003; Lai, 2003; Quest et al., 2004) and the reader is referred to these reviews for a comprehensive and detailed discussion of lipid rafts. Evidence suggests that cholesterol condenses the packing of sphingolipid molecules and this microdomain forms a separate lipid-ordered phase in the exofacial leaflet of the membrane (Brown and London, 1998; Simons and Ikonen, 2000). Lipid rafts are thought to be involved in signal transduction, protein sorting, and may be factors in several different diseases. There has been substantial interest in lipid rafts in brain, both with respect to normal functioning and with certain neurodegenerative diseases. Lipid rafts were reported to be involved in maintenance of neuronal structure and function (Hering et al., 2003), and it was shown in another study that SNARE proteins were enriched in rafts, including the cholesterol-binding protein synaptophysin (Chamberlain et al., 2001). Lipid rafts contain the cellular prion protein and its scrapie isoform (Naslavsky et al., 1997). Data have been reported on localization of APP and Aβ in lipid rafts and these studies are discussed in ❷ Sect. 3. Both apoE genotype and increasing age altered synaptosomal lipid raft structural components (Igbavboa et al., 2005). These differences were most evident for the lipid raft protein markers alkaline phosphatase and flotillin-1 in comparison to the lipid markers sphingomyelin and cholesterol. Lipid rafts of young apoE4 mice were more similar to those of older mice with respect to alkaline phosphatase activity and flotillin-1 abundance as compared with young apoE3 mice. Cholesterol levels of lipid rafts did increase with age in both genotypes. The mechanism of raft formation is not well understood. Potential explanations for raft formation include preference of cholesterol for the saturated acyl chains of sphingolipids compared with glycerophospholipids and the dynamic interactions of protein–lipid and protein–protein linkages (Lai, 2003). An additional mechanism has been proposed whereby proteins are encased in a shell of cholesterol and sphingolipid and this "lipid shell" is delivered to cholesterol–sphingolipid membrane domains (Anderson and Jacobson, 2002).

While there have been a sizeable number of studies on what have been described as lipid rafts, there are many unanswered questions pertaining to these lipid domains. There is no agreement on the shape, size, or lifetime of rafts in vivo (Lai, 2003). Lipid rafts have not been visualized in a cell in contrast to caveolae (Lai, 2003). However, in more recent studies using different biophysical techniques (e.g., FRET, particle tracking, fluorescence anisotropy, EPR) to determine the viscosity and diffusion parameters, information on lipid rafts in cells is inferred. These techniques do not actually provide an image of a raft but do allow an estimation of the size of lipid rafts ranging between 10 and 100 nm (Edidin, 2003; Lai, 2003). An intriguing observation made was that lipid rafts may be relatively unstable with a lifetime of less than a millisecond (Subczynski and Kusumi, 2003). If rafts exist for less than a millisecond then isolation of rafts as commonly done using density gradient centrifugation may be problematic with respect to the protein and lipid composition of the presumed raft fraction. In fact, a contentious issue is the method of isolating lipid rafts (Hooper, 1999; Brown and London, 2000; Edidin, 2003; Lai, 2003; Lichtenberg et al., 2005). The standard method is to use a cold detergent such as Triton X-100 and density gradient centrifugation. It has been argued that the use of detergents may actually induce formation of detergent-resistant lipid domains and not be representative of membrane structures (Lichtenberg et al., 2005). In addition, it has also been observed that different detergent/lipid ratios and starting materials can influence the lipid and protein composition, making comparisons among studies difficult (Edidin, 2003). The use of nondetergent methods has been suggested (Brown and London, 2000), and clearly differences are seen both qualitatively and quantitatively in proteins and lipids when a detergent method is employed in contrast to a nondetergent method using brain synaptosomes (Eckert et al., 2003).

Whereas lipid rafts have not been visualized, caveolae were detected by electron microscopy over 50 years ago and are 50–100 nm invaginations in the plasma membrane (Palade, 1953; Yamada, 1955). Caveolae are flask-like structures in membranes, which are enriched in cholesterol and sphingolipids and contain the protein caveolin as seen in ❷ *Figure 7-2*, panel B. Functionally, caveolae are involved in endocytosis, signal transduction, and cholesterol homeostasis (Anderson and Jacobson, 2002; Fielding and Fielding, 2003). Caveolins are a protein family consisting of caveolin-1 and caveolin-2, which are expressed in numerous cell types, and caveolin-3, primarily limited to muscle cells (Anderson, 1993; Lisanti et al., 1994). Caveolin-1 was identified in rat astrocytes and electron microscopy revealed caveolae in astrocyte membranes (Cameron et al., 1997; Teixeira et al., 1999). There is some debate as to whether caveolin are present in neurons. Caveolin mRNA was not detected in rat hippocampal neurons (Cameron et al., 1997) and the caveolin-1 protein was not seen in rat forebrain SPM (Wu et al., 1997). However, both caveolin-1 mRNA and protein were found in primary rat hippocampal neurons and caveolin-1 protein was reported in mouse primary hippocampal neurons (Bu et al., 2003; Gaudreault et al., 2004). An explanation for the discrepancies between the two sets of studies is not clear. It is possible that studies reporting caveolin-1 in neurons may have had some astrocytes present. There have not been any reports of caveolae in neurons in contrast to caveolae observed in astrocytes (Cameron et al., 1997).

4   Cholesterol and Brain Pathophysiology

4.1 Niemann–Pick Type C Disease, Malformation Syndromes, and Huntington's Disease

Cholesterol plays many roles in the brain, and it is required for optimal functioning. In some instances, the regulation of this sterol is altered leading to neuropathophysiology. Two of the most striking examples where aberrant cholesterol homeostasis underlies pathology are malformation syndromes resulting from inborn errors of cholesterol synthesis and Niemann–Pick type C (NPC) disease. Malformation syndromes comprise at least five syndromes in which inborn errors of cholesterol synthesis occur during development (Porter, 2002). Smith–Lemli–Opitz syndrome (SLOS) is one of the best studied malformation syndromes and is characterized by mental retardation, microcephaly, and other features. SLOS is due to a deficit in cholesterol synthesis resulting from mutations in the gene for the protein 3β-hydroxysterol Δ^7-reductase (DHCR7) (Porter, 2002). This protein converts 7-dehydrocholesterol to cholesterol. Cholesterol deficiency can result in structural and functional cell impairment, but it has also been proposed that the accumulation of precursor sterols may have pathophysiological consequences in malformation syndromes (Porter, 2002).

NPC is an autosomal recessive lipid storage disease caused by mutations in the NPC1 protein (Vance et al., 2005). It has been estimated that 95% of individuals with NPC have a dysfunctional NPC1 protein and approximately 5% have mutations in NPC2. Accumulation of lipids including cholesterol, gangliosides, and other lipids in the endocytic pathway is characteristic of NPC (Vanier et al., 1983; Blanchette-Mackie et al., 1988). Cholesterol accumulation occurs in both peripheral and neural cells but pathophysiology is greatest in brain (Suresh et al., 1998). It has been proposed that NPC1 is involved in cholesterol trafficking but neither the specific function of this protein is well understood nor the function of NPC2. As pointed out in a recent review (Vance et al., 2005), the association between cholesterol abundance in the endosomal pathway and neurodegeneration has not been clearly substantiated. Instead, an alterative hypothesis was proposed implicating a deficit in cholesterol in other cell organelles, resulting from the accumulation in the endosomal pathway (Vance et al., 2005). There is emerging albeit small number of studies linking impairment of cholesterol synthesis with Huntington's disease (HD) (Sipione et al., 2002; Valenza et al., 2005). A microarray analysis of clonal striatal cells expressing different fragments of huntingtin, a protein involved in HD, and expression of genes regulating lipid metabolism including cholesterol metabolism were observed (Sipione et al., 2002). In a follow-up study of human HD samples, expression levels of mRNAs for HMG-CoA reductase, cytochrome P450 lanosterol 14α-demethylase, and 7-dehydroxcholesterol reductase were reduced in the striatum and cerebral cortex as compared with control levels. Similar findings were observed in a mouse model of HD (Valenza et al., 2005). The reduction in gene activity was attributed to a decrease in the transcription factor SREBP. Earlier studies of lipid composition in brain tissue and skin fibroblasts, however, did not observe differences in cholesterol levels (Norton et al., 1978) or synthesis (Maltese, 1984) in patients with HD compared with control individuals. Further work is needed to establish a linkage between cholesterol homeostasis and HD.

4.2 Increasing Age and Cholesterol Homeostasis

Aging is not considered a disease but there are certainly changes in brain structure and function with increasing age (Teter and Finch, 2004). To that end, it has been previously proposed that cholesterol increases in neuronal membranes, leading to alterations in membrane structure and function (Cutler et al., 2004). In a review of studies on aging and brain cholesterol, the conclusion was that changes in brain cholesterol levels have not been consistently observed (Wood and Schroeder, 1988). The lack of agreement on brain aging and cholesterol may be due in part to the brain area examined, whole brain preparation versus a membrane preparation. The majority of studies on aging and brain cholesterol have examined age differences in the total amounts of brain cholesterol whereas age differences could occur in the amounts of cholesterol domains. As discussed in the section on TCD, the asymmetric distribution of cholesterol in SPM of aged mice was reduced compared with younger mice, in the absence of changes in the total amount of SPM cholesterol (Igbavboa et al., 1996). In addition, it was reported that cholesterol content of lipid rafts was greater in 24-month-old mice expressing either human apoE3 or apoE4 as compared with 2- and 12-month-old mice (Igbavboa et al., 2005). Whether bulk brain cholesterol abundance increases with age is not established, but as mentioned earlier in this chapter, brain dolichol levels are dramatically increased with age but the consequences of this increase are not known. Dolichol has been reported to increase in aged rat brains in the absence of an increase in cholesterol. FPP is a precursor for both cholesterol and dolichol, involving separate pathways (❯ *Figure 7-1*), and the aged-related increase in dolichol may be due to an upregulation in enzymes associated with that specific pathway.

4.3 Alzheimer's Disease

Several different lines of evidence point to a potential role of cholesterol in AD (Burns and Duff, 2002; Michikawa, 2003; Wood et al., 2003; Wolozin, 2004). Some but not all epidemiological studies report that patients taking statins were at a lower risk of developing AD than subjects not taking statins (Jick et al., 2000; Wolozin et al., 2000; Heart Protection Study Collaborative Group, 2002; Shepherd et al., 2002). ApoE, as discussed earlier, is a major carrier of cholesterol in brain (Mahley et al., 1984; Pitas et al., 1987b; Mauch et al., 2001), and individuals with the apoE4 allele are at greater risk of developing AD compared with individuals with the apoE2 or -3 alleles (Poirier et al., 1993b; Saunders et al., 1993). There is a large body of experimental data showing interplay between cholesterol and Aβ, a protein thought to be an important contributor to neurodegeneration, which occurs with AD. Cholesterol levels modulate APP expression and

Aβ production (Bodovitz and Klein, 1996; Howlands et al., 1998; Simons et al., 1998; Runz et al., 2002). Conversely, Aβ alters cellular cholesterol dynamics, particularly cholesterol trafficking in astrocytes and neurons, which could certainly impact on cell function (Puttfarcken et al., 1997; Beffert et al., 1998; Liu et al., 1998; LaDu et al., 2000, 2001; Igbavboa et al., 2003). It was reported that a high-cholesterol diet in a transgenic mouse expressing APP/PS1 increased Aβ load (Refolo et al., 2000). Cholesterol levels in brain of the cholesterol diet group were significantly higher compared with the control group, with a mean difference of 1.92 mg/g between the two groups. On the other hand, the mean difference between the two groups for plasma cholesterol was 101.81 mg/dl. As discussed earlier, plasma cholesterol levels and brain cholesterol levels are not in equilibrium. Certainly the plasma and brain cholesterol levels in the aforementioned study support this conclusion. Furthermore, it has been shown that statin administration to guinea pigs reduced Aβ levels but did not reduce brain cholesterol levels (Fassbender et al., 2001), which would suggest that alterations in total brain cholesterol are not involved in Aβ production.

If dietary administration of cholesterol does not appreciably increase brain cholesterol levels then what is the explanation for the changes observed in Aβ dynamics? Perhaps changes in cholesterol domains may be the pivotal factor in APP and Aβ dynamics. Statin-induced redistribution of cholesterol between the exofacial and cytofacial leaflets of mouse SPM was associated with APP processing (Burns et al., 2004). APP as well as Aβ and presenilin-1 have been found to be located in lipid raft fractions (Bouillot et al., 1996; Lee et al., 1998; Morishima-Kawashima and Ihara, 1998; Hayashi et al., 2000). Caveolin-3 was upregulated in astrocytes nearby senile plaques in brain tissue of patients with AD and brain tissue of mice which overexpress human APP with the Swedish mutation (Nishiyama et al., 1999), suggesting possible involvement of caveolae. However, arguing against the location of APP in lipid rafts or caveolae were results showing that APP and BACE1 were situated in more fluid regions of membranes in contrast to cholesterol-enriched regions of the hippocampus of patients with AD and mice expressing wild-type human APP (Abad-Rodriguez et al., 2004). It was concluded in this study that neuronal loss and not accumulation of cholesterol increases amyloidogenesis. Most explanations for effects of cholesterol levels on APP and Aβ have centered on cholesterol abundance in the brain. Perhaps some compound outside of brain could be influencing APP and Aβ. To date, no compound has been identified. A potential candidate is a group of cholesterol metabolites such as oxysterols (Heverin et al., 2005). Under normal conditions oxysterols are present in trace amounts but it is reasonable to expect that dietary administration of cholesterol could increase their abundance. Oxysterols in contrast to cholesterol can partition into membranes including the BBB and it was recently reported that uptake into the brain of the oxysterol 27-hydroxycholesterol from the peripheral circulation was observed in both humans and rats (Heverin et al., 2005). Whether oxysterols originating outside of brain and crossing the BBB may contribute to effects of high-cholesterol diets on Aβ dynamics is yet to be determined. While plasma oxysterols may possibly act on Aβ dynamics, these molecules would not explain the effects of statins in reducing APP and Aβ levels. Statins have cholesterol-independent effects involving reduction of isoprenoids, leading to less prenylated proteins, which could be a factor in reducing APP and Aβ levels. Statins inhibited the inflammatory effects of Aβ, which were due to reduced isoprenoid levels in contrast to a reduction in cholesterol in microglia cells (Cordle and Landreth, 2005).

The experimental findings on cholesterol–APP/Aβ interaction are not in agreement as to the contribution of cholesterol. This lack of agreement is also observed in epidemiological studies. Some have proposed that elevated cholesterol levels may be a risk factor for AD (Sparks et al., 2002; Puglielli et al., 2003). However, in a review of studies on serum and brain cholesterol levels the conclusion reached was that there was no consistent support for elevated cholesterol levels as a risk factor for AD (Wood et al., 2005). Actually such a conclusion is not surprising when consideration is given to the number of AD patients versus the number of individuals with hypercholesterolemia. The number of patients in the U.S. with AD is estimated at 4.5 million (Hebert et al., 2003) and the estimated number of American adults with cholesterol values of 200 mg/dl and higher is 105 million (CDC/NCHS, 2003), and of this number 37 million have cholesterol levels of 240 mg/dl higher. If elevated cholesterol is a risk factor for AD then there should be more individuals with AD. Granted this conclusion is a broad generalization and does not take into account factors such as age differences, lipoprotein profiles, and other disorders associated with hypercholesterolemia. Perhaps there is a subset of individuals with elevated cholesterol levels who are at risk for AD.

For example, it has been reported that elevated cholesterol levels between 40–55 years of age may be predictive of subsequent development of AD (Pappolla et al., 2003). A significant association was seen between amyloid load and total serum cholesterol levels in the 40- to 55-year-old age group compared with older individuals where no association was observed. Hypercholesterolemia may be more pathological in middle aged individuals than in older individuals. Interestingly, a recent study found that high cholesterol levels in late life were predictive of a reduced risk of dementia (Mielke et al., 2005). It was suggested in this study that the timing of cholesterol determination may be an important factor in an association between cholesterol levels and dementia.

5 Conclusion

Cholesterol is absolutely necessary for optimal brain function. Either too much cholesterol or too little can disrupt neuronal structure and function. While there are similarities in cholesterol dynamics in brain and outside of brain, there are major differences in the brain (ratio of unesterified cholesterol to esterified cholesterol, apolipoprotein and lipoprotein distribution, and production of the oxysterol 24S-hydroxycholesterol), making the actions of cholesterol unique in the central nervous system. The contribution of oxysterols to cell function in the brain is not well understood for either sterols enriched in the brain or those derived from plasma. The role of isoprenoid compounds (dolichol, GGPP, FPP) on brain cell function requires further study and the levels of GGPP and FPP in brain will need to be determined in order to understand the contribution of these potentially important compounds.

Increasing attention is being given to brain cholesterol domains and their role in cell function. Cholesterol is asymmetrically distributed between the two membrane leaflets. A majority of the studies that have reported changes in TCD have shown that the percent of cholesterol in the exofacial leaflet is increased and the cytofacial leaflet cholesterol is reduced. An explanation for what would appear to be a one-directional movement of cholesterol has not been forthcoming. Potential mechanisms may involve lipid and protein composition, lipid packing, and membrane curvature. Another question pertains to the functional significance of TCD. In some instances (i.e., increasing age, alcohol consumption, apoE4 isoform, apoE-null), the alterations in TCD could be interpreted as pathophysiological with respect to the membrane. On the other hand, statins have similar effects on TCD and their role is generally viewed as neuroprotective. Lipid rafts have attracted considerable attention. However, there are concerns regarding whether lipid rafts actually are present in vivo and on their size, shape, lifetime, and methods of isolation. Technological advancements (e.g., three-dimensional structure, optics, improved fluorescent cholesterol analogues) will have to be made in order to confirm lipid rafts as a biological entity (Lai, 2003).

Aberrant cholesterol homeostasis is clearly a factor in the pathophysiology of malformation syndromes resulting from inborn errors of cholesterol synthesis and NPC disease in the central nervous system. There is some evidence that abnormal cholesterol dynamics may be involved in HD and neuronal dysfunction occurring with increasing age but more work is needed to establish the contribution of cholesterol in these conditions. AD is another disease where cholesterol may be a factor in promoting neurodegeneration. However, this topic is not without controversy and it remains to be established as to the role of cholesterol in AD.

Finally, Brown and Goldstein in their Nobel address indicated that ever since its discovery cholesterol has "exerted an almost hypnotic fascination for scientists from the most diverse areas of science and medicine." This comment certainly rings true for those of us studying the regulation and function of this fascinating molecule in brain.

Acknowledgments

This work was supported by grants from the National Institutes of Health AG-23524, AG-18357, NATO Collaborative Linkage Grant (980136), and resources/facilities of the Minneapolis VA Medical Center.

References

Abad-Rodriguez J, Ledesma MD, Craessaerts K, Perga S, Medina M, et al. 2004. Neuronal membrane cholesterol loss enhances amyloid peptide generation. J Cell Biol 167: 953-960.

Agranoff BW. 1989. Lipids. Basic Neurochemistry: Molecular, Cellular, and Medical Aspects. Siegel G, Agranoff B, Albers RW, Molinoff P, editors. New York: Raven Press, Ltd. pp. 91-107.

Anderson RGW. 1993. Caveolae: Where incoming and outgoing messengers meet. Proc Natl Acad Sci USA 90: 10909-10913.

Anderson RGW, Jacobson K. 2002. A role for lipid shells in targeting proteins to caveolae, rafts, and other lipid domains. Science 296: 1821-1825.

Andersson M, Appelkvist EL, Kristensson K, Dallner G. 1987. Distribution of dolichol and dolichyl phosphate in human brain. J Neurochem 49: 685-691.

Arismendi-Morillo G, Castellano A. 2005. Tumoral microblood vessels and vascular microenvironment in human astrocytic tumors. A transmission electron microscopy study. J Neuro-Oncol 73: 211-217.

Beffert U, Aumont N, Dea D, Lussier-Cacan S, Davignon J, et al. 1998. β-amyloid peptides increase the binding and internalization of apolipoprotein E to hippocampal neurons. J Neurochem 70: 1458-1466.

Björkhem I, Diczfalusy U. 2002. Oxysterols. Arterioscler Thromb Vasc Biol 22: 734-742.

Blanchette-Mackie EJ, Dwyer NK, Amende LM, Kruth HS, Butler JD, et al. 1988. Type-C Niemann–Pick disease: Low density lipoprotein uptake is associated with premature cholesterol accumulation in the Golgi complex and excessive cholesterol storage in lysosomes. Proc Natl Acad Sci USA 85: 8022-8026.

Bodovitz S, Klein WL. 1996. Cholesterol modulates α-secretase cleavage of amyloid precursor protein. J Biol Chem 271: 4436-4440.

Bogman K, Peyer A-K, Török M, Küsters E, Drewe J. 2001. HMG-CoA reductase inhibitors and P-glycoprotein modulation. Br J Pharmacol 132: 1183-1192.

Bouillot C, Prochiantz A, Rougon G, Allinquant B. 1996. Axonal amyloid precursor protein expressed by neurons in vitro is present in a membrane fraction with caveolae-like properties. J Biol Chem 271: 7640-7644.

Boyles JK, Pitas RE, Wilson E, Mahley RW, Taylor JM. 1985. Apolipoprotein E associated with astrocytic glia of the central nervous system and with nonmyelinating glia of the peripheral nervous system. J Clin Invest 76: 1501-1513.

Brown DA, London E. 1998. Functions of lipid rafts in biological membranes. Annu Rev Cell Dev Biol 14: 111-136.

Brown DA, London E. 2000. Structure and function of sphingolipid- and cholesterol-rich membrane rafts. J Biol Chem 275: 17221-17224.

Bu J, Bruckner SR, Sengoku T, Geddes JW, Estus S. 2003. Glutamate regulates caveolin expression in rat hippocampal neurons. J Neurosci Res 72: 185-190.

Burns M, Duff K. 2002. Cholesterol in Alzheimer's disease and tauopathy. Ann NY Acad Sci 977: 367-375.

Burns MP, Igbavboa U, Wood WG, Duff K. 2004. Common effects of statins on CNS cholesterol and APP processing. Abstract Viewer/Itinerary Planner, Society for Neuroscience 716.4.

Buttini M, Yu GQ, Shockley K, Huang Y, Jones B, et al. 2002. Modulation of Alzheimer-like synaptic and cholinergic deficits in transgenic mice by human apolipoprotein E depends on isoform, aging, and overexpression of amyloid β peptides but not on plaque formation. J Neurosci 22: 10539-10548.

Cameron PL, Ruffin JW, Bollag R, Rasmussen H, Cameron RS. 1997. Identification of caveolin and caveolin-related proteins in the brain. J Neurosci 17: 9520-9535.

CDC/NCHS 2003. Cholesterol status among adults in the United States. National Health and Nutrition Examination Survey, CDC/NCHS.

Chamberlain LH, Burgoyne RD, Gould GW. 2001. SNARE proteins are highly enriched in lipid rafts in PC12 cells: Implications for the spatial control of exocytosis. Proc Natl Acad Sci USA 98: 5619-5624.

Chung YM, Bae YS, Lee SY. 2003. Molecular ordering of ROS production, mitochondrial changes, and caspase activation during sodium salicylate-induced apoptosis. Free Radic Biol Med 34: 434-442.

Connor J, Schroit AJ. 1990. Aminophospholipid translocation in erythrocytes: Evidence for the involvement of a specific transporter and an endofacial protein. Biochemistry 29: 37-43.

Cordle A, Landreth G. 2005. 3-hydroxy-3-methylglutaryl-coenzyme A reductase inhibitors attenuate β-amyloid-induced microglial inflammatory responses. J Neurosci 25: 299-307.

Crisby M, Rahman SMA, Sylvén C, Winblad B, Schultzberg M. 2004. Effects of high-cholesterol diet on gliosis in apolipoprotein E knockout mice Implications for Alzheimer's disease and stroke. Neurosci Lett 369: 87-92.

Cutler RG, Kelly J, Storie K, Pedersen WA, Tammara A, et al. 2004. Involvement of oxidative stress-induced abnormalities in ceramide and cholesterol metabolism in brain aging and Alzheimer's disease. Proc Natl Acad Sci USA 101: 2070-2075.

Dam H. 1958. Historical introduction to cholesterol. Chemistry, Biochemistry and Pathology. Cook RP, editor. New York: Academic Press; pp. 1-14.

Dekroon RM, Armati PJ. 2003. The endosomal trafficking of apolipoprotein E3 and E4 in cultured human brain neurons and astrocytes. Neurobiol Dis 8: 78-89.

Diaz C, Schroit AJ. 1996. Role of translocases in the generation of phosphatidylserine asymmetry. J Membr Biol 151: 1-9.

Dietschy JM. 1997. Overview of cholesterol and lipoprotein metabolism in the brain, liver and extrahepatic organs. Nutr Metab Cardiovasc Dis 7: 162-168.

Dietschy JM, Turley SD. 2004. Cholesterol metabolism in the central nervous system during early development and in the mature animal. J Lipid Res 45: 1375-1397.

Dougherty RM, Galli C, Ferro-Luzzi A, Iacono JM. 1987. Lipid and phospholipid fatty acid composition of plasma, red blood cells, and platelets and how they are affected by dietary lipids: A study of normal subjects from, Italy, Finland, and the USA. Am J Clin Nuer 45: 443-455.

Eckert GP, Igbavboa U, Müller WE, Wood WG. 2003. Lipid rafts of purified mouse brain synaptosomes prepared with or without detergent reveal different lipid and protein domains. Brain Res 962: 144-150.

Eckert GP, Kirsch C, Müller WE. 2001. Differential effects of lovastatin treatment on brain cholesterol levels in normal and apoE-deficient mice. Neuroreport 12: 883-887.

Edidin M. 2003. The state of lipid rafts: From model membranes to cells. Annu Rev Biophys Biomol Struct 32: 257-283.

Fagan AM, Holtzman DM. 2000. Astrocyte lipoproteins, effects of apoE on neuronal function, and role of apoE in amyloid-β deposition in vivo. Microsc Res Tech 50: 297-304.

Fagan AM, Holtzman DM, Munson G, Mathur T, Schneider D, et al. 1999. Unique lipoproteins secreted by primary astrocytes from wild type, apoE(−/−), and human apoE transgenic mice. J Biol Chem 274: 30001-30007.

Fassbender K, Simons M, Bergmann C, Stroick M, Lutjohann D, et al. 2001. Simvastatin strongly reduces levels of Alzheimer's disease β-amyloid peptides Aβ 42 and Aβ 40 in vitro and in vivo. Proc Natl Acad Sci USA 98: 5856-5861.

Fielding CJ, Fielding PE. 2003. Relationship between cholesterol trafficking and signaling in rafts and caveolae. Biochim Biophys Acta 1610: 219-228.

Garrigues A, Escargueil AE, Orlowski S. 2002. The multidrug transporter, P-glycoprotein, actively mediates cholesterol redistribution in the cell membrane. Proc Natl Acad Sci USA 99: 10347-10352.

Gaudreault SB, Chabot C, Gratton J-P, Poirier J. 2004. The caveolin scaffolding domain modifies 2-amino-3-hydroxy-5-methyl-4-isoxazole propionate receptor binding properties by inhibiting phospholipase A₂ activity. J Biol Chem 279: 356-362.

Gong JS, Kobayashi M, Hayashi H, Zou K, Sawamura N, et al. 2002. Apolipoprotein E (ApoE) isoform-dependent lipid release from astrocytes prepared from human apoE3 and apoE4 knockin mice. J Biol Chem 277: 29919-29926.

Harr SD, Uint L, Hollister R, Hyman BT, Mendez AJ. 1996. Brain expression of apolipoproteins E, J, and A-I in Alzheimer's disease. J Neurochem 66: 2429-2435.

Hayashi H, Campenot RB, Vance DE, Vance JE. 2004. Glial lipoproteins stimulate axon growth of central nervous system neurons in compartmented cultures. J Biol Chem 279: 14009-14015.

Hayashi H, Igbavboa U, Hamanaka H, Kobayashi M, Fujita SC, et al. 2002. Cholesterol is increased in the exofacial leaflet of synaptic plasma membranes of human apolipoprotein E4 knockin mice. Neuroreport 13: 383-386.

Hayashi H, Mizuno T, Michikawa M, Haass C, Yanagisawa K. 2000. Amyloid precursor protein in unique cholesterol-rich microdomains different from caveolae-like domains. Biochim Biophys Acta 1483: 81-90.

Heart Protection Study Collaborative Group 2002. MRC/BHF Heart Protection Study of cholesterol lowering with simvastatin in 20536 high-risk individuals: A randomised placebo-controlled trial. Lancet 360: 7-22.

Hebert LE, Scherr PA, Bienias JL, Bennett DA, Evans DA. 2003. Alzheimer disease in the US population: Prevalence estimates using the 2000 census. Arch Neurol 60: 1119-1122.

Hering H, Lin CC, Sheng M. 2003. Lipid rafts in the maintenance of synapses, dendritic spines, and surface AMPA receptor stability. J Neurosci 23: 3262-3271.

Heverin M, Meaney S, Lütjohann D, Diczfalusy U, Wahren J, et al. 2005. Crossing the barrier: Net flux of 27-hydroxycholesterol into the human brain. J Lipid Res 46: 1047-1052.

Holstein SA, Hohl RJ. 2004. Isoprenoids: Remarkable diversity of form and function. Lipids 39: 293-309.

Holtzman DM. 2004. In vivo effects of ApoE and clusterin on amyloid-β metabolism and neuropathology. J Mol Neurosci 23: 247-254.

Holtzman DM, Pitas RE, Kilbridge J, Nathan B, Mahley RW, et al. 1995. Low-density lipoprotein receptor-related protein mediates apolipoprotein E-dependent neurite outgrowth in a central nervous system-derived neuronal cell line. Proc Natl Acad Sci USA 92: 9480-9484.

Hooper NM. 1999. Detergent-insoluble glycosphingolipid/cholesterol-rich membrane domains, lipid rafts, and caveolae (Review). Mol Mem Biol 16: 145-156.

Howlands DS, Trusko SP, Savage MJ, Reaume AG, Lang DM, et al. 1998. Modulation of secreted β-amyloid precursor protein and amyloid β peptide in brain by cholesterol. J Biol Chem 273: 16576-16582.

Huang Y, Weisgraber KH, Mucke L, Mahley RW. 2004. Apolipoprotein E: Diversity of cellular origins, structural and biophysical properties, and effects in Alzheimer's disease. J Mol Neurosci 23: 189-204.

Igbavboa U, Avdulov NA, Chochina SV, Wood WG. 1997. Transbilayer distribution of cholesterol is modified in brain synaptic plasma membranes of knockout mice deficient in the low-density lipoprotein receptor, apolipoprotein E, or both proteins. J Neurochem 69: 1661-1667.

Igbavboa U, Avdulov NA, Schroeder F, Wood WG. 1996. Increasing age alters transbilayer fluidity and cholesterol asymmetry in synaptic plasma membranes of mice. J Neurochem 66: 1717-1725.

Igbavboa U, Eckert GP, Malo TM, Studniski A, Johnson LNA, et al. 2005. Murine synaptosomal lipid raft protein and lipid composition are altered by expression of human apoE3 and 4 and by increasing age. J Neurol Sci 229–230: 225-232.

Igbavboa U, Hamilton J, Kim H-Y, Sun GY, Wood WG. 2002. A new role for apolipoprotein E: Modulating transport of polyunsaturated phospholipid molecular species in synaptic plasma membranes. J Neurochem 80: 255-261.

Igbavboa U, Pidcock JM, Johnson LNA, Malo TM, Studniski A, et al. 2003. Cholesterol distribution in the Golgi complex of DITNC1 astrocytes is differentially altered by fresh and aged amyloid β-peptide$_{1-42}$. J Biol Chem 278: 17150-17157.

Ingelsson M, Jesneck J, Irizarry MC, Hyman BT, Rebeck GW. 2004. Lack of association of the cholesterol 24-hydroxylase (CYP46) intron 2 polymorphism with Alzheimer's disease. Neurosci Lett 367: 228-231.

Jick H, Zornberg GL, Jick SS, Seshadri S, Drachman DA. 2000. Statins and the risk of dementia. Lancet 356: 1627-1631.

Johnson-Anuna LN, Eckert GP, Keller JH, Igbavboa U, Franke C, et al. 2005. Chronic administration of statins alters multiple gene expression patterns in mouse cerebral cortex. J Pharmacol Exp Ther 312: 786-793.

Jordán J, Galindo MF, Miller RJ, Reardon CA, Getz GS, et al. 1998. Isoform-specific effect of apolipoprotein E on cell survival and β-amyloid-induced toxicity in rat hippocampal pyramidal neuronal cultures. J Neurosci 18: 195-204.

Kabara JJ. 1973. A critical review of brain cholesterol metabolism. Prog Brain Res 40: 363-382.

Kirsch C, Eckert GP, Müller WE. 2003. Statin effects on cholesterol micro-domains in brain plasma membranes. Biochem Pharmacol 65: 843-856.

Koch S, Donarski N, Goetze K, Kreckel M, Stuerenburg H-J, et al. 2001. Characterization of four lipoprotein classes in human cerebrospinal fluid. J Lipid Res 42: 1143-1151.

La Du MJ, Shah JA, Reardon CA, Getz GS, Bu G, et al. 2000. Apolipoprotein E receptors mediate the effects of β-amyloid on astrocyte cultures. J Biol Chem 275: 33974-33980.

La Du MJ, Shah JA, Reardon CA, Getz GS, Bu G, et al. 2001. Apolipoprotein E and apolipoprotein E receptors modulate Aβ-induced glial neuroinflammatory responses. Neurochem Int 39: 427-434.

Lai EC. 2003. Lipid rafts make for slippery platforms. J Cell Biol 162: 365-370.

Lee S-J, Liyanage U, Bickel PE, Xia W, Lansbury PT, et al. 1998. A detergent-insoluble membrane compartment contains amyloid-β in vivo. Nat Med 4: 730-734.

Lichtenberg D, Goñi FM, Heerklotz H. 2005. Detergent-resistant membranes should not be identified with membrane rafts. Trends Biochem Sci 30: 430-436.

Lisanti MP, Scherer PE, Tang Z, Sargiacomo M. 1994. Caveolae, caveolin, and caveolin-rich membrane domains: A signaling hypothesis. Trends Cell Biol 4: 231-235.

Liu Y, Peterson DA, Schubert D. 1998. Amyloid-β peptide alters intracellular vesicle trafficking and cholesterol homeostasis. Proc Natl Acad Sci USA 95: 13266-13271.

Lund EG, Guileyardo JM, Russell DW. 1999. cDNA cloning of cholesterol 24-hydroxylase, a mediator of cholesterol homeostasis in the brain. Proc Natl Acad Sci USA 96: 7238-7243.

Lutjohann D, Breuer O, Ahlborg G, Nennesmo I, Siden A, et al. 1996. Cholesterol homeostasis in human brain: Evidence for an age-dependent flux of 24S-hydroxycholesterol from the brain into the circulation. Proc Natl Acad Sci USA 93: 9799-9804.

Lütjohann D, Stroick M, Bertsch T, Kühl S, Lindenthal B, et al. 2004. High doses of simvastatin, pravastatin, and cholesterol reduce brain cholesterol synthesis in guinea pigs. Steroids 69: 431-438.

Ma J, Brewer H, Potter H. 1996. Alzheimer Aβ neurotoxicity: Promotion by anti-chymotrypsin, apoE4; inhibition by Aβ-related peptides. Neurobiol Aging 17: 773-780.

Mahley RW. 1988. Apolipoprotein E: Cholesterol transport protein with expanding role in cell biology. Science 240: 622-630.

Mahley RW, Innerarity TL, Rall SC Jr, Weisgraber KH. 1984. Plasma lipoproteins: Apolipoprotein structure and function. J Lipid Res 25: 1277-1294.

Maltese WA. 1984. Cholesterol synthesis in cultured skin fibroblasts from patients with Huntington's disease. Biochem Med 32: 144-150.

Masliah E, Mallory M, Ge N, Alford M, Veinbergs I, et al. 1995. Neurodegeneration in the central nervous system of apoE-deficient mice. Exp Neurol 136: 107-122.

Masliah E, Mallory M, Veinbergs I, Miller A, Samuel W. 1996. Alternations in apolipoprotein E expression during aging and neurodegeneration. Prog Neurobiol 50: 493-503.

Mauch DH, Nägler K, Schumacher S, Göritz C, Müller E-C, et al. 2001. CNS synaptogenesis promoted by glia-derived cholesterol. Science 294: 1354-1357.

Mcfarlane SI, Muniyappa R, Francisco R, Sowers JR. 2002. Pleiotropic effects of statins: Lipid reduction and beyond. J Clin Endocrinol Metab 87: 1451-1458.

Michikawa M. 2003. The role of cholesterol in pathogenesis of Alzheimer's disease: Dual metabolic interaction between amyloid β-protein and cholesterol. Mol Neurobiol 27: 1-12.

Mielke MM, Zandi PP, Sjögren M, Gustafson D, Östling S, et al. 2005. High total cholesterol levels in late life associated with a reduced risk of dementia. Neurology 64: 1689-1695.

Mitter D, Reisinger C, Hinz B, Hollmann S, Yelamanchili SV, et al. 2003. The synaptophysin/synaptobrevin interaction critically depends on the cholesterol content. J Neurochem 84: 35-42.

Miyata M, Smith JD. 1996. Apolipoprotein E allele-specific antioxidant activity and effects on cytotoxicity by oxidative insults and β-amyloid peptides. Nat Genet 14: 55-61.

Moore SA, Yoder E, Murphy S, Dutton GR, Spector AA. 1991. Astrocytes not neurons produce docosahexaenoic acid 22:6-ω-3 and arachidonic acid 20:4-ω6. J Neurochem 56: 518-524.

Morishima-Kawashima M, Ihara Y. 1998. The presence of amyloid β-protein in the detergent-insoluble membrane compartment of human neuroblastoma cells. Biochemistry 37: 15247-15253.

Naslavsky N, Stein R, Yanai A, Friedlander G, Taraboulos A. 1997. Characterization of detergent-insoluble complexes containing the cellular prion protein and scrapie isoform. J Biol Chem 272: 6324-6331.

Nathan BP, Jiang Y, Wong GK, Shen F, Brewer GJ, et al. 2002. Apolipoprotein E4 inhibits and apolipoprotein E3 promotes neurite outgrowth in cultured adult mouse cortical neurons through the low-density lipoprotein receptor-related protein. Brain Res 928: 96-105.

Ng Ying Kin NM, Palo J, Haltia M, Wolfe LS. 1983. High levels of brain dolichols in neuronal ceroid-lipofuscinosis and senescence. J Neurochem 40: 1465-1473.

Nishiyama K, Trapp BD, Ikezu T, Ransohoff RM, Tomita T, et al. 1999. Caveolin-3 upregulation activates β-secretase-mediated cleavage of the amyloid precursor protein in Alzheimer's disease. J Neurosci 19: 6538-6548.

North P, Fleischer S. 1983. Alteration of synaptic membrane cholesterol/phospholipid ratio using a lipid transfer protein. J Biol Chem 258(2): 1242-1253.

Norton WT, Igbal K, Tiffany C, Tellez-Nagel I. 1978. Huntington disease: Normal lipid composition of purified neuronal perikarya and whole cortex. Neurology 28: 812-816.

Oda T, Pasinetti GM, Osterburg HH, Anderson C, Johnson SAFCE. 1994. Purification and characterization of brain clusterin. Biochem Biophys Res Commun 204: 1131-1136.

Ohyama Y, Meaney S, Heverin M, Ekström L, Brafman A, et al. 2006. Studies on the transcriptional regulation of cholesterol24-hydroxylase (9CYP46A1): Marked insensitivity towards different regulatory axes. J Biol Chem 281: 3810-3820.

Op den Kamp JAF. 1979. Lipid asymmetry in membranes. Annu Rev Biochem 48: 47-71.

Palade GE. 1953. Fine structure of blood capillaries. J Appl Phys 24: 1424-1436.

Papassotiropoulos A, Wollmer MA, Tsolaki M, Brunner F, Molyva D, et al. 2005. A cluster of cholesterol-related genes confers susceptibility for Alzheimer's disease. J Clin Psychiatry 66: 940-947.

Pappolla MA, Bryant-Thomas T, Herbert D, Pacheco J, Fabra Garcia M, et al. 2003. Mild hypercholesterolemia is an early risk factor for the development of Alzheimer amyloid pathology. Neurology 61: 199-205.

Pitas RE, Boyles JK, Lee SH, Foss D, Mahley RW. 1987a. Astrocytes synthesize apolipoprotein E and metabolize apolipoprotein E-containing lipoproteins. Biochim Biophys Acta 917: 148-161.

Pitas RE, Boyles JK, Lee SH, Hui D, Weisgraber KH. 1987b. Lipoproteins and their receptors in the central nervous system. Characterization of the lipoproteins in cerebrospinal fluid and identification of apolipoprotein B, E (LDL) receptors in the brain. J Biol Chem 262: 14352-14360.

Poirier J. 1994. Apolipoprotein E in animal models of CNS injury and in Alzheimer's disease. Trends Neurosci 17: 525-530.

Poirier J. 2005. Apolipoprotein E, cholesterol transport, and synthesis in sporadic Alzheimer's disease. J Mol Neurosci 26: 355-361.

Poirier J, Baccichet A, Dea D, Gauthier S. 1993a. Cholesterol synthesis and lipoprotein reuptake during synaptic remodelling in hippocampus in adult rats. Neuroscience 55: 81-90.

Poirier J, Davignon J, Bouthillier D, Kogan S, Bertrand P, et al. 1993b. Apolipoprotein E polymorphism and Alzheimer's disease. Lancet 342: 697-699.

Porn MI, Tenhunen J, Slotte JP. 1991. Increased steroid hormone secretion in mouse Leydig tumor cells after induction of cholesterol translocation by sphingomyelin degradation. Biochim Biophys Acta 1093: 7-12.

Porter FD. 2002. Malformation syndromes due to inborn errors of cholesterol synthesis. J Clin Invest 110: 715-724.

Puglielli L, Tanzi RE, Kovacs DM. 2003. Alzheimer's disease: The cholesterol connection. Nat Neurosci 6: 345-351.

Pullarkat RK, Reha H. 1982. Accumulation of dolichols in brains of elderly. J Biol Chem 257: 5991-5993.

Puttfarcken PS, Manelli AM, Falduto MT, Getz GS, La Du MJ. 1997. Effect of apolipoprotein E on neurite outgrowth and β-amyloid-induced toxicity in developing rat primary hippocampal cultures. J Neurochem 68: 760-769.

Quarles RH, Morell P, McFarlin DE. 1989. Diseases involving myelin. Basic Neurochemistry: Molecular, Cellular, and Medical Aspects. Siegel G, Agranoff B, Albers RW, Molinoff P, editors. New York: Raven Press; pp. 697-713.

Quest AFG, Leyton L, Párraga M. 2004. Caveolins, caveolae, and lipid rafts in cellular transport, signaling, and disease. Biochem Cell Biol 82: 129-144.

Rall SC Jr, Weisgraber KH, Mahley RW. 1982. Human apolipoprotein E: The complete amino acid sequence. J Biol Chem 257: 4171-4178.

Ramsey RB, Nicholas HJ. 1972. Brain lipids. Adv Lipid Res 10: 143-232.

Rao AM, Igbavboa U, Semotuk M, Schroeder F, Wood WG. 1993. Kinetics and size of cholesterol lateral domains in synaptosomal membranes: Modification by sphingomyelinase and effects on membrane enzyme activity. Neurochem Int 23: 45-52.

Rebeck GW. 2004. Cholesterol efflux as a critical component of Alzheimer's disease pathogenesis. J Mol Neurosci 23: 219-224.

Refolo LM, Pappolla MA, Malester B, LaFrancois J, Bryant-Thomas T, et al. 2000. Hypercholesterolemia accelerates the Alzheimer's amyloid pathology in a transgenic mouse model. Neurobiol Dis 7: 321-331.

Rip JW, Rupar CA, Ravi K, Carroll KK. 1985. Distribution, metabolism, and function of dolichol and polyprenols. Prog Lipid Res 24: 269-309.

Roelofsen B. 1982. Phospholipases as tools to study the localization of phospholipids in biological membranes. A critical review. J Toxicol 1(1): 87-197.

Roheim PS, Carey M, Forte T, Vega GL. 1979. Apolipoproteins in human cerebrospinal fluid. Proc Natl Acad Sci USA 76: 4646-4649.

Runz H, Rietdorf J, Tomic I, de Bernard M, Beyreuther K, et al. 2002. Inhibition of intracellular cholesterol transport alters presenilin localization and amyloid precursor protein processing in neuronal cells. J Neurosci 22: 1679-1689.

Saunders AM, Strittmatter WJ, Schmechel D, St. George-Hyslop PH, Pericak-Vance MA, et al. 1993. Association of apolipoprotein E allele E4 with late-onset familial and sporadic Alzheimer's disease. Neurology 43: 1467-1472.

Schachter D, Abbott RE, Cogan U, Flamm M. 1983. Lipid fluidity of the individual hemileaflets of human erythrocyte membranes. Ann NY Acad Sci 414: 19-28.

Schinkel AH. 1997. The physiological function of drug-transporting P-glycoproteins. Semin Cancer Biol 8: 161-170.

Schroeder F, Frolov AA, Murphy EJ, Atshaves BP, Pu L, et al. 1996. Recent advances in membrane cholesterol domain dynamics and intracellular cholesterol trafficking. Proc Soc Exp Biol Med 213: 150-177.

Schroeder F, Morrison WJ, Gorka C, Wood WG. 1988. Trans-bilayer effects of ethanol on fluidity of brain membrane leaflets. Biochim Biophys Acta 946: 85-94.

Schroeder F, Nemecz G, Wood WG, Morrot G, Ayraut-Jarrier M, et al. 1991. Transmembrane distribution of sterol in the human erythrocyte. Biochim Biophys Acta 1066: 183-192.

Shepherd J, Blauw GJ, Murphy MB, Bollen ELEM, Buckley BM, et al. 2002. Pravastatin in elderly at risk of vascular disease (PROSPER): A randomised controlled trial. Lancet 360: 1623-1630.

Simons K, Ikonen E. 2000. How cells handle cholesterol. Science 290: 1721-1726.

Simons M, Keller P, Destrooper B, Beyreuther K, Dotti CG, et al. 1998. Cholesterol depletion inhibits the generation of β-amyloid in hippocampal neurons. Proc Natl Acad Sci USA 95: 6460-6464.

Sipione S, Rigamonti D, Valenza M, Zuccato C, Conti L, et al. 2002. Early transcriptional profiles in huntingtin-inducible striatal cells by microarray analyses. Hum Mol Genet 15: 1953-1965.

Slotte JP, Bierman EL. 1988. Depletion of plasma-membrane sphingomyelin rapidly alters the distribution of cholesterol between plasma membranes and intracellular cholesterol pools in cultured fibroblasts. Biochem J 250: 653-658.

Sparks DL, Connor DJ, Browne PJ, Lopez JE, Sabbagh MN. 2002. HMG-CoA reductase inhibitors (statins) in the treatment of Alzheimer's disease and why it would be ill-advised to use one that crosses the blood–brain barrier. J Nutr Health Aging 6: 324-331.

Srere PA, Chaikoff IL, Treitman SS, Burstein LS. 1950. The extrahepatic synthesis of cholesterol. J Biol Chem 182: 629-634.

Subczynski WK, Kusumi A. 2003. Dynamics of raft molecules in the cell and artificial membranes: Approaches by pulse EPR spin labeling and single molecule optical microscopy. Biochim Biophys Acta 1610: 231-243.

Sun Y, Wu S, Bu G, Onifade MK, Patel SN, et al. 1998. Glial fibrillary acidic protein–apolipoprotein E (apoE) transgenic mice: Astrocyte-specific expression and differing biological effects of astrocyte-secreted apoE3 and apoE4 lipoproteins. J Neurosci 18: 3261-3272.

Suresh S, Yan Z, Patel RC, Patel YC, Patel SC. 1998. Cellular cholesterol storage in the Niemann–Pick disease type C mouse is associated with increased expression and defective processing of apolipoprotein D. J Neurochem 70: 242-251.

Teixeira A, Chaverot N, Schröder C, Strosberg AD, Couraud P-O, et al. 1999. Requirement of caveolae microdomains in extracellular signal-regulated kinase and focal adhesion kinase activation induced by endothelin-1 in primary astrocytes. J Neurochem 72: 120-128.

Teter B, Finch CE. 2004. Caiban's heritance and the genetics of neuronal aging. Trends Neurosci 27: 627-632.

Teter B, Xu PT, Gilbert JR, Roses AD, Galasko D, et al. 2002. Defective neuronal sprouting by human apolipoprotein E4 is a gain-of-negative function. J Neurosci Res 68: 331-336.

Thiele C, Hannah MJ, Fahrenholz F, Huttner WB. 2000. Cholesterol binds to synaptophysin and is required for biogenesis of synaptic vesicles. Nat Cell Biol 2: 42-49.

Titov VN. 1997. Structure of Apo A-I high density lipoproteins: A review. Biochemistry (Moscow) 62: 3-19.

Tong H, Holstein SA, Hohl RJ. 2005. Simultaneous determination of farnesyl and geranylgeranyl pyrophosphate levels in cultured cells. Anal Biochem 336: 51-59.

Tosi MR, Bottura G, Lucchi P, Reggiani A, Trinchero A, et al. 2003. Cholesteryl esters in human malignant neoplasms. Int J Mol Med 11: 95-98.

Turley SD, Dietschy JM. 1997. Regional variation in cholesterol synthesis and low-density lipoprotein transport in the brain of the fetus, newborn, and adult animal. Nutr Metab Cardiovasc Dis 7: 195-201.

Valenza M, Rigamonti D, Goffredo D, Zuccato C, Fenu S, et al. 2005. Dysfunction of the cholesterol biosynthetic pathway in Huntington's disease. J Neurosci 25: 9932-9939.

Vance DE, Van den Bosch H. 2001. Cholesterol in the year 2000. Biochim Biophys Acta 1529: 1-8.

Vance JE, Hayashi H, Karten B. 2005. Cholesterol homeostasis in neurons and glial cells. Semin Cell Dev Biol 16: 193-212.

Vanier MT, Rousson R, Louisot P. 1983. Chromatofocusing of skin fibroblast sphingomyelinase: Alterations in Niemann–Pick disease type C shared by GM1-gangliosidosis. Clin Chim Acta 130: 155-161.

Waelsch H, Sperry WM, Stoyanoff VA. 1940. Lipid metabolism in brain during myelination. J Biol Chem 135: 297-302.

Wassmann S, Laufs U, Bäumer AT, Müller K, Konkol C, et al. 2001. Inhibition of geranylgeranylation reduces angiotensin II-mediated free radical production in vascular smooth cells: Involvement of angiotensin AT1 receptor expression Rac1 GTPase. Mol Pharmacol 59: 646-654.

Weisgraber KH, Rall SC, Mahley RW. 1981. Human E apoprotein heterogeneity cysteine–arginine interchanges in the amino acid sequence of the apo-E isoforms. J Biol Chem 256: 9077-9083.

White F, Nicoll JA, Roses AD, Horsburgh K. 2001. Impaired neuronal plasticity in transgenic mice expressing human apolipoprotein E4 compared to E3 in a model of entorhinal cortex lesion. Neurobiol Dis 8: 611-625.

Wolfe LS, Ng Ying Kin NM, Palo J, Bergeron C, Kotila M, et al. 1985. Dolichols are elevated in brain tissue from Alzheimer's disease, but not in urinary sediment from Alzheimer's disease and Down's syndrome. Neurochem Pathol 3: 213-221.

Wolozin B. 2004. Cholesterol, statins, and dementia. Curr Opin Lipidol 15: 667-672.

Wolozin B, Kellman W, Ruosseau P, Celesia GG, Siegel G. 2000. Decreased prevalence of Alzheimer disease associated with 3-hydroxy-3-methyglutaryl coenzyme A reductase inhibitors. Arch Neurol 57: 1439-1443.

Wood WG, Schroeder F. 1988. Membrane structure in aged humans and animals. Central Nervous System Disorders of Aging: Clinical Intervention and Research. Strong R, Wood WG, Burke WJ, editors. New York: Raven Press; pp. 199-209.

Wood WG, Eckert GP, Igbavboa U, Müller WE. 2003. Amyloid β-peptide interactions with membranes and cholesterol: Causes or casualties of Alzheimer's disease. Biochim Biophys Acta 1610: 281-290.

Wood WG, Gorka C, Schroeder F. 1989a. Acute and chronic effects of ethanol on transbilayer membrane domains. J Neurochem 52: 1925-1930.

Wood WG, Sun GY, Schroeder F. 1989b. Membrane properties of dolichol in different age groups of mice. Chem Phys Lipids 51: 219-226.

Wood WG, Gorka C, Williamson LS, Strong R, Sun AY, et al. 1986. Dolichol alters dynamic and static properties of mouse synaptosomal plasma membranes. FEBS Lett 205 (1): 25-28.

Wood WG, Igbavboa U, Eckert GP, Johnson-Anuna LN, Müller WE. 2005. Is hypercholesterolemia a risk factor for Alzheimer's disease? Mol Neurobiol 31: 185-192.

Wood WG, Igbavboa U, Rao AM, Schroeder F, Avdulov NA. 1995. Cholesterol oxidation reduces Ca^{2+}/Mg^{2+}-ATPase activity, interdigitation, and increases fluidity of brain synaptic plasma membranes. Brain Res 683: 36-42.

Wood WG, Rao AM, Igbavboa U, Semotuk M. 1993. Cholesterol exchange and lateral cholesterol pools in synaptosomal membranes of pair-fed control and chronic ethanol-treated mice. Alcohol Clin Exp Res 17: 345-350.

Wood WG, Schroeder F, Avdulov NA, Chochina SV, Igbavboa U. 1999. Recent advances in brain cholesterol dynamics: Transport, domains and Alzheimer's disease. Lipids 34: 225-234.

Wood WG, Schroeder F, Hogy L, Rao AM, Nemecz G. 1990. Asymmetric distribution of a fluorescent sterol in synaptic plasma membranes: Effects of chronic ethanol consumption. Biochim Biophys Acta 1025: 243-246.

Wood WG, Schroeder F, Igbavboa U, Avdulov NA, Chochina SV. 2002. Brain membrane cholesterol domains, aging, and amyloid β-peptides. Neurobiol Aging 23: 685-694.

Wu C, Butz S, Ying Ys, Anderson RGW. 1997. Tyrosine kinase receptors concentrated in caveolae-like domains from neuronal plasma membrane. J Biol Chem 272: 3554-3559.

Xu Q, Li YH, Cyras C, Sanan DA, Cordell B. 2000. Isolation and characterization of apolipoproteins from murine microglia. J Biol Chem 275: 31770-31777.

Yamada E. 1955. The fine structure of the gall bladder epithelium of the mouse. J Biophys Biochem Cytol 1: 445-458.

Ye S, Huang Y, Mullendorff K, Dong L, Giedt G, et al. 2005. Apolipoprotein (apo) E4 enhances amyloid-β peptide production in cultured neuronal cells: ApoE structure as a potential therapeutic target. Proc Natl Acad Sci USA 102: 18700-18705.

Zachowski A. 1993. Phospholipids in animal eukaryotic membranes: Transverse asymmetry and movement. Biophys J 294: 1-14.

8 Aquaporins in the Central Nervous System

M. C. Papadopoulos · S. Saadoun · A. S. Verkman

Abstract: The aquaporins (AQPs) are a family of water channels expressed in plasma membrane of many cell types. At least three aquaporins are expressed in the central nervous system (CNS): AQP1 in choroid plexus, AQP4 in astrocytes, including those at the blood–brain and brain–cerebrospinal fluid barriers, and AQP9 in a subset of astrocytes. Phenotype analysis of transgenic mice lacking aquaporins has provided evidence for involvement of AQP1 in cerebrospinal fluid production and AQP4 in cerebral water balance, astrocyte migration, and neural signal transduction. AQP4 null mice have reduced brain swelling and improved neurological outcome in models of cytotoxic brain edema including water intoxication, focal cerebral ischemia, and bacterial meningitis, but greater swelling in models of vasogenic (fluid leak) edema including cortical freeze-injury, brain tumor, brain abscess, and hydrocephalus. AQP4 deficiency slows astrocyte migration in response to a chemotactic stimulus in vitro, and AQP4 deletion impairs glial scar progression following injury in vivo. AQP4 null mice also manifest abnormalities in evoked potential responses and extracellular space K^+ dynamics that may be caused by impaired K^+ reuptake by AQP4-deficient astrocytes. Thus, aquaporins in the CNS have a variety of functions in brain water balance, glial cell migration, and neural signal transduction. Modulation of AQP4 expression or function may provide a novel therapeutic strategy for various CNS disorders including stroke, tumor, infection, hydrocephalus, epilepsy, and trauma.

List of Abbreviations: aCSF, Artificial cerebrospinal fluid; AQP, Aquaporin; CNS, Central nervous system; CSF, Cerebrospinal fluid; ECS, Extracellular space; EEG, Electroencephalogram; FITC, Fluorescein isothiocyanate; GABA, Gamma aminobutyric acid; $(-/-)$, Knockout mouse; OAPs, Orthogonal arrays of particles; $(+/+)$, Wildtype mouse

1   Introduction

Fluid movement among the vascular, parenchymal, and ventricular compartments in brain is of fundamental importance in normal brain physiology and clinically relevant pathological conditions. Brain edema plays a role in the pathophysiology of a wide range of central nervous system (CNS) abnormalities such as stroke, tumor, infection, hydrocephalus, and traumatic brain injury (Fishman, 1975). Edema produces elevated intracranial pressure, potentially leading to brain ischemia, herniation, and death. Despite a large body of empirical data on brain edema and its causes and consequences, current treatments for brain edema such as hyperosmolar agents and surgical decompression have changed little since their introduction more than 80 years ago (Weed and McKibben, 1919). The discovery of aquaporin (AQP) water channels had led to the first molecular-level information about water transporting mechanisms in brain, and as discussed in this chapter, new possibilities for the therapy of brain edema and other CNS abnormalities.

The aquaporins are a family of small ($\sim$30 kDa per monomer), hydrophobic integral membrane proteins that are expressed widely in the animal and plant kingdoms, with 13 members identified so far in mammals. The mammalian aquaporins are expressed in various epithelia and endothelia involved in fluid transport, as well as in cell types that are classically thought not to carry out fluid transport such as skin, fat, and urinary bladder cells. In most cell types, the aquaporins are expressed at the plasma membrane. The aquaporins have been the subject of intense study by structural biologists, with high-resolution structural data available for several water channels (Ringler et al., 1999; Murata et al., 2000; Ren et al., 2000, 2001; Sui et al., 2000, 2001; Verkman and Mitra, 2000; Engel and Stahlberg, 2002; Fujiyoshi et al., 2002; de Groot et al., 2003; Zampighi et al., 2003; Harries et al., 2004; Schenk et al., 2005). Aquaporin monomers contain six tilted α-helical domains forming a barrel-like structure, with inverted symmetry between the first and last three helices. Aquaporin monomers contain independent water pores, though the monomers are stably assembled in membranes as tetramers.

An extensive body of functional measurements in heterologous expression systems and native cells indicate that AQPs 1, 2, 4, 5, and 8 are primarily water selective, whereas AQPs 3, 7, and 9 (called "aquaglyceroporins") also transport glycerol and possibly other small solutes in the case of AQP9. Molecular dynamics simulations based on the AQP1 crystal structure suggest tortuous, single-file passage of water through a narrow pore of <0.3-nm size, in which steric and electrostatic factors prevent transport of protons and other small molecules (Tajkhorshid et al., 2002). The reader is referred to reviews for more details about the structure and function of aquaporins (Verkman and Mitra, 2000; Engel and Stahlberg, 2002; Fujiyoshi et al., 2002; Agre and Kozono, 2003).

This chapter is focused on the role of aquaporins in brain function, as deduced from expression and regulation studies, and from phenotype analysis of transgenic mice lacking brain aquaporins.

2 Physiological Roles of Aquaporins Outside the CNS

2.1 Epithelial Fluid Transport

Analysis of transgenic mice lacking specific aquaporins has provided considerable insight into the physiological roles of aquaporins (Verkman, 2005). ❷ *Figure 8-1* shows some of the mechanisms by which

❑ **Figure 8-1**
Mechanisms of aquaporin function outside of the CNS. (a) Reduced water permeability in glandular epithelium impairs active, near-isosmolar fluid transport by slowing osmotic water transport into the acinar lumen, producing hypertonic secretion. (b) Reduced transepithelial water permeability in kidney collecting duct impairs urinary concentrating ability by preventing osmotic equilibration of luminal fluid. (c) Aquaporin-facilitated water entry into protruding lamellipodia, accounting for aquaporin-dependent cell migration. (d) Reduced steady-state glycerol content in epidermis and stratum corneum following AQP3 deletion, accounting for reduced skin hydration in AQP3 deficiency. (e) Impaired AQP7-dependent glycerol escape from adipocytes resulting in intracellular glycerol accumulation and increased triglyceride content, accounting for progressive adipocyte hypertrophy in AQP7 deficiency

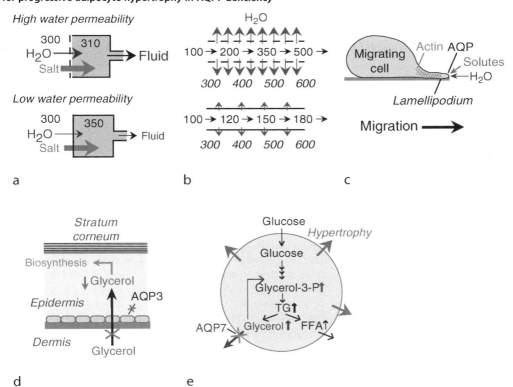

aquaporins are involved in important functions. Mice lacking several of the aquaporins (AQPs 1–4) manifest a defect in urinary concentrating ability. Impairment of active, near-isosmolar fluid absorption in kidney proximal tubule in AQP1 deficiency accounts in part for this defect. Near-isosmolar fluid secretion is impaired in salivary and airway submucosal gland in AQP5 deficiency, and for AQP1-dependent secretion of aqueous fluid by the ciliary epithelium and cerebrospinal fluid (CSF) by choroid plexus (see ❷ Sect. 4.1.2). The general paradigm from these findings is that high transepithelial water permeability permits rapid water transport in response to active transepithelial salt transport. As shown in ❷ Figure 8-1a, aquaporin deletion impairs osmotic equilibration, resulting in secretion of a reduced volume of relatively hypertonic fluid. ❷ Figure 8-1b depicts a second mechanism for involvement of aquaporins in mammalian physiology, in which the aquaporins facilitate passive, osmotically driven water transport. For example, osmotic extraction of water in kidney collecting duct increases urine osmolality in antidiuresis. Reduced collecting duct water permeability produced by aquaporin deficiency impairs osmotic equilibration and thus reduces urine osmolality.

2.2   Endothelial Functions

As discussed further in ❷ Sect. 4.3, a newly discovered role of aquaporins is in facilitating cell migration (Saadoun et al., 2005). ❷ Figure 8-1c shows the proposed mechanism. Actin cleavage and ion uptake at the tip of a lamellipodium create local osmotic gradients that drive the influx of water across the cell membrane. Water entry increases local hydrostatic pressure to cause cell membrane protrusion, creating space for actin polymerization and stabilization of the protrusion. Aquaporins in the region of membrane protrusions would enhance water entry and thus the dynamics of cell membrane protrusions and cell motility.

2.3   Role of Aquaglyceroporins

The above roles of aquaporins can be ascribed largely to their water-transporting function. There is now strong evidence that the aquaglyceroporins have unique biological roles that are related to their glycerol transport function. AQP3-facilitated glycerol transport in skin is an important determinant of epidermal and stratum corneum hydration (❷ Figure 8-1d). AQP3 is expressed strongly in the basal layer of keratinocytes in mammalian skin. Mice lacking AQP3 have reduced stratum corneum hydration and skin elasticity, delayed biosynthesis of the stratum corneum after removal by tape-stripping, and delayed wound healing. The mechanism responsible for the skin phenotype in AQP3 deficiency involves reduced epidermal cell skin glycerol permeability, resulting in reduced glycerol content in the stratum corneum and epidermis, with normal glycerol in dermis and serum. In support of this mechanism was the finding that glycerol replacement by topical or systemic routes corrected each of the skin phenotype abnormalities in AQP3 null mice (Hara and Verkman, 2003).

Another aquaglyceroporin, AQP7, is expressed in the plasma membrane of adipocytes. AQP7 null mice have a greater fat mass than wild-type mice as they age (Hara-Chikuma et al., 2005). Their adipocytes remarkably hypertrophy, and accumulate more glycerol and triglycerides than those in wild-type mice. Measurements in adipocytes of comparable size from younger mice showed reduced glycerol permeability in AQP7 deficiency and slowed glycerol release from minced fat tissue, without defects in lipolysis and lipogenesis. As depicted in ❷ Figure 8-1e, we proposed that the progressive triglyceride accumulation in AQP7-deficient adipocytes results from reduced plasma membrane glycerol permeability, and consequent increased steady-state glycerol and glycerol-3-phosphate concentrations, and increased triglyceride biosynthesis.

Thus, the aquaporins and their glycerol-transporting subset, the aquaglyceroporins, have a variety of functions in mammalian physiology. Many of the general paradigms about aquaporin function, such as in tissue swelling and cell migration, apply to CNS tissues as described in the next section. In addition, studies of aquaporins in the CNS have revealed new roles of aquaporins, as in neural signal transduction, which were predicted from studies in nonneural tissues.

3   Indirect Evidence for a Role of Aquaporins in the CNS

3.1   Aquaporin Expression in Brain

The sites of aquaporin expression provided clues about their functions in the CNS. Only AQPs 4 and 1 are strongly expressed in normal mouse brain (❯ *Figure 8-2a*) (Hasegawa et al., 1993; Nielsen et al., 1997; Rash et al., 1998), and similar aquaporin expression has recently been reported in normal human brain (Saadoun et al., 2002a, b; Lee et al., 2004; Mobasheri and Marples, 2004). AQP9 may also be weakly expressed, although its sites of expression remain controversial (see ❯ *Sect. 3.1.3*) (Badaut et al., 2002; Arima et al., 2003; Badaut and Regli, 2004). The expression of water channels is altered in several pathological conditions as will be discussed in ❯ *Sect. 3.3*.

3.1.1 Aquaporin-4

Immunohistochemical studies in rodent (Hasegawa et al., 1993; Rash et al., 1998) and human (Saadoun et al., 2002b; Lee et al., 2004) brains showed that AQP4 is strongly expressed in the glial limiting membrane

◻ Figure 8-2
Aquaporin expression in brain. (a) Only AQPs 1, 4, and 9 mRNAs (*arrowed*) are expressed in normal brain (mouse). AQP1 is strongly expressed in (b) choroid plexus epithelial cells (mouse), which form the border between CSF and blood. In human brain, AQP4 is found in (c) astrocyte foot processes around capillaries (*arrows*), and in (d) the glia limitans (*stars*), which is the boundary between brain and CSF. AQP1 and AQP4 immunostaining was visualized brown using diaminobenzidine, with cresyl violet counterstain

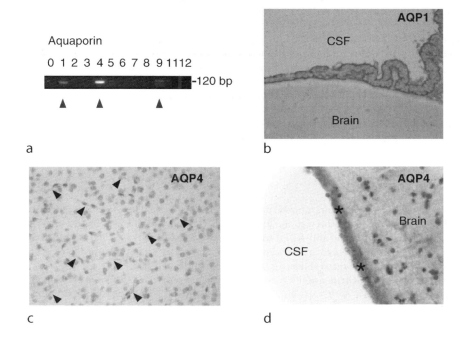

and astrocyte foot processes (❯ *Figure 8-2c* and *d*). The glial limiting membrane is comprised of densely packed astrocyte processes and is found under the pia matter at the border between brain parenchyma and subarachnoid CSF, and under the ependyma at the border between brain parenchyma and ventricular CSF. The ependymal epithelial cells, which line the ventricular wall, also express AQP4 in the basolateral plasma membranes (Frigeri et al., 1995; Nielsen et al., 1997; Rash et al., 1998). AQP4 expression is polarized in astrocyte foot processes that surround brain capillaries (Frigeri et al., 1995; Nielsen et al., 1997; Rash et al., 1998; Saadoun et al., 2002b), at the border between brain parenchyma and blood. High-resolution immunoelectron microscopy confirmed that AQP4 is concentrated in glial membranes facing the CSF–brain and blood–brain interfaces; AQP4 is not expressed in neurons or meningeal cells. The strong AQP4 expression at the border between major fluid compartments (blood and CSF) and brain parenchyma suggests that AQP4 may play an important role in the movement of water into and out of the brain. AQP4 is also found in astrocytes within the hypothalamic magnocellular nuclei (Jung et al., 1994; Nielsen et al., 1997), which are structures involved in osmoregulation. In the hypothalamus, AQP4 is expressed in astrocytic lamellae, which are in direct contact with vasopressin-secreting neurons. Although it has been suggested that AQP4 may be an important brain osmoreceptor (Jung et al., 1994), AQP4 null mice have normal osmoregulation apart from a minor defect in maximal urine concentrating ability (Ma et al., 1997).

Within the plasma membrane, AQP4 is a component of the regular square arrays seen by freeze-fracture electron microscopy, called orthogonal arrays of particles (OAPs). The involvement of AQP4 in OAP formation was originally proposed because of the expression of AQP4 in tissues known to contain OAPs (Frigeri et al., 1995), and it was later proven in heterologously expressing cell cultures (Yang et al., 1996) and from the absence of OAPs in AQP4 null mice (Verbavatz et al., 1997). Immunogold-label freeze-fracture electron microscopy confirmed the presence of AQP4 in OAPs in astrocyte foot processes in the brain (Nielsen et al., 1997; Rash et al., 1998).

3.1.2 Aquaporin-1

The choroid plexus forms the border between two major fluid compartments—CSF and blood. AQP1 is found in the ventricular-facing surface of choroid plexus epithelial cells in normal mouse (Oshio et al., 2005), rat (Masseguin et al., 2000; Speake et al., 2003), and human (Longatti et al., 2004; Mobasheri and Marples, 2004) brains (❯ *Figure 8-2b*). It has therefore been suggested that AQP1 plays a role in the production of CSF. Interestingly, AQP1 is not expressed in normal mouse brain endothelial cells, which are surrounded by astrocyte foot processes, although it is abundant in peripheral endothelia (Verkman, 2002; Saadoun et al., 2005). The lack of AQP1 from brain endothelia is in keeping with the low permeability of the blood–brain barrier to several substances. Interestingly, human brain tumor endothelial cells (Saadoun et al., 2002a) and cultured rodent cerebral endothelial cells (Dolman et al., 2005) express AQP1 protein, suggesting that in normal brain astrocytes might produce a factor that inhibits endothelial AQP1 expression.

3.1.3 Aquaporin-9

Unlike AQPs 4 and 1, AQP9 also transports small molecules, including glycerol, lactate, and urea (Ishibashi et al., 1998; Ko et al., 1999; Carbrey et al., 2003). However, a limitation in AQP9 immunohistochemical studies has been the lack of good anti-AQP9 antibodies and so uncertainty in reliability of localization data. In the brain, AQP9 immunoreactivity has been detected in tanycytes, which are nonciliated ependymal cells found in circumventricular organs (Elkjaer et al., 2000; Badaut et al., 2001; Nicchia et al., 2001; Badaut and Regli, 2004). It is not clear whether AQP9 is expressed in the subset of ciliated ependymal cells (Elkjaer et al., 2000; Badaut et al., 2001). AQP9 was also detected in cerebrovascular endothelia, astrocytes of the glia limitans, and white matter tracts (Elkjaer et al., 2000; Badaut et al., 2001; Nicchia et al., 2001; Badaut and

Regli, 2004). In contrast to AQP4, which is expressed primarily in the foot processes of astrocytes, AQP9 is reported to be expressed throughout the astrocyte cell bodies and processes in the brain. More recently, AQP9 has also been detected in catecholaminergic and glucose-sensitive neurons (Badaut and Regli, 2004), raising the possibility that AQP9 is involved in brain energy metabolism. According to the "lactate-shuttle" hypothesis, astrocytes take up glucose, metabolize it to lactate, and transport it to neurons, which use lactate as an energy substrate (Tsacopoulos and Magistretti, 1996). AQP9 is speculated to facilitate the transport of lactate from astrocytes to neurons, and so possibly its function in normal brain might be more related to lactate rather than water transport.

3.2   Aquaporin Expression in Spinal Cord

3.2.1 Aquaporin-4

In mouse spinal cord, AQP4 is present in both white and gray matter in a similar pattern as in brain, in pericapillary astrocyte foot processes, astrocyte foot processes adjacent to ependymal cells lining the central canal, and astrocyte processes comprising the glia limitans (Oshio et al., 2004). This suggests AQP4 involvement in water fluxes into and out of the spinal cord, as in brain. There is evidence of AQP4 expression in astrocyte processes in direct contact with neurons and synapses (Vitellaro-Zuccarello et al., 2005), raising the possibility that AQP4 may also modulate synaptic function in spinal cord.

3.2.2 Aquaporin-1

An interesting difference between mouse brain and spinal cord is the selective expression of AQP1 in neurons in the superficial dorsal horn of the spinal cord (Solenov et al., 2002), which is involved in the transmission of pain signals to the brain. C-fiber–related pain nociception was significantly reduced in AQP1 null mice in thermal tail flick and capsaicin injection studies, though perception of non-C-fiber pressure pain was not different from that in wild-type mice (Oshio et al., 2006). AQP1 has also been detected in neurons in cranial ganglia involved in nociception (Matsumoto et al., 2004). These findings suggest the possibility of AQP1 inhibitors as analgesics.

3.2.3 Aquaporin-9

Unlike brain, AQP9 is abundantly expressed in mouse spinal cord mostly in white matter where it colocalizes with radially arranged astrocytes (Oshio et al., 2004). As in brain astrocytes, AQP9 expression in spinal cord astrocytes is not polarized but is found throughout the astrocyte plasma membrane. It is not known why AQP9 is more prominent in spinal cord compared with brain. Because AQP9 is an aquaglyceroporin, it may play a role in lipid metabolism within the spinal cord, which is largely composed of fat-rich myelinated tracts.

3.3   Regulation of Aquaporin Expression

3.3.1 Aquaporin-4

Expression of AQP4 in rat brain is low before birth and increases steadily over the first 2 weeks after birth (Wen et al., 1999), which is associated with a decrease in extracellular space volume (Lehmenkuhler et al., 1993). Several studies have shown that AQP4 expression in brain is sensitive to brain edema caused by brain injury, providing indirect evidence for involvement of AQP4 in brain edema. AQP4 expression in astrocytes in vivo becomes upregulated in response to traumatic brain injury in rodents (Sun et al., 2003) and humans (Saadoun et al., 2003), focal cerebral ischemia in rodents (Taniguchi et al., 2000) and humans (Aoki et al., 2003), human malignant brain tumors (Saadoun et al., 2002b), rodent hyponatremia (Vajda et al., 2000), acute bacterial meningitis in mice (Papadopoulos and Verkman, 2005) and humans (Saadoun et al., 2003), and mouse staphylococcal brain abscess (Bloch et al., 2005). After the injury, AQP4 loses its polarity and becomes expressed throughout the astrocyte plasma membrane. In human brain tumors (❯ *Figure 8-3c* and *d*),

◻ Figure 8-3

Increased aquaporin immunoreactivity in human malignant brain tumors. (a) AQP1 is not found in normal cerebrovascular endothelium but is present in erythrocyte plasma membranes. (b) AQP1 is expressed in the vascular endothelium (*stars*) of brain tumors (adenocarcinoma). AQP4 expression in (c) region of reactive astrocytes (*arrows*) associated with metastatic brain carcinoma and (d) malignant cells within glioblastoma multiforme. AQP1 and AQP4 immunostaining was visualized brown using diaminobenzidine, with cresyl violet counterstain

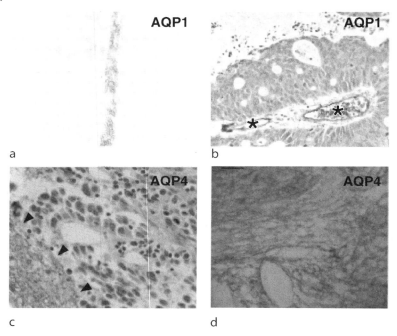

AQP4 protein expression correlates with the amount of edema (Saadoun et al., 2002b), and in rat focal cerebral ischemia the time course of increased AQP4 mRNA expression parallels brain edema (Taniguchi et al., 2000). Although brain edema is generally associated with upregulated AQP4 expression, AQP4 downregulation has been reported in some instances (Ke et al., 2001, 2002; Kiening et al., 2002). Recent evidence using AQP4 null mice suggests that AQP4 may increase the formation of cytotoxic (intracellular) brain edema but facilitate the elimination of vasogenic (extracellular) brain edema (Manley et al., 2000, 2004; Papadopoulos et al., 2002, 2004a, b; Bloch et al., 2005; Papadopoulos and Verkman, 2005) (see ❯ *Sects. 4.1.3* and ❯ *4.1.4*). In some cases, such as in brain tumors, which are associated with mainly vasogenic brain edema, the increased AQP4 expression may therefore be an adaptive response that facilitates the elimination of excess fluid. In other cases, such as cerebral ischemia, which primarily causes cytotoxic edema, upregulated AQP4 may be a maladaptive response that increases the rate of formation of brain edema. Interestingly, mannitol, an osmotic diuretic commonly used clinically to reduce intracranial pressure, stimulates the expression of AQPs 4 and 9 in mouse brain (Arima et al., 2003). This observation raises the possibility that AQP4 may mediate some of the brain edema–reducing effect of mannitol.

The molecular mechanisms responsible for increased brain AQP4 expression with development and injury are not understood, but p38 mitogen–activated protein kinase (Arima et al., 2003) and protein kinase C (Yamamoto et al., 2001) might be involved. The human AQP4 gene, located on chromosome 18, encodes proteins of 31 (M23 isoform) and 34 kDa (M1 isoform) that are produced by alternative splicing and separate promoters (Yang et al., 1995; Lu et al., 1996; Umenishi and Verkman, 1998). Both isoforms are expressed in the brain, but the smaller isoform is mainly found in other tissues. It is not known whether the M23 and M1 AQP4 isoforms become differentially expressed after brain injury. In transfected Chinese Hamster Ovary cells, M23 forms large orthogonal arrays containing more than 100 particles with frequent cross bridges, whereas M1 produces small arrays of less than 12 particles with no cross bridges (Furman et al., 2003). By changing the relative proportions of M1 versus M23 AQP4 isoform expression, it may be possible to change the pattern of water flow across the astrocyte membrane, analogous to changing the pattern of water flow in a showerhead. However, the functional significance of these observations remains unclear. It has been suggested that the degree of higher-order organization of AQP4 in OAPs influences single-channel osmotic water permeability (Yang et al., 1996, 1997; Silberstein et al., 2004).

3.3.2 Aquaporin-1

Although in normal brain AQP1 is found only in the choroid plexus, AQP1 becomes expressed in microvascular endothelium (❯ *Figure 8-3a* and *b*) and reactive astrocytes in human (Saadoun et al., 2002a) and rodent (Endo et al., 1999) malignant brain tumors. AQP1 expression in tumor endothelia may contribute to the increased blood–brain barrier water permeability of brain tumors. Recent data obtained using AQP1 null mice suggest that AQP1 expression in endothelial cells facilitates angiogenesis (Saadoun et al., 2005), which is essential for the rapid growth of malignant tumors (see ❯ *Sect. 4.3.2*). The expression of AQP1 in tumor vessels, but not in normal brain vessels, might be related to the absence of astrocytes in tumor, which might signal endothelial cells to inhibit AQP1 expression. This idea is supported by recent cell culture data showing that brain endothelia express AQP1 in the absence of astrocytes (Dolman et al., 2005). The nature of the communications between astrocytes and endothelial cells that regulate AQP1 expression in endothelia remain unknown.

3.3.3 Aquaporin-9

In response to focal brain ischemia, AQP9 becomes strongly expressed in some reactive astrocytes (Badaut et al., 2001). It has been suggested that AQP9, which can also transport lactate, may facilitate the elimination of excess lactate from the extracellular space into astrocytes during the reperfusion phase of ischemia (Badaut et al., 2001). This intriguing idea has not been experimentally validated.

Several molecules have been shown to regulate AQP9 expression, including protein kinases C and A, which reduce (Yamamoto et al., 2001) and increase (Yamamoto et al., 2002) AQP9 mRNA expression, respectively. P38 MAP-kinase has also been shown to be involved in increasing AQP9 expression after an osmotic stress (Arima et al., 2003).

Understanding the role of aquaporins in different pathologies is clinically important, for example in deciding whether an AQP4 activator/inducer or inhibitor is likely to reduce brain swelling. Such functional information cannot be obtained from descriptive expression or regulation studies; as discussed below, phenotype analysis of aquaporin null mice has greatly contributed to our understanding of the role of aquaporins in brain water homeostasis.

4   Evidence from Transgenic Mouse Models

4.1   Brain Fluid Balance

4.1.1 Introduction

The intracranial cavity (1.3–1.6 L) contains the brain parenchyma, which consists of intracellular (1.1–1.3 L in humans) and interstitial compartments (100–150 mL), CSF (75–100 mL), and blood (75–100 mL). Exchange of water between these compartments occurs at the blood–brain barrier, ventricular ependyma, glia limitans, choroid plexus, and arachnoid granulations. Osmotic gradients and hydrostatic pressure differences are the forces that drive water movement between the various compartments.

The accumulation of excess water in the brain parenchyma is termed brain edema. The two main types of brain edema are cytotoxic (intracellular) and vasogenic (extracellular) (Klatzo, 1987; Kimelberg, 1995). In many clinical conditions both types of edema coexist. Cytotoxic edema is seen early on following ischemic stroke, where the lack of energy substrates causes primarily astrocyte swelling by osmotic water flow (Kimelberg, 1995). Vasogenic edema is found in brain tumors, where destruction of the blood–brain barrier within the tumor bed allows excess fluid to enter the extracellular space of the brain parenchyma by hydrostatic forces (Klatzo, 1987). Because AQP4 controls the movement of water into and out of the brain parenchyma, it is expected to have a major role in cytotoxic and vasogenic brain edema (see ❷ *Sects. 4.1.3* and ❷ *4.1.4*).

The accumulation of excess water within the CSF compartment is termed hydrocephalus and is classified into noncommunicating (obstructive) and communicating. Obstructive hydrocephalus is caused by blockage in the flow pathway of CSF within the ventricular system (e.g., by a tumor), whereas communicating hydrocephalus is caused by damage to the arachnoid granulations that prevents CSF absorption (e.g., by subarachnoid blood). Rarely, hydrocephalus may be caused by CSF overproduction from a choroid plexus tumor. The expression of AQP1 in choroid plexus suggests its involvement in CSF secretion.

4.1.2 CSF Dynamics

In humans, CSF is produced primarily by the choroid plexus at a rate of ∼0.5 L a day (Brown et al., 2004). CSF is eliminated primarily down a hydrostatic pressure gradient through arachnoid granulations mostly into the sagittal venous sinus. The strong AQP1 expression in choroid plexus epithelium produces a fivefold higher osmotically induced water transport across the choroid plexus in wild-type versus AQP1 null mice. AQP1 null mice have a lower intracranial pressure than wild-type mice, with ∼25% reduced CSF production as measured using a dye dilution method (Oshio et al., 2005). As expected from the lack of AQP1 in the CSF outflow pathway, AQP1 null mice have normal CSF outflow. These findings provided the first functional evidence for involvement of AQP1 in CSF secretion. AQP1 inhibition might thus provide a new way of reducing CSF production rate in hydrocephalus, provided that AQP1 expression in choroid plexus does not become downregulated during hydrocephalus. Although AQP1 inhibition produces only a modest reduction in CSF production, AQP1 inhibitors may still be clinically useful in potentiating the effect of acetazolamide, which reduces CSF production by a different mechanism. Moreover, because intracranial compliance is nonlinear, a 25% reduction in CSF secretion produced enough drop in intracranial pressure to improve survival in the cortical freeze mouse model of brain injury (Oshio et al., 2005).

4.1.3 Cytotoxic Edema

Although a role for AQP4 in brain edema was suspected from regulation studies, the mechanisms of AQP4 involvement in cytotoxic versus vasogenic edema only became apparent from experiments with AQP4 null mice. In two models of cytotoxic edema, water intoxication and permanent focal ischemia (❷ *Figure 8-4*),

□ Figure 8-4

AQP4 deletion reduces cytotoxic brain edema. (a) Improved survival of AQP4 null mice (−/−) compared with wild type (+/+) following water intoxication produced by intraperitoneal injection of water (0.2-mL/g body weight). (b) (*Top*) Brain sections of mice at 24 h after ischemic stroke produced by permanent middle cerebral artery occlusion. Note midline shift and marked edema in brain from wild-type mice. (*Bottom*) Average hemispheric enlargement expressed as a percentage determined by image analysis of brain sections

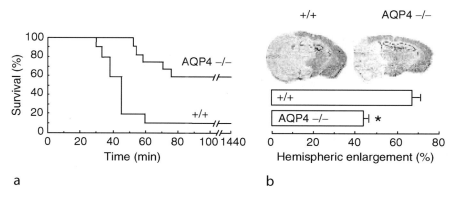

brain swelling was reduced in AQP4 null versus wild-type mice (Manley et al., 2000). Similar findings have been reported using α syntrophin (Amiry-Moghaddam et al., 2003) and dystrophin (Vajda et al., 2002) null mice, which have reduced brain AQP4 expression. Cytotoxic brain edema produced by Streptococcus pneumoniae was also reduced in AQP4 null mice (Papadopoulos and Verkman, 2005). Several outcome indices were used in these studies, including brain water content, intracranial pressure, ultrastructure, neurological score, and survival. AQP4 deletion is associated with reduced blood–brain barrier osmotic permeability (Papadopoulos and Verkman, 2005), suggesting that the mechanism by which AQP4 deletion limits cytotoxic brain swelling involves a reduction in the rate of entry of water into the brain. These findings suggest the possibility of AQP4 inhibitors as a novel means of reducing cytotoxic brain edema.

4.1.4 Vasogenic Edema

In contrast to the negative role of AQP4 in cytotoxic brain edema, AQP4 deletion increases vasogenic brain swelling following cortical freeze injury (❯ *Figure 8-5*), intraparenchymal fluid infusion, brain tumor (Papadopoulos et al., 2004a), and brain abscess (Bloch et al., 2005). Since insults that cause vasogenic brain edema damage the blood–brain barrier and the AQP4-rich astrocyte foot processes, the entry of excess water from the blood into the brain in vasogenic brain edema should be AQP4 independent. However, elimination of vasogenic edema fluid still occurs across AQP4-rich regions through the glia limitans into the subarachnoid CSF, across the ependyma into the ventricles, and through intact blood–brain barrier away from the lesion into the bloodstream. AQP4 deletion therefore increases vasogenic brain edema by reducing the rate of edema elimination. These data suggest that in vasogenic edema AQP4 inhibitors would aggravate brain swelling, whereas AQP4 activators/inducers are predicted to reduce brain swelling.

For many years, it has been thought that elimination of vasogenic edema fluid occurs by bulk flow through the extracellular space, primarily into CSF (Reulen et al., 1978, 1980; Tsuyumu et al., 1981; Wrba et al., 1997, 1998; Uhl et al., 1999). The finding that AQP4 facilitates the elimination of vasogenic edema fluid is therefore perplexing because it suggests that edema fluid may be eliminated from the extracellular space by a transcellular route (Papadopoulos et al., 2004a). Another possibility, however, is that AQP4

☐ **Figure 8-5**

AQP4 facilitates elimination of vasogenic brain edema in mice. Six hours after focal cortical freeze injury, AQP4 null mice (−/−) had (a) reduced intracranial pressure, and (b) lower % brain water content in the hemisphere ipsilateral and contralateral to the injury. Inset in (a) shows freeze-injured region demarcated by Evans blue staining. *$p < 0.01$, Data are mean ± SEM

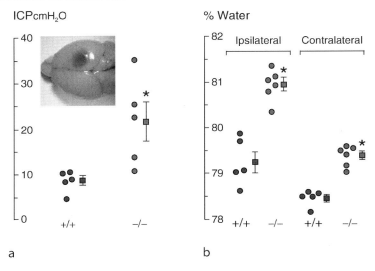

controls cell volume at the borders between brain parenchyma and CSF. According to this hypothesis, AQP4 deletion increases the size of astrocyte processes and ependymal cells, and reducing the space between them, which increases the resistance to outflow of extracellular edema fluid. Although these ideas have not been investigated in AQP4 null mice, enlarged astrocyte processes have been reported in mice lacking dystrophin that have reduced plasma membrane AQP4 expression (Nico et al., 2003).

4.1.5 Hydrocephalus

Hydrocephalus is caused by an imbalance in CSF production and absorption, resulting in excess ventricular fluid accumulation, depressed level of consciousness, and death if untreated (see ❷ *Sect. 4.1.1*). Current therapy for hydrocephalus involves surgical diversion of excess ventricular fluid, often by shunting into the peritoneal cavity. Although the molecular mechanisms of CSF production have been extensively investigated, little is known about CSF absorption (Keep et al., 1997; Brown et al., 2004; Redzic and Segal, 2004; Ennis and Keep, 2005). Recent evidence suggests AQP4-facilitated CSF absorption in hydrocephalus by a transparenchymal pathway into the cerebral vasculature (Bloch et al., 2006). For these experiments, a mouse model of hydrocephalus was created by injecting kaolin into the cisterna magna to obstruct CSF outflow pathways. Three days after kaolin injection, the resulting ventriculomegaly and elevated intracranial pressure were more marked in AQP4 null than wild-type mice, consistent with reduced CSF elimination in the AQP4 null mice. Brain parenchymal water content also increased 2–3% by 3 days, indicating backflow of CSF from the ventricles into the parenchymal extracellular space (ECS), analogous to the hydrocephalic edema seen in humans with acute hydrocephalus (Fishman, 1975). These results provide a rational basis for evaluation of AQP4 induction as a nonsurgical therapy to increase CSF absorption in hydrocephalus. Perhaps AQP4 induction can be combined with strategies to reduce CSF production, such as AQP1 inhibition (Oshio et al., 2005), for increased therapeutic benefit.

4.2   Neural Signal Transduction

The brain (ECS) comprises ~20% of brain tissue volume, consisting of a jellylike matrix in which neurons, glial cells, and blood vessels are embedded. The ECS contains ions, neurotransmitters, metabolites, peptides, and extracellular matrix molecules, forming the microenvironment for brain cells and the medium for nonsynaptic cell–cell communication. For example, neuroexcitability is accompanied by cellular K^+ release into the ECS and reuptake by glial cells. Several lines of evidence suggested the involvement of AQP4 in neural signal transduction. Based on the expression of AQP4 in epithelial cells adjacent to hair cells in rat inner ear, we initially investigated the involvement of AQP4 in auditory signal transduction (Li and Verkman, 2001). Auditory brainstem response thresholds were remarkably increased by >20 dB in AQP4 null mice compared to wild-type mice. Also, light-evoked potentials (b-wave amplitude measured by electroretinography) were reduced in AQP4 null mice (Li et al., 2002), consistent with the view that the AQP4-expressing Müller (glia-like) cells are functionally coupled to the transducing bipolar cells. In brain, seizure susceptibility in response to the convulsant (GABA antagonist) pentylenetetrazol was increased in AQP4 null mice (Binder et al., 2004b). More recently, in vivo EEG characterization of electrically induced seizures in the hippocampus indicated greater threshold and remarkably longer seizure duration in AQP4 null mice compared to wild-type mice (Binder et al., 2006). These phenotype observations suggested involvement of AQP4 in neural signal transduction, which we proposed could be related to AQP4-dependent K^+ dynamics in the ECS involving altered baseline ECS volume and K^+ reuptake from the ECS following neuroexcitation.

Evidence for an expanded ECS in AQP4 deficiency was obtained using a surface photobleaching method to measure the diffusion of fluorescently labeled macromolecules (Binder et al., 2004a; Papadopoulos et al., 2005). ECS in mouse brain was labeled by exposure of the intact dura to fluorescein dextran after craniectomy. Fluorescein-dextran diffusion was detected by fluorescence recovery after laser-induced cortical photobleaching using confocal optics. FITC-dextran diffusion was slowed approximately three-fold in brain ECS relative to solution. The cortical photobleaching approach was applied to problems of brain edema, seizure initiation, and AQP4 deficiency. Cytotoxic brain edema (produced by water intoxication) or seizure activity (produced by convulsants) slowed diffusion by more than tenfold and created dead-space microdomains in which free diffusion was prevented. FITC-dextran diffusion in brain ECS was significantly increased in AQP4 mice, indicating reduced "tortuosity" likely related to increased ECS volume.

Recent in vivo evidence was obtained for impaired K^+ reuptake from the ECS in AQP4 deficiency. A long-wavelength K^+-sensing fluorescent indicator, TAC-Red, was synthesized, which consisted of a triaza-cryptand K^+ ionophore coupled to a 3,6-bis(dimethylamino) xanthylium chromophore (Padmawar et al., 2005). The ECS of mouse brain surface was stained with TAC-Red by exposing the intact dura (after craniectomy) to artificial CSF (aCSF) containing TAC-Red. A pin prick model of cortical spreading depression produced propagating K^+ waves at the cortical surface. An approximately twofold slowed reuptake of K^+ was found in AQP4 null mice, though similar rates of K^+ release. We also found impaired K^+ reuptake from the ECS in vivo using K^+ sensitive microelectrodes and an electrical stimulation method (Binder et al., 2006); a similar conclusion was reported using hippocampal slices from α-syntrophin-deficient mice that manifest AQP4 mislocalization (Puwarawuttipanit et al., 2006). Thus, altered ECS volume and K^+ dynamics may account, at least in part, for the phenotype findings in AQP4 null mice. For example, the prolonged seizure duration in AQP4 null mice following electrical stimulation may be accounted for by the slowed K^+ reuptake into AQP4-expressing glial cells. However, the precise mechanisms relating AQP4 deficiency and altered neuroexcitability will require further investigation.

4.3   Cell Migration

4.3.1 Introduction

Cell migration is a complex multistep process that involves cell shape changes and rapid actin polymerization and depolymerization (Condeelis, 1993; Lauffenburger and Horwitz, 1996; Lambrechts et al., 2004). We recently showed aquaporin-facilitated cell migration in several different cell types, including mouse endothelia, Chinese Hamster Ovary cells, Fisher rat thyroid (Saadoun et al., 2005) cells, primary mouse cortical astrocytes (Saadoun et al., 2005), and kidney proximal tubule cells (Hara-Chikuma and Verkman, 2006). Here we discuss two brain processes that require cell migration: angiogenesis in brain tumors and glial scar formation following brain injury.

4.3.2 Angiogenesis in Brain Tumors

The observation that malignant melanoma grows faster in the brains of wild-type versus AQP1 null mice (Saadoun et al., 2005) suggests that AQP1 expression in endothelia of malignant human (Saadoun et al., 2002a) and rodent (Endo et al., 1999) brain tumors may facilitate angiogenesis, which is essential for rapid tumor growth (❷ *Figure 8-6*). The formation of new blood vessels within brain tumors requires multiple steps, including endothelial cell division, invasion of the extracellular matrix, migration, and tube formation. AQP1 is required during endothelial cell migration, but does not participate in the other steps of angiogenesis. AQP1 polarizes to the anterior end of the plasma membrane of migrating endothelial cells, where it facilitates the rapid formation of cell processes (lamellipodia and filopodia). Migrating AQP1 null endothelial cells form fewer processes at the leading end than wild-type endothelial cells because the formation of processes is probably associated with rapid water fluxes across the plasma membrane at the

◻ **Figure 8-6**

AQP1 deletion reduces the growth of tumors in mice. (a) Volume of malignant melanoma implanted (*left*) subcutaneously or (*right*) in brain (measured at 7 day postinjection), in wild-type (+/+) versus AQP1 null (−/−) mice. (b) (*Left*) Melanomas from wild-type mice have many capillaries and little necrosis, compared with (*right*) AQP4 null mice, which have few blood vessels and "islands" of viable tissue (*stars*) surrounded by necrotic regions (n). *$p < 0.01$, mean +/− SEM. In (b) the vessels were visualized brown by ILB$_4$/DAB staining with hematoxylin counterstain

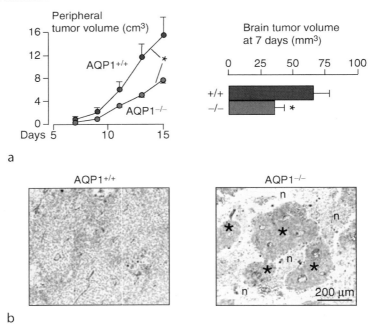

anterior end of the cell (Condeelis, 1993). The finding that AQP1 is important in the growth of brain tumors suggests that AQP1 inhibitors may have antitumor activity, by inhibiting the formation of new blood vessels.

4.3.3 Astrocyte Migration

Following traumatic brain injury, some astrocytes react by proliferating and migrating toward the site of injury (Bush et al., 1999; Pekny and Nilsson, 2005). These reactive astrocytes form multiple processes, which are densely packed around the site of injury. Reactive astrocytes have been shown to have increased AQP4 protein expression (Saadoun et al., 2002b, 2003; Aoki et al., 2003; Arima et al., 2003). Although reactive astrocytes are the main cell types that comprise the glial scar, other cell types, such as microglia, are also involved. Interestingly, it has recently been reported that reactive microglia also express AQP4 (Tomas-Camardiel et al., 2004). The glial scar has beneficial properties, such as repair of the damaged blood–brain barrier (Bush et al., 1999), as well as detrimental effects such as the inhibition of neuronal regeneration (Silver and Miller, 2004).

❯ *Figure 8-7* shows that loss of AQP4 expression in cultured mouse cortical astrocytes severely slows astrocyte migration speed. Similar to AQP1 in endothelial cells, AQP4 also polarizes to the leading edge of

❑ Figure 8-7

AQP4 deletion reduces astrocyte migration speed. (a) The Boyden migration assay. Astrocytes are plated on the porous filter in the top chamber, migrate toward a chemotactic stimulus, and attach to the undersurface of the filter in the bottom chamber. Nonmigrated cells are scraped off and the migrated astrocytes are stained blue and counted. (b) Wild-type (+/+) and AQP4 null (−/−) astrocytes that migrated through the porous filter in 6 h. (c) Summary of results. $^*p < 0.01$, mean ± SEM. Cells were stained with Coomassie blue

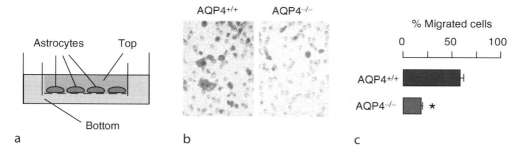

the plasma membrane of migrating astrocytes, where it may facilitate rapid transmembrane water fluxes responsible for cell shape changes. In a stab model of traumatic brain injury in vivo, AQP4 deletion was associated with impaired glial scar formation. These observations provide a novel explanation, which is unrelated to effects on brain edema, of why AQP4 becomes upregulated in astrocytes in response to brain damage: increased AQP4 expression accelerates the migration of reactive astrocytes toward the region of damage. Another intriguing observation is that the level of AQP4 protein expression in human astrocytoma cells directly correlates with the grade of malignancy (Saadoun et al., 2002b). We hypothesize that the high level of AQP4 expression in astrocytomas facilitates the migration of tumor cells, which may partly explain the highly infiltrative nature of these tumors. The association between AQP4 and astrocyte migration suggests that AQP4 inhibitors might reduce glial scarring and infiltration of malignant astrocytoma cells into surrounding brain.

5 Summary and Perspective

Studies of aquaporin expression and regulation, and phenotype analysis of mice lacking aquaporins, have indicated the involvement of aquaporins in several aspects of CNS function. AQP1 in choroid plexus facilitates secretion of CSF, though quantitatively the fraction of total choroidal, AQP1-dependent fluid secretion is modest. The role of AQP9 in the CNS is currently unclear. Phenotype analysis of AQP4 null mice has confirmed the involvement of AQP4 in cytotoxic brain edema, and provided strong evidence for unexpected roles of AQP4 in vasogenic brain edema, glial cell migration, and neural signal transduction. AQP4 facilitates water movement into and out of the brain in models of cytotoxic and vasogenic brain edema, predicting that AQP4 inhibition should reduce the accumulation of excess brain water in cytotoxic edema and that AQP4 induction/activation should reduce brain edema in vasogenic edema. Modulation of AQP4 expression or function is also predicted to modulate glial scar formation, which may be of clinical utility in traumatic injury, tumor, and infection. Interestingly, AQP4 appears also to play a key role in brain water and ion homeostasis during rapid neural activity, perhaps by altering baseline ECS volume and the kinetics of astroglial cell K^+ reuptake. The seizure phenotype data in AQP4 null mice suggest the possibility of AQP4 modulation in epilepsy therapy. The aquaporins thus provide a molecular-level mechanism for water movement into and out of the brain under normal and pathological conditions, and for astroglial cell migration and signaling functions. The identification of aquaporin inducers and inhibitors is thus of great importance not only in furthering animal studies of aquaporin functions in the CNS but as basis for the development of aquaporin-based drugs for several CNS pathologies.

References

Agre P, Kozono D. 2003. Aquaporin water channels: Molecular mechanisms for human diseases. FEBS Lett 555: 72-78.

Amiry-Moghaddam M, Otsuka T, Hurn PD, Traystman RJ, Haug FM, et al. 2003. An alpha-syntrophin-dependent pool of AQP4 in astroglial end-feet confers bidirectional water flow between blood and brain. Proc Natl Acad Sci USA 100: 2106-2111.

Aoki K, Uchihara T, Tsuchiya K, Nakamura A, Ikeda K, et al. 2003. Enhanced expression of aquaporin 4 in human brain with infarction. Acta Neuropathol (Berl) 106: 121-124.

Arima H, Yamamoto N, Sobue K, Umenishi F, Tada T, et al. 2003. Hyperosmolar mannitol simulates expression of aquaporins 4 and 9 through a p38 mitogen-activated protein kinase-dependent pathway in rat astrocytes. J Biol Chem 278: 44525-44534.

Badaut J, Regli L. 2004. Distribution and possible roles of aquaporin 9 in the brain. Neuroscience 129: 971-981.

Badaut J, Hirt L, Granziera C, Bogousslavsky J, Magistretti PJ, et al. 2001. Astrocyte-specific expression of aquaporin-9 in mouse brain is increased after transient focal cerebral ischemia. J Cereb Blood Flow Metab 21: 477-482.

Badaut J, Lasbennes F, Magistretti PJ, Regli L. 2002. Aquaporins in brain: Distribution, physiology, and pathophysiology. J Cereb Blood Flow Metab 22: 367-378.

Binder DK, Papadopoulos MC, Haggie PM, Verkman AS. 2004a. In vivo measurement of brain extracellular space diffusion by cortical surface photobleaching. J Neurosci 24: 8049-8056.

Binder DK, Oshio K, Ma T, Verkman AS, Manley GT. 2004b. Increased seizure threshold in mice lacking aquaporin-4 water channels. Neuroreport 15: 259-262.

Binder DK, Yao X, Sick TJ, Verkman AS, Manley GT. 2006. Increased seizure duration and slowed potassium kinetics in mice lacking aquaporin-4 water channels. Glia. 53: 631-636.

Bloch O, Papadopoulos MC, Manley GT, Verkman AS. 2005. Aquaporin-4 gene deletion in mice increases focal edema associated with staphylococcal brain abscess. J Neurochem 95: 254-262.

Bloch O, Manley GT, Verkman AS. 2006. Accelerated progression of kaolin-induced hydrocephalus in aquaporin-4 deficient mice. J Cereb Blood Flow Metab, in press.

Brown PD, Davies SL, Speake T, Millar ID. 2004. Molecular mechanisms of cerebrospinal fluid production. Neuroscience 129: 957-970.

Bush TG, Puvanachandra N, Horner CH, Polito A, Ostenfeld T, et al. 1999. Leukocyte infiltration, neuronal degeneration, and neurite outgrowth after ablation of scar-forming, reactive astrocytes in adult transgenic mice. Neuron 23: 297-308.

Carbrey JM, Gorelick-Feldman DA, Kozono D, Praetorius J, Nielsen S, et al. 2003. Aquaglyceroporin AQP9: Solute permeation and metabolic control of expression in liver. Proc Natl Acad Sci USA 100: 2945-2950.

Condeelis J. 1993. Life at the leading edge: The formation of cell protrusions. Annu Rev Cell Biol 9: 411-444.

de Groot BL, Engel A, Grubmuller H. 2003. The structure of the aquaporin-1 water channel: A comparison between cryo-electron microscopy and X-ray crystallography. J Mol Biol 325: 485-493.

Dolman D, Drndarski S, Abbott NJ, Rattray M. 2005. Induction of aquaporin 1 but not aquaporin 4 messenger RNA in rat primary brain microvessel endothelial cells in culture. J Neurochem 93: 825-833.

Elkjaer M, Vajda Z, Nejsum LN, Kwon T, Jensen UB, et al. 2000. Immunoloalization of AQP9 in liver, epididymis, testis, spleen, and brain. Biochem Biophys Res Commun 276: 1118-1128.

Kwon T, Endo M, Jain RK, Witwer B, Brown D. 1999. Water channel (aquaporin 1) expression and distribution in mammary carcinomas and glioblastomas. Microvasc Res 58: 89-98.

Engel A, Stahlberg H. 2002. Aquaglyceroporins: Channel proteins with a conserved core, multiple functions, and variable surfaces. Int Rev Cytol 215: 75-104.

Ennis SR, Keep RF. 2006. The effects of cerebral ischemia on the rat choroid plexus. J Cereb Blood Flow Metab 26: 675-683.

Fishman RA. 1975. Brain edema. N Engl J Med 293: 706-711.

Frigeri A, Gropper MA, Umenishi F, Kawashima M, Brown D, et al. 1995. Localization of MIWC and GLIP water channel homologs in neuromuscular, epithelial and glandular tissues. J Cell Sci 108: 2993-3002.

Fujiyoshi Y, Mitsuoka K, de Groot BL, Philippsen A, Grubmuller H, et al. 2002. Structure and function of water channels. Curr Opin Struct Biol 12: 509-515.

Furman CS, Gorelick-Feldman DA, Davidson KG, Yasumura T, Neely JD, et al. 2003. Aquaporin-4 square array assembly: Opposing actions of M1 and M23 isoforms. Proc Natl Acad Sci USA 100: 13609-13614.

Hara M, Verkman AS. 2003. Glycerol replacement corrects defective skin hydration, elasticity, and barrier function in aquaporin-3-deficient mice. Proc Natl Acad Sci USA 100: 7360-7365.

Hara-Chikuma M, Verkman AS. 2006. Aquaporin-1 facilitates epithelial cell migration in kidney proximal tubule. J Am Soc Nephrol 17: 39-45.

Hara-Chikuma M, Sohara E, Rai T, Ikawa M, Okabe M, et al. 2005. Progressive adipocyte hypertrophy in aquaporin-7-deficient mice: Adipocyte glycerol permeability as a novel regulator of fat accumulation. J Biol Chem 280: 15493-15496.

Harries WE, Akhavan D, Miercke LJ, Khademi S, Stroud RM. 2004. The channel architecture of aquaporin 0 at a 2.2-A resolution. Proc Natl Acad Sci USA 101: 14045-14050.

Hasegawa H, Zhang R, Dohrman A, Verkman AS. 1993. Tissue-specific expression of mRNA encoding rat kidney water channel CHIP28k by in situ hybridization. Am J Physiol 264: C237-C245.

Ishibashi K, Kuwahara M, Gu Y, Tanaka Y, Jung JS, Bhat RV, Preston GM, Guggino WB, Baraban JM, et al. 1994. Molecular characterization of an aquaporin cDNA from brain: Candidate osmoreceptor and regulator of water balance. Proc Natl Acad Sci USA 91: 13052-13056.

Ke C, Poon WS, Ng HK, Pang JC, Chan Y. 2001. Heterogeneous responses of aquaporin-4 in oedema formation in a replicated severe traumatic brain injury model in rats. Neurosci Lett 301: 21-24.

Ke C, Poon WS, Ng HK, Lai FM, Tang NL, et al. 2002. Impact of experimental acute hyponatremia on severe traumatic brain injury in rats: Influences on injuries, permeability of blood-brain barrier, ultrastructural features, and aquaporin-4 expression. Exp Neurol 178: 194-206.

Keep RF, Xiang J, Ulanski LJ, Brosius FC, Betz AL. 1997. Choroid plexus ion transporter expression and cerebrospinal fluid secretion. Acta Neurochir Suppl 70: 279-281.

Kiening KL, van Landeghem FK, Schreiber S, Thomale UW, von Deimling A, et al. 2002. Decreased hemispheric Aquaporin-4 is linked to evolving brain edema following controlled cortical impact injury in rats. Neurosci Lett 324: 105-108.

Kimelberg HK. 1995. Current concepts of brain edema. Review of laboratory investigations. J Neurosurg 83: 1051-1059.

Klatzo I. 1987. Pathophysiological aspects of brain edema. Acta Neuropathol (Berl) 72: 236-239.

Ko SB, Uchida S, Naruse S, Kuwahara M, Ishibashi K, et al. 1999. Cloning and functional expression of rAOP9L a new member of aquaporin family from rat liver. Biochem Mol Biol Int 47: 309-318.

Lambrechts A, Van Troys M, Ampe C. 2004. The actin cytoskeleton in normal and pathological cell motility. Int J Biochem Cell Biol 36: 1890-1909.

Lauffenburger DA, Horwitz AF. 1996. Cell migration: A physically integrated molecular process. Cell 84: 359-369.

Lee TS, Eid T, Mane S, Kim JH, Spencer DD, et al. 2004. Aquaporin-4 is increased in the sclerotic hippocampus in human temporal lobe epilepsy. Acta Neuropathol (Berl) 108: 493-502.

Lehmenkuhler A, Sykova E, Svoboda J, Zilles K, Nicholson C. 1993. Extracellular space parameters in the rat neocortex and subcortical white matter during postnatal development determined by diffusion analysis. Neuroscience 55: 339-351.

Li J, Verkman AS. 2001. Impaired hearing in mice lacking aquaporin-4 water channels. J Biol Chem 276: 31233-31237.

Li J, Patil RV, Verkman AS. 2002. Mildly abnormal retinal function in transgenic mice without Muller cell aquaporin-4 water channels. Invest Ophthalmol Vis Sci 43: 573-579.

Longatti PL, Basaldella L, Orvieto E, Fiorindi A, Carteri A. 2004. Choroid plexus and aquaporin-1: A novel explanation of cerebrospinal fluid production. Pediatr Neurosurg 40: 277-283.

Lu M, Lee MD, Smith BL, Jung JS, Agre P, et al. 1996. The human AQP4 gene: Definition of the locus encoding two water channel polypeptides in brain. Proc Natl Acad Sci USA 93: 10908-10912.

Ma T, Yang B, Gillespie A, Carlson EJ, Epstein CJ, et al. 1997. Generation and phenotype of a transgenic knockout mouse lacking the mercurial-insensitive water channel aquaporin-4. J Clin Invest 100: 957-962.

Manley GT, Fujimura M, Ma T, Noshita N, Filiz F, et al. 2000. Aquaporin-4 deletion in mice reduces brain edema after acute water intoxication and ischemic stroke. Nat Med 6: 159-163.

Manley GT, Binder DK, Papadopoulos MC, Verkman AS. 2004. New insights into water transport and edema in the central nervous system from phenotype analysis of aquaporin-4 null mice. Neuroscience 129: 983-991.

Masseguin C, Corcoran M, Carcenac C, Daunton NG, Guell A, et al. 2000. Altered gravity downregulates aquaporin-1 protein expression in choroid plexus. J Appl Physiol 88: 843-850.

Matsumoto I, Nagamatsu N, Arai S, Emori Y, Abe K. 2004. Identification of candidate genes involved in somatosensory functions of cranial sensory ganglia. Brain Res Mol Brain Res 126: 98-102.

Mobasheri A, Marples D. 2004. Expression of the AQP-1 water channel in normal human tissues: A semiquantitative study using tissue microarray technology. Am J Physiol Cell Physiol 286: C529-C537.

Murata K, Mitsuoka K, Hirai T, Walz T, Agre P, et al. 2000. Structural determinants of water permeation through aquaporin-1. Nature 407: 599-605.

Nicchia GP, Frigeri A, Nico B, Ribatti D, Svelto M. 2001. Tissue distribution and membrane localization of aquaporin-9 water channel: Evidence for sex-linked differences in liver. J Histochem Cytochem 49: 1547-1556.

Nico B, Frigeri A, Nicchia GP, Corsi P, Ribatti D, et al. 2003. Severe alterations of endothelial and glial cells in the blood-brain barrier of dystrophic mdx mice. Glia 42: 235-251.

Nielsen S, Nagelhus EA, Amiry-Moghaddam M, Bourque C, Agre P, et al. 1997. Specialized membrane domains for water transport in glial cells: High-resolution immunogold cytochemistry of aquaporin-4 in rat brain. J Neurosci 17: 171-180.

Oshio K, Binder DK, Yang B, Schecter S, Verkman AS, et al. 2004. Expression of aquaporin water channels in mouse spinal cord. Neuroscience 127: 685-693.

Oshio K, Watanabe H, Song Y, Verkman AS, Manley GT. 2005. Reduced cerebrospinal fluid production and intracranial pressure in mice lacking choroid plexus water channel Aquaporin-1. FASEB J 19: 76-78.

Oshio K, Watanabe H, Yan D, Verkman AS, Manley GT. 2006. Impaired pain sensation in mice lacking aquaporin-1 water channels. Biochem Biophys Res Commun, 341: 1022-1028.

Padmawar P, Yao X, Bloch O, Manley GT, Verkman AS. 2005. K+ waves in brain cortex visualized using a long-wavelength K+-sensing fluorescent indicator. Nat Methods 2: 825-827.

Papadopoulos MC, Verkman AS. 2005. Aquaporin-4 gene disruption in mice reduces brain swelling and mortality in pneumococcal meningitis. J Biol Chem 280: 13906-13912.

Papadopoulos MC, Krishna S, Verkman AS. 2002. Aquaporin water channels and brain edema. Mt Sinai J Med 69: 242-248.

Papadopoulos MC, Manley GT, Krishna S, Verkman AS. 2004a. Aquaporin-4 facilitates reabsorption of excess fluid in vasogenic brain edema. FASEB J 18: 1291-1293.

Papadopoulos MC, Saadoun S, Binder DK, Manley GT, Krishna S, et al. 2004b. Molecular mechanisms of brain tumor edema. Neuroscience 129: 1011-1020.

Papadopoulos MC, Binder DK, Verkman AS. 2005. Enhanced macromolecular diffusion in brain extracellular space in mouse models of vasogenic edema measured by cortical surface photobleaching. FASEB J 19: 425-427.

Pekny M, Nilsson M. 2005. Astrocyte activation and reactive gliosis. Glia 50: 427-434.

Puwarawuttipanit W, Bragg AD, Frydenlund DS, Mylonakou MN, Nagelhus EA, et al. 2006. Differential effect of alpha-syntrophin knockout on aquaporin-4 and Kir4.1 expression in retinal macroglial cells in mice. Neuroscience 137: 165-175.

Rash JE, Yasumura T, Hudson CS, Agre P, Nielsen S. 1998. Direct immunogold labeling of aquaporin-4 in square arrays of astrocyte and ependymocyte plasma membranes in rat brain and spinal cord. Proc Natl Acad Sci USA 95: 11981-11986.

Redzic ZB, Segal MB. 2004. The structure of the choroid plexus and the physiology of the choroid plexus epithelium. Adv Drug Deliv Rev 56: 1695-1716.

Ren G, Cheng A, Reddy V, Melnyk P, Mitra AK. 2000. Three-dimensional fold of the human AQP1 water channel determined at 4 A resolution by electron crystallography of two-dimensional crystals embedded in ice. J Mol Biol 301: 369-387.

Ren G, Reddy VS, Cheng A, Melnyk P, Mitra AK. 2001. Visualization of a water-selective pore by electron crystallography in vitreous ice. Proc Natl Acad Sci USA 98: 1398-1403.

Reulen HJ, Tsuyumu M, Tack A, Fenske AR, Prioleau GR. 1978. Clearance of edema fluid into cerebrospinal fluid. A mechanism for resolution of vasogenic brain edema. J Neurosurg 48: 754-764.

Reulen HJ, Tsuyumu M, Prioleau G. 1980. Further results concerning the resolution of vasogenic brain edema. Adv Neurol 28: 375-381.

Ringler P, Borgnia MJ, Stahlberg H, Maloney PC, Agre P, et al. 1999. Structure of the water channel AqpZ from Escherichia coli revealed by electron crystallography. J Mol Biol 291: 1181-1190.

Saadoun S, Papadopoulos MC, Davies DC, Bell BA, Krishna S. 2002a. Increased aquaporin 1 water channel expression in human brain tumors. Br J Cancer 87: 621-623.

Saadoun S, Papadopoulos MC, Davies DC, Krishna S, Bell BA. 2002b. Aquaporin-4 expression is increased in oedematous human brain tumors. J Neurol Neurosurg Psychiatry 72: 262-265.

Saadoun S, Papadopoulos MC, Krishna S. 2003. Water transport becomes uncoupled from K^+ siphoning in brain contusion, bacterial meningitis, and brain tumors: Immunohistochemical case review. J Clin Pathol 56: 972-975.

Saadoun S, Papadopoulos MC, Hara-Chikuma M, Verkman AS. 2005. Impairment of angiogenesis and cell migration by targeted aquaporin-1 gene disruption. Nature 434: 786-792.

Schenk AD, Werten PJ, Scheuring S, de Groot BL, Muller SA, et al. 2005. The 4.5 A structure of human AQP2. J Mol Biol 350: 278-289.

Silberstein C, Bouley R, Huang Y, Fang P, Pastor-Soler N, et al. 2004. Membrane organization and function of M1 and M23 isoforms of aquaporin-4 in epithelial cells. Am J Physiol Renal Physiol 287: F501-F511.

Silver J, Miller JH. 2004. Regeneration beyond the glial scar. Nat Rev Neurosci 5: 146-156.

Solenov EI, Vetrivel L, Oshio K, Manley GT, Verkman AS. 2002. Optical measurement of swelling and water transport in spinal cord slices from aquaporin null mice. J Neurosci Methods 113: 85-90.

Speake T, Freeman LJ, Brown PD. 2003. Expression of aquaporin 1 and aquaporin 4 water channels in rat choroid plexus. Biochim Biophys Acta 1609: 80-86.

Sui H, Walian PJ, Tang G, Oh A, Jap BK. 2000. Crystallization and preliminary X-ray crystallographic analysis of water channel AQP1. Acta Crystallogr D Biol Crystallogr 56: 1198-1200.

Sui H, Han BG, Lee JK, Walian P, Jap BK. 2001. Structural basis of water-specific transport through the AQP1 water channel. Nature 414: 872-878.

Sun MC, Honey CR, Berk C, Wong NL, Tsui JK. 2003. Regulation of aquaporin-4 in a traumatic brain injury model in rats. J Neurosurg 98: 565-569.

Tajkhorshid E, Nollert P, Jensen MO, Miercke LJ, O'Connell J, et al. 2002. Control of the selectivity of the aquaporin water channel family by global orientational tuning. Science 296: 525-530.

Taniguchi M, Yamashita T, Kumura E, Tamatani M, Kobayashi A, et al. 2000. Induction of aquaporin-4 water channel mRNA after focal cerebral ischemia in rat. Brain Res Mol Brain Res 78: 131-137.

Tomas-Camardiel M, Venero JL, de Pablos RM, Rite I, Machado A, et al. 2004. In vivo expression of aquaporin-4 by reactive microglia. J Neurochem 91: 891-899.

Tsacopoulos M, Magistretti PJ. 1996. Metabolic coupling between glia and neurons. J Neurosci 16: 877-885.

Tsuyumu M, Reulen HJ, Prioleau G. 1981. Dynamics of formation and resolution of vasogenic brain oedema. I. Measurement of oedema clearance into ventricular CSF. Acta Neurochir (Wien) 57: 1-13.

Uhl E, Wrba E, Nehring V, Chang RC, Baethmann A, et al. 1999. Technical note: A new model for quantitative analysis of brain oedema resolution into the ventricles and the subarachnoid space. Acta Neurochir (Wien) 141: 89-92.

Umenishi F, Verkman AS. 1998. Isolation and functional analysis of alternative promoters in the human aquaporin-4 water channel gene. Genomics 50: 373-377.

Vajda Z, Promeneur D, Doczi T, Sulyok E, Frokiaer J, et al. 2000. Increased aquaporin-4 immunoreactivity in rat brain in response to systemic hyponatremia. Biochem Biophys Res Commun 270: 495-503.

Vajda Z, Pedersen M, Fuchtbauer EM, Wertz K, Stodkilde-Jorgensen H, et al. 2002. Delayed onset of brain edema and mislocalization of aquaporin-4 in dystrophin-null transgenic mice. Proc Natl Acad Sci USA 99: 13131-13136.

Verbavatz JM, Ma T, Gobin R, Verkman AS. 1997. Absence of orthogonal arrays in kidney, brain and muscle from transgenic knockout mice lacking water channel aquaporin-4. J Cell Sci 110: 2855-2860.

Verkman AS. 2002. Aquaporin water channels and endothelial cell function. J Anat 200: 617-627.

Verkman AS. 2005. Novel roles of aquaporins revealed by phenotype analysis of knockout mice. Rev Physiol Biochem Pharmacol 155: 31-55.

Verkman AS, Mitra AK. 2000. Structure and function of aquaporin water channels. Am J Physiol Renal Physiol 278: F13-F28.

Vitellaro-Zuccarello L, Mazzetti S, Bosisio P, Monti C, De Biasi S. 2005. Distribution of Aquaporin 4 in rodent spinal cord: Relationship with astrocyte markers and chondroitin sulfate proteoglycans. Glia 51: 148-159.

Weed LH, McKibben PS. 1919. Experimental alteration of brain bulk. Am J Physiol 48: 531-538.

Wen H, Nagelhus EA, Amiry-Moghaddam M, Agre P, Ottersen OP, et al. 1999. Ontogeny of water transport in rat brain: Postnatal expression of the aquaporin-4 water channel. Eur J Neurosci 11: 935-945.

Wrba E, Nehring V, Chang RC, Baethmann A, Reulen HJ, et al. 1997. Quantitative analysis of brain edema resolution into the cerebral ventricles and subarachnoid space. Acta Neurochir Suppl 70: 288-290.

Wrba E, Nehring V, Baethmann A, Reulen HJ, Uhl E. 1998. Resolution of experimental vasogenic brain edema at different intracranial pressures. Acta Neurochir Suppl 71: 313-315.

Yamamoto N, Sobue K, Miyachi T, Inagaki M, Miura Y, et al. 2001. Differential regulation of aquaporin expression in astrocytes by protein kinase C. Brain Res Mol Brain Res 95: 110-116.

Yamamoto N, Sobue K, Fujita M, Katsuya H, Asai K. 2002. Differential regulation of aquaporin-5 and -9 expression in astrocytes by protein kinase A. Brain Res Mol Brain Res 104: 96-102.

Yang B, Ma T, Verkman AS. 1995. cDNA cloning, gene organization, and chromosomal localization of a human mercurial insensitive water channel. Evidence for distinct transcriptional units. J Biol Chem 270: 22907-22913.

Yang B, Brown D, Verkman AS. 1996. The mercurial insensitive water channel (AQP-4) forms orthogonal arrays in stably transfected Chinese hamster ovary cells. J Biol Chem 271: 4577-4580.

Yang B, van Hoek AN, Verkman AS. 1997. Very high single channel water permeability of aquaporin-4 in baculovirus-infected insect cells and liposomes reconstituted with purified aquaporin-4. Biochemistry 36: 7625-7632.

Zampighi GA, Kreman M, Lanzavecchia S, Turk E, Eskandari S, et al. 2003. Structure of functional single AQP0 channels in phospholipid membranes. J Mol Biol 325: 201-210.

9 Peptide Mediators of the Brain Endothelium

B. Kis · Y. Ueta · D. W. Busija

Abstract: Cerebral endothelial cells are the major cellular component of the blood–brain barrier, which separates the brain microenvironment from the circulating blood and is responsible for the maintenance of the ionic and metabolic homeostasis of the brain parenchyma. Cerebral endothelial cells are a rich source of peptide mediators which act as autocrine or paracrine factors and influence the resistance vessels in the cerebral circulation, blood–brain barrier transport features and the behavior of the cellular elements of the blood. Targeting the production of these peptide mediators or their receptors provides a useful therapeutic approach during injuries or inflammatory processes in the brain and the cerebral vasculature. In this review we summarize current knowledge of peptide mediators produced by cerebral endothelial cells, such as adrenomedullin, angiotensin, endothelin and several others as well as their role in the regulation of blood–brain barrier functions and cerebral vascular control.

List of Abbreviations: ACE, angiotensin converting enzyme; AD, Alzheimer's disease; AM, adrenomedullin; AT, angiotensin receptor; BBB, blood–brain barrier; cAMP, cyclic adenosine monophosphate; CEC, cerebral endothelial cell; CGRP, calcitonin gene-related peptide; CNS, central nervous system; CRLR, calcitonin receptor-like receptor; CSF, cerebrospinal fluid; DNA, deoxyribonucleic acid; eNOS, endothelial nitric oxide synthase; ET, endothelin; GM-CSF, granulocyte-macrophage colony-stimulating factor; HIF, hypoxia inducible factor-1; HIV, human immunodeficiency virus; ICAM-1, intercellular adhesion molecule-1; IL, interleukin; LFA, leukocyte function-associated antigen; MCP, monocyte chemoattractant protein; MHC, major histocompatibility complex; MIP, macrophage inflammatory protein; mRNA, messenger ribonucleic acid; NGF, Nerve growth factor; NK, neurokinin; NO, nitric oxide; NOS, nitric oxide synthase; NPY, neuropeptide Y; P-gp, P-glycoprotein; PKC, protein kinase C; RAMP, receptor-activity modifying protein; RANTES, regulated upon activation normal T cell expressed and secreted; RT-PCR, reverse transcriptase-polymerase chain reaction; SHR, stroke-prone spontaneously hypertensive rat; SP, substance P; TNF, tumor necrosis factor; VIP, vasoactive intestinal polypeptide; VSMC, vascular smooth muscle cells

1 Introduction

Endothelial cells form the continuous innermost layer of the blood vessels providing an antithrombotic surface toward the circulating blood. Endothelial cells express receptors, which respond to different mediators and also control the vascular tone and blood flow through secretion of diverse vasoactive substances (Burnstock and Ralevic, 1994). Although cerebral endothelial cells (CECs) share many common properties of the peripheral endothelium (Joo, 1996; Rubin and Staddon, 1999), they have a unique morphological and functional feature, the formation of the blood–brain barrier (BBB). The BBB contributes to the stability of the brain parenchymal microenvironment by strictly controlling the traffic of molecules and cells between the blood and the central nervous system (CNS) (Joo, 1996; Rubin and Staddon, 1999). The brain endothelium is also an important component of the BBB in which fundamental changes occur during the inflammatory, infectious, and immune-mediated diseases of the CNS (Andjelkovic and Pachter, 1998).

The BBB phenotype of CECs is induced by the astroglial environment (Janzer and Raff, 1987). Although the effect of neurons on the induction of some specific CEC properties has been described [for review see Bauer and Bauer, (2000)], the effect of astroglia on CECs is more prominent. Several BBB parameters are upregulated when CECs are cocultured with astroglia or cultured in astrocyte-conditioned medium, such as the expression and localization of tight junction proteins occludin, claudin-1, ZO-1 are increased, as well as the number of tight junction strands (Wolburg et al., 1994). These changes in CECs lead to a major increase in transendothelial electrical resistance (Rubin et al., 1991; Cecchelli et al., 1999). Astroglia also augment the expression and activity of specific BBB transporters and enzymes (Deli and Joo, 1996; Cecchelli et al., 1999). Despite the large number of studies, the molecular mechanisms of astrocyte signaling to CECs, membrane interactions, and/or secreted factors are still not fully understood (Rubin and Staddon, 1999).

The cerebral microvascular endothelium, like other endothelial layers, is capable of producing several substances mediating endothelium-dependent vasorelaxation or vasoconstriction (Kontos et al., 1990), regulate the BBB permeability (Joo and Klatzo, 1989), and play a role in the regulation of cell–cell interactions during inflammatory and immunological processes (Andjelkovic and Pachter, 1998). The chemical nature of these mediators produced by CECs ranges from gaseous anorganic molecules [e.g., nitric oxide (Morin and Stanboli, 1993)] through lipid mediators [e.g., prostaglandins (Moore et al., 1988; Kis et al., 1999)] to peptides. In this chapter, we summarize current knowledge of peptide mediators produced by CECs.

2 Adrenomedullin

Adrenomedullin (AM) was originally isolated from human pheochromocytoma, and the initial reports suggested that the adrenal medulla, ventricle, kidney, and lung have the highest levels of expression of AM messenger ribonucleic acid (mRNA) (Kitamura et al., 1993; Sakata et al., 1993). However, since the discovery that the AM gene expression is 20–40-fold higher in endothelial cells than even in the adrenal medulla (Sugo et al., 1994), this peptide has been regarded as an important secretory product of vascular endothelium together with nitric oxide, endothelins, and prostanoids.

The high AM production in peripheral endothelial cells (Sugo et al., 1994; Isumi et al., 1998) made it probable that CECs could be an important source of AM in the cerebral microcirculation. However, the first report did not support this hypothesis; Sugo et al. (1994) found very low AM production by cultured bovine CECs, which represented only a few percent of the AM production of rat aortic endothelial cells. Moreover, this observation about the low AM production of CECs later was supported by Ladoux and Frelin (2000), who described weak AM mRNA expression in clones of rat CECs. It should be mentioned, however, that the CECs in these studies were at very high-passage number (10–20 passages) (Sugo et al., 1994; Ladoux and Frelin, 2000), which might alter the original phenotype of the primary cells (Goetz et al., 1985; Shi and Audus, 1994).

In contrast to these experiments, Kis et al. (2002) found unexpectedly high AM production in primary cultures of rat CECs both at the peptide and at the mRNA levels. Rat CECs had AM production at about one magnitude higher than reported for other primary cells [for review see Minamino et al. (2002)]. Thus, data available indicate that rat CECs synthesize and secrete AM at the highest rate measured. The high AM production of rat CECs was further induced by astrocyte-derived factors because significantly elevated AM production was detected in the culture medium of primary rat CECs cocultured with astrocytes or cultured in astrocyte-conditioned medium (Kis et al., 2002). AM production of rat CECs could not be induced by cytokines, bacterial lipopolysaccharide, and thrombin (Kis et al., 2002), which are the most powerful inducers of AM release in peripheral endothelial cells (Isumi et al., 1998). AM was secreted primarily but not exclusively at the luminal (blood) side of CEC monolayers (Kis et al., 2002). Contrary to AM, endothelin-1 (ET-1), a vasoconstrictor peptide, is secreted mostly toward the abluminal (brain) side of bovine CECs (Dehouck et al., 1997; Isumi et al., 1998).

AM immunoreactivity was not detectable (Kis et al., 2002) or was very week in brain microvessels (Serrano et al., 2000, 2002). The weak AM immunoreactivity in brain endothelial cells and the high and time-dependently increased level of AM in the culture medium (Kis et al., 2002) suggest that most of the AM formed by rat CECs is immediately secreted, as it happens in peripheral endothelial cells (Sugo et al., 1994; Isumi et al., 1998). These observations also suggest that immunochemistry is probably not the optimal method to study AM production by cerebral endothelium.

In rat, the AM concentration in the jugular vein was about 50% higher than that in the carotid artery and also a 50% higher level of AM was found in the venous plasma effluxed from the brain than that from peripheral organs (Kis et al., 2002) These in vivo observations independently support the in vitro findings that CECs have a very high AM production. Previously, no significant difference was observed between AM levels in the venous blood from kidney, lung, adrenal gland, and the systemic arterial blood of rats (Hwang and Tang, 2000). However, a significantly lower concentration in the left ventricle and aorta compared to venous side of the circulation was reported in some studies, and it was also shown that the lung is the major site of AM clearance in humans (Nishikimi et al., 1994, 2000). We can conclude that the cerebral circulation has an exceptionally high AM concentration due to the significantly elevated basal AM secretion by brain endothelial cells, which is induced by astrocyte-derived factors.

When injected intravenously, AM acts predominantly in organs and tissues in which the AM gene is highly expressed, which suggests that AM is functioning as a local autocrine and/or paracrine hormone (Hinson et al., 2000). This view raises the possibility that AM released by rat CECs acts primarily on AM receptors present in the cerebral endothelium itself and on adjacent cells. Two receptors have been proposed to have specific AM-binding properties. These receptors are combinations of calcitonin receptor-like receptor (CRLR) with either the receptor-activity modifying protein 2 (RAMP-2) or RAMP-3 (McLatchie et al., 1998). On the other hand, the combination of CRLR with RAMP-1 defines the calcitonin gene-related peptide receptor 1 (CGRP1) (McLatchie et al., 1998). The second messenger associated with AM receptor activation is the elevation of intracellular cAMP (Smith et al., 2002).

AM receptor components, CRLR, RAMP-2, and RAMP-3 as well as CGRP1 were detected on isolated rat cerebral microvessels (Kobayashi et al., 2000) and cultured rat CECs (Kis et al., 2002) by RT-PCR. RAMP-2 showed the highest expression, followed by RAMP-3 and RAMP-1, and exogenous AM increased the intracellular cAMP concentration in rat CECs, suggesting the existence of functional AM receptors on these cells (Kis et al., 2002). Although astrocyte-derived factors increased the AM production of rat CECs, they did not change the expression of the AM receptor components in rat CECs (Kis et al., 2002). Oliver et al. (2002) reported the same expression pattern of RAMPs in human cerebral vasculature.

The following findings that (1) CECs secrete exceptionally high amount of AM; (2) the AM concentration in the cerebral circulation is significantly higher than in other part of the body; (3) both isolated cerebral microvessels (Kobayashi et al., 2000) and cultured rat CECs (Kis et al., 2002) express mRNA of functional AM receptor components and exhibit a dose-dependent increase in cAMP concentration after administration of exogenous AM (Kis et al., 2002); and (4) cAMP is an important second messenger in the regulation of BBB functions (Rubin and Staddon, 1999), suggested a function for AM as an autocrine and/or paracrine regulator of BBB.

The experiments of Kis et al. (2001b, 2003) provided evidence that AM has cAMP-like effects on specific BBB functions in vitro. Exogenous AM increased transendothelial electrical resistance and reduced endothelial permeability for the low-molecular weight sodium fluorescein, which suggests a tightening of intercellular junctions. AM also decreased endothelial fluid phase endocytosis and activated the P-glycoprotein (P-gp) efflux pump in cultures of rat CECs (Kis et al., 2001b). Treatment with both the AM receptor antagonist, AM_{22-52}, and the AM antisense oligonucleotide, decreased the basal intracellular cAMP level in rat CECs (Kis et al., 2002). Michibata et al. (1998) have reported that neutralization of endogenous AM by monoclonal antibodies reduced the basal cAMP production in bovine aortic endothelial cells. It was also shown that antisense treatment significantly reduces the AM production in primary rat CECs and decreases transendothelial electrical resistance (Kis et al., 2001b). It is remarkable that the basal intracellular cAMP concentration is the highest in rat CECs followed by GP8-immortalized rat CECs and human umbilical vein endothelial cells, which corresponds to the AM production of these cells (Kis et al., 2002). These observations suggest that AM, as an autocrine mediator, plays an important role in the maintenance of basal intra-endothelial cAMP levels and appears to be an autocrine inducer of BBB functions of CECs via the activation of the adenylate cyclase enzyme. Moreover, astrocyte-derived factors increased the AM production by primary rat CECs suggesting that AM is involved in the astrocytic regulation of the BBB phenotype (Janzer and Raff, 1987; Rubin and Staddon, 1999). Therefore, AM appears to be a physiological link between astrocyte-derived factors, cAMP, and the induction and maintenance of the BBB properties by CECs.

Besides the regulation of CEC permeability, cAMP is also important in the regulation of the permeability of other endothelial and epithelial cells of the body (Michel and Curry, 1999). Interestingly, AM knockout homozygous mice die at midgestation with extreme hydrops fetalis and cardiovascular abnormalities including severe hemorrhages and pericardial effusions (Shindo et al., 2000; Caron and Smithies, 2001). These findings suggest a more general role for AM as an endothelium-derived autocrine hormone in the regulation of endothelial permeability in the body.

The vasodilator effect of AM in the cerebral circulation is supported by several observations [for review see Kis et al. (2001a)]. Greater sensitivity to AM was found in canine basilar arteries than in renal, coronary, and femoral arteries (Nakamura et al., 1995). Robust vasodilator responses to AM were seen in dog (Baskaya et al., 1995; Nakamura et al., 1995; Wang et al., 1995), rat (Wang et al., 1995; Nishimura and Suzuki, 1997), and human (Sams et al., 2000) cerebral arteries as well as in rat cerebral arterioles (Lang et al., 1997;

Mori et al., 1997). Moreover, AM induced increases in cerebral (Dogan et al., 1997; Takao et al., 1999) and vertebral (Baskaya et al., 1995) blood flow. The vasodilator effects of AM may be dependent on at least two mechanisms, a direct action of AM on vascular smooth muscle cells (VSMCs) coupled to the accumulation of intracellular cAMP (Ishizaka et al., 1994), and an indirect mechanism involving the stimulation of NO production (Hirata et al., 1995). However, in rat cerebral arterioles Lang et al. (1997) demonstrated a role for both ATP-sensitive and calcium-dependent potassium channels in dilator response to AM.

The observations that AM is secreted in large amount by brain endothelium, the high AM concentration in the cerebral circulation (Kis et al., 2002) and the expression of AM receptors in the cerebral vasculature (Moreno et al., 1999; Kobayashi et al., 2000; Ladoux and Frelin, 2000; Sams et al., 2000; Kis et al., 2002; Oliver et al., 2002) raises the possibility that AM might have a role in the maintenance of resting tone of cerebral vessels and might be important in the physiological regulation of cerebral hemodynamics.

Hypoxia increases AM production in cultured rat cerebral (Ladoux and Frelin, 2000), bovine carotid (Saito et al., 2001), and human coronary artery endothelial cells (Nakayama et al., 1999). Serrano et al. (2002) demonstrated an increase in AM expression in cortical neurons and in perivascular structures that may represent glial elements or pericytes as well as in endothelial cells. There are several mechanisms by which ischemia may increase AM expression. One of them involves the hypoxia inducible factor-1 (HIF-1) which binds to the DNA motifs known as hypoxia-responsive elements and influences gene expression (Caro, 2001). Several hypoxia-responsive elements have been found in human and mouse AM genes (Garayoa et al., 2000). Another mechanism for increased AM expression could be the augmentation of AM mRNA stability that takes place during hypoxia (Garayoa et al., 2000; Ladoux and Frelin, 2000). Exogenous AM administration increased the barrier phenotype in monolayers of CECs (Kis et al., 2001b), which may suggest that increased AM production can play a protective role in the maintenance of BBB integrity during hypoxia.

As a cerebral vasodilator, it would be expected that excess production of AM may lead to improved postischemic neurological outcome. Consistent with this view, Dogan et al. (1997) and Watanabe et al. (2001) reported beneficial effects of intravenous administration of AM in focal cerebral ischemia in rats. AM tended to suppress the reduction in regional cerebral blood flow after middle cerebral artery occlusion and inhibited the increase in myeloperoxidase activity (i.e., decreased the number of infiltrating neutrophils) in the ischemic area, which led to significantly decreased brain injury (Dogan et al., 1997; Watanabe et al., 2001).

AM is suspected to participate in the pathologic mechanism of subarachnoid hemorrhage. Plasma concentrations of AM were increased in patients suffering from subarachnoid hemorrhage throughout the study period (Kikumoto et al., 1998; Fujioka et al., 2000), and AM levels correlated with the clinical condition of patients (Kikumoto et al., 1998). However, in these studies no relationship was found between plasma AM concentration and the onset of cerebral vasospasm (Kikumoto et al., 1998; Fujioka et al., 2000), a major cause of delayed brain ischemia after subarachnoid hemorrhage (Kassell et al., 1985). On the other hand, Wijdicks et al. (2001) reported significant correlation between increased levels of circulating AM and the presence of vasospasm. Patients with symptomatic vasospasm had significantly higher levels of AM in CSF than those without vasospasm, and while the AM concentration in CSF increased with time in response to brain ischemia, this increase was unrelated to the plasma concentrations (Fujioka et al., 2000). It was suggested that the elevated plasma AM concentrations may be the consequence of increased sympathetic activity after subarachnoid hemorrhage (Benedict and Loach, 1978), which could stimulate vascular tissue to secrete AM into the circulation (Benedict and Loach, 1978; Ishimitsu et al., 1994). The relationship between AM and subarachnoid hemorrhage needs to be explored further in the laboratory and in a larger series of patients with subarachnoid hemorrhage.

3 Angiotensins

The renin–angiotensin system is classically viewed as a complex blood-borne hormonal system in which substrate (angiotensinogen) and enzyme (renin) are released into the circulation from the liver and kidney, respectively (Lavoie and Sigmund, 2003). The resulting product, the decapeptide angiotensin I is biologically inactive and is cleaved by the angiotensin converting enzyme (ACE) in blood and on endothelial cells to release the effector octapeptide angiotensin II (Lavoie and Sigmund, 2003). Angiotensin II exerts is biological actions via binding to either the type 1 (AT$_1$) or the type 2 (AT$_2$) receptor; both receptors appear to be G-protein–coupled (Kaschina and Unger, 2003).

Recent studies indicate the presence of a functioning endogenous angiotensin system in the CNS, which contains the same components of the renin-angiotensin cascade as the peripheral tissues and blood (Davisson, 2003). CECs are active components of the angiotensin system of the brain; like other endothelial cells, they produce ACE (Gimbrone et al., 1979; Hamming et al., 2004) and very recently Robbins et al. (unpublished observations) demonstrated the presence of angiotensinogen and renin in CECs. CECs express AT$_1$ receptors (Rose and Audus, 1999; Ito et al., 2001), which plays important role in cerebrovascular pathologies. Intracerebroventricular administration of angiotensin II increased BBB permeability (Grubb and Raichle, 1981) and internal carotid infusion of low dose of angiotensin II reduced cerebral blood flow (Kramar et al., 1997). Cerebral edema was prevented and reduced in stroke-prone spontaneously hypertensive rats (SHR) treated with either the AT$_1$ receptor antagonist losartan or the ACE inhibitor enalapril (Blezer et al., 2001). Losartan treatment also attenuated BBB permeability in diabetic hypertension presumably due to its protective effect on endothelial cells (Kaya et al., 2003). AT$_1$ receptor stimulation decreased (Yamakawa et al., 2003), while AT$_1$ receptor antagonist treatment normalized endothelial nitric oxide synthase (eNOS) expression in cerebral microvessels of SHRs (Yamakawa et al., 2003; Ando et al., 2004), decreased intercellular adhesion molecule-1 (ICAM-1) expression, and ameliorated endothelial injury in the cerebral cortex of SHRs (Takemori et al., 2000; Ito et al., 2001; Ando et al., 2004). Rose and Audus (1999) demonstrated that AT$_1$ receptors also mediate angiotensin II uptake and transport by CECs.

Besides angiotensin II, other angiotensin peptides, such as angiotensin III [Ang-(2–8)], angiotensin IV [Ang-(3–8)], and angiotensin-(1–7), also have important biological activities (Ardaillou, 1997). Angiotensin IV and especially angiotensin-(1–7) have become an angiotensin of interest in the past few years because its cardiovascular actions counteract those of angiotensin II (Santos et al., 2000). This is also true for the cerebrovascular system where AT$_1$ receptor activation by angiotensin II is associated with vasoconstriction (Edvinsson et al., 1979) and reductions in CBF (Kramar et al., 1997), while AT$_4$ receptor activation by angiotensin IV results in increases in CBF (Kramar et al., 1997) and angiotensin-(1–7) receptor activation by angiotensin-(1–7) dilate cerebral arteries (Meng and Busija, 1993; Feterik et al., 2000).

4 Bradykinin

Kinins are peptide hormones, which are locally released by kallikrein-mediated proteolysis from their precursors, the kininogens (Bhoola et al., 1992). The broad spectrum of their actions is mediated by B$_1$ and B$_2$ kinin receptors (Blaukat, 2003). Bradykinin and kallidin preferentially bind to B$_2$ receptors, whereas the carboxy-terminally truncated kinins desArg^9-bradykinin and desArg^{10}-kallidin have a high affinity to B$_1$ receptors (Blaukat, 2003). In contrast to the B$_2$ receptor that is constitutively expressed in many tissues, B$_1$ is almost undetectable but is upregulated under pathophysiological conditions such as tissue injury and inflammation (Marceau et al., 1997). Kinin receptors are coupled to G-proteins leading to an activation of phospholipase C and subsequent generation of second messengers diacylglycerol and inositol-1,4,5-trisphosphate leading to protein kinase C (PKC) activation and intracellular calcium level elevation (Blaukat, 2003).

Bradykinin is one of the most important products of a series of pathophysiological processes that occurs following tissue injury. The CNS contains all of the components of the kallikrein–kinin system and there is growing evidence that the kinin system has important effects not only in the periphery but also within the CNS following injury, disease, infection, and inflammation (Walker et al., 1995).

Bradykinin plays important role in cerebrovascular pathologies (Wahl et al., 1999), especially, in brain edema formation (Raichle and Grubb, 1978; Unterberg et al., 1984). Although bradykinin production has not been studied in CECs, we can assume that they are able to synthesize bradykinin similar to peripheral endothelium (Wiemer et al., 1991, 1994). In some brain regions, kallikrein seems to be specifically localized within and surrounding blood vessels (Kitagawa et al., 1991). The B$_2$ receptor is expressed constitutively on

CECs both at luminal and abluminal membranes (Wahl et al., 1999). The B_1 receptor could not be detected on resting CECs, but it was expressed upon stimulation with interferon-γ (Prat et al., 2000). Selective opening of the BBB for small tracers (Na-fluorescein, MW: 376) has been found in cats during cortical superfusion or intra-arterial application of bradykinin (Unterberg et al., 1984). This leakage is mediated by B_2 receptors of CECs and results from an opening of tight junctions (Zausinger, 2003). An increase of the bradykinin concentration in the interstitial space of the brain up to concentrations which induce extravasation, dilatation, and edema formation has been found under several pathological conditions (Wahl et al., 1999).

Bradykinin receptors of the CECs are targeted therapeutically by both with agonists and antagonists. B_2 receptor agonists are being developed for clinical use to open the BBB transiently for delivery of therapeutic agents to the brain, particularly, antitumor drugs (Emerich et al., 2001). Because bradykinin is associated with brain edema and inflammation after CNS ischemia or injury, B_2 receptor antagonists are being designed for treating the consequences of neurotrauma (Zausinger, 2003).

5 Cytokines

Cytokines are soluble polypeptide mediators that serve to communicate with leukocytes as well as with cells of other tissues and organs. CECs have been shown to express receptors for cytokines (Van Dam et al., 1996; Konsman et al., 2004) and respond to cytokine exposure. Cytokines have been found to alter the permeability of brain vascular endothelium in vitro (Burke-Gaffney and Keenan, 1993; de Vries et al., 1996) and in vivo (Megyeri et al., 1992). They also upregulate the expression of class I and II MHC antigens (Male and Pryce, 1988) and adhesion molecules in CECs (Wong and Dorovini-Zis, 1992; Male et al., 1994), therefore, facilitate the adhesion of inflammatory cells to cerebral endothelium. Cytokines stimulate the secretion of various vasoactive and pro-inflammatory mediators from CECs, including prostaglandins (de Vries et al., 1995) and endothelins (Skopal et al., 1998).

Endothelial cells are not only a target for cytokines but can actively produce and secrete a variety of cytokines in response to various stimuli. CECs have been reported to produce interleukin-1β (IL-1β) (Fabry et al., 1993; Bourdoulous et al., 1995; Corsini et al., 1996; Zhang et al., 1998), IL-6 (Fabry et al., 1993; Rott et al., 1993; Bourdoulous et al., 1995; Lou et al., 1996; Zidovetzki et al., 1998; Etienne et al., 1999; Reyes et al., 1999), IL-8 (Bourdoulous et al., 1995; Lou et al., 1996; Lee et al., 2003), tumor necrosis factor-α (TNF-α) (Freyer et al., 1999), transforming growth factor-β (Grammas and Ovase, 2002), granulocyte-macrophage colony-stimulating factor (GM-CSF) (Hart et al., 1992), and chemokines (Shukaliak and Dorovini-Zis, 2000; Omari et al., 2004). Cytokines are present at very low level in resting CECs, but their expression dramatically increases after stimulation. Cytokines expressed by peripheral vascular endothelial cells are known to be key players in regulating the recruitment of leukocytes to the sites of tissue inflammation (Imhof and Dunon, 1995; Mantovani et al., 1997). Cytokine production by CECs emphasizes the active participation of brain microvascular endothelium in inflammatory reactions of the CNS.

Inflammatory mechanisms are thought to contribute to the pathogenesis of neurodegenerative diseases, such as Alzheimer's disease (AD), especially in the later stages (Akiyama et al., 2000). Grammas and Ovase (2001) demonstrated that cerebral microvessels from AD patients release significantly higher levels of IL-1β, IL-6, TNF-α, and monocyte chemoattractant protein (MCP-1) compared to microvessels from non-AD control individuals. These authors later demonstrated the important role of cerebrovascular transforming growth factor-β in the pathogenesis of AD (Grammas and Ovase, 2002). These results suggest that the cerebral microcirculation contributes inflammatory mediators to the milieu of the brain in AD and may be involved in the subsequent neuronal pathogenesis in this disorder.

Chemokines are a subclass of cytokines that induce activation and directional migration of leukocytes (Rollins, 1997). β-chemokines play an important role in the recruitment of mononuclear cells during inflammatory conditions of the CNS such as experimental allergic encephalomyelitis and multiple sclerosis (Simpson et al., 1998; Ransohoff, 1999). CECs have been reported to be potential sources of β-chemokines

(Shukaliak and Dorovini-Zis, 2000). Members of the β-chemokine subfamily include "regulated upon activation normal T cell expressed and secreted" peptide (RANTES), MCP-1, macrophage inflammatory protein-1α (MIP-1α), and MIP-1β. All four members have been shown to activate and induce chemotaxis of T lymphocytes and monocytes/macrophages (Rollins, 1997). TNF-α, interferon-γ, and CD40 ligand (CD40L) stimulate the production of RANTES, MCP-1, MIP-1α, and MIP-1β (Omari et al., 2004) in CECs. Increased β-chemokine production may then lead to further activation of leukocytes and increase their binding to cerebral EC adhesion molecules, which are similarly upregulated by cytokines (Omari and Dorovini-Zis, 2003), and thus increase their recruitment through the compromised BBB.

6 Endothelins

The first endothelin, ET-1, was isolated from the medium of cultured aortic endothelial cells (Yanagisawa et al., 1988). However, the endothelial cells are not the only source of ETs in the body; their production has been found in many different tissues (Hunley and Kon, 2001). Three members of the ET family have been described, ET-1, -2, -3, each of them is encoded by a distinct gene. All isoforms contain 21 amino acids and posses two intramolecular disulfide bridges (Hunley and Kon, 2001). Of the three isoforms, the most widely distributed, best studied, and most powerful is ET-1. The human ET-1 synthesis begins with the translation of the prepro-ET-1 mRNA into a 212-amino acid prepro peptide that undergoes proteolytic cleavage by a specific endopeptidase to release a 38-amino acid intermediary structure, termed "big" ET-1 (Russell and Davenport, 1999). Big ET-1 is cleaved to the mature ET-1 either intracellularly or extracellularly by one of several ET-converting enzymes (Turner et al., 1998). Big ET-1 has only 1% of the contractile activity of the mature peptide in vivo, stressing the importance of ET converting enzymes. The processing of the other two preproisoforms proceeds in a parallel fashion. Two ET receptors have been described in mammals, ET_A and ET_B, both of which are G-protein–coupled receptors (Ohlstein et al., 1996). The most generalized signal transduction pathway following ET exposure is the phospholipase C—phosphatidyl inositol cascade. The receptors show different relative affinities for the three ET isoforms. The ET_A receptor is characterized by the rank order affinity ET-1 = ET-2 ≫ ET-3, while ET_B receptor shows equal affinity toward all three isopeptides (Ohlstein et al., 1996).

Because of their high vasoconstrictor potency and long-lasting effects, ETs have excited great interest in the field of cardiovascular research. Recent studies emphasize its important role in systemic and pulmonary hypertension, congestive heart failure, obstructive pulmonary diseases, renal failure, and insulin resistance (Hunley and Kon, 2001; Miller et al., 2002). ETs also play an important role in cerebrovascular regulation and are involved in the pathogenesis of brain injuries during cerebral ischemia and subarachnoid hemorrhage (Armstead, 2004; Zimmermann and Seifert, 2004).

CECs like other endothelium produce ET (Yoshimoto et al., 1990, 1991; Dehouck et al., 1997) and also contain ET-converting enzyme (Vatter et al., 2002). They express both ET_A (Stanimirovic et al., 1994; Kawai et al., 1997) and ET_B receptors; the latter are immunolocalized to both the luminal and abluminal surfaces of the capillary endothelium (Hartz et al., 2004). In CECs ET_A receptors are linked to phospholipase C and phospholipase A_2 activation (Stanimirovic et al., 1994). Stimulation of ET_B activated nitric oxide synthase and PKC in CECs (Hartz et al., 2004). Interestingly, the ET produced by CECs is released mainly to the basal side (corresponding to the brain side) and not to the apical side (corresponding to the vascular lumen side) (Yoshimoto et al., 1991; Dehouck et al., 1997). This observation indicate that ET-1 constricts arterioles locally at the same place where it is produced, by acting on the underlying layers of smooth muscle cells, which express ET_A receptors (Takenaka et al., 1993). Yoshimoto et al. (1991) demonstrated that CECs produce less ET-1 under low-oxygen pressure and that they produce more ET-1 under low-carbon dioxide pressure. These results may suggest that the negative feedback regulation of cerebral blood flow through oxygen and carbon dioxide pressure is mediated by ET-1 produced locally by cerebral microvascular endothelia (Yoshimoto et al., 1991).

In pathological condition, release of excessive ET from CECs or surrounding tissues can contribute to the formation of cerebral edema. Endothelin has been reported to increase BBB permeability in vivo (Miller et al., 1996; Narushima et al., 2003) and inhibit P-gp–mediated efflux transport function of CECs in isolated cerebral capillaries (Hartz et al., 2004). Matsuo et al. (2001) showed that 1-h middle cerebral artery occlusion in rat provides sufficient stimulation to elevate the ET-1 level in the damaged brain and administration of an ET_A antagonist resulted in significant reduction of brain injury and plasma extravasation after ischemia/reperfusion injury. These findings clearly suggest the involvement of ET-1 in the pathogenesis of brain edema accompanying cerebrovascular injury (Volpe and Cosentino, 2000).

The results of current clinical and experimental investigations support the hypothesis that ET-1 is a major cause of cerebral vasospasm after subarachnoid hemorrhage (Chow et al., 2002; Juvela, 2002; Zimmermann and Seifert, 2004). Cerebral vasospasm occurring after subarachnoid hemorrhage is still the leading cause of death and disability in patients with ruptured aneurysms. Despite extensive experimental and clinical investigation, the etiology and pathophysiology of cerebral vasospasm are poorly understood (Zimmermann and Seifert, 1998). In concert with a number of other vasoactive factors, however, ETs may substantially contribute to the disturbed equilibrium of vasoconstriction and vasorelaxation under the pathophysiological situation of subarachnoid hemorrhage. A number of experimental studies demonstrate the preventive and/or therapeutic potentials of ET receptor antagonists in vivo and in vitro, support the hypothesis that ET is a major cause of cerebral vasospasm after subarachnoid hemorrhage (Seifert et al., 1995; Juvela, 2000).

7 Substance P

Substance P (SP) belongs to the tachykinin neuropeptide family. These neuropeptides share the carboxy-terminal sequence Phe-X-Gly-Leu-Met-NH_2, where X is an aromatic (Tyr or Phe) or hydrophobic (Val or Ile) amino acid (Almeida et al., 2004). This common sequence is essential for the tachykinin's receptor interaction and activation, whereas the distinct amino-terminal sequences of the tachykinins provide their receptor subtype specificity. In mammals, two separate genes encode the tachykinins designated preprotachykinin I and preprotachykinin II (Nawa et al., 1984). The preprotachykinin I gene can express four distinct forms of mRNA through alternative splicing, two of which (the β and γ forms) encode synthesis of both SP and neurokinin A, while the other two, the α and δ forms, encode SP only (Nawa et al., 1984).

Tachykinin effects on target cells are mediated by at least three specific receptors, the neurokinin-1 (NK1), NK2, and NK3 receptors (Nakanishi, 1991; Almeida et al., 2004). These receptors are members of G-protein–coupled receptor superfamily (Nakanishi, 1991; Almeida et al., 2004). Although SP can activate each of the tachykinin receptors, it preferentially activates the NK1 (Nakanishi, 1991; Almeida et al., 2004). Agonist stimulation of the NK1 receptor in many tissue and cell types causes activation of phospholipase C, which catalyzes the hydrolysis of phosphoinositides into inositol 1,4,5-trisphosphate and diacylglycerol. These second messengers are then available for the mobilization of calcium from internal reticular stores and for the activation of PKC.

Although SP is most famous for its dominant role in the neurogenic inflammation (Foreman, 1987) and was originally described as a peptide of neuronal origin, studies have demonstrated its production by many other cell types. Thus, SP is produced by the endothelium of peripheral organs (Loesch and Burnstock, 1988; Ralevic et al., 1990) and also in the cerebral endothelium of rats (Milner et al., 1995; Cioni et al., 1998; Annunziata et al., 2002), bovines (Linnik and Moskowitz, 1989), and humans (Linnik and Moskowitz, 1989; Gorelova et al., 1996).

In the periphery, SP elicits local vasodilatation and alters vascular permeability, thus enhancing the delivery and accumulation of leukocytes to tissues for the expression of local immune responses (Pernow, 1983). SP can specifically stimulate the chemotaxis of lymphocytes, monocytes, neutrophils, and fibroblasts (Pernow, 1983). Moreover, the SP-induced release of inflammatory mediators stimulates further leukocyte recruitment, thereby amplifying the inflammatory response (Lambrecht, 2001).

SP has similar role in the cerebral microcirculation. It was demonstrated that SP is present at low expression levels in unstimulated brain endothelium and is upregulated after stimulation with proinflammatory cytokines IL-1β and TNF-α (Cioni et al., 1998; Annunziata et al., 2002). These cytokines induced specific SP-precursor mRNA transcription in brain endothelial cells suggesting an action on encoding gene expression. IL-1β and TNF-α are known to increase BBB permeability (Megyeri et al., 1992; Burke-Gaffney and Keenan, 1993; de Vries et al., 1996), and Annunziata et al. (2002) demonstrated that SP mediates the TNF-α and IFN-γ-induced BBB permeability increase and associated morphological changes of cerebral endothelium. SP is synthesized and released by cytokine-stimulated brain endothelium and binds to NK1 receptors on endothelial cells (Stumm et al., 2001), triggering an autocrine circuit (Cioni et al., 1998). Like in other cells, the NK1 receptor stimulation leads to the activation of PKC in CECs (Catalan et al., 1989). However, SP-related vasodilation is due to production of nitric oxide (Busija and Chen, 1992). SP upregulates class II MHC antigens on rat brain endothelium (Annunziata et al., 2002), which highlights a possible involvement of SP in enhancing antigen presentation by brain endothelium. SP has been also found to increase lymphocyte adhesion to brain endothelium, acting as a chemotactic molecule and upregulating ICAM-1 expression (Vishwanath and Mukherjee, 1996; Annunziata et al., 2002). ICAM-1 is a member of immunoglobulin family involved in firm adhesion of lymphocytes to endothelium through binding to its natural receptor LFA-1 (Rothlein et al., 1986). During inflammatory and autoimmune processes of the CNS the cytokine-induced SP secretion by brain endothelial cells may augment stimulation of immunocompetent cells, which in turn increases the production/release of proinflammatory cytokines leading to a self-perpetuating feed-forward immunoregulatory loop in the cerebral microcirculation.

SP seems to have a role in the CNS invasion by human immunodeficiency virus-1 (HIV-1). Annunziata et al. (1998) demonstrated that the HIV-1 envelope protein gp120 increased the permeability of rat brain endothelial cells to albumin in a dose-dependent manner. Spantide, a powerful SP antagonist as well as anti-SP polyclonal antibody, completely blocked the gp120-induced increase in albumin permeability. Brain endothelial cells, exposed to gp120, displayed cell surface immunoreactivity for SP, suggesting that SP is secreted by brain endothelium in response to gp120 stimulation and binds to brain endothelial cells through a receptor-mediated mechanism leading to increased BBB permeability.

Stumm et al. (2001) found increased NK1 receptor expression in cerebral endothelium of the ischemic brain after middle cerebral artery occlusion. Their results suggest that the induction of NK1 receptor in cerebral endothelium contributes to the impairment of the BBB in the ischemic brain, which causes edema formation and increased leukocyte diapedesis, important components of the pathophysiology of stroke.

Taken together, all these findings suggest that SP production in cerebral endothelium plays a central role in the breakdown of the BBB during ischemia and inflammatory processes of the CNS. Thus, specifically targeting tachykinin receptors may be a promising therapy against ischemic cerebrovascular diseases and in inflammatory brain injuries.

8 Miscellaneous Peptide Mediators of the Cerebral Endothelium

In this section, we will briefly describe several peptide mediators, which are produced by CECs, but whose roles in physiologic or pathologic processes in the cerebral microcirculation are not extensively investigated and are poorly understood.

CECs produce complement proteins (C1 inhibitor, factor H, factor B, C4), and the production of these proteins are upregulated by interferon-γ (Vastag et al., 1998). These data indicate that complement proteins are expressed locally by the brain microvessels and may modulate the inflammatory responses of brain tissue.

Nerve growth factor (NGF), a member of the family of neurotrophins, is the first and best-characterized neurotrophic factor (Levi-Montalcini et al., 1996). Recent evidence shows that NGF may also be an important angiogenic factor. In the brain, NGF induces arteriogenesis and promotes the enlargement of preexisting capillaries in newborn rats (Calza et al., 2001) and selectively enhances arteriole formation in response to ischemia (Turrini et al., 2002). The study of Moser et al. (2004) showed that rat brain capillary endothelial cells proliferate in response to NGF, produce and secrete NGF and express NGF receptors, and that NGF secretion is enhanced after inflammatory stimulation. NGF may thus be an important autocrine or paracrine growth factor of brain capillary endothelial cells, which can regulate endothelial proliferation and angiogenesis.

Neuropeptide Y (NPY) is a transmitter of the cerebrovascular sympathetic nerves that causes cerebral artery constriction and reductions in cerebral blood flow (Hokfelt et al., 1998). NPY is widely distributed in the brain where it appears to regulate regional blood flow in addition to its many other regulatory roles (e.g., anxiety and mood, cognition and learning, eating behavior, endocrine function, and central cardio-vascular regulation) (Hokfelt et al., 1998). NPY acts on a family of G-protein–coupled receptors (Y_1 through Y_6) (Michel et al., 1998). Although the production of NPY in CECs has not been described, peripheral endothelial cells synthesize NPY and "NPY-converting enzyme" dipeptidyl peptidase IV which terminates the Y_1 activity of NPY (Zukowska-Grojec et al., 1998). Therefore, CECs could be a source of NPY and a site of NPY metabolism in the cerebral circulation. Interestingly, NPY is a potent angiogenic factor acting on the Y_2 receptors of endothelial cells (Zukowska-Grojec et al., 1998).

The occurrence of vasoactive intestinal polypeptide (VIP) in the perivascular plexus of cerebral vessels and its actions as a vasodilator is well known (Paspalas and Papadopoulos, 1998). In newborn piglets, mRNA and protein for VIP and VIP receptor-associated protein were found in CECs, whereas the endothelium of adult animals did not express VIP mRNA or native VIP protein but does express the VIP receptor (Lange et al., 1999). Because VIP has been reported to stimulate mitogenesis and induce secretion of trophic factors (Brenneman et al., 1990), it was suggested that VIP acts in an autocrine fashion to stimulate angiogenesis in the developing brain (Lange et al., 1999).

Vasopressin immunoreactivity was demonstrated in CECs (Loesch et al., 1993). CECs express V1 vasopressin receptor (Hess et al., 1991), and it has been reported that vasopressin increases the BBB permeability to water (Raichle and Grubb, 1978).

9 Summary

CECs are a rich source of peptide mediators, which act as autocrine or paracrine factors and influence the resistance vessels in the cerebral circulation, BBB transport features, and the behavior of the cellular elements of the blood. Targeting the production of or receptors for these peptide mediators provides a useful therapeutic approach during injuries or inflammatory processes in the brain and the cerebral vasculature.

Acknowledgments

The work in the authors' labs was supported by Grant-in-Aid for JSPS Fellows (No.98260 and S-02167 for B. K.) and for Scientific Research on Priority Areas (B) (No.10218210 for Y.U.) and Exploratory Research (No.14667020 for YU) from the Ministry of Education, Culture, Sports, Science and Technology, Japan, and by grants from NIH (HL-30260, HL-66074, HL-65380, HL-77731, DK-62372 for D.W.B.) and AHA Bugher Foundation Award (0270114N for D.W.B.).

References

Akiyama H, Barger S, Barnum S, Bradt B, Bauer J, et al. 2000. Inflammation and Alzheimer's disease. Neurobiol Aging 21: 383-421.

Almeida TA, Rojo J, Nieto PM, Pinto FM, Hernandez M, et al. 2004. Tachykinins and tachykinin receptors: Structure and activity relationships. Curr Med Chem 11: 2045-2081.

Andjelkovic AV, Pachter JS. 1998. Central nervous system endothelium in neuroinflammatory neuroinfectious and neurodegenerative disease. J Neurosci Res 51: 423-430.

Ando H, Zhou J, Macova M, Imboden H, Saavedra JM. 2004. Angiotensin II AT1 receptor blockade reverses pathological hypertrophy and inflammation in brain microvessels of spontaneously hypertensive rats. Stroke 35: 1726-1731.

Annunziata P, Cioni C, Toneatto S, Paccagnini E. 1998. HIV-1 gp120 increases the permeability of rat brain endothelium cultures by a mechanism involving substance P. Aids 12: 2377-2385.

Annunziata P, Cioni C, Santonini R, Paccagnini E. 2002. Substance P antagonist blocks leakage and reduces activation of cytokine-stimulated rat brain endothelium. J Neuroimmunol 131: 41-49.

Ardaillou R. 1997. Active fragments of angiotensin II: Enzymatic pathways of synthesis and biological effects. Curr Opin Nephrol Hypertens 6: 28-34.

Armstead WM. 2004. Endothelins and the role of endothelin antagonists in the management of posttraumatic vasospasm. Curr Pharm Des 10: 2185-2192.

Baskaya MK, Suzuki Y, Anzai M, Seki Y, Saito K, et al. 1995. Effects of adrenomedullin calcitonin gene-related peptide and amylin on cerebral circulation in dogs. J Cereb Blood Flow Metab 15: 827-834.

Bauer HC, Bauer H. 2000. Neural induction of the blood-brain barrier: Still an enigma. Cell Mol Neurobiol 20: 13-28.

Benedict CR, Loach AB. 1978. Sympathetic nervous system activity in patients with subarachnoid hemorrhage. Stroke 9: 237-244.

Bhoola KD, Figueroa CD, Worthy K. 1992. Bioregulation of kinins: Kallikreins kininogens and kininases. Pharmacol Rev 44: 1-80.

Blaukat A. 2003. Structure and signalling pathways of kinin receptors. Andrologia 35: 17-23.

Blezer EL, Nicolay K, Koomans HA, Joles JA. 2001. Losartan versus enalapril on cerebral edema and proteinuria in stroke-prone hypertensive rats. Am J Hypertens 14: 54-61.

Bourdoulous S, Bensaid A, Martinez D, Sheikboudou C, Trap I, et al. 1995. Infection of bovine brain microvessel endothelial cells with Cowdria ruminantium elicits IL-1 beta -6, and -8 mRNA production and expression of an unusual MHC class II DQ alpha transcript. J Immunol 154: 4032-4038.

Brenneman DE, Nicol T, Warren D, Bowers LM. 1990. Vasoactive intestinal peptide: A neurotrophic releasing agent and an astroglial mitogen. J Neurosci Res 25: 386-394.

Burke-Gaffney A, Keenan AK. 1993. Modulation of human endothelial cell permeability by combinations of the cytokines interleukin-1 alpha/beta tumor necrosis factor-alpha and interferon-gamma. Immunopharmacology 25: 1-9.

Burnstock G, Ralevic V. 1994. New insights into the local regulation of blood flow by perivascular nerves and endothelium. Br J Plast Surg 47: 527-543.

Busija DW, Chen J. 1992. Effects of trigeminal neurotransmitters on piglet pial arterioles. J Dev Physiol 18: 67-72.

Calza L, Giardino L, Giuliani A, Aloe L, Levi-Montalcini R. 2001. Nerve growth factor control of neuronal expression of angiogenetic and vasoactive factors. Proc Natl Acad Sci USA 98: 4160-4165.

Caro J. 2001. Hypoxia regulation of gene transcription. High Alt Med Biol 2: 145-154.

Caron KM, Smithies O. 2001. Extreme hydrops fetalis and cardiovascular abnormalities in mice lacking a functional Adrenomedullin gene. Proc Natl Acad Sci USA 98: 615-619.

Catalan RE, Martinez AM, Aragones MD, Fernandez I. 1989. Substance P stimulates translocation of protein kinase C in brain microvessels. Biochem Biophys Res Commun 164: 595-600.

Cecchelli R, Dehouck B, Descamps L, Fenart L, Buee-Scherrer VV, et al. 1999. In vitro model for evaluating drug transport across the blood-brain barrier. Adv Drug Deliv Rev 36: 165-178.

Chow M, Dumont AS, Kassell NF. 2002. Endothelin receptor antagonists and cerebral vasospasm: An update. Neurosurgery 51: 1333-1341; discussion 1342.

Cioni C, Renzi D, Calabro A, Annunziata P. 1998. Enhanced secretion of substance P by cytokine-stimulated rat brain endothelium cultures. J Neuroimmunol 84: 76-85.

Corsini E, Dufour A, Ciusani E, Gelati M, Frigerio S, et al. 1996. Human brain endothelial cells and astrocytes produce IL-1 beta but not IL-10. Scand J Immunol 44: 506-511.

Davisson RL. 2003. Physiological genomic analysis of the brain renin-angiotensin system. Am J Physiol 285: R498-R511.

de Vries HE, Hoogendoorn KH, van Dijk J, Zijlstra FJ, van Dam AM, et al. 1995. Eicosanoid production by rat cerebral endothelial cells: Stimulation by lipopolysaccharide interleukin-1 and interleukin-6. J Neuroimmunol 59: 1-8.

de Vries HE, Blom-Roosemalen MC, van Oosten M, de Boer AG, van Berkel TJ, et al. 1996. The influence of cytokines on the integrity of the blood-brain barrier in vitro. J Neuroimmunol 64: 37-43.

Dehouck MP, Vigne P, Torpier G, Breittmayer JP, Cecchelli R, et al. 1997. Endothelin-1 as a mediator of endothelial cell-pericyte interactions in bovine brain capillaries. J Cereb Blood Flow Metab 17: 464-469.

Deli MA, Joo F. 1996. Cultured vascular endothelial cells of the brain. Keio J Med 45: 183-198; discussion 198–189.

Dogan A, Suzuki Y, Koketsu N, Osuka K, Saito K, et al. 1997. Intravenous infusion of adrenomedullin and increase in regional cerebral blood flow and prevention of ischemic brain injury after middle cerebral artery occlusion in rats. J Cereb Blood Flow Metab 17: 19-25.

Edvinsson L, Hardebo JE, Owman C. 1979. Effects of angiotensin II on cerebral blood vessels. Acta Physiol Scand 105: 381-383.

Emerich DF, Dean RL, Osborn C, Bartus RT. 2001. The development of the bradykinin agonist labradimil as a means to increase the permeability of the blood-brain barrier: From concept to clinical evaluation. Clin Pharmacokinet 40: 105-123.

Etienne S, Bourdoulous S, Strosberg AD, Couraud PO. 1999. MHC class II engagement in brain endothelial cells induces protein kinase A-dependent IL-6 secretion and phosphorylation of cAMP response element-binding protein. J Immunol 163: 3636-3641.

Fabry Z, Fitzsimmons KM, Herlein JA, Moninger TO, Dobbs MB, et al. 1993. Production of the cytokines interleukin 1 and 6 by murine brain microvessel endothelium and smooth muscle pericytes. J Neuroimmunol 47: 23-34.

Feterik K, Smith L, Katusic ZS. 2000. Angiotensin-(1–7) causes endothelium-dependent relaxation in canine middle cerebral artery. Brain Res 873: 75-82.

Foreman JC. 1987. Peptides and neurogenic inflammation. Br Med Bull 43: 386-400.

Freyer D, Manz R, Ziegenhorn A, Weih M, Angstwurm K, et al. 1999. Cerebral endothelial cells release TNF-alpha after stimulation with cell walls of Streptococcus pneumoniae and regulate inducible nitric oxide synthase and ICAM-1 expression via autocrine loops. J Immunol 163: 4308-4314.

Fujioka M, Nishio K, Sakaki T, Minamino N, Kitamura K. 2000. Adrenomedullin in patients with cerebral vasospasm after aneurysmal subarachnoid hemorrhage. Stroke 31: 3079-3083.

Garayoa M, Martinez A, Lee S, Pio R, An WG, et al. 2000. Hypoxia-inducible factor-1 (HIF-1) up-regulates adrenomedullin expression in human tumor cell lines during oxygen deprivation: A possible promotion mechanism of carcinogenesis. Mol Endocrinol 14: 848-862.

Gimbrone MA, Jr, Majeau GR, Atkinson WJ, Sadler W, Cruise SA. 1979. Angiotensin-converting enzyme activity in isolated brain microvessels. Life Sci 25: 1075-1083.

Goetz IE, Warren J, Estrada C, Roberts E, Krause DN. 1985. Long-term serial cultivation of arterial and capillary endothelium from adult bovine brain. In Vitro Cell Dev Biol 21: 172-180.

Gorelova E, Loesch A, Bodin P, Chadwick L, Hamlyn PJ, et al. 1996. Localisation of immunoreactive factor VIII nitric oxide synthase substance P endothelin-1 and 5-hydroxytryptamine in human postmortem middle cerebral artery. J Anat 188 (Pt 1): 97-107.

Grammas P, Ovase R. 2001. Inflammatory factors are elevated in brain microvessels in Alzheimer's disease. Neurobiol Aging 22: 837-842.

Grammas P, Ovase R. 2002. Cerebrovascular transforming growth factor-beta contributes to inflammation in the Alzheimer's disease brain. Am J Pathol 160: 1583-1587.

Grubb RL, Jr., Raichle ME. 1981. Intraventricular angiotensin II increases brain vascular permeability. Brain Res 210: 426-430.

Hamming I, Timens W, Bulthuis ML, Lely AT, Navis GJ, et al. 2004. Tissue distribution of ACE2 protein the functional receptor for SARS coronavirus. A first step in understanding SARS pathogenesis. J Pathol 203: 631-637.

Hart MN, Fabry Z, Love-Homan L, Keiner J, Sadewasser KL, et al. 1992. Brain microvascular smooth muscle and endothelial cells produce granulocyte macrophage colony-stimulating factor and support colony formation of granulocyte-macrophage-like cells. Am J Pathol 141: 421-427.

Hartz AM, Bauer B, Fricker G, Miller DS. 2004. Rapid regulation of P-glycoprotein at the blood-brain barrier by endothelin-1. Mol Pharmacol 66: 387-394.

Hess J, Jensen CV, Diemer NH. 1991. The vasopressin receptor of the blood-brain barrier in the rat hippocampus is linked to calcium signalling. Neurosci Lett 132: 8-10.

Hinson JP, Kapas S, Smith DM. 2000. Adrenomedullin a multifunctional regulatory peptide. Endocr Rev 21: 138-167.

Hirata Y, Hayakawa H, Suzuki Y, Suzuki E, Ikenouchi H, et al. 1995. Mechanisms of adrenomedullin-induced vasodilation in the rat kidney. Hypertension 25: 790-795.

Hokfelt T, Broberger C, Zhang X, Diez M, Kopp J, et al. 1998. Neuropeptide Y: Some viewpoints on a multifaceted peptide in the normal and diseased nervous system. Brain Res Brain Res Rev 26: 154-166.

Hunley TE, Kon V. 2001. Update on endothelins—biology and clinical implications. Pediatr Nephrol 16: 752-762.

Hwang IS, Tang F. 2000. Peripheral distribution and gene expression of adrenomedullin in the rat: Possible source of blood adrenomedullin. Neuropeptides 34: 32-37.

Imhof BA, Dunon D. 1995. Leukocyte migration and adhesion. Adv Immunol 58: 345-416.

Ishimitsu T, Nishikimi T, Saito Y, Kitamura K, Eto T, et al. 1994. Plasma levels of adrenomedullin a newly identified hypotensive peptide in patients with hypertension and renal failure. J Clin Invest 94: 2158-2161.

Ishizaka Y, Tanaka M, Kitamura K, Kangawa K, Minamino N, et al. 1994. Adrenomedullin stimulates cyclic AMP formation in rat vascular smooth muscle cells. Biochem Biophys Res Commun 200: 642-646.

Isumi Y, Shoji H, Sugo S, Tochimoto T, Yoshioka M, et al. 1998. Regulation of adrenomedullin production in rat endothelial cells. Endocrinology 139: 838-846.

Ito H, Takemori K, Suzuki T. 2001. Role of angiotensin II type 1 receptor in the leucocytes and endothelial cells of brain microvessels in the pathogenesis of hypertensive cerebral injury. J Hypertens 19: 591-597.

Janzer RC, Raff MC. 1987. Astrocytes induce blood-brain barrier properties in endothelial cells. Nature 325: 253-257.

Joo F. 1996. Endothelial cells of the brain and other organ systems: Some similarities and differences. Prog Neurobiol 48: 255-273.

Joo F, Klatzo I. 1989. Role of cerebral endothelium in brain oedema. Neurol Res 11: 67-75.

Juvela S. 2000. Plasma endothelin concentrations after aneurysmal subarachnoid hemorrhage. J Neurosurg 92: 390-400.

Juvela S. 2002. Plasma endothelin and big endothelin concentrations and serum endothelin-converting enzyme activity following aneurysmal subarachnoid hemorrhage. J Neurosurg 97: 1287-1293.

Kaschina E, Unger T. 2003. Angiotensin AT1/AT2 receptors: Regulation signalling and function. Blood Press 12: 70-88.

Kassell NF, Sasaki T, Colohan AR, Nazar G. 1985. Cerebral vasospasm following aneurysmal subarachnoid hemorrhage. Stroke 16: 562-572.

Kawai N, Yamamoto T, Yamamoto H, McCarron RM, Spatz M. 1997. Functional characterization of endothelin receptors on cultured brain capillary endothelial cells of the rat. Neurochem Int 31: 597-605.

Kaya M, Kalayci R, Kucuk M, Arican N, Elmas I, et al. 2003. Effect of losartan on the blood-brain barrier permeability in diabetic hypertensive rats. Life Sci 73: 3235-3244.

Kikumoto K, Kubo A, Hayashi Y, Minamino N, Inoue S, et al. 1998. Increased plasma concentration of adrenomedullin in patients with subarachnoid hemorrhage. Anesth Analg 87: 859-863.

Kis B, Szabo CA, Paticza J, Krizbai IA, Mezei Z, et al. 1999. Vasoactive substances produced by cultured rat brain endothelial cells. Eur J Pharmacol 368: 35-42.

Kis B, Abraham CS, Deli MA, Kobayashi H, Wada A, et al. 2001a. Adrenomedullin in the cerebral circulation. Peptides 22: 1825-1834.

Kis B, Deli MA, Kobayashi H, Abraham CS, Yanagita T, et al. 2001b. Adrenomedullin regulates blood-brain barrier functions in vitro. Neuroreport 12: 4139-4142.

Kis B, Kaiya H, Nishi R, Deli MA, Abraham CS, et al. 2002. Cerebral endothelial cells are a major source of adrenomedullin. J Neuroendocrinol 14: 283-293.

Kis B, Snipes JA, Deli MA, Abraham CS, Yamashita H, et al. 2003. Chronic adrenomedullin treatment improves blood-brain barrier function but has no effects on expression of tight junction proteins. Acta Neurochir Suppl 86: 565-568.

Kitagawa A, Kizuki K, Moriya H, Kudo M, Noguchi T. 1991. Localization of kallikrein in rat pineal glands. Endocrinol Jpn 38: 109-112.

Kitamura K, Kangawa K, Kawamoto M, Ichiki Y, Nakamura S, et al. 1993. Adrenomedullin: A novel hypotensive peptide isolated from human pheochromocytoma. Biochem Biophys Res Commun 192: 553-560.

Kobayashi H, Minami S, Yamamoto R, Masumoto K, Yanagita T, et al. 2000. Adrenomedullin receptors in rat cerebral microvessels. Brain Res Mol Brain Res 81: 1-6.

Konsman JP, Vigues S, Mackerlova L, Bristow A, Blomqvist A. 2004. Rat brain vascular distribution of interleukin-1 type-1 receptor immunoreactivity: Relationship to patterns of inducible cyclooxygenase expression by peripheral inflammatory stimuli. J Comp Neurol 472: 113-129.

Kontos HA, Wei EP, Kukreja RC, Ellis EF, Hess ML. 1990. Differences in endothelium-dependent cerebral dilation by bradykinin and acetylcholine. Am J Physiol 258: H1261-1266.

Kramar EA, Harding JW, Wright JW. 1997. Angiotensin II- and IV-induced changes in cerebral blood flow. Roles of AT1, AT2, and AT4 receptor subtypes. Regul Pept 68: 131-138.

Ladoux A, Frelin C. 2000. Coordinated Up-regulation by hypoxia of adrenomedullin and one of its putative receptors (RDC-1) in cells of the rat blood-brain barrier. J Biol Chem 275: 39914-39919.

Lambrecht BN. 2001. Immunologists getting nervous: Neuropeptides dendritic cells and T cell activation. Respir Res 2: 133-138.

Lang MG, Paterno R, Faraci FM, Heistad DD. 1997. Mechanisms of adrenomedullin-induced dilatation of cerebral arterioles. Stroke 28: 181-185.

Lange D, Funa K, Ishisaki A, Bauer R, Wollina U. 1999. Autocrine endothelial regulation in brain stem vessels of newborn piglets. Histol Histopathol 14: 821-825.

Lavoie JL, Sigmund CD. 2003. Minireview: Overview of the renin-angiotensin system—an endocrine and paracrine system. Endocrinology 144: 2179-2183.

Lee TH, Avraham HK, Jiang S, Avraham S. 2003. Vascular endothelial growth factor modulates the transendothelial migration of MDA-MB-231 breast cancer cells through regulation of brain microvascular endothelial cell permeability. J Biol Chem 278: 5277-5284.

Levi-Montalcini R, Skaper SD, Dal Toso R, Petrelli L, Leon A. 1996. Nerve growth factor: From neurotrophin to neurokine. Trends Neurosci 19: 514-520.

Linnik MD, Moskowitz MA. 1989. Identification of immunoreactive substance P in human and other mammalian endothelial cells. Peptides 10: 957-962.

Loesch A, Burnstock G. 1988. Ultrastructural localisation of serotonin and substance P in vascular endothelial cells of rat femoral and mesenteric arteries. Anat Embryol (Berl) 178: 137-142.

Loesch A, Domer FR, Alexander B, Burnstock G. 1993. Electron-immunocytochemistry of peptides in endothelial cells of rabbit cerebral vessels following perfusion with a perfluorocarbon emulsion. Brain Res 611: 333-337.

Lou J, Dayer JM, Grau GE, Burger D. 1996. Direct cell/cell contact with stimulated T lymphocytes induces the expression of cell adhesion molecules and cytokines by human brain microvascular endothelial cells. Eur J Immunol 26: 3107-3113.

Male D, Pryce G. 1988. Synergy between interferons and monokines in MHC induction on brain endothelium. Immunol Lett 17: 267-271.

Male D, Rahman J, Pryce G, Tamatani T, Miyasaka M. 1994. Lymphocyte migration into the CNS modelled in vitro:

Roles of LFA-1, ICAM-1 and VLA-4. Immunology 81: 366-372.

Mantovani A, Bussolino F, Introna M. 1997. Cytokine regulation of endothelial cell function: From molecular level to the bedside. Immunol Today 18: 231-240.

Marceau F, Larrivee JF, Saint-Jacques E, Bachvarov DR. 1997. The kinin B1 receptor: An inducible G protein coupled receptor. Can J Physiol Pharmacol 75: 725-730.

Matsuo Y, Mihara S, Ninomiya M, Fujimoto M. 2001. Protective effect of endothelin type A receptor antagonist on brain edema and injury after transient middle cerebral artery occlusion in rats. Stroke 32: 2143-2148.

McLatchie LM, Fraser NJ, Main MJ, Wise A, Brown J, et al. 1998. RAMPs regulate the transport and ligand specificity of the calcitonin- receptor-like receptor. Nature 393: 333-339.

Megyeri P, Abraham CS, Temesvari P, Kovacs J, Vas T, et al. 1992. Recombinant human tumor necrosis factor alpha constricts pial arterioles and increases blood-brain barrier permeability in newborn piglets. Neurosci Lett 148: 137-140.

Meng W, Busija DW. 1993. Comparative effects of angiotensin-(1–7) and angiotensin II on piglet pial arterioles. Stroke 24: 2041-2044; discussion 2045.

Michel CC, Curry FE. 1999. Microvascular permeability. Physiol Rev 79: 703-761.

Michel MC, Beck-Sickinger A, Cox H, Doods HN, Herzog H, et al. 1998. XVI. International Union of Pharmacology recommendations for the nomenclature of neuropeptide Y peptide YY and pancreatic polypeptide receptors. Pharmacol Rev 50: 143-150.

Michibata H, Mukoyama M, Tanaka I, Suga S, Nakagawa M, et al. 1998. Autocrine/paracrine role of adrenomedullin in cultured endothelial and mesangial cells. Kidney Int 53: 979-985.

Miller RD, Monsul NT, Vender JR, Lehmann JC. 1996. NMDA- and endothelin-1-induced increases in blood-brain barrier permeability quantitated with Lucifer yellow. J Neurol Sci 136: 37-40.

Miller AW, Tulbert C, Puskar M, Busija DW. 2002. Enhanced endothelin activity prevents vasodilation to insulin in insulin resistance. Hypertension 40: 78-82.

Milner P, Bodin P, Loesch A, Burnstock G. 1995. Interactions between sensory perivascular nerves and the endothelium in brain microvessels. Int J Microcirc Clin Exp 15: 1-9.

Minamino N, Kikumoto K, Isumi Y. 2002. Regulation of adrenomedullin expression and release. Microsc Res Tech 57: 28-39.

Moore SA, Spector AA, Hart MN. 1988. Eicosanoid metabolism in cerebromicrovascular endothelium. Am J Physiol 254: C37-C44.

Moreno MJ, Cohen Z, Stanimirovic DB, Hamel E. 1999. Functional calcitonin gene-related peptide type 1 and adrenomedullin receptors in human trigeminal ganglia brain vessels and cerebromicrovascular or astroglial cells in culture. J Cereb Blood Flow Metab 19: 1270-1278.

Mori Y, Takayasu M, Suzuki Y, Shibuya M, Yoshida J, et al. 1997. Effects of adrenomedullin on rat cerebral arterioles. Eur J Pharmacol 330: 195-198.

Morin AM, Stanboli A. 1993. Nitric oxide synthase in cultured endothelial cells of cerebrovascular origin: Cytochemistry. J Neurosci Res 36: 272-279.

Moser KV, Reindl M, Blasig I, Humpel C. 2004. Brain capillary endothelial cells proliferate in response to NGF express NGF receptors and secrete NGF after inflammation. Brain Res 1017: 53-60.

Nakamura K, Toda H, Terasako K, Kakuyama M, Hatano Y, et al. 1995. Vasodilative effect of adrenomedullin in isolated arteries of the dog. Jpn J Pharmacol 67: 259-262.

Nakanishi S. 1991. Mammalian tachykinin receptors. Annu Rev Neurosci 14: 123-136.

Nakayama M, Takahashi K, Murakami O, Shirato K, et al. 1999. Induction of adrenomedullin by hypoxia in cultured human coronary artery endothelial cells. Peptides 20: 769-772.

Narushima I, Kita T, Kubo K, Yonetani Y, Momochi C, et al. 2003. Highly enhanced permeability of blood-brain barrier induced by repeated administration of endothelin-1 in dogs and rats. Pharmacol Toxicol 92: 21-26.

Nawa H, Kotani H, Nakanishi S. 1984. Tissue-specific generation of two preprotachykinin mRNAs from one gene by alternative RNA splicing. Nature 312: 729-734.

Nishikimi T, Kitamura K, Saito Y, Shimada K, Ishimitsu T, et al. 1994. Clinical studies on the sites of production and clearance of circulating adrenomedullin in human subjects. Hypertension 24: 600-604.

Nishikimi T, Matsuoka H, Shimada K, Matsuo H, Kangawa K. 2000. Production and clearance sites of two molecular forms of adrenomedullin in human plasma. Am J Hypertens 13: 1032-1034.

Nishimura Y, Suzuki A. 1997. Relaxant effects of vasodilator peptides on isolated basilar arteries from stroke-prone spontaneously hypertensive rats. Clin Exp Pharmacol Physiol 24: 157-161.

Ohlstein EH, Elliott JD, Feuerstein GZ, Ruffolo RR, Jr. 1996. Endothelin receptors: Receptor classification novel receptor antagonists and potential therapeutic targets. Med Res Rev 16: 365-390.

Oliver KR, Wainwright A, Edvinsson L, Pickard JD, Hill RG. 2002. Immunohistochemical localization of calcitonin receptor-like receptor and receptor activity-modifying proteins in the human cerebral vasculature. J Cereb Blood Flow Metab 22: 620-629.

Omari KM, Chui R, Dorovini-Zis K. 2004. Induction of beta-chemokine secretion by human brain microvessel endothelial cells via CD40/CD40L interactions. J Neuroimmunol 146: 203-208.

Omari KM, Dorovini-Zis K. 2003. CD40 expressed by human brain endothelial cells regulates CD4+ T cell adhesion to endothelium. J Neuroimmunol 134: 166-178.

Paspalas CD, Papadopoulos GC. 1998. Ultrastructural evidence for combined action of noradrenaline and vasoactive intestinal polypeptide upon neurons astrocytes and blood vessels of the rat cerebral cortex. Brain Res Bull 45: 247-259.

Pernow B. 1983. Substance P. Pharmacol Rev 35: 85-141.

Prat A, Biernacki K, Pouly S, Nalbantoglu J, Couture R, et al. 2000. Kinin B1 receptor expression and function on human brain endothelial cells. J Neuropathol Exp Neurol 59: 896-906.

Raichle ME, Grubb RL, Jr. 1978. Regulation of brain water permeability by centrally-released vasopressin. Brain Res 143: 191-194.

Ralevic V, Milner P, Hudlicka O, Kristek F, Burnstock G. 1990. Substance P is released from the endothelium of normal and capsaicin-treated rat hind-limb vasculature in vivo by increased flow. Circ Res 66: 1178-1183.

Ransohoff RM. 1999. Mechanisms of inflammation in MS tissue: Adhesion molecules and chemokines. J Neuroimmunol 98: 57-68.

Reyes TM, Fabry Z, Coe CL. 1999. Brain endothelial cell production of a neuroprotective cytokine interleukin-6, in response to noxious stimuli. Brain Res 851: 215-220.

Rollins BJ. 1997. Chemokines. Blood 90: 909-928.

Rose JM, Audus KL. 1999. AT1 receptors mediate angiotensin II uptake and transport by bovine brain microvessel endothelial cells in primary culture. J Cardiovasc Pharmacol 33: 30-35.

Rothlein R, Dustin ML, Marlin SD, Springer TA. 1986. A human intercellular adhesion molecule (ICAM-1) distinct from LFA-1. J Immunol 137: 1270-1274.

Rott O, Tontsch U, Fleischer B, Cash E. 1993. Interleukin-6 production in "normal" and HTLV-1 tax-expressing brain-specific endothelial cells. Eur J Immunol 23: 1987-1991.

Rubin LL, Hall DE, Porter S, Barbu K, Cannon C, et al. 1991. A cell culture model of the blood-brain barrier. J Cell Biol 115: 1725-1735.

Rubin LL, Staddon JM. 1999. The cell biology of the blood-brain barrier. Annu Rev Neurosci 22: 11-28.

Russell FD, Davenport AP. 1999. Secretory pathways in endothelin synthesis. Br J Pharmacol 126: 391-398.

Saito T, Itoh H, Chun TH, Fukunaga Y, Yamashita J, et al. 2001. Coordinate regulation of endothelin and adrenomedullin secretion by oxidative stress in endothelial cells. Am J Physiol 281: H1364-1371.

Sakata J, Shimokubo T, Kitamura K, Nakamura S, Kangawa K, et al. 1993. Molecular cloning and biological activities of rat adrenomedullin a hypotensive peptide. Biochem Biophys Res Commun 195: 921-927.

Sams A, Knyihar-Csillik E, Engberg J, Szok D, Tajti J, et al. 2000. CGRP and adrenomedullin receptor populations in human cerebral arteries: In vitro pharmacological and molecular investigations in different artery sizes. Eur J Pharmacol 408: 183-193.

Santos RA, Campagnole-Santos MJ, Andrade SP. 2000. Angiotensin-(1-7): an update. Regul Pept 91: 45-62.

Seifert V, Loffler BM, Zimmermann M, Roux S, Stolke D. 1995. Endothelin concentrations in patients with aneurysmal subarachnoid hemorrhage. Correlation with cerebral vasospasm delayed ischemic neurological deficits and volume of hematoma. J Neurosurg 82: 55-62.

Serrano J, Uttenthal LO, Martinez A, Fernandez AP, Martinez de Velasco J, et al. 2000. Distribution of adrenomedullin-like immunoreactivity in the rat central nervous system by light and electron microscopy. Brain Res 853: 245-268. bin/cas/tree/store/bres/cas_sub/browse/browse.cgi?year=2000&volume=2853&issue=2002&aid=16136.

Serrano J, Alonso D, Encinas JM, Lopez JC, Fernandez AP, et al. 2002. Adrenomedullin expression is up-regulated by ischemia-reperfusion in the cerebral cortex of the adult rat. Neuroscience 109: 717-731.

Shi F, Audus KL. 1994. Biochemical characteristics of primary and passaged cultures of primate brain microvessel endothelial cells. Neurochem Res 19: 427-433.

Shindo T, Kurihara H, Maemura K, Kurihara Y, Kuwaki T, et al. 2000. Hypotension and resistance to lipopolysaccharide-induced shock in transgenic mice overexpressing adrenomedullin in their vasculature. Circulation 101: 2309-2316.

Shukaliak JA, Dorovini-Zis K. 2000. Expression of the beta-chemokines RANTES and MIP-1 beta by human brain microvessel endothelial cells in primary culture. J Neuropathol Exp Neurol 59: 339-352.

Simpson JE, Newcombe J, Cuzner ML, Woodroofe MN. 1998. Expression of monocyte chemoattractant protein-1 and other beta-chemokines by resident glia and inflammatory cells in multiple sclerosis lesions. J Neuroimmunol 84: 238-249.

Skopal J, Turbucz P, Vastag M, Bori Z, Pek M, et al. 1998. Regulation of endothelin release from human brain microvessel endothelial cells. J Cardiovasc Pharmacol 31 (Suppl 1): S370-372.

Smith DM, Coppock HA, Withers DJ, Owji AA, Hay DL, et al. 2002. Adrenomedullin: Receptor and signal transduction. Biochem Soc Trans 30: 432-437.

Stanimirovic DB, Bertrand N, McCarron R, Uematsu S, Spatz M. 1994. Arachidonic acid release and permeability changes induced by endothelins in human cerebromicrovascular endothelium. Acta Neurochir Suppl (Wien) 60 (Suppl): 71-75.

Stumm R, Culmsee C, Schafer MK, Krieglstein J, Weihe E. 2001. Adaptive plasticity in tachykinin and tachykinin receptor expression after focal cerebral ischemia is differentially linked to gabaergic and glutamatergic cerebrocortical circuits and cerebrovenular endothelium. J Neurosci 21: 798-811.

Sugo S, Minamino N, Kangawa K, Miyamoto K, Kitamura K, et al. 1994. Endothelial cells actively synthesize and secrete adrenomedullin. Biochem Biophys Res Commun 201: 1160-1166.

Takao M, Tomita M, Tanahashi N, Kobari M, Fukuuchi Y. 1999. Transient vasodilatory effects of adrenomedullin on cerebral parenchymal microvessels in cats. Neurosci Lett 268: 147-150.

Takemori K, Ito H, Suzuki T. 2000. Effects of the AT1 receptor antagonist on adhesion molecule expression in leukocytes and brain microvessels of stroke-prone spontaneously hypertensive rats. Am J Hypertens 13: 1233-1241.

Takenaka K, Kishino J, Arita H, Okano Y, Sakai N, et al. 1993. Biological activity of the endothelin family in cultured basilar arterial smooth muscle cells. Neurol Res 15: 29-32.

Turner AJ, Barnes K, Schweizer A, Valdenaire O. 1998. Isoforms of endothelin-converting enzyme: Why and where? Trends Pharmacol Sci 19: 483-486.

Turrini P, Gaetano C, Antonelli A, Capogrossi MC, Aloe L. 2002. Nerve growth factor induces angiogenic activity in a mouse model of hindlimb ischemia. Neurosci Lett 323: 109-112.

Unterberg A, Wahl M, Baethmann A. 1984. Effects of bradykinin on permeability and diameter of pial vessels in vivo. J Cereb Blood Flow Metab 4: 574-585.

Van Dam AM, De Vries HE, Kuiper J, Zijlstra FJ, De Boer AG, et al. 1996. Interleukin-1 receptors on rat brain endothelial cells: A role in neuroimmune interaction? FASEB J 10: 351-356.

Vastag M, Skopal J, Kramer J, Kolev K, Voko Z, et al. 1998. Endothelial cells cultured from human brain microvessels produce complement proteins factor H factor B C1 inhibitor and C4. Immunobiology 199: 5-13.

Vatter H, Mursch K, Zimmermann M, Zilliken P, Kolenda H, et al. 2002. Endothelin-converting enzyme activity in human cerebral circulation. Neurosurgery 51: 445-451; discussion 451-442.

Vishwanath R, Mukherjee R. 1996. Substance P promotes lymphocyte-endothelial cell adhesion preferentially via LFA-1/ICAM-1 interactions. J Neuroimmunol 71: 163-171.

Volpe M, Cosentino F. 2000. Abnormalities of endothelial function in the pathogenesis of stroke: The importance of endothelin. J Cardiovasc Pharmacol 35: S45-48.

Wahl M, Gorlach C, Hortobagyi T, Benyo Z. 1999. Effects of bradykinin in the cerebral circulation. Acta Physiol Hung 86: 155-160.

Walker K, Perkins M, Dray A. 1995. Kinins and kinin receptors in the nervous system. Neurochem Int 26: 1-16; discussion 17-26.

Wang X, Yue TL, Barone FC, White RF, Clark RK, et al. 1995. Discovery of adrenomedullin in rat ischemic cortex and evidence for its role in exacerbating focal brain ischemic damage. Proc Natl Acad Sci USA 92: 11480-11484.

Watanabe K, Takayasu M, Noda A, Hara M, Takagi T, et al. 2001. Adrenomedullin reduces ischemic brain injury after transient middle cerebral artery occlusion in rats. Acta Neurochir (Wien) 143: 1157-1161.

Wiemer G, Fink E, Linz W, Hropot M, Scholkens BE, et al. 1994. Furosemide enhances the release of endothelial kinins nitric oxide and prostacyclin. J Pharmacol Exp Ther 271: 1611-1615.

Wiemer G, Scholkens BA, Becker RH, Busse R. 1991. Ramiprilat enhances endothelial autacoid formation by inhibiting breakdown of endothelium-derived bradykinin. Hypertension 18: 558-563.

Wijdicks EF, Heublein DM, Burnett JC, Jr. 2001. Increase and uncoupling of adrenomedullin from the natriuretic peptide system in aneurysmal subarachnoid hemorrhage. J Neurosurg 94: 252-256.

Wolburg H, Neuhaus J, Kniesel U, Krauss B, Schmid EM, et al. 1994. Modulation of tight junction structure in blood-brain barrier endothelial cells. Effects of tissue culture second messengers and cocultured astrocytes. J Cell Sci 107: 1347-1357.

Wong D, Dorovini-Zis K. 1992. Upregulation of intercellular adhesion molecule-1 (ICAM-1) expression in primary cultures of human brain microvessel endothelial cells by cytokines and lipopolysaccharide. J Neuroimmunol 39: 11-21.

Yamakawa H, Jezova M, Ando H, Saavedra JM. 2003. Normalization of endothelial and inducible nitric oxide synthase expression in brain microvessels of spontaneously hypertensive rats by angiotensin II AT1 receptor inhibition. J Cereb Blood Flow Metab 23: 371-380.

Yanagisawa M, Kurihara H, Kimura S, Tomobe Y, Kobayashi M, et al. 1988. A novel potent vasoconstrictor peptide produced by vascular endothelial cells. Nature 332: 411-415.

Yoshimoto S, Ishizaki Y, Kurihara H, Sasaki T, Yoshizumi M, et al. 1990. Cerebral microvessel endothelium is producing endothelin. Brain Res 508: 283-285.

Yoshimoto S, Ishizaki Y, Sasaki T, Murota S. 1991. Effect of carbon dioxide and oxygen on endothelin production by cultured porcine cerebral endothelial cells. Stroke 22: 378-383.

Zausinger S. 2003. Bradykinin receptor antagonists in cerebral ischemia and trauma. IDrugs 6: 970-975.

Zhang Z, Chopp M, Goussev A, Powers C. 1998. Cerebral vessels express interleukin 1beta after focal cerebral ischemia. Brain Res 784: 210-217.

Zidovetzki R, Wang JL, Chen P, Jeyaseelan R, Hofman F. 1998. Human immunodeficiency virus Tat protein induces interleukin 6 mRNA expression in human brain endothelial cells via protein kinase C- and cAMP-dependent protein kinase pathways. AIDS Res Hum Retroviruses 14: 825-833.

Zimmermann M, Seifert V. 1998. Endothelin and subarachnoid hemorrhage: An overview. Neurosurgery 43: 863-875; discussion 875–866.

Zimmermann M, Seifert V. 2004. Endothelin receptor antagonists and cerebral vasospasm. Clin Auton Res 14: 143-145.

Zukowska-Grojec Z, Karwatowska-Prokopczuk E, Rose W, Rone J, Movafagh S, et al. 1998. Neuropeptide Y: A novel angiogenic factor from the sympathetic nerves and endothelium. Circ Res 83: 187-195.

10   Na$^+$, K$^+$-ATPase in the Brain: Structure and Function

G. Rodríguez de Lores Arnaiz

Abstract: Maintenance of the Na$^+$ and K$^+$ gradients between the intracellular and extracellular compartments of animal cells is a prerequisite for basic cellular homeostasis and for diverse functions of specialized cells. Na$^+$, K$^+$-ATPase (sodium- and potassium-activated adenosine 5'-triphosphatase), also called Na$^+$ pump or Na$^+$, K$^+$-pump, is an ubiquitous membrane transport protein in mammalian cells, responsible to establish and maintain high K$^+$ and low Na$^+$ concentration in the cytoplasm; it is essential for normal resting membrane potentials and diverse cellular activities. As all ATPases, it hydrolyzes ATP and occludes ions within the membrane inserted segment of the protein during the translocation process. This system couples the hydrolysis of one molecule of ATP to exchange three sodium for two potassium ions, thus maintaining the normal gradient of these cations in animal cells. It acts as an electrogenic ion transporter, which is autophosphorylated on an aspartic acid residue by the gamma phosphate group of the ATP molecule that it hydrolyzes. Oxidative metabolism is very active in brain, where large amounts of chemical energy as ATP molecules are consumed, mostly required to maintain cellular Na$^+$/K$^+$ gradients that underlie resting and action potentials, which are involved in nerve impulse propagation, neurotransmitter release and cation homeostasis.

Na$^+$, K$^+$-ATPase is an olygomeric enzyme consisting of α and β subunits, both required for enzyme function. The α subunit is the catalytic one which crosses ten times the membrane; the binding sites for ATP and the inhibitor ouabain as well as ion occlusion occur in this subunit. Three isoforms with cell-type and development-specific expression patterns are present in brain. Subunits $\alpha 1$, $\alpha 2$, and $\alpha 3$ bind ouabain with low, intermediate and high affinity, respectively; the last two isoforms are associated to neurons whereas the first is related to glial cells. The β subunit regulates the activity and conformational stability of the α subunit, is highly glycosylated and presents a single-transmembrane span. It seems to participate in the modulation of enzyme affinity for K$^+$ and Na$^+$ and is important for ATP hydrolysis, ion transport, and binding of inhibitors such as ouabain. This subunit must interact with α subunit in order to accomplish ion transport. In association with the $\alpha\beta$ dimmer there is a third subunit which belongs to the FXYD family proteins. It modulates transport function of the enzyme, seems not essential for functional Na$^+$, K$^+$-ATPase but most likely plays a regulatory role in a tissue-specific manner. These small proteins are considered as channels or regulators of ion channels; they are hydrophobic type I proteins with a single-transmembrane span. The mammalian FXYD proteins from FXYD1 to FXYD7 exhibit tissue-specific distribution. FXYD7 is expressed exclusively in the brain, it is associated with $\alpha 1$-β isozymes and is most likely involved in neuronal excitability. Phospholemman (FXYD1) is highly expressed in selected structures in the CNS.

Due to changing physiological needs, diverse regulatory mechanisms are operative to ensure not only appropriate expression of Na$^+$, K$^+$-ATPase but also required enzyme activity. Multiple mechanisms can regulate Na$^+$, K$^+$-ATPase activity, coherent with the diverse functional roles in different conditions, which leads this protein to be vulnerable to pathogenic insults and a target for therapeutics. Besides its dependence for ATP, this enzyme activity is regulated by phosphorylation state, endogenous ouabain-like substances, neurotransmitters, oxidant stress such as reactive oxygen species, and diverse peptides.

In addition to pumping ions, Na$^+$, K$^+$-ATPase seems to act as a signal transducer. Binding of ouabain to Na$^+$, K$^+$-ATPase changes the interaction of the enzyme with neighboring membrane proteins inducing the formation of multiple signaling modules, leading to Src kinase activation, transactivation of the epidermal growth factor receptor and enhanced formation of reactive oxygen species. Interaction of such signals results in the activity of several other cascades, including phospholipase C activation. The inhibition of Src blocks many of the ouabain-activated signaling pathways. Src binds to Na$^+$, K$^+$-ATPase directly and ouabain modulates the interaction between Na$^+$, K$^+$-ATPase and Src, leading to Src activation. The possibility that signaling Na$^+$, K$^+$-ATPase is concentrated in an separate pool on the plasma membrane has been advanced and potential interaction between Na$^+$, K$^+$-ATPase and caveolins studied, due to enzyme concentration in caveloae/rafts.

Apoptosis has been recognized in a wide range of disease states, and Na$^+$, K$^+$-ATPase deficiency seems to be a contributor to apoptosis and pathogenesis. Physiological concentration of intracellular K$^+$ acts as a repressor of apoptotic effectors. The pro-apoptotic disruption of K$^+$ homeostasis can be mediated by over-activated K$^+$ channels or ionotropic glutamate receptor, accompanied by decreased K$^+$ uptake provoked by Na$^+$, K$^+$-ATPase disfunction.

Na$^+$, K$^+$-ATPase activity is reduced or is insufficient to maintain adequate ionic balances during and after episodes of hypoglycemia, ischemia or epilepsy, as well as after administration of excitotoxins like glutamate agonists. Besides, a relationship between endogenous Na$^+$, K$^+$-ATPase inhibitors with central dysfunction as occurs in Parkinson's disease, CNS glioma, schizophrenia and epilepsy has been established.

List of Abbreviations: DARPP-32, dopamine- and cAMP-regulated phosphoprotein of 32 kDa; HPLC, high performance liquid chromatography; Na$^+$, K$^+$-ATPase, sodium- and potassium-activated adenosine 5'-triphosphatase; PKC, protein kinase C ; PP1, protein phosphatase 1

1   Introduction

Maintenance of the Na$^+$ and K$^+$ gradients between the intracellular and extracellular compartments of animal cells is a prerequisite for basic cellular homeostasis and for diverse functions of specialized cells.

Sodium- and potassium-activated adenosine 5'-triphosphatase (Na$^+$, K$^+$-ATPase), discovered by Skou (1957), also called Na$^+$ pump or Na$^+$, K$^+$-pump, is an ubiquitous membrane transport protein in mammalian cells, responsible to establish and maintain high-K$^+$ and low-Na$^+$ concentration in the cytoplasm; it is essential for normal resting membrane potentials and diverse cellular activities.

As all ATPases, it hydrolyzes ATP and occludes ions within the membrane inserted segment of the protein during the translocation process, thus the ionophore is accessible from one membrane side at any given time. This system couples the hydrolysis of one molecule of ATP to exchange three sodium for two potassium ions, thus maintaining the normal gradient of these cations in animal cells. It acts as an electrogenic ion transporter, which is autophosphorylated on an aspartic acid residue by the γ phosphate group of the ATP molecule that it hydrolyzes (Albers and Siegel, 1999; Scheiner-Bobis, 2002).

2   Brain Na$^+$, K$^+$-ATPase Function

The Na$^+$ pump regulates K$^+$ entry with Na$^+$ exit from the neuron and therefore is responsible for Na$^+$/K$^+$ equilibrium maintenance through neuronal membranes; this mechanism is essential in the normal cell cycle, cell-volume regulation, osmotic balance, nervous system differentiation as well as in the maintenance and restoration of the resting membrane potential in excitable cells. Likewise, ion gradients formed due to Na$^+$, K$^+$-ATPase activity are required for Na$^+$-coupled transport of nutrients and amino acids into the cells (Stahl, 1986).

Oxidative metabolism is very active in brain, where large amounts of chemical energy as ATP molecules are consumed. It is mostly required to maintain cellular Na$^+$/K$^+$ gradients that underlie resting and action potentials, which are involved in nerve impulse propagation, neurotransmitter release, and cation homeostasis (Albers and Siegel, 1999).

Na$^+$, K$^+$-ATPase concentrates in surrounding membranes of nerve endings (Rodríguez de Lores Arnaiz et al., 1967), a crucial site in neurotransmission. The involvement of Na$^+$, K$^+$-ATPase in diverse biological processes is often studied employing ouabain and related cardiac glycosides, which proved to behave as selective and powerful inhibitors (Albers and Siegel, 1999).

In comparison with its environment, every living cell is negatively charged and thus cell environment constitute a battery able to perform work. The cell uses this electrochemical gradient to provide itself with nutrients, either ionic or nonionic, from the surrounding medium and to extrude metabolites and ions from its interior. In this way, intracellular medium composition remains constant while allowing adaptation to permanent environment changes (Scheiner-Bobis, 2002).

Since the Na$^+$ pump is responsible for the establishment and maintenance of this electrochemical gradient in animal cells, it is obviously essential for neuronal communication. Besides, the resulting electrochemical Na$^+$ gradient from its activity is the driving force behind secondary transport systems. Na$^+$, K$^+$-ATPase is an ion transporter crucial not only for neural but also for glial physiology by direct electrogenic activity and regulation of ion gradients.

In order to maintain neuronal cytoplasmic Ca^{2+} concentration one-ten thousand times lower that in the extracellular millieu, two mechanisms are operative. One of them is a calcium pump and the other is a Na$^+$/Ca^{2+} exchanger. The latter is dependent on functional Na$^+$, K$^+$-ATPase in a process inhibited by omitting Na$^+$ and including ouabain (Putney, 1999). Therefore, failure of the Na$^+$, K$^+$-pump leads to depletion of intracellular K$^+$, accumulation of intracellular free Ca^{2+} by activation of voltage-gated Ca^{2+} channels, and reversion of the Na$^+$/Ca^{2+} exchanger (DiPolo and Beaugé, 1991; Xiao et al., 2002).

The Na$^+$, K$^+$-ATPase presents two conformational states, E$_1$ and E$_2$, characterized by their particular interactions with sodium and potassium ions, ATP, and ouabain as well as by their behavior in tryptic cleavage experiments. To explain the sequence of reactions involved in Na$^+$/K$^+$ transport, several models have been proposed, including that referred to as the Albers-Post scheme, based on biochemical analysis of partial reactions of the pump, for example, kinetics of phosphorylation/dephosphorylation (❷ *Figure 10-1*). Other models include cooperate interaction between enzyme subunits (Scheiner-Bobis, 2002).

A particular characteristic of the Na$^+$, K$^+$-ATPase is its ability to hydrolyze phosphoesters and phosphoanhydrides in the presence of potassium ions, the so-called K$^+$-stimulated phosphatase activity, which is ouabain sensitive. However, Na$^+$, K$^+$-ATPase or K$^+$-*p*-nitrophenylphosphatase activities may not always provide the same information since differences in subcellular distribution (Rodríguez de Lores Arnaiz et al., 1967) in Km values as well as in sensitivity to ouabain and fluoride (Yoshida et al., 1969) have been observed.

3   Brain Na$^+$, K$^+$-ATPase Structure

Na$^+$, K$^+$-ATPase is an olygomeric enzyme consisting of α and β subunits, both required for enzyme function.

The α subunit is the catalytic one with a relative molecular mass of about 100–113 kDa, depending on the presence of different isoforms: α1, α2, α3, or α4, the latter identified only in testis (Shamraj and Lingrel, 1994). The α subunit crosses ten times the membrane, forming transmembrane domains M1–M10; both the N and C termini are localized on the cytosolic side; the binding sites for ATP and the inhibitor ouabain as well as ion occlusion occur in this subunit (Antolovic et al., 1991). Its three isoforms in brain have cell-type and development-specific expression patterns. The α2 isoform is widely expressed in neurons in late gestation but is primarily expressed in astrocytes in adult brain; most interesting mice lacking the α2 isoform fail to survive after birth (Moseley et al., 2003).

The β subunit regulates the activity and conformational stability of the α subunit (Eakle et al., 1994; Chow and Forte, 1995); it is highly glycosylated, has a relative molecular mass of roughly 60 kDa, and the mass of the protein moiety is 36–38 kDa. It presents a single-transmembrane span with the N terminus localized on the intracellular membrane side (Malik et al., 1996; Blanco and Mercer, 1998). The β subunit seems to participate in the modulation of enzyme affinity for K$^+$ and Na$^+$ (Jaisser et al., 1992; Lutsenko and Kaplan, 1993) and is important for ATP hydrolysis, ion transport, and binding of inhibitors such as ouabain. This subunit must interact with α subunit in order to accomplish ion transport (Scheiner-Bobis, 2002).

Regarding β subunit isoforms, β2 type is related to glial cells as an adhesion cell molecule; it is expressed where β1 isoform is absent, including astrocytes and tissues in the central nervous system (glia, choroid plexus, arachnoid membrane), showing specialized ion-translocating characteristics (Schmalzing et al., 1992; Scheiner-Bobis, 2002).

In mammals, four genes (α1–α4) encode the α subunit and three genes (β1–β3) encode the β subunit (Blanco and Mercer, 1998). In the nervous system, all α and β isoforms are expressed; α1 is ubiquitously distributed with highest expression levels in kidney, α2 predominates in skeletal muscle, brain, and heart, and α3 seems to be the most abundant form in brain, although it is also present in heart. According to temporal and spatial expression in the brain, the various α and β isoforms may be expressed in the same cell type (McGrail et al., 1991; Watts et al., 1991).

Subunits α1, α2, and α3 bind ouabain with low, intermediate, and high affinity, respectively; the last two isoforms are associated to neurons whereas the first is related to glial cells (Sweadner, 1989; Berrebi-Bertrand et al., 1990; McGrail et al., 1991).

□ Figure 10-1

The mechanism of the ATP-dependent Na$^+$ pump. The sequence of reaction steps is indicated by the *large arrows*. *Left*: Pump molecules are in the E$_1$ conformation, which has high affinity for Na$^+$ and ATP and low affinity for K$^+$. Ionophoric sites are accessible only from the cytoplasmic side. *Step 1*: K$^+$ is discharged as metabolic energy is added to the system by ATP binding. *Step 2*: Three Na$^+$ bind and the enzyme is reversibly phosphorylated. *Step 3*: The conformational transition from E$_1$-P to E$_2$-P, shown at the *top*, is the "power stroke" of the pump during which the ionophoric sites with their three bound Na$^+$ become accessible to the extracellular side and decrease their affinity for Na$^+$. Part of the free energy of the enzyme acylphosphate has been dissipated in this process. *Right*: Pump molecules are in the E$_2$ conformation. *Step 4*: Three Na$^+$ dissociate from E$_2$-P. *Step 5*: Two K$^+$ bind and more free energy is dissipated as the enzyme acylphosphate is hydrolyzed. At this point, the two K$^+$ become tightly bound ("occluded"). *Step 6*: E$_2$ reverts to E$_1$ carrying the K$^+$ to the cytoplasmic side. From Albers and Siegel (1999) with permission of the authors and the publisher

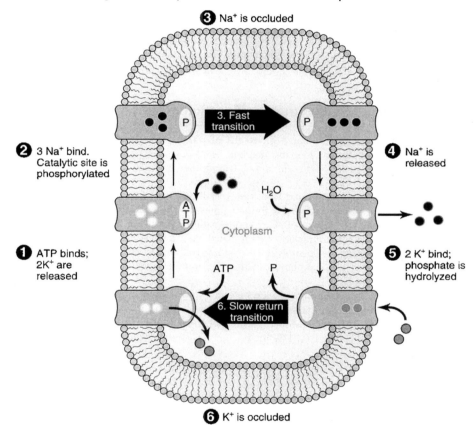

Since all three α-subunit isoforms are present in neurons from the neostriatum, isoform specificity for neurotransmitter-dependent regulation of Na$^+$, K$^+$-ATPase activity has been suggested (Teixeira et al., 2003).

In association with the αβ dimmer, there is a third subunit with a mass of 7–11 kDa belonging to the FXYD family proteins. It modulates transport function of the enzyme (Beguin et al., 1997), seems not essential for functional Na$^+$, K$^+$-ATPase but most likely plays a regulatory role in a tissue-specific manner (Therien and Blostein, 2000; Scheiner-Bobis, 2002).

3.1   FXYD Proteins

These small proteins are considered as channels or regulators of ion channels (Sweadner and Rael, 2000). The FXYD proteins act as tissue-specific regulators of the Na$^+$, K$^+$-ATPase; they are hydrophobic type I proteins with a single-transmembrane span containing an extracellular invariant sequence. These proteins are not an integral part of the Na$^+$, K$^+$-ATPase, but their function is to modulate catalytic enzyme properties by molecular interactions with specific enzyme domains (Sweadner and Rael, 2000; Cornelius and Mahmmoud, 2003).

The mammalian FXYD proteins from FXYD1 to FXYD7 exhibit tissue-specific distribution (Geering et al., 2003). FXYD7 is expressed exclusively in the brain, it bears N-terminal, posttranslationally added modifications on threonine residues, such as O-glycosylations, important for protein stabilization. It is associated with α1-β isozymes and is most likely involved in neuronal excitability (Beguin et al., 2002; Crambert et al., 2003).

Phospholemman (FXYD1) is highly expressed in selected structures in the CNS. Phospholemman antibodies precipitate all three Na$^+$, K$^+$-ATPase α subunit isoforms (α1–α3) from cerebellum, indicating that the interaction is not specific to a particular α isoform and that phospholemman is present in both neurons and glia (Feschenko et al., 2003).

4   Methodology to Study Structure/Function of Na$^+$, K$^+$-ATPase

Ideas regarding active transport are based on results of transport physiology, protein chemistry, and heterologous expression of mutant proteins (Kaplan, 2002). Crystallographic studies have shown that this enzyme crystallizes in such a way so to allow $\alpha\beta$ protomers to be in close contact inter se (Skriver et al., 1989).

Mutagenesis, proteolytic cleavage, and transition metal-catalyzed cleavages have provided abundant evidence about residues involved in binding of sodium, potassium, and magnesium ions and ATP as well as in changes which accompany E$_1$-E$_2$ or E$_1$-P–E$_2$-P conformational transitions (Jorgensen et al., 2003).

Tryptic removal of the hydrophilic part of the isolated Na$^+$, K$^+$-ATPase indicates that the remaining C-terminal, membrane-spanning segment, is able to occlude Na$^+$ or Rb$^+$ (the K$^+$ analog) (Shainskaya and Karlish, 1994), showing that the ionophore consists of membrane-spanning domains (Scheiner-Bobis, 2002).

Diverse mutants by substitution of acidic amino acids within the membrane-spanning domains were analyzed, to observe that this substitution does not always have a marked effect in the affinity for Na$^+$ or K$^+$ or alters its electrical properties (Jewell-Motz and Lingrel, 1993; Van Huysse et al., 1993; Vilsen, 1993). However, in same cases, alterations on K$^+$ but not on Na$^+$ recognition were recorded (Vilsen, 1993; Kuntzweiler et al., 1996).

5   Enzyme Regulation

Due to changing physiological needs, diverse regulatory mechanisms are operative to ensure not only appropriate expression of Na$^+$, K$^+$-ATPase but also required enzyme activity.

Multiple mechanisms can regulate Na$^+$, K$^+$-ATPase activity, coherent with the diverse functional roles in different conditions, which leads this protein to be vulnerable to pathogenic insults and a target for therapeutics (Hollenberg and Graves, 1996; Therien and Blostein, 2000). Besides its dependence for ATP, this enzyme activity is regulated by phosphorylation state (Therien and Blostein, 2000), endogenous ouabain-like substances (Budzikowski et al., 1998; Rodríguez de Lores Arnaiz, 2000; Lichtstein and Rosen, 2001; Bagrov et al., 2002), neurotransmitters (Hernández, 1992), oxidant stress such as reactive oxygen species (Kourie, 1998), and diverse peptides (Rodríguez de Lores Arnaiz and López Ordieres, 2003).

5.1   Regulation by Phosphorylation/Dephosphorylation

Protein phosphorylation is a key process in biological regulation that involves a protein kinase, a protein phosphatase, and a substrate protein. The kinases catalyze the transfer of the terminal γ phosphate of ATP to the hydroxyl moiety in the corresponding amino acid residue in a reaction requiring Mg^{2+}. In turn, protein phosphatases catalyze the cleavage of this phosphoester bond through hydrolysis. At nervous system level, protein phosphorylation is the major molecular mechanism through which the function of neural proteins is regulated in response to extracellular signals, including response to neurotransmitter stimuli; it is the major mechanism of neural plasticity, including memory processing (Nestler and Greengard, 1999).

Phosphorylation of Na$^+$, K$^+$-ATPase catalytic subunit inhibits enzyme activity (Bertorello et al., 1991); accordingly, inhibition of protein kinase C (PKC) restores enzyme activity (Hermenegildo et al., 1992, 1993). Dephosphorylation of Na$^+$, K$^+$-ATPase is mediated by calcineurin, a serine/threonine phosphatase involved in a wide range of cellular responses to Ca^{2+} mobilizing signals, in the regulation of neuronal excitability by controlling the activity of ion channels, in the release of neurotransmitters and hormones, in synaptic plasticity, and gene transcription (Yakel, 1997; Rusnak and Mertz, 2000). Likewise, changes in dopamine- and cAMP-regulated phosphoprotein of 32 kDa (DARPP-32) activity would lead to altered protein phosphatase 1 (PP1) activity and hence to modified Na$^+$, K$^+$-ATPase dephosphorylation (Li et al., 1995; Greengard, 2001) (❯ Figure 10-2).

5.2   Endogenous Modulators

Findings of Na$^+$, K$^+$-ATPase modulation by diverse molecules may provide an explanation to understand regulatory mechanisms involved not only in normal but also in pathological conditions. The search for possible modulation of Na$^+$ pump by neuroactive substances including neurotransmitters has been the aim of diverse studies, and results recorded have been summarized (Rodríguez de Lores Arnaiz, 1983, 1992; Goto et al., 1992; Hernández, 1992). The term endobain was proposed for endogenous ouabain-like substances (Rodríguez de Lores Arnaiz, 1993) and gathered information was reviewed (Rodríguez de Lores Arnaiz, 2000).

Taking into account their chemical nature, endogenous Na$^+$, K$^+$-ATPase modulators may be grouped into steroids (identical or closely resembling ouabain) and nonsteroids (of diverse structure). Digitalis-like factors are endogenous mammalian cardenolides with structural features similar to plant-derived digitalis compounds, which may act as effectors of ion-transport activity through interaction with Na$^+$, K$^+$-ATPase.

Factors very similar to ouabain have been isolated from human plasma (Hamlyn et al., 1991; Mathews et al., 1991) and rat hypothalamus (Ferrandi et al., 1992; Yamada et al., 1992), whereas a factor which differs from ouabain in biophysical properties has been purified from bovine hypothalamus (Sancho, 1998).

Na$^+$ pump inhibitors of the bufodienolide type of cardiotonic steroids have been identified in human cataractous lens (Lichtstein et al., 1993), human urine after acute myocardial infarction (Bagrov et al., 1998), and bovine adrenal glands (Schneider et al., 1998).

A plasma Na$^+$ pump inhibitor that enhances cardiovascular function is a steroidal ouabain isomer secreted by the adrenal cortex (Hamlyn et al., 1998); most interestingly, adrenal cells have the necessary machinery for de novo biosynthesis of digitalis-like factors (Qazzaz et al., 2004).

An ouabain isomer is present in bovine hypothalamus (Tymiak et al., 1993), which was attributed to the same substance present in human plasma (Zhao et al., 1995).

From human urine, two ouabain-displacing compounds have been purified, one of them closely resembling ouabain whereas the other one is indistinguishable from digoxin (Goto and Yamada, 1998).

Ouabain has been detected in plasma (Ludens et al., 1991; Butt et al., 1997), hypothalamic and medullary neurons (Budzikowski et al., 1998), and bovine adrenal glands (Schneider et al., 1998). Ouabain has been isolated and identified in human blood as well as in bovine adrenal glands and hypothalamus; it circulates in elevated concentrations in Caucasians presenting elevated blood pressure (Schoner, 2000).

☐ Figure 10-2

Signaling pathways in the neostriatum. Activation of several neurotransmitter receptors regulate DARPP-32 phosphorylation. On one hand, pathways involving activation of adenylyl cyclase and PKA or guanylyl cyclase and PKG lead to DARPP-32 phosphorylation. On the other hand, pathways which increase intracellular Ca^{2+} activate protein phosphatase activity, namely protein PP2B, Ca^{2+}/calmodulin-dependent protein phosphatase or calcineurin. Activated PP2B dephosphorylates DARPP-32. Phosphorylation of DARPP-32 converts it from an inactive molecule into a very potent inhibitor of PP1. PP1 controls phosphorylation state and activity of ion pumps, voltage-gated ion channels, neurotransmitter receptors, and transcription factors. The phosphorylation state of DARPP-32 is also regulated by centrally acting drugs, including antipsychotics and drugs of abuse. NKA, Na$^+$, K$^+$-ATPase, L- and N/P-Ca^{2+}, L type, and N/P type Ca^{2+} channels. For full description, see Greengard (2001). From Greengard (2001) with permission of the author and the publisher

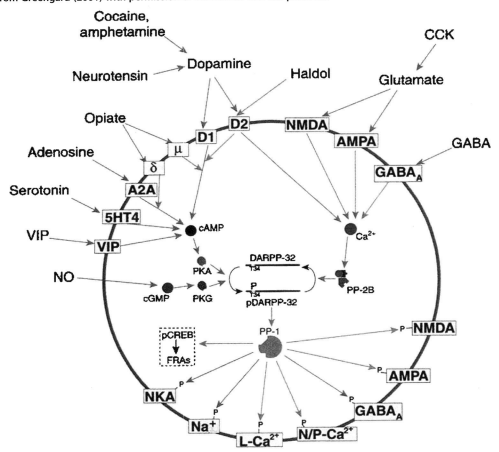

Morphine or buprenorphine stimulate synaptosome Na$^+$, K$^+$-ATPase activity, an effect prevented by opioid antagonist naloxone, and accordingly blocked by either μ or μ1 antagonists or by Pertussis toxin, indicating involvement of μ-opioid receptors and G(i/o) proteins (Masocha et al., 2002).

Regarding nonsteroid modulators, low-MW substances, either nonpeptidic (Fishman, 1979; Shimoni et al., 1984) or peptidic (Akagawa et al., 1984) have been described. Another ouabain-like factor unrelated to ouabain has been identified in human urine and proved to be chemically a vanadium diascorbate adduct (Kramer et al., 1998). Among nonsteroid factors, endobain E is highly hydrophilic, nonlipidic, nonpeptidic, and anionic in nature, acid stable but alkali labile (Rodríguez de Lores Arnaiz and Peña, 1995); it differs from ouabain in high performance liquid chromatography (HPLC) retention time, chromatographic behavior, and UV spectra (Peña and Rodríguez de Lores Arnaiz, 1997), and it contains ascorbic acid and another unidentified compound (Rodríguez de Lores Arnaiz et al., 2003).

5.2.1 Classical Neurotransmitters and Neuropeptides as Enzyme Modulators

Some neurotransmitters are able to modify Na$^+$, K$^+$-ATPase activity when added in vitro during the enzyme assay (Stahl, 1986; Wu, 1986). Catecholamines norepinephrine and dopamine modify synaptosomal membrane Na$^+$, K$^+$-ATPase activity. They behave as enzyme inhibitors or stimulators, according to the absence or presence of a brain soluble fraction during enzyme assay (Rodríguez de Lores Arnaiz and Mistrorigo, 1978; Rodríguez de Lores Arnaiz, 1983).

A wide variety of peptides exerting specific functions in different tissues are present in neurons and are synthesized by them, conforming a broad family of active neuropeptides both at central and peripheral nervous systems (Mains and Eipper, 1999). Some of them, like insulin (Bojorge and Rodríguez de Lores Arnaiz, 1987), neurotensin (López Ordieres and Rodríguez de Lores Arnaiz, 2000, 2001), and calcitonin (Rodríguez de Lores Arnaiz and López Ordieres, 1997), exhibit in vitro inhibitory effect on synaptosomal membrane Na$^+$, K$^+$-ATPase activity whereas others, like substance P (Lachowicz and Janiszewska, 1985) and Angiotensin-(1–7) (López Ordieres et al., 1998), stimulate enzyme activity. An ouabain-like hexapeptide, complementary to an ouabain binding site on the Na$^+$, K$^+$-ATPase, exhibits activity in a digitalis bioassay (Mulchahey et al., 1999).

Na$^+$, K$^+$-ATPase, neurotransmitter receptors, as well as neuropeptide receptors are all molecular entities inserted in synaptic region membranes and probably contiguous; therefore, it is tempting to speculate that when a given classical neurotransmitter and/or a neuropeptide are/is released, a molecular interaction is favored between the corresponding specific receptor(s) and this enzyme. Diverse examples provided by the literature support the notion that neuropeptide receptors play major roles in diverse peptide effects on ion transport at synaptic level (Rodríguez de Lores Arnaiz and López Ordieres, 2003). Taking into account that Na$^+$, K$^+$-ATPase is a ubiquitous membrane-bound enzyme, the possibility of its regulation by released active substances at diverse neuron sites seems tenable.

6   Na$^+$, K$^+$-ATPase as a Signal Transducer

In addition to pumping ions, Na$^+$, K$^+$-ATPase seems to act as a signal transducer (Haas et al., 2000). Binding of ouabain to Na$^+$, K$^+$-ATPase changes the interaction of the enzyme with neighboring membrane proteins inducing the formation of multiple signaling modules, leading to Src kinase activation, transactivation of the epidermal growth factor receptor, and enhanced formation of reactive oxygen species (Xie, 2003). Interaction of such signals results in the activity of several other cascades, including phospholipase C activation (Xie and Askari, 2002). Multiple protein kinase cascades became activated, including mitogen-activated protein kinases and PKC isozymes in a cell-specific manner. Likewise, mitochondrial production of reactive oxygen species is activated, and intracellular Ca^{2+} concentration is regulated. Cross talk among the activated pathways may result in changes in the expression of a number of genes (Xie and Cai, 2003).

The inhibition of Src blocks many of the ouabain-activated signaling pathways. Src binds to Na$^+$, K$^+$-ATPase directly and ouabain modulates the interaction between Na$^+$, K$^+$-ATPase and Src leading to Src activation. The possibility that signaling Na$^+$, K$^+$-ATPase is concentrated in a separate pool on the plasma membrane has been advanced and potential interaction between Na$^+$, K$^+$-ATPase and caveolins studied, due to enzyme concentration in caveolae/rafts (Xie, 2003; Wang et al., 2004).

In rat cardiac myocytes and renal cells, a cascade of events seems to occur following ouabain interaction with a minor fraction of Na$^+$, K$^+$-ATPase. After Na$^+$ pump inhibition by ouabain, intracellular Na$^+$ concentration increases with a subsequent gradual enhancement or oscillations in intracellular Ca^{2+}

concentration. At present, it is not clear whether such increase in intracellular Ca^{2+} concentration is part of or a result of the cascade, or alternatively, a totally independent phenomenon (Hansen, 2003). This process most likely involves stimulation of a clathrin-dependent endocytosis pathway that translocates Na$^+$, K$^+$-ATPase to intracellular compartments, suggesting a role of endocytosis in ouabain-induced signal transduction (Liu et al., 2004).

Inhibition of Na$^+$, K$^+$-ATPase by ouabain results in phosphatidylinositol turnover enhancement in rat cerebral cortex, an effect markedly higher in neonatal than in adult brain (Balduini and Costa, 1990; Calviño et al., 2001). Similarly, phosphatidylinositol turnover increase results with an endogenous ouabain-like substance termed endobain E (Rodríguez de Lores Arnaiz, 2000), an effect recorded in neonatal but not in adult rat cerebral cortex (Calviño et al., 2001). Taking into account the above-mentioned findings, endobain E could well act as a physiological inducer of the signaling system.

7   Ion Homeostasis, Apoptosis, and Hybrid Death

Apoptosis has been recognized in a wide range of disease states, and Na$^+$, K$^+$-ATPase deficiency seems to be a contributor to apoptosis and pathogenesis; accordingly, experimental evidence indicates that Na$^+$, K$^+$-ATPase alteration exerts a unique role in cell death, including apoptosis either alone or concurrent with necrosis (hybrid death) (Yu, 2003a).

Ouabain induces concentration-dependent neuronal death, triggering transient neuronal cell swelling followed by cell shrinkage, accompanied by intracellular Ca^{2+} and Na$^+$ increase, K$^+$ decrease, caspase-3 activation, cytochrome C release, and DNA fragmentation. Neuronal death associated with Na$^+$ pump failure implies concurrent apoptotic and necrotic components mediated by intracellular depletion of K$^+$ and accumulation of Ca^{2+} and Na$^+$, respectively. Hybrid death induced by ouabain seems to be a distinct form of cell death related to brain injury due to inadequate energy supply and disrupted ion homeostasis (Xiao et al., 2002).

Studies performed in cortical neurons in culture show that apoptotic insults, such as serum deprivation, staurosporin, and C2-ceramide, impair Na$^+$, K$^+$-ATPase activity concomitant with depletion of intracellular ATP and production of reactive oxygen species (Wang et al., 2003).

Whereas Ca^{2+} influx and Ca^{2+} accumulation lead to cell necrosis, excessive K$^+$ efflux with concomitant intracellular K$^+$ depletion are early key steps in apoptosis. Interestingly, physiological concentration of intracellular K$^+$ acts as a repressor of apoptotic effectors. The pro-apoptotic disruption of K$^+$ homeostasis can be mediated by over-activated K$^+$ channels or ionotropic glutamate receptor, accompanied by decreased K$^+$ uptake provoked by Na$^+$, K$^+$-ATPase disfunction (Yu, 2003b).

8   Na$^+$, K$^+$-ATPase Disfunction and Pathological States

Na$^+$, K$^+$-ATPase activity is reduced or is insufficient to maintain adequate ionic balances during and after episodes of hypoglycemia, ischemia, or epilepsy, as well as after administration of excitotoxins like glutamate agonists. At presynaptic level, Na$^+$, K$^+$-ATPase inhibition impairs the Na$^+$ gradient, which drives the uptake of acidic amino acids and a variety of other neurotransmitters, resulting in reuptake blockade and stimulation release of glutamate and other neurotransmitters that modulate glutamate neurotoxicity (Lees, 1991).

A relationship between central dysfunction with digoxin and the isoprenoid pathway has been established. Among such disorders, Parkinson's disease, CNS glioma, schizophrenia, and epilepsy may be mentioned in which digoxin, an endogenous Na$^+$, K$^+$-ATPase inhibitor secreted by the hypothalamus, is elevated concomitant with a decrease in red blood cell membrane Na$^+$, K$^+$-ATPase activity. Digoxin can also modify other neuroactive substances, thus contributing to membrane Na$^+$, K$^+$-ATPase inhibition. A central role of hypothalamic digoxin in conscious perception, neuroimmunoendocrine integration, as well as cellular function coordination has been proposed (Kurup and Kurup, 2002).

Expression of Na$^+$, K$^+$-ATPase mRNA levels was analyzed by in situ hybridization in the superior frontal cortex and cerebellum of Alzheimer's disease subjects. In Alzheimer's disease cases, increases in α1-mRNA are related to increased reactive gliosis whereas decreases in α3-mRNA are greatly accelerated (Chauhan et al., 1997).

Acute focal cerebral ischemia is associated with decreased Na⁺, K⁺-ATPase activity; therefore, early detection and localization of potentially reversible ischemic cerebral edema are essential for clinical applications (Mintorovitch et al., 1994). Focal cerebral ischemia results in a decrease in Na⁺, K⁺-ATPase activity and in changes in affinity of the enzyme ouabain sites. Although all three α isoforms are present, only two sites for ouabain are detected. It has been suggested that ischemia induces intrinsic modifications in Na⁺, K⁺-ATPase, resulting in perturbations of membrane integrity and/or association of the α isoforms (Jamme et al., 1997).

Na⁺, K⁺-ATPase activity of synaptic plasma membranes in adult and aged animals is enhanced by ischemia, more markedly in adult than in aged animals; persistance of changes during the recirculating times indicate the delayed postischemic suffering of the brain (Villa et al., 2002).

Mutations in the Na⁺, K⁺-ATPase pump gene ATP1A2 are associated with familial hemiplegic migraine and benign familial infantile convulsions (Vanmolkot et al., 2003).

Ouabain-like activity in the CNS correlates with diverse pathophysiological conditions. In spontaneously hypertensive and in Dahl salt-sensitive rats, ouabain concentration enhancement was observed, which appears to be responsible for increased sympathoexcitation, decreased sympathoinhibition, desensitized arterial baroreflex function, and development of hypertension (Leenen et al., 1993,1994 ; Huang and Leenen, 1995). Congestive heart failure has been associated with marked enhancement of both peripheral and brain ouabain-like activity (Leenen et al., 1995), most likely mediating the increase in resting sympathetic tone and sympathoexcitatory responses to stress. A decrease in brain Na⁺, K⁺-ATPase expression and activity at 1 week postnatal suprarenal constriction may contribute to hypertension while the increase in the α2/α3 brain expression and activity at 4 weeks is most likely a compensatory response to established hypertension (Chow et al., 2002).

8.1 Na⁺, K⁺-ATPase, Behavior, and Psychiatric Diseases

Clinical studies have shown enzyme activity changes in patients with bipolar and unipolar mood disorders (Bagrov et al., 2002). A reduction in Na⁺, K⁺-ATPase activity has been associated with depressive disorders and was also observed in hippocampus of rats subjected to an experimental model of depression (Gamaro et al., 2003).

A model for mood-cycle regulation has been proposed that involves steroid hormones by means of Na⁺, K⁺-ATPase regulation; this hypothesis contends that steroid hormones inhibit Na⁺, K⁺-ATPase activity in hypothalamus, directly or through their conversion into digitalis-like compounds, which in turn, stimulate β-endorphin secretion, normally leading to elevated mood (Traub and Lichtstein, 2000).

Administration of Na⁺, K⁺-ATPase inhibitors antagonize the antinociceptive effect of morphine in mice, an effect independent of opioid receptors (Masocha et al., 2003).

Inhibition of Na⁺, K⁺-ATPase activity leads not only to edema and cell death in the CNS but also impairs learning and memory, and several sex steroid hormones protect against neuronal cell damage and disfunction of learning and memory. It was observed that 17β estradiol and testosterone ameliorate amnesia induced by ouabain, a nongenomic effect independent of radical scavenging action (Sato et al., 2004).

9 Concluding Remarks

Na⁺, K⁺-ATPase activity is essential for multiple neuron functions. At synaptic membrane level, cross talk between macromolecules seems to be possible. It may occur between two neurotransmitter receptors or between a neurotransmitter receptor and an enzyme molecule such as Na⁺, K⁺-ATPase.

Evidence for close interaction between Na⁺, K⁺-ATPase activity and a single or two receptor entities have been reviewed. Neurotransmitter receptors involved include preferentially glutamatergic receptors, several catecholaminergic and serotonergic type receptors, cholinergic muscarinic and GABAergic receptors, as well as diverse neuropeptide receptors (Rodríguez de Lores Arnaiz, 2002). Whether Na$^+$, K$^+$-ATPase regulation modulates receptor activity or vice versa is an open question. In either case, it is tenable that vicinal rather than distant regulation takes place at the synaptic membrane (Rodríguez de Lores Arnaiz, 2002). In these membranes, Na$^+$, K$^+$-ATPase (Rodríguez de Lores Arnaiz et al., 1967) and neurotransmitter receptors (De Robertis, 1983) are highly concentrated in such a way that these macromolecules might well interact since they are most likely contiguously located.

Dimerization of G-protein–coupled receptors has been demonstrated. This is a molecular cross talk between signaling molecules, which may involve homodimerization as well as heterodimerization either between different receptor subtypes or between distinct G-protein–coupled receptors (Bai, 2004). On the basis of this notion, it may be speculated that dimerization could occur either between a subunit of Na$^+$, K$^+$-ATPase and a subunit of a G-protein–coupled neurotransmitter receptor or between a Na$^+$, K$^+$-ATPase subunit and a G-protein–coupled peptide receptor, leading to a wide variety of effects or to diverse cascade reactions involved in physiological and pathological conditions.

Acknowledgments

The author is chief investigator from Consejo Nacional de Investigaciones Científicas y Técnicas (CONICET). This work was supported by grants from Agencia Nacional de Promoción Científica y Tecnológica, CONICET, and Universidad de Buenos Aires, Argentina.

References

Akagawa K, Hara N, Tsukada Y. 1984. Partial purification and properties of the inhibitors of Na$^+$, K$^+$-ATPase and ouabain-binding in bovine central nervous system. J Neurochem 42: 775-780.

Albers RW, Siegel GJ. 1999. Membrane transport. Basic Neurochemistry, 6th edn. Siegel GJ, Agranoff BW, Albers RW, Fisher SK, Uhler MD, editors. Philadelphia: Lippincott-Raven; pp. 95-118.

Antolovic R, Bruller HJ, Bunk S, Linder D, Schoner W. 1991. Epitope mapping by amino-acid-sequence-specific antibodies reveals that both ends of the alpha subunit of Na$^+$/K($^+$)-ATPase are located on the cytoplasmic side of the membrane. Eur J Biochem 199: 195-202.

Bagrov AY, Fedorova OV, Dmitrieva RI, Howald WN, Hunter AP, et al. 1998. Characterization of a urinary bufodienolide Na$^+$, K$^+$-ATPase inhibitor in patients after acute myocardial infarction. Hypertension 31: 1097-1103.

Bagrov AY, Bagrov YY, Fedorova OV, Kashkin VA, Patkina NA, et al. 2002. Endogenous digitalis-like ligands of the sodium pump: possible involvement in mood control and ethanol addiction. Eur Neuropsychopharmacol 12: 1-12.

Bai M. 2004. Dimerization of G-protein-coupled receptors: roles in signal transduction. Cell Signal 16: 175-186.

Balduini W, Costa LG. 1990. Characterization of ouabain-induced phosphoinositide hydrolysis in brain slices of the neonatal rat. Neurochem Res 15: 1023-1029.

Beguin P, Wang X, Firsov D, Puoti A, Claeys D, et al. 1997. The gamma subunit is a specific component of the Na, K-ATPase and modulates its transport function. EMBO J. 16: 4250-4260.

Beguin P, Crambert G, Monnet-Tschudi F, Uldry M, Horisberger JD, et al. 2002. FXYD7 is a brain-specific regulator of NaK-ATPase alpha 1-beta isozymes. EMBO J 21: 3264-3273.

Berrebi-Bertrand I, Maixent JM, Christe G, Leleièvre LG. 1990. Two active Na$^+$/K$^+$-ATPases of high affinity for ouabain in adult rat brain membranes. Biochim Biophys Acta 1021: 148-156.

Bertorello AM, Aperia A, Walaas SI, Nairn AC, Greengard P. 1991. Phosphorylation of the catalytic subunit of Na$^+$, K$^+$-ATPase inhibits the activity of the enzyme. Proc Natl Acad Sci USA 88: 11359-1362.

Blanco G, Mercer RW. 1998. Isozymes of the Na-K-ATPase: heterogeneity in structure diversity in function. Am J Physiol-Renal Physiol 275: F633-F650.

Bojorge G, Rodríguez de Lores Arnaiz G. 1987. Insulin modifies Na$^+$, K$^+$-ATPase activity of synaptosomal membranes and whole homogenates prepared from rat cerebral cortex. Neurochem Int 11: 11-16.

Budzikowski AS, Leenen FH. 1998. Brain "ouabain", a neurosteroid mediates sympathetic hyperactivity in salt-sensitive hypertension. Clin Exp Hypertens 20: 119-140.

Butt AN, Semra YK, Ho CS, Swaminathan R. 1997. Effect of high salt intake on plasma and tissue concentration of endogenous ouabain-like substance in the rat. Life Sci 61: 2367-2373.

Calviño MA, Peña C, Rodríguez de Lores Arnaiz G. 2001. An endogenous Na$^+$, K$^+$-ATPase inhibitor enhances phosphoinositide hydrolysis in neonatal but not in adult rat brain cortex. Neurochem Res 26: 1253-1259.

Chauhan NB, Lee JM, Siegel GJ. 1997. NaK-ATPase mRNA levels and plaque load in Alzheimer's disease. J Mol Neurosci 9: 151-166.

Chow DC, Forte JG. 1995. Functional significance of the beta-subunit for heterodimeric P-type ATPases. J Exp Biol 198: 1-17.

Chow MK, Shao Q, Ren B, Leenen FH, Van Huysse JW. 2002. Changes in brain Na, K-ATPase isoform expression and enzymatic activity after aortic constriction. Brain Res 944: 124-134.

Cornelius F, Mahmmoud YA. 2003. Functional modulation of the sodium pump: the regulatory proteins "Fixit". News Physiol Sci 18: 119-124.

Crambert G, Beguin P, Uldry M, Monnet-Tschudi F, Horisberger JD, et al. 2003. FXYD7, the first brain- and isoform-specific regulator of Na, K-ATPase: biosynthesis and function of its posttranslational modifications. Ann N Y Acad Sci 986: 444-448.

De Robertis E. 1983. The synaptosome. Two decades of cell fractionation of the brain. Intern Brain Res Org Monogr Ser 10: 1-10.

DiPolo R, Beaugé L. 1991. Regulation of Na–Ca exchange. An overview. Ann N Y Acad Sci 639: 100-111.

Eakle KA, Kabalin MA, Wang SG, Farley RA. 1994. The influence of beta subunit structure on the stability of Na$^+$/K$^+$-ATPase complexes and interaction with K$^+$. J Biol Chem 269: 6550-6557.

Ferrandi M, Minotti E, Salardi S, Florio M, Bianchi G, et al. 1992. Ouabain-like factor in Milan hypertensive rats. Am J Physiol-Renal Physiol 263: F739-F748.

Feschenko MS, Donnet C, Wetzel RK, Asinovski NK, Jones LR, et al. 2003. Phospholemman a single-span membrane protein is an accessory protein of Na, K-ATPase in cerebellum and choroid plexus. J Neurosci 23: 2161-2169.

Fishman MC. 1979. Endogenous digitalis-like activity in mammalian brain. Proc Natl Acad Sci USA 76: 4661-4663.

Gamaro GD, Streck EL, Matte C, Prediger ME, Wyse AT, et al. 2003. Reduction of hippocampal Na$^+$, K$^+$-ATPase activity in rats subjected to an experimental model of depression. Neurochem Res 28: 1339-1344.

Geering K, Beguin P, Garty H, Karlish S, Fuzesi M, et al. 2003. FXYD proteins: new tissue- and isoform-specific regulators of NaK-ATPase. Ann N Y Acad Sci 986: 388-394.

Goto A, Yamada K. 1998. Purification of endogenous digitalis-like factors from normal human urine. Clin Exp Hypertens 20: 551-556.

Goto A, Yamada K, Yagi N, Yoshioka M, Sugimoto T. 1992. Physiology and pharmacology of endogenous digitalis-like factors. Pharmacol Rev 44: 377-399.

Greengard P. 2001. The neurobiology of slow synaptic transmission. Science 294: 1024-1030.

Haas M, Askari A, Xie Z. 2000. Involvement of Src and epidermal growth factor receptor in the signal-transducing function of Na$^+$/K$^+$-ATPase. J Biol Chem 275: 27832-27837.

Hamlyn JM, Blaustein MP, Bova S, DuCharme DW, Harris DW, et al. 1991. Identification and characterization of an ouabain-like compound from human plasma. Proc Natl Acad Sci USA 88: 6259-6263.

Hamlyn JM, Lu ZR, Manunta P, Ludens JH, Kimura K, et al. 1998. Observations on the nature biosynthesis secretion and significance of endogenous ouabain. Clin Exp Hypertens 20: 523-533.

Hansen O. 2003. No evidence for a role in signal-transduction of Na$^+$/K$^+$-ATPase interaction with putative endogenous ouabain. Eur J Biochem 270: 1916-1919.

Hermenegildo C, Felipo V, Miñana MD, Grisolía S. 1992. Inhibition of protein kinase C restores Na$^+$, K$^+$-ATPase activity in sciatic nerve of diabetic mice. J Neurochem 58: 1246-1249.

Hermenegildo C, Felipo V, Miñana MD, Romero FJ, Grisolía S. 1993. Sustained recovery of Na(+)-K(+)-ATPase activity in the sciatic nerve of diabetic mice by administration of H7 or calphostin C inhibitors of PKC. Diabetes 42: 257-262.

Hernández RJ. 1992. Na(+)-K(+)-ATPase regulation by neurotransmitters. Neurochem Int 20: 1-10.

Hollenberg NK, Graves SW. 1996. Endogenous sodium pump inhibition: current status and therapeutic opportunities. Prog Drug Res 46: 9-42.

Huang BS, Leenen FHH. 1995. Brain ouabain sodium and arterial baroreflex in spontaneous hypertensive rats. Hypertension 25 (Pt. 2): 814-817.

Jaisser F, Horisberger JD, Rossier BC. 1992. The beta subunit modulates potassium activation of the Na–K pump. Ann N Y Acad Sci 671: 113-119.

Jamme I, Petit E, Gerbi A, Maixent JM, Mac Kenzie ET, et al. 1997. Changes in ouabain affinity of Na+, K+-ATPase during focal cerebral ischaemia in the mouse. Brain Res 774: 123-130.

Jewell-Motz EA, Lingrel JB. 1993. Site-directed mutagenesis of the Na, K-ATPase: consequences of substitutions of negatively-charged amino acids localized in the transmembrane domains. Biochemistry 32: 13523-13530.

Jorgensen PL, Hakansson KO, Karlish SJ. 2003. Structure and mechanism of Na, K-ATPase: functional sites and their interactions. Annu Rev Physiol 65: 817-849.

Kaplan JH. 2002. Biochemistry of Na, K-ATPase. Annu Rev Biochem 71: 511-535.

Kramer HJ, Krampitz G, Bäcker A, Meyer-Lehnert H. 1998. Ouabain-like factors in human urine: identification of a Na–K-ATPase inhibitor as vanadium-diascorbate adduct. Clin Exp Hypertens 20: 557-571.

Kourie JI. 1998. Interaction of reactive oxygen species with ion transport mechanisms. Am J Physiol-Cell Physiol 275: C1-C24.

Kuntzweiler TA, Arguello JM, Lingrel JB. 1996. Asp804 and Asp808 in the transmembrane domain of the Na, K-ATPase alpha subunit are cation coordinating residues. J Biol Chem 271: 29682-29687.

Kurup RK, Kurup PA. 2002. Central role of hypothalamic digoxin in conscious perception neuroimmunoendocrine integration and coordination of cellular function: relation to hemispheric dominance. Int J Neurosci 112: 705-739.

Lachowicz L, Janiszewska G. 1985. Role of theophylline during the action of SP in vitro on the activity of synaptosomal membrane ATPase (EC 3.6.1.3) from different areas of rat brain. Gen Pharmacol 16: 149-152.

Leenen FH, Harmsen E, Yu H, Ou C. 1993. Effects of dietary sodium on central and peripheral ouabain-like activity in spontaneously hypertensive rats. Am J Physiol-Heart Physiol 264: H2051-H2055.

Leenen FH, Harmsen E, Yu H. 1994. Dietary sodium and central vs. peripheral ouabain-like activity in Dahl salt-sensitive vs. salt-resistant rats. Am J Physiol-Heart Physiol 267: H1916-H1920.

Leenen FH, Huang BS, Yu H, Yuan B. 1995. Brain "ouabain" mediates sympathetic hyperactivity in congestive heart failure. Circ Res 77: 993-1000.

Lees GJ. 1991. Inhibition of sodium-potassium-ATPase: a potentially ubiquitous mechanism contributing to central nervous system neuropathology. Brain Res Brain Res Rev 16: 283-300.

Li D, Aperia A, Celsi G, da Cruz e Silva EF, Greengard P, et al. 1995. Protein phosphatase-1 in the kidney: evidence for a role in the regulation of medullary Na(+)-K(+)-ATPase. Am J Physiol 269: F673-F680.

Lichtstein D, Rosen H. 2001. Endogenous digitalis-like Na$^+$, K$^+$-ATPase inhibitors and brain function. Neurochem Res 26: 971-978.

Lichtstein D, Gati I, Samuelov S, Berson D, Rozenman Y, et al. 1993. Identification of digitalis-like compounds in human cataractous lenses. Eur J Biochem 216: 261-268.

Liu J, Kesiry R, Periyasamy SM, Malhotra D, Xie Z, et al. 2004. Ouabain induces endocytosis of plasmalemmal Na/K-ATPase in LLC-PK 1 cells by a clathrin-dependent mechanism. Kidney Int 66: 227-241.

López Ordieres MG, Rodríguez de Lores Arnaiz G. 2000. Neurotensin inhibits neuronal Na$^+$, K$^+$-ATPase activity through high affinity peptide receptor. Peptides 21: 571-576.

López Ordieres MG, Rodríguez de Lores Arnaiz G. 2001. K$^+$-p-nitrophenyl-phosphatase inhibition by neurotensin involves high affinity neurotensin receptor: influence of potassium concentration and enzyme phosphorylation. Regul Pept 101: 183-187.

López Ordieres MG, Gironacci M, Rodríguez de Lores Arnaiz G, Peña C. 1998. Effect of angiotensin-(1–7) on ATPase activities in several tissues. Regul Pept 77: 135-139.

Ludens JH, Clark MA, DuCharme DW, Harris DW, Lutzke BS, et al. 1991. Purification of an endogenous digitalislike factor from human plasma for structural analysis. Hypertension 17: 923-929.

Lutsenko S, Kaplan JH. 1993. An essential role for the extracellular domain of the Na, K-ATPase beta-subunit in cation occlusion. Biochemistry 32: 6737-6743.

Mains RE, Eipper BA. 1999. Peptides. Basic Neurochemistry, 6th edn. Siegel GJ, Agranoff BW, Albers RW, Fisher SK, Uhler MD, editors. Philadelphia: Lippincott-Raven; pp. 363-382.

Malik N, Canfield VA, Beckers MC, Gros P, Levenson R. 1996. Identification of the mammalian Na, K-ATPase beta 3 subunit. J Biol Chem 271: 22754-22758.

Masocha W, González LG, Baeyens JM, Agil A. 2002. Mechanisms involved in morphine-induced activation of synaptosomal Na$^+$, K$^+$-ATPase. Brain Res 957: 311-319.

Masocha W, Horvath C, Agil A, Ocana M, Del Pozo E, et al. 2003. Role of Na$^+$, K$^+$-ATPase in morphine-induced antinociception. J Pharmacol Exp Ther 306: 1122-1128.

Mathews WR, DuCharme DW, Hamlyn JM, Harris DW, Mandel F, et al. 1991. Mass spectral characterization of an endogenous digitalislike factor from human plasma. Hypertension 17: 930-935.

McGrail KM, Phillips JM, Sweadner KJ. 1991. Immunofluorescent localization of three Na, K-ATPase isozymes in the rat central nervous system: both neurons and glia express more than one Na, K-ATPase. J Neurosci 11: 381-391.

Mintorovitch J, Yang GY, Shimizu H, Kucharczyk J, Chan PH, et al. 1994. Diffusion-weighted magnetic resonance imaging of acute focal cerebral ischemia: comparison of signal intensity with changes in brain water and Na(+), K(+)-ATPase activity. J Cereb Blood Flow Metab 14: 332-336.

Moseley AE, Lieske SP, Wetzel RK, James PF, He S, et al. 2003. The Na, K-ATPase alpha 2 isoform is expressed in neurons and its absence disrupts neuronal activity in newborn mice. J Biol Chem 278: 5317-5324.

Mulchahey JJ, Nagy G, Neill JD. 1999. A molecular recognition hypothesis for nonpeptides: Na+ K+ ATPase and endogenous digitalis-like peptides. Cell Mol Life Sci 55: 653-662.

Nestler EJ, Greengard P. 1999. Serine and threonine phosphorylation. Basic Neurochemistry, 6th edn. Philadelphia: Lippincott-Raven; pp. 471-495.

Peña C, Rodríguez de Lores Arnaiz G. 1997. Differential properties between an endogenous brain Na⁺, K⁺-ATPase inhibitor and ouabain. Neurochem Res 22: 379-383.

Putney JW Jr. 1999. Calcium. Basic Neurochemistry, 6th edn. Siegel GJ, Agranoff BW, Albers RW, Fisher SK, Uhler MD, editors. Philadelphia: Lippincott-Raven; pp. 453-469.

Qazzaz HM, Cao Z, Bolanowski DD, Clark BJ, Valdes R Jr. 2004. De novo biosynthesis and radiolabeling of mammalian digitalis-like factors. Clin Chem 50: 612-620.

Rodríguez de Lores Arnaiz G. 1983. Neuronal Na⁺, K⁺-ATPase and its regulation by catecholamines. Intern Brain Res Org Monogr Ser 10: 147-158.

Rodríguez de Lores Arnaiz G. 1992. In search of synaptosomal Na⁺, K⁺-ATPase regulators. Mol Neurobiol 6: 359-375.

Rodríguez de Lores Arnaiz G. 1993. An endogenous factor which interacts with synaptosomal membrane Na⁺, K⁺-ATPase activation by K⁺. Neurochem Res 18: 655-661.

Rodríguez de Lores Arnaiz G. 2000. How many endobains are there? Neurochem Res 25: 1421-1430.

Rodríguez de Lores Arnaiz G. 2002. Interplay between Na⁺, K⁺-ATPase and neurotransmitter receptors. Current Topics in Neurochemistry Research Trends, Vol. 3., Richard R, editor. Trivandrum, India: Research Trends; pp. 189-198.

Rodríguez de Lores Arnaiz G, Mistrorigo de Pacheco M. 1978. Regulation of (Na⁺, K⁺) adenosine triphosphatase of nerve ending membranes: action of norepinephrine and a soluble factor. Neurochem Res 3: 733-744.

Rodríguez de Lores Arnaiz G, Peña C. 1995. Characterization of synaptosomal membrane Na⁺, K⁺-ATPase inhibitors. Neurochem Int 27: 319-327.

Rodríguez de Lores Arnaiz G, López Ordieres MG. 1997. A study of calcitonin effect on synaptosomal membrane enzymes. Peptides 18: 613-615.

Rodríguez de Lores Arnaiz G, López Ordieres MG. 2003. Neuropeptides and CNS Na⁺, K⁺-ATPase. Current Topics in Peptide & Protein Research Research Trends, Vol. 5. Richard R, editor. Trivandrum, India: Research Trends; pp. 75-85.

Rodríguez de Lores Arnaiz G, Alberici M, De Robertis E. 1967. Ultrastructural and enzymic studies of cholinergic and non-cholinergic synaptic membranes isolated from brain cortex. J Neurochem 14: 215-225.

Rodríguez de Lores Arnaiz G, Herbin T, Peña C. 2003. A comparative study between a brain Na⁺, K⁺-ATPase

inhibitor (endobain E) and ascorbic acid. Neurochem Res 28: 903-910.

Rusnak F, Mertz P. 2000. Calcineurin: form and function. Physiol Rev 80: 1483-1521.

Sancho JM. 1998. A non-ouabain Na/K ATPase inhibitor isolated from bovine hypothalamus. Its relation to hypothalamic ouabain. Clin Exp Hypertens 20: 535-542.

Sato T, Tanaka K, Ohnishi Y, Teramoto T, Irifune M, et al. 2004. Effects of steroid hormones on (Na⁺, K⁺)-ATPase activity inhibition-induced amnesia on the step-through passive avoidance task in gonadectomized mice. Pharmacol Res 49: 151-159.

Scheiner-Bobis G. 2002. The sodium pump. Its molecular properties and mechanism of ion transport. Eur J Biochem 269: 2424-2433.

Schmalzing G, Kroner S, Schachner M, Gloor S. 1992. The adhesion molecule on glia (AMOG/beta 2) and alpha 1 subunits assemble to functional sodium pumps in Xenopus oocytes. J Biol Chem 267: 20212-20216.

Schneider R, Wray V, Nimtz M, Lehmann WD, Kirch U, et al. 1998. Bovine adrenals contain in addition to ouabain a second inhibitor of the sodium pump. J Biol Chem 273: 784-792.

Schoner W. 2000. Ouabain a new steroid hormone of adrenal gland and hypothalamus. Exp Clin Endocrinol Diabetes 108: 449-454.

Shainskaya A, Karlish SJ. 1994. Evidence that the cation occlusion domain of Na/K-ATPase consists of a complex of membrane-spanning segments. Analysis of limit membrane-embedded tryptic fragments. J Biol Chem 269: 10780-10789.

Shamraj OI, Lingrel JB. 1994. A putative fourth Na+, K(+)-ATPase alpha-subunit gene is expressed in testis. Proc Natl Acad Sci USA 91: 12952-12956.

Shimoni Y, Gotsman M, Deutsch J, Kachalsky S, and Lichtstein D. 1984. Endogenous ouabain-like compound increases heart muscle contractility. Nature 307: 369-371.

Skou J. 1957. The influence of some cations on an adenosine triphosphatase from peripheral nerves. Biochim Biophys Acta 23: 394-401.

Skriver E, Maunsbach AB, Hebert H, Scheiner-Bobis G, Schoner W. 1989. Two-dimensional crystalline arrays of NaK-ATPase with new subunit interactions induced by cobalt-tetrammine-ATP. J Ultrastruct Mol Struct Res 102: 189-195.

Stahl W. 1986. The NaK-ATPase of nervous tissue. Neurochem Int 8: 449-476.

Sweadner KJ. 1989. Isozymes of Na⁺, K⁺-ATPase. Biochim Biophys Acta 988: 185-220.

Sweadner KJ, Rael E. 2000. The FXYD gene family of small ion transport regulators or channels: cDNA sequence protein signature sequence and expression. Genomics 68: 41-56.

Teixeira VL, Katz AI, Pedemonte CH, Bertorello AM. 2003. Isoform-specific regulation of Na$^+$, K$^+$-ATPase endocytosis and recruitment to the plasma membrane. Ann N Y Acad Sci 986: 587-594.

Therien AG, Blostein R. 2000. Mechanisms of sodium pump regulation. Am J Physiol-Cell Physiol 279: C541-C566.

Traub N, Lichtstein D. 2000. The mood cycle hypothesis: possible involvement of steroid hormones in mood regulation by means of Na$^+$, K$^+$-ATPase inhibition. J Basic Clin Physiol Pharmacol 11: 375-394.

Tymiak AA, Norman JA, Bolgar M, Di Donato GC, Lee H, et al. 1993. Physicochemical characterization of a ouabain isomer isolated from bovine hypothalamus. Proc Natl Acad Sci USA 90: 8189-8193.

Van Huysse JW, Jewell EA, Lingrel JB. 1993. Site-directed mutagenesis of a predicted cation binding site of Na, K-ATPase. Biochemistry 32: 819-826.

Vanmolkot KR, Kors EE, Hottenga JJ, Terwindt GM, Haan J, et al. 2003. Novel mutations in the Na$^+$, K$^+$-ATPase pump gene ATP1A2 associated with familial hemiplegic migraine and benign familial infantile convulsions. Ann Neurol 54: 360-366.

Villa RF, Gorini A, Hoyer S. 2002. ATPases of synaptic plasma membranes from hippocampus after ischemia and recovery during ageing. Neurochem Res 27: 861-870.

Vilsen B. 1993. Glutamate 329 located in the fourth transmembrane segment of the alpha-subunit of the rat kidney Na+, K+-ATPase is not an essential residue for active transport of sodium and potassium ions. Biochemistry 32: 13340-13349.

Wang XQ, Xiao AY, Sheline C, Hyrc K, Yang A, et al. 2003. Apoptotic insults impair Na$^+$, K$^+$-ATPase activity as a mechanism of neuronal death mediated by concurrent ATP deficiency and oxidant stress. J Cell Sci 116: 2099-2110.

Wang H, Haas M, Liang M, Cai T, Tian J, et al. 2004. Ouabain assembles signaling cascades through the caveolar Na+/K+-ATPase. J Biol Chem 279: 17250-17259.

Watts AG, Sánchez-Watts G, Emanuel JR, Levenson R. 1991. Cell-specific expression of mRNAs encoding Na+, K(+)-ATPase alpha- and beta-subunit isoforms within the rat central nervous system. Proc Natl Acad Sci USA 88: 7425-7429.

Wu PH. 1986. Na$^+$, K$^+$-ATPase in nervous tissue. Neuromethods Enzymes. Boulton AA, Baker GB, Wu PH, editors. Clifton, NJ: Humana Press; pp. 451-502.

Xiao AY, Wei L, Xia S, Rothman S, Yu SP. 2002. Ionic mechanism of ouabain-induced concurrent apoptosis and necrosis in individual cultured cortical neurons. J Neurosci 22: 1350-1362.

Xie Z. 2003. Molecular mechanisms of Na/K-ATPase-mediated signal transduction. Ann N Y Acad Sci 986: 497-503.

Xie Z, Askari A. 2002. Na(+)/K(+)-ATPase as a signal transducer. Eur J Biochem 269: 2434-2439.

Xie Z, Cai T. 2003. Na+-K+-ATPase-mediated signal transduction: from protein interaction to cellular function. Mol Interv 3: 157-168.

Yakel JL. 1997. Calcineurin regulation of synaptic function: from ion channels to transmitter release and gene transcription. Trends Pharmacol Sci 18: 124-134.

Yamada HM, Naruse M, Naruse K, Demura H, Takahashi H, et al. 1992. Histological study on ouabain immunoreactivities in the mammalian hypothalamus. Neurosci Lett 141: 143-146.

Yoshida H, Nagai K, Ohashi T, Nakagawa Y. 1969. K$^+$-dependent phosphatase activity observed in the presence of both adenosine triphosphate and Na$^+$. Biochim Biophys Acta 171: 178-185.

Yu SP. 2003a. Na$^+$, K$^+$-ATPase: the new face of an old player in pathogenesis and apoptotic/hybrid cell death. Biochem Pharmacol 66: 1601-1609.

Yu SP. 2003b. Regulation and critical role of potassium homeostasis in apoptosis. Prog Neurobiol 70: 363-386.

Zhao N, Lo L, Berova N, Nakanishi K, Tymiak AA, et al. 1995. Na, K-ATPase inhibitors from bovine hypothalamus and human plasma are different from ouabain: nanogram scale CD structural analysis. Biochemistry 34: 9893-9896.

11 Na$^+$/Ca^{2+} Exchangers and Ca^{2+} Transport in Neurons

J. Lytton

Abstract: The Na$^+$/Ca^{2+} exchanger transports Na$^+$ in exchange for Ca^{2+} ions across the plasma membrane. This action influences both membrane excitability and Ca^{2+} homeostasis in different neuronal environments, such as dendrite, soma, and axon. The direction of transport is determined by the relative orientation of the Na$^+$ and Ca^{2+} gradients, the membrane potential, and the number of ions bound and transported. Under typical physiological conditions in neurons, the Na$^+$/Ca^{2+} exchanger mostly extrudes Ca^{2+} from the cytoplasm in exchange for Na$^+$ entry, thereby generating an accompanying inward current. However, the exchanger may also participate in Ca^{2+} entry associated with specific signaling events. Additionally, during periods of ischemia and/or excitotoxic stimulation, the exchanger reverses, allowing Ca^{2+} entry that contributes to cellular damage. The Na$^+$/Ca^{2+} exchanger is encoded by a family of homologous gene products that are expressed with distinct patterns in different brain regions. Two major branches of the gene family are expressed in brain, one that encodes transporters exchanging Na$^+$ ions for only Ca^{2+} ion (NCX) and the other that exchanges Na$^+$ ions for both Ca^{2+} and K$^+$ (NCKX). The NCX branch has three known members, NCX1 (*SLC8A1*), NCX2 (*SLC8A2*), and NCX3 (*SLC8A3*), while the NCKX branch has five known members, NCKX1 (*SLC24A1*) through NCKX5 (*SLC24A5*). Unique, but overlapping, patterns of expression of these different gene products suggest that they each subserve unique physiological roles. Most of the members of the NCX and NCKX gene families have only been identified recently using molecular cloning or bioinformatic tools, and thus their unique contributions to Ca^{2+} homeostasis and neuronal physiology are only beginning to be understood.

List of Abbreviations: CAX, H$^+$/Ca^{2+}-exchanger; CCX, cation/Ca^{2+}-exchanger; ER, endoplasmic reticulum; LTD, long-term depression; LTP, long-term potentiation; NCKX, Na$^+$/(Ca^{2+}+K$^+$)-exchanger; NCX, Na$^+$/Ca^{2+}-exchanger; NMDA, *N*-methyl-D-aspartate; PMCA, plasma membrane Ca^{2+}-ATPase; PSD95, post-synaptic density protein of 95kDa; ROC, receptor-operated channel; SERCA, sarcoplasmic or endoplasmic reticulum Ca^{2+}-ATPase; SMOC, second messenger-operated channel; SOC, store-operated channel; SR, sarcoplasmic reticulum; VCX, vacuolar H$^+$/Ca^{2+}-exchanger; VOC, voltage-operated channel

1 Neuronal Ca^{2+} Homeostasis

Ca^{2+} ion is a highly versatile intracellular second messenger, and changes in its cytosolic concentration ([Ca^{2+}]$_i$) control a large number of cellular processes involved in almost all aspects of brain function, including neurotransmitter release, synaptic plasticity, neurite outgrowth, growth cone behavior, and cell death (Berridge et al., 2000). Indeed, Ca^{2+} signals can lead paradoxically to diametrically-opposed responses within the same cell. For example, long-term potentiation (LTP) and long-term depression (LTD) are both induced in hippocampal neurons by activation of NMDA-receptor Ca^{2+} channels. While a short, marked elevation in [Ca^{2+}]$_i$ close to the membrane is thought to underlie LTP, a sustained, but modest, increment in [Ca^{2+}]$_i$ leads to LTD (Augustine et al., 2003). Observations of this kind have led to the conclusion that specificity of the ubiquitous Ca^{2+} signal lies in complex and organized spatial and temporal patterns of changing [Ca^{2+}]$_i$ (Berridge et al., 2003) as well as in the nature of the downstream targets.

Ca^{2+} cannot be metabolized, as other second messengers can, and so its concentration is controlled primarily by transport across the membranes of intracellular compartments (such as the endoplasmic reticulum and the mitochondrion) and the plasma membrane (❷ *Figure 11-1*). Cells possess a complex array of different Ca^{2+}-transporting mechanisms that can be conceptually divided into those that contribute to rises in [Ca^{2+}]$_i$, the "on" reactions, and lowering of [Ca^{2+}]$_i$, the "off" reactions (Berridge et al., 2000). A rise in [Ca^{2+}]$_i$ is triggered by cell signaling events, such as membrane depolarization, which leads to the opening of plasma membrane voltage-gated Ca^{2+} channels; ligand binding that can trigger the opening of a receptor-operated channel such as the NMDA-receptor; ligand–receptor interactions that lead to the activation of second messenger pathways and subsequently either the opening of second messenger-operated channels, such as cyclic-nucleotide-gated channels in the plasma membrane, or the InsP$_3$-receptor channel in the endoplasmic reticulum. Emptying of the intracellular Ca^{2+} stores can lead to further Ca^{2+} release and the activation of cell surface entry via store-operated channels, thus propagating the Ca^{2+} signal throughout the cell (Berridge et al., 2003).

◻ **Figure 11-1**

Calcium transport pathways. Molecular pathways that mediate an increase in cytoplasmic [Ca^{2+}] – so called "on" reactions – are shown in the upper part of the figure with arrows pointing toward cytoplasmic Ca^{2+}, while those pathways that lower cytoplasmic [Ca^{2+}] – so called "off" reactions – are shown in the lower part of the figure with arrows leading away from cytoplasmic Ca^{2+}. ER/SR, endoplasmic reticulum/sarcoplasmic reticulum; SOC, store-operated channel (possible interaction with the ER-associated inositoltrisphosphate receptor Ca^{2+} channel (IP$_3$R) is shown with a grey double-headed arrow); ROC, receptor-operated channel (e.g., NMDA-receptor glutamate channel); VOC, voltage-operated channel (e.g., L-type Ca^{2+} channel); SMOC, second messenger-operated channel (e.g., cyclic nucleotide-gated channel); RyR, ryanodine-receptor Ca^{2+} channel of the ER/SR; SERCA, sarcoplasmic or endoplasmic reticulum Ca^{2+}-ATPase pump; Muni, mitochondrial electrogenic Ca^{2+} uniporter; Mncx, mitochondrial Na$^+$/Ca^{2+}-exchanger; PMCA, plasma membrane Ca^{2+}-ATPase pump; NCX, Na$^+$/Ca^{2+}-exchanger (K$^+$-independent); NCKX, Na$^+$/(Ca^{2+}+K$^+$)-exchanger (K$^+$-dependent)

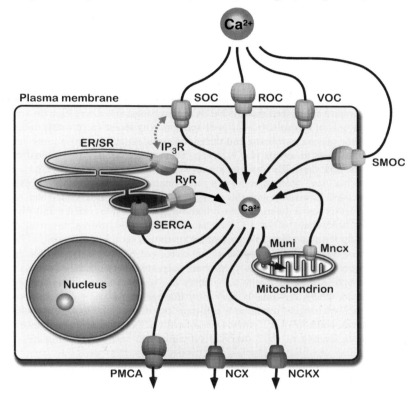

During and following a Ca^{2+} signal, [Ca^{2+}]$_i$ is lowered by contributions from intracellular calcium-binding proteins, such as calbindins and parvalumbin, and by transport across membranes via the ATP-dependent Ca^{2+} pumps of the plasma membrane (PMCA) and the endoplasmic reticulum (SERCA), the electrophoretic uptake of Ca^{2+} into mitochondria, and Na$^+$-gradient driven Ca^{2+} efflux through the Na$^+$/Ca^{2+} exchanger. The architecture of a Ca^{2+} signal depends upon the integrated activities of these various on- and off-reactions, including their individual properties and activation and inhibition profiles. For example, sudden opening of a voltage-gated Ca^{2+} channel can generate a very large, but highly localized, signal that leads to synaptic vesicle fusion. On the other hand, activation of second-messenger pathways can be prolonged depending on the sustained binding of a ligand to its receptor, which can result in cyclical, wavelike patterns of Ca^{2+} release and reuptake into the endoplasmic reticulum that propagate for large distances within and even between cells (Augustine et al., 2003; Berridge et al., 2003).

Ca^{2+} signals can be further modulated by the molecular organization of the component proteins involved. A variety of scaffolding proteins, including PSD95, homer, and shank, are thought to link together channels, transporters, and downstream signaling components into macromolecular complexes, thus altering the kinetics of the Ca^{2+} signal and the organization of the sensing mechanisms (Berridge et al., 2003).

The specificity of the Ca^{2+} signal then lies in the unique and precise collection of different signaling and transport molecules expressed in a particular cell, their relative spatial location, the balance of their activities, and the manner in which the Ca^{2+} signal is initiated. Although the regulation of Ca^{2+} homeostasis is quite robust, pathological disturbances can cause it to go awry. The resulting dysregulation of Ca^{2+} concentration has extreme consequences, resulting in cell damage and death that are a prelude to the pathological consequences of diseased states such as stroke and neurodegeneration (Rizzuto and Pozzan, 2003).

2 Na$^+$/Ca^{2+} Exchange: A Key Ca^{2+}-Efflux Mechanism

Studies in several different systems almost four decades ago uncovered a reciprocal relation between Na$^+$ and Ca^{2+} with respect to both concentration and flux across cell membranes. These observations led to the conclusion that a coupled countertransport system specific for Na$^+$ and Ca^{2+} existed in the plasma membrane—called "Na$^+$/Ca^{2+} exchange". This finding established the physiological importance of Na$^+$/Ca^{2+} exchanger as a mechanism contributing to the control of Ca^{2+} homeostasis, and launched the study of the protein molecules underlying this essential activity (Blaustein and Lederer, 1999).

Functional studies have established that the Na$^+$/Ca^{2+} exchanger has a very high capacity to transport Ca^{2+} but is activated only at cytosolic [Ca^{2+}]$_i$ well above resting levels. In contrast, the ATP-dependent Ca^{2+} pumps of both the plasma membrane and the endoplasmic reticulum have a more limited transport capacity but are active closer to resting [Ca^{2+}]$_i$ levels. These observations have resulted in the generally accepted view that the ATP-dependent pumps are responsible for removing cytosolic Ca^{2+} under basal conditions, while the Na$^+$/Ca^{2+} exchanger plays a more important role when [Ca^{2+}]$_i$ rises substantially (Wanaverbecq et al., 2003). Consistent with this view, Na$^+$/Ca^{2+}-exchanger levels are high in those regions of neurons where Ca^{2+} flux across the membrane is high such as at synapses (Reuter and Porzig, 1995; Papa et al., 2003). It seems likely that the Na$^+$/Ca^{2+} exchanger is primarily involved in extruding Ca^{2+} under these conditions to help terminate a signaling event and maintain Ca^{2+} homeostasis.

There is evidence, however, indicating that the exchanger plays a different role under different circumstances (❷ *Figure 11-2*). For example, it has been suggested that in certain neurons the glutamate-induced Ca^{2+}-signal is at least partly due to Ca^{2+} entry via "reverse" Na$^+$/Ca^{2+}-exchange activity (Hoyt et al., 1998; Kiedrowski, 1999). Presumably Na$^+$-entry through ionotropic glutamate receptors in close proximity to Na$^+$/Ca^{2+} exchangers results in a sufficient elevation in the local ion gradients to reverse the Na$^+$/Ca^{2+} exchanger and allow Ca^{2+} entry. Unregulated Ca^{2+} entry via this mechanism is thought to be a major mechanism leading to Ca^{2+} overload subsequent to excitotoxic stimulation and ischemia (Li et al., 2000).

Recent evidence suggests another possible role for Na$^+$/Ca^{2+} exchange in receptor signaling. The neuronal signaling molecules serotonin and orexin both cause depolarization of their target neurons, a response that appears to be induced by activation of an inward Na$^+$/Ca^{2+}-exchange current, as Ca^{2+} is extruded through the Na$^+$/Ca^{2+} exchanger, probably subsequent to local calcium release from intracellular stores (Eriksson et al., 2001, 2002; Burdakov et al., 2003; Wu et al., 2004).

Thus, just as the Ca^{2+} ion serves to regulate many different physiological events, the Na$^+$/Ca^{2+} exchange itself plays different roles in different locations and at different times. Insight into this complexity of function is beginning to emerge with the molecular analysis of Na$^+$/Ca^{2+}-exchanger expression.

3 Na$^+$/Ca^{2+} Exchange: Identification of the Protein Molecule

The application of classical biochemical membrane protein techniques to investigation of the Na$^+$/Ca^{2+} exchanger (Reeves and Sutko, 1979) allowed several groups to partially purify proteins associated with

■ Figure 11-2
The direction of Na$^+$/Ca^{2+}-exchanger Ca^{2+} flux depends upon local ion concentrations. The Ca^{2+} efflux mode is activated when cytoplasmic [Ca^{2+}] rises (e.g., via the opening of plasma membrane voltage-operated or receptor-operated Ca^{2+} channels, or signaling events that open RyR and/or IP$_3$R channels of the ER/SR). The Ca^{2+} influx mode is activated when cytosolic [Na$^+$] rises, for example, through entry via glutamate-operated or store-operated nonselective channels. Note that standing concentration gradients can exist between the submembrane space underlying the Na$^+$/Ca^{2+}-exchanger and the bulk cytoplasm. Thus, changes in either [Ca^{2+}] or [Na$^+$] that are sufficient to activate the exchanger may not be evident in measurements of global cytosolic concentrations

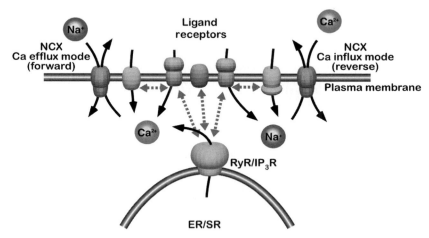

Na$^+$/Ca^{2+}-exchange activity from heart membranes, and prepare antibody reagents. Assisted by these approaches, Philipson's group identified a 120-kDa protein of canine cardiac sarcolemmal membranes, and its 70-kDa proteolytic product, as the Na$^+$/Ca^{2+} exchanger (Philipson et al., 1988). Using expression cloning techniques in combination with biochemistry and immunology, Philipson's laboratory was then successful in the molecular cloning of the canine cardiac Na$^+$/Ca^{2+} exchanger, a landmark achievement published in *Science* in 1990, which confirmed the identity of the Na$^+$/Ca^{2+} exchanger (Nicoll et al., 1990). The cardiac Na$^+$/Ca^{2+}-exchanger gene, NCX1 (*SLC8A1*), encodes a protein of about 120 kDa comprised of a short hydrophobic amino terminus, thought to serve as a signal peptide, followed by a hydrophilic extracellular glycosylated loop, a hydrophobic transmembrane region, a large hydrophilic cytosolic loop, and a final carboxyl terminal hydrophobic transmembrane region (❯ *Figure 11-3*)

At roughly the same time that the cardiac Na$^+$/Ca^{2+} exchanger was being characterized, studies in retinal rod photoreceptors revealed a Na$^+$/Ca^{2+}-exchange mechanism responsible for controlling cytosolic Ca^{2+} in rod outer segments. Electrophysiological and biochemical studies of rod Na$^+$/Ca^{2+} exchange revealed that, unlike cardiac Na$^+$/Ca^{2+} exchanger, the rod Na$^+$/Ca^{2+} exchanger catalyzed the exchange of Na$^+$ for both Ca^{2+} and K$^+$ (Cervetto et al., 1989; Schnetkamp et al., 1989). Eventually solubilization and reconstitution studies allowed purification of the bovine rod photoreceptor Na$^+$/(Ca^{2+}+K$^+$) exchanger, which was identified as a ~220-kDa protein (Cook and Kaupp, 1988). The gene encoding this protein was then cloned in 1992 by Cook's laboratory (Reiländer et al., 1992). As expected from the functional differences, the rod photoreceptor Na$^+$/Ca^{2+} exchanger is encoded by a different gene than is the cardiac exchanger. This gene, NCKX1 (*SLC24A1*), encodes a protein with a similar membrane architecture compared to NCX1, although the extracellular and cytosolic loops are of dramatically different length. Surprisingly, since these molecules share both a mechanistic similarity and a similar topology pattern, their amino acid sequence similarity is limited to only two short hydrophobic stretches, now known to be evolutionarily conserved across phyla, and termed the "α-repeats" (❯ *Figure 11-3*).

◻ **Figure 11-3**

Topology models for NCX-type and NCKX-type Na$^+$/Ca^{2+} exchangers. The predicted folding of each class of protein with respect to the membrane, based on hydropathy analysis and experimental data, is shown. The cylinders labeled M0 (putative signal peptide, removed co- or posttranslationally) to M11 indicate transmembrane helices, with the exception of M6 that was originally proposed to span the membrane but later modeled to be cytoplasmic. The conserved α- and β-repeat regions are boxed and labeled. The N terminus (N) and C terminus (C) of the mature protein as well as sites of glycosylation (CHO), alternative splicing, calcium binding, and the exchange-inhibitory peptide (XIP) sequence are also indicated. Reproduced from Lytton J. 2004. Membrane transporters: Na/Ca exchangers. Encyclopedia of Biological Chemistry, Vol. 2, pp 631–636, with permission from Elsevier

NCX-type

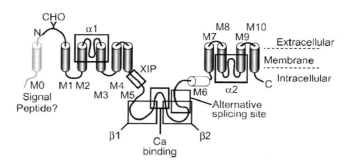

NCKX-type

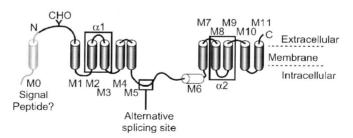

4 Emergence of a Gene Superfamily

The cloning of the canine cardiac Na$^+$/Ca^{2+} exchanger NCX1 led to an immediate explosion in the molecular analysis of the field. NCX1 genes were described from several different animal species, and alternatively spliced NCX1 transcripts encoding different protein isoforms were identified in many other tissues. Soon molecular cloning approaches revealing new, structurally related genes that defined a family composed of NCX1 and two other members, NCX2 (*SLC8A2*) and NCX3 (*SLC8A3*), whose products display about 70% amino acid identity with one another (Li et al., 1994; Nicoll et al., 1996b). NCX3 is also subject to alternative splicing, in a similar location as NCX1.

Advance in the molecular analysis of the Na$^+$/(Ca^{2+}+K$^+$)-exchanger family was not as rapid, but eventually a second gene NCKX2 (*SLC24A2*) was identified through molecular cloning techniques, followed by the identification of NCKX3 (*SLC24A3*) and NCKX4 (*SLC24A4*) using bioinformatic tools (Tsoi et al., 1998; Kraev et al., 2001; Li et al., 2002). Most recently, NCKX5 has been identified as a gene involved in regulating pigmentation (Lamason et al., 2005). Another gene, NCKX6, originally identified as a member of the NCKX family (Cai and Lytton, 2004a, b), has now been reclassified as belonging to a different branch, dubbed CCX, of the overall cation/Ca^{2+}-exchange superfamily tree and may have unique functional properties (see later).

Shortly following the cloning of NCX1, it was recognized that the protein contains two regions of internal similarity, the "α-repeats" and the "β-repeats" (❯ Figure 11-3). The α-repeats, lying one in each half of the molecule, suggest an ancient gene-duplication event (Schwarz and Benzer, 1997). As noted earlier, the α-repeats are the only regions of significant similarity between NCX and NCKX exchangers. Querying the databases using the α-repeat motif identifies a large number of genes in species ranging from higher vertebrates, invertebrates, plants, yeast, bacteria, and archaea (❯ Figure 11-4). The proteins encoded by all these genes contain two homologous α-repeat motifs, each within a hydrophobic region, suggesting these are all membrane transporters. Phylogenetic analysis of these sequences reveals five major branches in the superfamily tree (Cai and Lytton, 2004a). In some cases, such as the NCX, NCKX, or CAX branches, the function of at least one member of the clade has been determined. In other cases, the sequences are quite divergent, and the functions of the encoded proteins have not been determined directly but are presumed to involve cation exchange of some kind, for example, Ca^{2+}/H$^+$ or Mg^{2+}/H$^+$ exchange. Mammals appear to

◻ Figure 11-4

Phylogenetic tree of the cation/Ca^{2+} exchanger superfamily. The evolutionary relation between 147 unique sequences is shown as a phylogentic tree based on the combined similarities of the two hydrophobic regions of each protein. A qualitatively similar pattern is obtained if the entire sequence from each protein is used for the analysis. Five major groups are defined and named after the previously characterized representative members from each group (YRBG, CAX, NCX, and NCKX), or temporarily assigned the name CCX for the group containing NCKX6. For visual reference, several proteins with assigned names have been highlighted: the YRBG protein from *Escherichia coli* (gi|26249782) (EcoYRBG); the vacuolar Ca^{2+}/H$^+$ exchanger from *Saccharomyces cerevisiae* (gi|1139591) (VCX); Ca^{2+}/H$^+$ exchangers from *Arabidopsis thaliana* (gi|9256741 and gi|1488267) (AthCAX1 and 2); the SLC8 gene family members from *Homo sapiens* (gi|10863913, gi|37551974, and gi|22087483) (NCX1–3); the SLC24 gene family members from *Homo sapiens* (gi|14785323, gi|13640164, gi|14717396, gi|21702721, and gi|45504369) (NCKX1–5); a member of the newly defined CCX branch of the superfamily (gi|25269331) (NCKX6). Modified from Cai and Lytton (2004) with permission from Oxford University Press

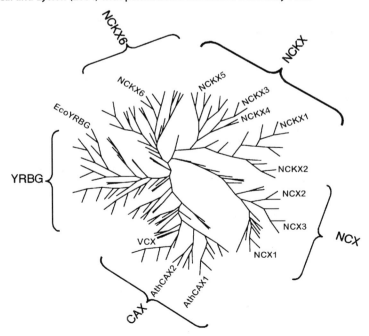

express multiple members of the NCX and NCKX branches of the superfamily. In addition, one member of the newly described CCX branch (NCKX6 or NCLX) is present at low levels in various mammalian tissues, but will not be discussed further here.

5 Patterns of NCX and NCKX Expression

NCX1 is variably expressed in almost all mammalian tissues, with the highest level found in heart, brain, and kidney. The predominant NCX1 transcript in each of these three tissues corresponds to a different alternatively spliced species and encodes a protein product that differs in a short region of the cytoplasmic loop (Kofuji et al., 1994; Lee et al., 1994). NCX2 is expressed at high levels in the brain, but not at significant levels elsewhere, while NCX3 is present only in skeletal muscle and at lower levels in selected brain regions (Quednau et al., 1997).

Within the brain, NCX family members have unique, but overlapping, patterns of expression. NCX1 is expressed most broadly throughout the cortex, hippocampus, thalamus, and cerebellum and is present in both neurons and glial cells. Interestingly, the alternatively spliced isoform present in neurons is different from that expressed in glia (He et al., 1998) (see later). NCX2 is the most abundantly expressed family member but restricted more to the hippocampus, striatum, and thalamus. NCX3 expression is the most restricted, with transcripts found mainly in the hippocampus and cerebellum. At the protein level, NCX2 appears more strongly associated with neuronal cell bodies and proximal dendrites, while NCX1 and NCX3 appear to be present in more distal dendritic and axonal processes as well as in glial cells (Papa et al., 2003).

NCKX1 is expressed almost exclusively in the eye, where the protein is present in the outer segments of rod photoreceptors. NCKX2 is expressed at high abundance in neurons throughout the brain (Tsoi et al., 1998). In the eye, NCKX2 had been identified in cone photoreceptors and retinal ganglion cells (Prinsen et al., 2000). Other tissues express much lower levels of NCKX2, which might be restricted to neurons that innervate those tissues. NCKX3 and NCKX4 are both abundantly expressed in brain and are also broadly distributed in a number of other tissues (Kraev et al., 2001; Li et al., 2002). NCKX5 is expressed highly in skin and retinal pigmented epithelium, and at lower levels in other tissues, including brain (Lamason et al., 2005).

In brain, NCXK2 is expressed at high levels in many regions, including cortex, hippocampus, thalamus, pontine nucleus, and cerebellum (Tsoi et al., 1998) (❷ *Figure 11-5*). The protein appears to be restricted to the dendritic region of hippocampal pyramidal neurons (Li et al., 2006) and axonal termini in others (Kim et al., 2003). NCKX4 is the most broadly distributed isoform that is present throughout brain probably in both neurons and glial cells (Li et al., 2002). NCKX3 has the most restricted neuronal pattern, present with a strikingly laminar distribution in cortex, in the CA3 neurons of the hippocampus and highest in various thalamic nuclei (Kraev et al., 2001). So far, neither NCKX3 nor NCKX4 have been identified at the protein level.

The mechanisms responsible for the distinct patterns of expression for both NCX and NCKX gene products in the brain have not yet been clearly elucidated. Expression of both NCX1 and NCKX2 is controlled by alternative promoters (Barnes et al., 1997; Nicholas et al., 1998; Scheller et al., 1998; Sharon et al., 2002). In the case of NCX1, these promoters provide tissue-specific and transcription factor–specific regulation of expression (Cheng et al., 1999; Nicholas and Philipson, 1999). In cultured neurons, pathways related to changing $[Ca^{2+}]_i$ play an important role in controlling the expression of the different NCX genes, suggesting that the activity and firing pattern of neurons may be central in determining the pattern of NC(K)X expression (Li et al., 2000; Gabellini et al., 2003). Similar studies have not yet been performed on the NCKX genes.

6 Structure of the NCX and NCKX Proteins

The overall architecture for proteins in the NCX and NCKX branches of the calcium-cation exchanger superfamily is conserved (❷ *Figure 11-3*). The amino terminus is hydrophobic and probably cleaved off co- or posttranslationally (Durkin et al., 1991; Sahin-Toth et al., 1995; Kang and Schnetkamp, 2003)

◻ Figure 11-5

NCKX transcript distribution in mouse brain. In situ hybridization using digoxigenen-labeled antisense probes specific for the indicated NCKX gene product was performed on parasagittal sections of mouse brain. Reproduced from Lytton et al. 2002. K-dependent Na/Ca exchangers in the brain. Ann N Y Acad Sci 976: 382–393, with permission of the New York Academy of Sciences

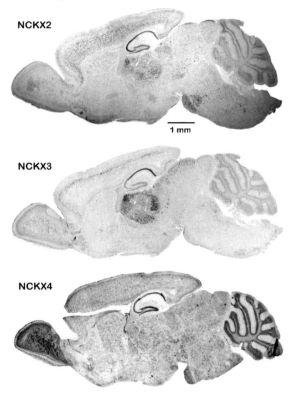

resulting in the subsequent hydrophilic amino-terminal loop of the mature protein being translocated to the extracellular space where it is glycosylated. This loop is followed by two hydrophobic regions interrupted by a large hydrophilic loop situated in the cytoplasm. The hydrophobic regions are modeled as clusters of transmembrane-spanning segments and are quite well conserved within each branch of the superfamily (i.e., NCX and NCKX). Indeed, each hydrophobic region contains one copy of the highly conserved α-repeat. The two large hydrophilic loops are not well conserved, and these regions contain sequences that contribute to the unique regulatory properties of the different exchanger isoforms.

The arrangement of transmembrane-spanning helices within each hydrophobic region has been a focus of much attention, as this part of the protein contains the ion binding and translocation sites. The current model is based both on hydropathy analysis and on experiments using cysteine-scanning mutagenesis and antibody epitope insertion, most of which have focused on NCX1 (Cook et al., 1998; Iwamoto et al., 1999; Nicoll et al., 1999). These experiments revealed that the two α-repeat regions have oppositely oriented topologies with respect to the membrane. Accessibility data suggests that part of each α-repeat forms a membrane reentrant loop structure (Iwamoto et al., 2000). The α-repeats come into close physical proximity with one another in the intact protein (Qiu et al., 2001). Many of the conserved amino acids in the α-repeat have been demonstrated to be important for transport function, supporting the notion that these regions are part of the ion binding and translocation pathway (Nicoll et al., 1996a; Ottolia et al., 2005). Studies on the NCKX2 protein are largely consistent with this model (Kinjo et al., 2003;

Winkfein et al., 2003; Kang et al., 2005a; Kinjo et al., 2005). Additionally, an aspartic acid residue within the α-2 repeat, conserved in all NCKX proteins but replaced with an asparagine in the NCX proteins, has been shown to be essential for K$^+$-dependency of NCKX2 (Kang et al., 2005b). However, there is no clear evidence that the α-repeats form reentrant loops in NCKX2. In addition, the NCKX2 carboxyl terminus resides outside the cell (Cai et al., 2002), while the NCX1 carboxyl terminus is intracellular (Nicoll et al., 1999).

The central hydrophilic cytoplasmic loop of NCX1 has been demonstrated to be important in mediating regulation of the exchanger. The exchanger is activated by micromolar concentrations of Ca^{2+}, stimulated by acidic phospholipids and other amphipathic molecules, and inhibited by high concentrations of cytosolic Na$^+$ (Matsuoka et al., 1993). An amphipathic sequence, denoted the eXchange Inhibitory Peptide (XIP), near the amino-terminal end of the loop appears to play an important role in both acidic phospholipid activation and Na$^+$-inhibition (Matsuoka et al., 1997). Two clusters of acidic amino acids near the center of the loop contribute to a Ca^{2+}-binding site or sites that are critical for NCX1 activity (Matsuoka et al., 1995). There is evidence that these different modes of regulation interact. The site of diversity introduced by alternative splicing of the NCX1 gene lies just downstream from the Ca^{2+}-binding motifs. Two mutually exclusive exons, one expressed primarily in cardiomyocytes and neurons and the other in nonexcitable cells, are combined with several cassette-type exons to form tissue-specific isoforms (Kofuji et al., 1994; Lee et al., 1994). Amino acids in this region of the protein appear to be involved in protein–protein interactions important for the different regulatory behaviors (Maack et al., 2005). This fact suggests that a difference in regulation is an important component of the tissue-specific NCX1 isoforms (Dunn et al., 2002; Dyck et al., 1999). In the brain, this would impart different properties to NCX1 expressed in neurons compared to NCX1 expressed in glial cells. Recent evidence indicates that the potent NCX1 inhibitor, SEA0400, acts through modulating regulation of the exchanger, suggesting the cytoplasmic loop may also be an important site for pharmacological intervention (Bouchard et al., 2004; Iwamoto et al., 2004). Recently the structure of part of the large central and cytoplasmic regulatory loop of NCX1, comprising the two β-repeats, was solved by NMR spectrometry (Hilge et al., 2006). This key advance is a critical step toward understanding the molecular mechanism(s) that underlie both regulation of NCX1, and inhibition by various pharmacological agents, such as SEA0400.

The cytoplasmic loops of other NCX or NCKX family members have not been investigated in so much detail as with NCX1, largely because less is known about regulation of these proteins. Both NCX2 and NCX3 are activated by cytoplasmic Ca^{2+} but are mostly unaffected by other factors that influence NCX1 activity (Linck et al., 1998). NCKX1, but not the other NCKX family members, has an unusually long loop as a consequence of a simple tandem repeat structure. It is possible that this region serves an important role in protein–protein interactions that organize rod photoreceptor signaling events (Bauer, 2002). Several of the NCKX family members are subject to alternative splicing that changes a short region toward the amino-terminal end of the cytoplasmic loop. The consequences of these differences on transport function have not been extensively studied.

7 Function of NCX and NCKX Proteins

Na$^+$/Ca^{2+} exchangers, as their name implies, couple the movement of Na$^+$ ions in one direction to Ca^{2+} ions in the other. Cardiac NCX1 has been demonstrated to transport three (or possibly four) Na$^+$ ions in exchange for one Ca^{2+} ion (Blaustein and Lederer, 1999; Fujioka et al., 2000; Dong et al., 2002). Rod NCKX1 and recombinant NCKX2 have been established to transport four Na$^+$ in exchange for both one Ca^{2+} and one K$^+$ (Cervetto et al., 1989; Schnetkamp et al., 1989; Dong et al., 2001; Szerencsei et al., 2001). The stoichiometry of the other NCX and NCKX family members has not been determined but is likely to be similar to their studied counterparts. The generally accepted model for an exchange process, now illuminated by an increasing number of molecular structures (Huang et al., 2003; Yernool et al., 2004), involves a single ion binding and transport site whose accessibility alternates across the membrane barrier. This site, which is likely formed by transmembrane portions of the protein that lie within the plane of the bilayer, can be occupied in the case of Na$^+$/Ca^{2+} exchangers either by three or four Na$^+$ ions or by one Ca^{2+} ion (and in the case of NCKX exchangers, one K$^+$ ion as well) but cannot be occupied by both Na$^+$ and Ca^{2+} ions simultaneously to yield a complex that allows ion transport. The gates that guard access to this ion-binding site must be locked (one closed and one open), until the site is fully occupied. Only then can both gates close simultaneously, creating an "occluded" state that subsequently opens to one side of the membrane or to the other but never to both sides simultaneously (❷ *Figure 11-6*). This model explains the observations that the Na$^+$/Ca^{2+} exchanger can catalyze Na$^+$/Na$^+$ exchange, Ca^{2+}/Ca^{2+} [or in the case of NCKX,

◻ **Figure 11-6**
Alternating access model to describe ion transport through the Na$^+$/Ca^{2+}-exchanger. The grey sphere indicates the full complement of transported ions required to form the occluded state (centre). For NCKX1 or 2, this would correspond to either 4 Na$^+$ ions or one Ca^{2+} ion and one K$^+$ ion. Ion liganding contacts are provided by regions of the two α-repeats, here modeled as oppositely oriented and rotationally symmetrical segments comprising a transmembrane helix with a break in the middle followed by a short helical pair forming a reentrant loop (in each cartoon, α-1 is on the left with an extracellularly oriented reentrant loop, while α-2 is on the right with an intracellularly oriented reentrant loop). The occluded state can resolve to one side of the membrane or the other, but not to both simultaneously

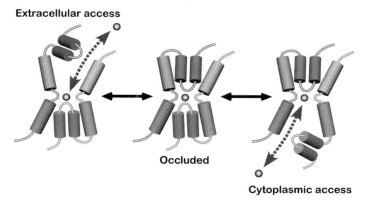

(Ca^{2+}+K$^+$)/(Ca^{2+}+K$^+$)] exchange as well as Na$^+$/Ca^{2+} exchange.

$\quad$ The direction of ion movement through the exchanger is determined by the net sum of electrochemical ion gradients across the membrane and the number of ions that bind to the transport site (Blaustein and Lederer, 1999). For example, assuming that NCX1 exchanges three Na$^+$ for one Ca^{2+}, then at roughly physiological concentrations of these ions (extracellular and intracellular [Na$^+$] of 150 mM and 10 mM and [Ca^{2+}] of 1.3 mM and 0.1 μM, respectively), the exchanger will extrude Ca^{2+} from the cell until the membrane potential rises above −34 mV. Thus, during a short interval at the peak of an action potential, NCX1 is expected to reverse and let Ca^{2+} into the cell. During an ischemic episode, however, local gradients of Na$^+$ run down and the membrane potential dissipates. Under these conditions, NCX1 would reverse and allow chronic Ca^{2+} entry. NCKX proteins couple four Na$^+$ and one K$^+$ ions to the movement of Ca^{2+} and thus would be expected to extrude Ca^{2+} over a broader range of ionic gradients and membrane potentials. For example, using the physiological concentrations of Na$^+$ and Ca^{2+} noted above and extracellular and intracellular [K$^+$] of 5 and 150 mM, respectively, an NCKX exchanger would extrude Ca^{2+} until the membrane potential rose above +121 mV. Thus NCKX would act to extrude Ca^{2+} even at the peak of an action potential and possibly even during a mild ischemic episode.

$\quad$ While the *direction* of flux is dictated by thermodynamic considerations, the *magnitude* of the flux is determined by kinetic factors. These include the speed of enzyme turnover, saturation of the transport sites, and regulation of activity, mediated by a number of factors (Blaustein and Lederer, 1999). The NCX1 protein has a very high maximum rate of turnover but its activity at resting concentrations of cytosolic

Ca^{2+} is limited by only partial occupancy of the transport sites (Hilgemann, 1996). Ca^{2+} also mediates a regulatory effect by binding to sites on the cytoplasmic loop of the exchanger, which must be occupied for activity. These combined Ca^{2+} dependencies mean that NCX1 has significant activity only when [Ca^{2+}]$_i$ reaches 1–10 μM, well above resting levels (Chernysh et al., 2004). Recent studies suggest that this Ca^{2+}-dependent regulation takes place on a beat-to-beat time scale in a cardiac myocyte (Ottolia et al., 2004). Rapid Ca^{2+} regulation of NCX1 would also be expected to modify exchanger activity in a neuron. Indeed, stimulation of Na$^+$/Ca^{2+}-exchange activity, probably via the Ca^{2+}-regulatory mechanism, has been implicated in the action of various ligand–receptor combinations and leads to a depolarizing current (Eriksson et al., 2001, 2002; Burdakov et al., 2003). Similar Ca^{2+}-binding sites and regulation have also been found for the NCX2 and NCX3 proteins.

In addition to regulation by Ca^{2+}, NCX1 activity is also modulated by other factors in a complex fashion through the central cytosolic loop (Shigekawa and Iwamoto, 2001). High concentrations of cytoplasmic Na$^+$ cause inactivation, while acidic phospholipids and ATP, through phosphorylation of phosphatidyl-inositol, activate the exchanger (Hilgemann et al., 1992a, b; Hilgemann and Ball, 1996). Na$^+$ inactivation and acidic phospholipid activation both appear to involve the XIP region of the central cytoplasmic loop, although the mechanisms are not well understood (Matsuoka et al., 1997; He et al., 2000). Moreover, either higher [Ca^{2+}]$_i$ or acidic phospholipid treatment prevent Na$^+$-dependent inhibition, suggesting interaction among all the regulatory events. NCX2, but not NCX3, also responds to treatment with ATP, suggesting it may share these modes of regulation (Linck et al., 1998). Activation of various kinase pathways has been shown to influence NCX1 and NCX3 activity, but there is little convincing evidence for direct phosphorylation (Iwamoto et al., 1998). Recent studies indicate that NCX1 may be part of a much larger macromolecular complex (Lencesova et al., 2004), and that calcineurin interacts to inhibit NCX1 function (Katanosaka et al., 2005), suggesting that complex protein–protein interactions may be involved in regulatory influences on exchanger function.

In comparison with heart NCX1, the rod photoreceptor exchanger NCKX1 appears to turnover more slowly (Friedel et al., 1991; Hilgemann, 1996). NCKX1 has a high apparent affinity for cytosolic Ca^{2+} and would be expected to drive Ca^{2+} down to very low levels. This is not observed in rod photoreceptors, however, suggesting that NCKX1 activity may be regulated (Schnetkamp and Szerencsei, 1993). While there is no detailed evidence documenting regulation, it has been observed that the cyclic nucleotide-gated channel is physically associated with NCKX1 (Bauer and Drechsler, 1992). This complex is thus a good candidate for such regulation, particularly since the channel and exchanger interact functionally through their respective roles in modulating Ca^{2+} homeostasis (Bauer, 2002). Little else is known regarding regulation of the other NCKX family members.

8 Physiological Roles for NCX and NCKX Proteins

Multiple roles for Na$^+$/Ca^{2+}-exchange function have been proposed as mentioned earlier. The principal role of NCX1 appears to be the rapid extrusion of high concentrations of Ca^{2+} that has entered neurons through surface channels, or has been released from the endoplasmic reticulum. This action terminates Ca^{2+} signaling events and helps to protect cells from Ca^{2+} overload (Blaustein and Lederer, 1999). Due to the electrogenic nature of a 3 Na$^+$ for 1 Ca^{2+} exchange process, Na$^+$/Ca^{2+}-exchanger activity in Ca^{2+} extrusion mode generates a depolarizing current. Such a current may play a role in shaping the action potential, at least in restricted surfaces of neurons where Na$^+$/Ca^{2+}-exchanger expression is high and may be critical for subsequent downstream signaling events (Eriksson et al., 2001; Burdakov et al., 2003).

NCX1 can be induced to mediate Ca^{2+} entry by relatively modest changes in local ion gradients and/or membrane potential. It is thought that Ca^{2+} entering this way may be employed to elevate cytoplasmic [Ca^{2+}]$_i$ during signaling events (Hoyt et al., 1998; Kiedrowski, 1999) or may be used to load endoplasmic reticulum stores in a process that sensitizes the stores for subsequent release (Arnon et al., 2000).

During periods of ischemia, ion gradients and the membrane potential collapse and extracellular pH changes dramatically (Hansen and Zeuthen, 1981). These changes result in the inappropriate release of the neurotransmitter glutamate, which accumulates to high levels and then acts on its receptor to initiate further cationic fluxes. This "excitotoxic" stimulation causes the entry into neurons of large quantities of Ca^{2+}. The role that Na$^+$/Ca^{2+} exchangers play in this process—contributing to the Ca^{2+} overload or protecting against it—has been the subject of much controversy. The collapse of the Na$^+$ gradient and the membrane potential would be expected—on theoretical grounds—to promote Ca^{2+} entry via reverse-mode operation of the exchanger. Inhibitor studies used in vitro under these conditions support this model (Kiedrowski et al., 2004). However, later on during any possible subsequent reperfusion recovery phase, Na$^+$/Ca^{2+}-exchange activity would be expected to remove Ca^{2+} that had entered earlier, and hence be neuroprotective. The importance of this role in ischemic models has been emphasized in animal studies (Pignataro et al., 2004a, b). The role of Na$^+$/Ca^{2+} exchangers during ischemia is further complicated by recent observations that the Ca^{2+}-activated protease, calpain impairs the ability of the neurons to extrude Ca^{2+} and cleaves both NCX1 and NCX3 (Bano et al., 2005). The effect of calpain proteolysis on the function of NCX1 or NCX3 is not known. Cleavage of these molecules might inhibit their function or might activate them by relieving inhibitory regulation, as observed with trypsin. The in vitro conditions used in these studies do not reproduce in vivo ionic conditions during ischemia, and so it is not clear if calpain cleavage acts as a feedback mechanism to prevent Na$^+$/Ca^{2+}-exchanger–mediated Ca^{2+} entry, or a feedforward mechanism to prevent Ca^{2+} extrusion and exacerbate damage, during an ischemic episode in vivo.

The specific relative roles of the three NCX family members have not been clearly established in brain. Their overlapping patterns of expression and overlapping functional similarity suggest that they play similar roles either in different neuronal populations or at different subcellular sites. The major gene product expressed in brain, NCX2, has been knocked out in mice, which results in enhanced performance in several hippocampal-dependent learning and memory tasks. This result supports the idea that NCX2 plays a predominant role in Ca^{2+} clearance at pre- and postsynaptic sites in the hippocampus (Jeon et al., 2003). NCX3 knockout mice have also been generated, but their pathology appears to be restricted largely to defects in muscle fibers and at the neuromuscular junction rather than within CNS neurons (Sokolow et al., 2004). NCX1 knockout mice die as embryos (Pott et al., 2004), and neuron-specific NCX1 knockouts have not yet been reported.

Knowledge of the specific roles for members of the NCKX family is only beginning to emerge. In the rod photoreceptors, NCKX1 plays a critical role in maintaining Ca^{2+} homeostasis, especially in the dark when the membrane is depolarized and the Na$^+$ gradient is low (Schnetkamp, 2004). Under these circumstances the 4 Na$^+$/(1 Ca^{2+}+K$^+$)-coupling ratio provides the thermodynamic power needed to maintain Ca^{2+} efflux and homeostasis. Parallel arguments for brain neurons would suggest that NCKX gene products might be expressed in neurons, or compartments of those neurons, where particularly high and frequent depolarizing pulses are anticipated. Under these conditions only a Na$^+$/Ca^{2+} exchanger that operates with the NCKX stoichiometry would be able to maintain Ca^{2+} homeostasis and protect against overload. This concept has been examined by determining the coordinated expression of NCKX (and NCX) isoforms with various channels or receptors (Sergeeva et al., 2003, 2004). Knockout of the NCKX2 gene in mice (Li et al., 2006) has recently revealed a profound deficit in hippocampal LTP, and associated deficits in motor learning and memory. These data are in striking contrast to observations from the NCX2 knockout mouse (Jeon et al., 2003). The opposite effect on hippocampal function induced by knocking out NCX2 or NCKX2 supports the concept that these different transporters must make unique spatial and temporal contributions to neuronal Ca^{2+} homeostasis. Recent studies on zebrafish have revealed a totally unexpected role for the NCKX5 protein in the development of pigmentation (Lamason et al., 2006). Furthermore, a major polymorphism in the NCKX5 gene is associated with the lighter pigmentation of humans of northern European ancestry compared to the darker complexion of African or Asian populations. It is thought that NCKX5, in contrast to the other members of the NCKX family, is expressed on melanosome granule membranes rather than at the cell surface. Precisely how NCKX5 function affects the development of pigment granules remains to be determined.

These recent studies emphasize how much is still to be learned about the physiological functions of NCX and NCKX molecules. It is anticipated that further studies of this nature will provide fascinating novel and exciting discoveries in the years ahead.

9 Concluding Remarks

Ca^{2+} homeostasis plays a complex and varied role in neuronal signaling. At least six different Na$^+$/Ca^{2+} exchanger gene products, belonging to both the NCX (SLC8) and NCKX (SLC24) gene families, display overlapping but distinct patters of neuronal expression in brain. Elucidating the unique individual physiological roles for each of the NCX and NCKX protein molecules continues to be an active and fertile area of research that is likely to provide exciting novel insights in the near future.

References

Arnon A, Hamlyn JM, Blaustein MP. 2000. Ouabain augments Ca$^{(2+)}$ transients in arterial smooth muscle without raising cytosolic Na$^{(+)}$. Am J Physiol Heart Circ Physiol 279 (2): H679-H691.

Augustine GJ, Santamaria F, Tanaka K. 2003. Local calcium signaling in neurons. Neuron 40 (2): 331-346.

Bano D, Young KW, Guerin CJ, Lefeuvre R, Rothwell NJ, et al. 2005. Cleavage of the plasma membrane Na$^+$/Ca^{2+} exchanger in excitotoxicity. Cell 120 (2): 275-285.

Barnes KV, Cheng G, Dawson MM, Menick DR. 1997. Cloning of cardiac kidney and brain promoters of the feline ncx1 gene. J Biol Chem 272 (17): 11510-11517.

Bauer PJ. 2002. Binding of the retinal rod Na$^+$/Ca^{2+}-K$^+$ exchanger to the cGMP-gated channel indicates local Ca(2+)-signaling in vertebrate photoreceptors. Ann N Y Acad Sci 976: 325-334.

Bauer PJ, Drechsler M. 1992. Association of cyclic GMP-gated channels and Na$^{(+)}$-Ca$^{(2+)}$-K$^+$ exchangers in bovine retinal rod outer segment plasma membranes. J Physiol 451: 109-131.

Berridge MJ, Lipp P, Bootman MD. 2000. The versatility and universality of calcium signaling. Nat Rev Mol Cell Biol 1 (1): 11-21.

Berridge MJ, Bootman MD, Roderick HL. 2003. Calcium signalling: Dynamics homeostasis and remodeling. Nat Rev Mol Cell Biol 4 (7): 517-529.

Blaustein MP, Lederer WJ. 1999. Sodium/calcium exchange: Its physiological implications. Physiol Rev 79: 763-854.

Bouchard R, Omelchenko A, Le HD, Choptiany P, Matsuda T, et al. 2004. Effects of SEA0400 on mutant NCX1.1 Na$^+$-Ca2$^+$ exchangers with altered ionic regulation. Mol Pharmacol 65 (3): 802-810.

Burdakov D, Liss B, Ashcroft FM. 2003. Orexin excites GABAergic neurons of the arcuate nucleus by activating the sodium–calcium exchanger. J Neurosci 23 (12): 4951-4957.

Cai X, Lytton J. 2004a. The cation/Ca^{2+} exchanger superfamily: Phylogenetic analysis and structural implications. Mol Biol Evol 21(9): 1692-1703.

Cai X, Lytton J. 2004b. Molecular cloning of a sixth member of the K$^+$-dependent Na$^+$/Ca^{2+} exchanger gene family NCKX6. J Biol Chem 279 (7): 5867-5876.

Cai X, Zhang K, Lytton J. 2002. Topological studies of the rat brain K(+)-dependent Na$^{(+)}$/Ca$^{(2+)}$ exchanger NCKX2 Ann N Y Acad Sci 976: 90-93.

Cervetto L, Lagnado L, Perry RJ, Robinson DW, McNaughton PA. 1989. Extrusion of calcium from rod outer segments is driven by both sodium and potassium gradients. Nature 337: 740-743.

Cheng G, Hagen TP, Dawson ML, Barnes KV, Menick DR. 1999. The role of GATA CArG E-box and a novel element in the regulation of cardiac expression of the Na$^+$-Ca^{2+} exchanger gene. J Biol Chem 274 (18): 12819-12826.

Chernysh O, Condrescu M, Reeves JP. 2004. Calcium-dependent regulation of calcium efflux by the cardiac sodium calcium exchanger. Am J Physiol Cell Physiol 287 (3) C797-806.

Cook NJ, Kaupp UB. 1988. Solubilization, purification and reconstitution of the sodium-calcium exchanger from bovine retinal rod outer segments. J Biol Chem 263 (23) 11382-11388.

Cook O, Low W, Rahamimoff H. 1998. Membrane topology of the rat brain Na$^+$-Ca^{2+} exchanger. Biochim Biophys Acta 1371 (1): 40-52.

Dong H, Light PE, French RJ, Lytton J. 2001. Electrophysiological characterization and ionic stoichiometry of the rat brain K$^+$-dependent Na$^+$/Ca^{2+} exchanger NCKX2. J Biol Chem 276 (28): 25919-25928.

Dong H, Dunn J, Lytton J. 2002. Stoichiometry of the cardiac Na$^+$/Ca^{2+} exchanger NCX1.1 measure in transfected HEK cells. Biophys J 82 (4): 1943-1952.

Dunn J, Elias CL, Le HD, Omelchenko A, Hryshko LV, et al. 2002. The molecular determinants of ionic regulatory differences between brain and kidney Na$^+$/Ca^{2+} exchanger (NCX1) isoforms. J Biol Chem 277 (37): 33957-33962.

Durkin JT, Ahrens DC, Pan YCE, Reeves JP. 1991. Purification and amino-terminal sequence of the bovine cardiac sodium calcium exchanger: Evidence for the presence of a signal sequence. Arch Biochem Biophys 290: 369-375.

Dyck C, Omelchenko A, Elias CL, Quednau BD, Philipson KD, et al. 1999. Ionic regulatory properties of brain and kidney splice variants of the NCX1 Na$^{(+)}$-Ca$^{(2+)}$ exchanger. J Gen Physiol 114 (5): 701-711.

Eriksson KS, Stevens DR, Haas HL. 2001. Serotonin excites tuberomammillary neurons by activation of Na$^{(+)}$/Ca$^{(2+)}$-exchange. Neuropharmacology 40 (3): 345-351.

Eriksson KS, Sergeeva OA, Stevens DR, Haas HL. 2002. Neurotransmitter-induced activation of sodium-calcium exchange causes neuronal excitation. Ann N Y Acad Sci 976: 405-407.

Friedel U, Wolbring G, Wohlfart P, Cook NJ. 1991. The sodium-calcium exchanger of bovine rod photoreceptors: K$^+$-dependence of the purified and reconstituted protein. Biochim Biophys Acta 1061: 247-252.

Fujioka Y, Komeda M, Matsuoka S. 2000. Stoichiometry of Na$^+$-Ca^{2+} exchange in inside-out patches excised from guinea-pig ventricular myocytes. J Physiol (Lond) 523 (Pt. 2): 339-351.

Gabellini N, Bortoluzzi S, Danieli GA, Carafoli E. 2003. Control of the Na$^+$/Ca^{2+} exchanger 3 promoter by cyclic adenosine monophosphate and Ca^{2+} in differentiating neurons. J Neurochem 84 (2): 282-293.

Hansen AJ, Zeuthen T. 1981. Extracellular ion concentrations during spreading depression and ischemia in the rat brain cortex. Acta Physiol Scand 113 (4): 437-445.

He S, Ruknudin A, Bambrick LL, Lederer WJ, Schulze DH. 1998. Isoform-specific regulation of the Na$^+$/Ca^{2+} exchanger in rat astrocytes and neurons by PKA. J Neurosci 18 (13): 4833-4841.

He Z, Feng S, Tong Q, Hilgemann DW, Philipson KD. 2000. Interaction of PIP(2) with the XIP region of the cardiac Na/Ca exchanger. Am J Physiol Cell Physiol 278 (4): C661-C666.

Hilge M, Aelen J, Vuister GW. 2006. Ca^{2+} regulation in the Na$^+$/Ca^{2+} exchanger involves two markedly different Ca^{2+} sensors. Mol Cell 22 (1): 15-25.

Hilgemann DW. 1996. Unitary cardiac Na$^+$, Ca^{2+} exchange current magnitudes determined from channel-like noise and charge movements of ion transport. Biophys J 71 (2): 759-768.

Hilgemann DW, Ball R. 1996. Regulation of cardiac Na$^+$, Ca^{2+} exchange and KATP potassium channels by PIP2. Science 273 (5277): 956-959.

Hilgemann DW, Collins A, Matsuoka S. 1992a. Steady-state and dynamic properties of cardiac sodium-calcium exchange secondary modulation by cytoplasmic calcium and ATP. J Gen Physiol 100: 933-961.

Hilgemann DW, Matsuoka S, Nagel GA, Collins A. 1992b. Steady-state and dynamic properties of cardiac sodium-calcium exchange Sodium-dependent inactivation. J Gen Physiol 100: 905-932.

Hoyt KR, Arden SR, Aizenman E, Reynolds IJ. 1998. Reverse Na$^+$/Ca^{2+} exchange contributes to glutamate-induced intracellular Ca^{2+} concentration increases in cultured rat forebrain neurons. Mol Pharmacol 53 (4): 742-749.

Huang Y, Lemieux MJ, Song J, Auer M, Wang DN. 2003. Structure and mechanism of the glycerol-3-phosphate transporter from Escherichia coli. Science 301 (5633): 616-620.

Iwamoto T, Pan Y, Nakamura TY, Wakabayashi S, Shigekawa M. 1998. Protein kinase C-dependent regulation of Na$^+$/Ca^{2+} exchanger isoforms NCX1 and NCX3 does not require their direct phosphorylation. Biochemistry 37 (49): 17230-17238.

Iwamoto T, Nakamura TY, Pan Y, Uehara A, Imanaga I, et al. 1999. Unique topology of the internal repeats in the cardiac Na$^+$/Ca^{2+} exchanger. FEBS Lett 446 (2–3): 264-268.

Iwamoto T, Uehara A, Imanaga I, Shigekawa M. 2000. The Na$^+$/Ca^{2+} exchanger NCX1 has oppositely oriented reentrant loop domains that contain conserved aspartic acids whose mutation alters its apparent Ca^{2+} affinity. J Biol Chem 275 (49): 38571-38580.

Iwamoto T, Kita S, Uehara A, Imanaga I, Matsuda T, et al. 2004. Molecular determinants of Na$^+$/Ca^{2+} exchange (NCX1) inhibition by SEA0400. J Biol Chem 279 (9): 7544-7553.

Jeon D, Yang YM, Jeong MJ, Philipson KD, Rhim H, et al. 2003. Enhanced learning and memory in mice lacking Na$^+$/Ca^{2+} exchanger 2. Neuron 38 (6): 965-976.

Kang K, Schnetkamp PP. 2003. Signal sequence cleavage and plasma membrane targeting of the retinal rod NCKX1 and cone NCKX2 Na$^+$/Ca^{2+}–K$^+$ exchangers. Biochemistry 42 (31): 9438-9445.

Kang KJ, Kinjo TG, Szerencsei RT, Schnetkamp PP. 2005a. Residues contributing to the Ca2+ and K+ binding pocket of the NCKX2 Na$^+$/Ca^{2+}-K$^+$ exchanger. J Biol Chem 280 (8): 6823-6833.

Kang KJ, Shibukawa Y, Szerencsei RT, Schnetkamp PP. 2005b. Substitution of a single residue, Asp575, renders the NCKX2 K$^+$-dependent Na$^+$/Ca^{2+} exchanger independent of K$^+$. J Biol Chem 280 (8): 6834-6839.

Katanosaka Y, Iwata Y, Kobayashi Y, Shibasaki F, Wakabayashi S, et al. 2005. Calcineurin inhibits Na$^+$/Ca^{2+} exchange in phenylephrine-treated hypertrophic cardiomyocytes. J Biol Chem 280 (7): 5764-5772.

Kiedrowski L. 1999. N-methyl-D-aspartate excitotoxicity: Relationships among plasma membrane potential Na$^{(+)}$/Ca$^{(2+)}$ exchange mitochondrial Ca$^{(2+)}$ overload and cytoplasmic concentrations of Ca$^{(2+)}$, H$^{(+)}$, and K$^{(+)}$. Mol Pharmacol 56 (3): 619-632.

Kiedrowski L, Czyz A, Baranauskas G, Li XF, Lytton J. 2004. Differential contribution of plasmalemmal Na/Ca exchange isoforms to sodium-dependent calcium influx and NMDA excitotoxicity in depolarized neurons. J Neurochem 90 (1): 117-128.

Kim MH, Lee SH, Park KH, Ho WK. 2003. Distribution of K$^+$-dependent Na$^+$/Ca^{2+} exchangers in the rat supraoptic magnocellular neuron is polarized to axon terminals. J Neurosci 23 (37): 11673-11680.

Kinjo TG, Szerencsei RT, Winkfein RJ, Kang K, Schnetkamp PP. 2003. Topology of the retinal cone NCKX2 Na/Ca-K exchanger. Biochemistry 42 (8): 2485-2491.

Kinjo TG, Kang K, Szerencsei RT, Winkfein RJ, Schnetkamp PP. 2005. Site-directed disulfide mapping of residues contributing to the Ca$^{(2+)}$ and K$^{(+)}$ binding pocket of the NCKX2 Na$^{(+)}$/Ca$^{(2+)}$-K$^{(+)}$ exchanger. Biochemistry 44 (21): 7787-7795.

Kofuji P, Lederer WJ, Schulze DH. 1994. Mutually exclusive and cassette exons underlie alternatively spliced isoforms of the Na/Ca exchanger. J Biol Chem 269: 5145-5149.

Kraev A, Quednau BD, Leach S, Li XF, Dong H, et al. 2001. Molecular cloning of a third member of the potassium-dependent sodium-calcium exchanger gene family NCKX3. J Biol Chem 276 (25): 23161-23172.

Lamason RL, Mohideen MA, Mest JR, Wong AC, Norton HL, Aros MC, Jurynec MJ, Mao X, Humphreville VR, Humbert JE, Sinha S, Moore JL, Jagadeeswaran P, Zhao W, Ning G, Makalowska I, McKeigue PM, O'donnell D, Kittles R, Parra EJ, Mangini NJ, Grunwald DJ, Shriver MD, Canfield VA, Cheng KC. 2005. SLC24A5, a putative cation exchanger, affects pigmentation in zebrafish and humans. Science 310 (5755): 1782-1786.

Lee S-L, Yu ASL, Lytton J. 1994. Tissue-specific expression of Na/Ca exchanger isoforms. J Biol Chem 269: 14849-14852.

Lencesova L, O'Neill A, Resneck WG, Bloch RJ, Blaustein MP. 2004. Plasma membrane-cytoskeleton-endoplasmic reticulum complexes in neurons and astrocytes. J Biol Chem 279 (4): 2885-2893.

Li L, Guerini D, Carafoli E. 2000. Calcineurin controls the transcription of Na$^+$/Ca^{2+} exchanger isoforms in developing cerebellar neurons. J Biol Chem 275 (27): 20903-20910.

Li S, Jiang Q, Stys PK. 2000. Important role of reverse Na$^{(+)}$-Ca$^{(2+)}$ exchange in spinal cord white matter injury at physiological temperature. J Neurophysiol 84 (2): 1116-1119.

Li XF, Kiedrowski L, Tremblay F, Fernandez FR, Perizzolo M, Winkfein RJ, Turner RW, Bains JS, Rancourt DE, Lytton J. 2006. Importance of K$^+$-dependent Na$^+$/Ca^{2+}-exchanger 2, NCKX2, in motor learning and memory. J Biol Chem 281 (10): 6273-6282.

Li XF, Kraev AS, Lytton J. 2002. Molecular cloning of a fourth member of the potassium-dependent sodium-calcium exchanger gene family NCKX4. J Biol Chem 277 (50): 48410-48417.

Li Z, Matsuoka S, Hryshko LV, Nicoll DA, Bersohn MM, et al. 1994. Cloning of the NCX2 isoform of the plasma membrane Na–Ca exchanger. J Biol Chem 269: 17434-17439.

Linck B, Qiu Z, He Z, Tong Q, Hilgemann DW, et al. 1998. Functional comparison of the three isoforms of the Na$^+$/Ca^{2+} exchanger (NCX1, NCX2, NCX3). Am J Physiol Cell Physiol 274 (2; Pt. 1): C415-C423.

Maack C, Ganesan A, Sidor A, O'Rourke B. 2005. Cardiac sodium–calcium exchanger is regulated by allosteric calcium and exchanger inhibitory peptide at distinct sites. Circ Res 96 (1): 91-99.

Matsuoka S, Nicoll DA, Reilly RF, Hilgemann DW, Philipson KD. 1993. Initial localization of regulatory regions of the cardiac sarcolemmal Na$^{(+)}$-Ca^{2+} exchanger. Proc Natl Acad Sci USA 90 (9): 3870-3874.

Matsuoka S, Nicoll DA, Hryshko LV, Levitsky DO, Weiss JN, et al. 1995. Regulation of the cardiac Na$^+$-Ca^{2+} exchanger by Ca^{2+}. Mutational analysis of the Ca^{2+}-binding domain. J Gen Physiol 105: 403-420.

Matsuoka S, Nicoll DA, He Z, Philipson KD. 1997. Regulation of cardiac Na$^{(+)}$-Ca^{2+} exchanger by the endogenous XIP region. J Gen Physiol 109 (2): 273-286.

Nicholas SB, Philipson KD. 1999. Cardiac expression of the Na$^{(+)}$/Ca$^{(2+)}$ exchanger NCX1 is GATA factor dependent. Am J Physiol Heart Circ Physiol 277 (1; Pt. 2): H324-H330.

Nicholas SB, Yang W, Lee SL, Zhu H, Philipson KD, et al. 1998. Alternative promoters and cardiac muscle cell-specific expression of the Na$^+$/Ca^{2+} exchanger gene. Am J Physiol Heart Circ Physiol 274 (1; Pt. 2): H217-H232.

Nicoll DA, Longoni S, Philipson KD. 1990. Molecular cloning and functional expression of the cardiac NaCa-exchanger. Science 250: 562-565.

Nicoll DA, Hryshko LV, Matsuoka S, Frank JS, Philipson KD. 1996a. Mutation of amino acid residues in the putative transmembrane segments of the cardiac sarcolemmal Na$^+$-Ca^{2+} exchanger. J Biol Chem 271 (23): 13385-13391.

Nicoll DA, Quednau BD, Qui Z, Xia Y-R, Lusis AJ, et al 1996b. Cloning of a third mammalian Na$^+$-Ca^{2+} exchanger NCX2. J Biol Chem 271 (40): 24914-24921.

Nicoll DA, Ottolia M, Lu L, Lu Y, Philipson KD. 1999. A new topological model of the cardiac sarcolemmal Na$^+$-Ca^{2+} exchanger. J Biol Chem 274 (2): 910-917.

Ottolia M, Philipson KD, John S. 2004. Conformational changes of the Ca$^{(2+)}$ regulatory site of the Na$^{(+)}$-Ca$^{(2+)}$ exchanger detected by FRET. Biophys J 87 (2): 899-906.

Ottolia M, Nicoll DA, Philipson KD. 2005. Mutational analysis of the alpha-1 repeat of the cardiac Na$^{(+)}$-Ca^{2+} exchanger. J Biol Chem 280 (2): 1061-1069.

Papa M, Canitano A, Boscia F, Castaldo P, Sellitti S, et al. 2003. Differential expression of the Na$^+$-Ca^{2+} exchanger transcripts and proteins in rat brain regions. J Comp Neurol 461 (1): 31-48.

Philipson KD, Longoni S, Ward R. 1988. Purification of the cardiac Na–Ca exchange protein. Biochim Biophys Acta 945: 298-306.

Ignataro G, Gala R, Cuomo O, Tortiglione A, Giaccio L, et al. 2004a. Two sodium/calcium exchanger gene products NCX1 and NCX3, play a major role in the development of permanent focal cerebral ischemia. Stroke 35 (11): 2566-2570.

Ignataro G, Tortiglione A, Scorziello A, Giaccio L, Secondo A, et al. 2004b. Evidence for a protective role played by the Na$^+$/Ca^{2+} exchanger in cerebral ischemia induced by middle cerebral artery occlusion in male rats. Neuropharmacology 46 (3): 439-448.

Ott C, Goldhaber JI, Philipson KD. 2004. Genetic manipulation of cardiac Na$^+$/Ca^{2+} exchange expression. Biochem Biophys Res Commun 322 (4): 1336-1340.

Prinsen CF, Szerencsei RT, Schnetkamp PPM. 2000. Molecular cloning and functional expression of the potassium-dependent sodium-calcium exchanger from human and chicken retinal cone photoreceptors. J Neurosci 20 (4): 1424-1434.

Qiu Z, Nicoll DA, Philipson KD. 2001. Helix packing of functionally important regions of the cardiac Na$^{(+)}$-Ca$^{(2+)}$ exchanger. J Biol Chem 276(1): 194-199.

Quednau BD, Nicoll DA, Philipson KD. 1997. Tissue specificity and alternative splicing of the Na$^+$/Ca^{2+} exchanger isoforms NCX1, NCX2, and NCX3 in rat. Am J Physiol Cell Physiol 272 (4; Pt. 1): C1250-C1261.

Reeves JP, Sutko JL. 1979. Sodium-calcium ion exchange in cardiac membrane vesicles. Proc Natl Acad Sci USA 76: 590-594.

Reiländer H, Achilles A, Friedel U, Maul G, Lottspeich F, et al. 1992. Primary structure and functional expression of the Na/CaK-exchanger from bovine rod photoreceptors. EMBO J 11: 1689-1695.

Reuter H, Porzig H. 1995. Localization and functional significance of the Na/Ca exchagner in presynaptic boutons of hippocampal cells in culture. Neuron 15: 1077-1084.

Rizzuto R, Pozzan T. 2003. When calcium goes wrong: Genetic alterations of a ubiquitous signaling route. Nat Genet 34 (2): 135-141.

Sahin-Toth M, Nicoll DA, Frank JS, Philipson KD, Friedlander M. 1995. The cleaved N-terminal signal sequence of the cardiac Na$(+)$-Ca2+ exchanger is not required for functional membrane integration. Biochem Biophys Res Commun 212 (3): 968-974.

Scheller T, Kraev A, Skinner S, Carafoli E. 1998. Cloning of the multipartite promoter of the sodium-calcium exchanger gene NCX1 and characterization of its activity in vascular smooth muscle cells. J Biol Chem 273 (13): 7643-7649.

Schnetkamp PP. 2004. The SLC24 Na$^+$/Ca^{2+}-K$^+$ exchanger family: Vision and beyond. Pflugers Arch 447 (5): 683-688.

Schnetkamp PPM, Szerencsei RT. 1993. Intracellular Ca^{2+} sequestration and release in intact bovine retinal rod outer segments role in inactivation of Na-Ca$^+$K exchange. J Biol Chem 268 (17): 12449-12457.

Schnetkamp PPM, Basu DK, Szerencsei RT. 1989. Na$^+$-Ca^{2+} exchange in bovine rod outer segments requires and transports K$^+$. Am J Physiol Cell Physiol 257 (1; Pt. 1): C153-C157.

Schwarz EM, Benzer S. 1997. *Calx* a sodium-calcium exchanger gene of *Drosophila melanogaster*. Proc Natl Acad Sci USA 94: 10249-10254.

Sergeeva OA, Amberger BT, Eriksson KS, Scherer A, Haas HL. 2003. Co-ordinated expression of 5-HT2C receptors with the NCX1 Na$^+$/Ca^{2+} exchanger in histaminergic neurons. J Neurochem 87 (3): 657-664.

Sergeeva OA, Amberger BT, Vorobjev VS, Eriksson KS, Haas HL. 2004. AMPA receptor properties and coexpression with sodium-calcium exchangers in rat hypothalamic neurons. Eur J Neurosci 19 (4): 957-965.

Sharon D, Yamamoto H, McGee TL, Rabe V, Szerencsei RT, et al. 2002. Mutated alleles of the rod and cone Na-Ca$^+$K-exchanger genes in patients with retinal diseases. Invest Ophthalmol Vis Sci 43 (6): 1971-1979.

Shigekawa M, Iwamoto T. 2001. Cardiac Na$^{(+)}$-Ca$^{(2+)}$ exchange: Molecular and pharmacological aspects. Circ Res 88 (9): 864-876.

Sokolow S, Manto M, Gailly P, Molgo J, Vandebrouck C, et al. 2004. Impaired neuromuscular transmission and skeletal muscle fiber necrosis in mice lacking Na/Ca exchanger 3. J Clin Invest 113 (2): 265-273.

Szerencsei RT, Prinsen CF, Schnetkamp PP. 2001. Stoichiometry of the retinal cone Na/Ca-K exchanger heterologously expressed in insect cells: Comparison with the bovine heart Na/Ca exchanger. Biochemistry 40 (20): 6009-6015.

Tsoi M, RheeK-H, Bungard D, Li X-F, Lee S-L, et al. 1998. Molecular cloning of a novel potassium-dependent sodium-calcium exchanger from rat brain. J Biol Chem 273: 4115-4162.

Wanaverbecq N, Marsh SJ, Al-Qatari M, Brown DA. 2003. The plasma membrane calcium-ATPase as a major mechanism for intracellular calcium regulation in neurones from the rat superior cervical ganglion. J Physiol 550 (Pt. 1): 83-101.

Winkfein RJ, Szerencsei RT, Kinjo TG, Kang K, Perizzolo M, et al. 2003. Scanning mutagenesis of the alpha repeats and of the transmembrane acidic residues of the human retinal cone Na/Ca-K exchanger. Biochemistry 42 (2): 543-552.

Wu M, Zaborszky L, Hajszan T, van den Pol AN, Alreja M. 2004. Hypocretin/orexin innervation and excitation of identified septohippocampal cholinergic neurons. J Neurosci 24 (14): 3527-3536.

Yernool D, Boudker O, Jin Y, Gouaux E. 2004. Structure of a glutamate transporter homologue from Pyrococcus horikoshii. Nature 431(7010): 811-818.

Ion Pumps and Ion Transporters in Neural Membranes

12 Glutamate-Induced Neuronal Death and Na^+/Ca^{2+} Exchange

L. Kiedrowski

Abstract: When Na$^+$, K$^+$-ATPase operation is compromised while ionotropic glutamate receptors are activated, the Na$^+$ and K$^+$ concentration gradients across neuronal plasma membranes rapidly collapse. This leads to the reversal of plasmalemmal Na$^+$/Ca^{2+} exchangers, i.e., to Ca^{2+} influx via the reversed exchangers. Two such exchanger families are expressed in the brain, K$^+$-dependent (NCKX) and K$^+$-independent (NCX). Studies performed in vitro showed that in depolarized neurons with elevated cytosolic [Na$^+$], both NCX and NCKX reverse and mediate toxic Ca^{2+} influx. Since analogous mechanisms very likely operate in the ischemic brain, the postischemic recovery of brain function could be improved by preventing NCX and NCKX reversal during ischemia. Inhibitors of NCX reversal are already available and improve brain recovery from ischemia. One may predict that an even better outcome could be reached if NCKX reversal were also prevented. However, to date, no inhibitors of NCKX reversal have been developed.

1   Plasmalemmal Na$^+$/Ca^{2+} Exchangers in the Brain

Two families of plasmalemmal Na$^+$/Ca^{2+} exchangers, K$^+$-dependent (NCKX) and K$^+$-independent (NCX), are expressed in the central nervous system and play an important role in Ca^{2+} homeostasis. Using the electrochemical Na$^+$ (in the case of NCX) or Na$^+$ and K$^+$ (in the case of NCKX) gradients established by Na$^+$, K$^+$-ATPase as the source or energy, the exchangers transport Ca^{2+} across the plasma membrane (for reviews see Blaustein and Lederer, 1999; Philipson and Nicoll, 2000; Schnetkamp, 2004).

The NCX family includes NCX1 (Nicoll et al., 1990; Kofuji et al., 1992), NCX2 (Li et al., 1994), and NCX3 (Nicoll et al., 1996), whereas the NCKX family includes NCKX1 (Reiländer et al., 1992), NCKX2 (Tsoi et al., 1998), NCKX3 (Kraev et al., 2001), NCKX4 (Li et al., 2002), NCKX5 (Schnetkamp, 2004), and NCKX6 (Cai and Lytton, 2004) isoforms. Alternative splicing of NCX1 and NCX3 (Quednau et al., 1997), NCKX1 (Poon et al., 2000), and NCKX2 (Prinsen et al., 2000) provides an additional level of heterogeneity in these proteins.

NCX and NCKX isoforms are expressed in distinct brain regions and cells (Yu and Colvin, 1997; Tsoi et al., 1998; Sakaue et al., 2000; Kraev et al., 2001; Li et al., 2002; Papa et al., 2003) in a developmentally regulated manner (Sakaue et al., 2000; Polumuri et al., 2002; Li and Lytton, 2002). NCKX isoforms are preferentially expressed in neurons (Kiedrowski et al., 2002), although NCKX1 unlike other NCKXs is abundantly expressed only in the retina (Poon et al., 2000). Within single neurons, NCX and NCKX isoforms, such as NCX1 (Juhaszova et al., 2000) or NCKX2 (Kim et al., 2003), are highly expressed in nerve terminals.

1.1 Stoichiometry of NCX and NCKX Exchange

While there is consensus regarding NCKX stoichiometry, 4 Na$^+$/(1 Ca^{2+} + 1 K$^+$) (Cervetto et al., 1989; Schnetkamp et al., 1989; Szerencsei et al., 2001; Dong et al., 2001), that of NCX remains a matter of debate. Although a 3 Na$^+$/1 Ca^{2+} (3:1) ratio for NCX operation was accepted for some time (Blaustein and Lederer, 1999), a 4 Na$^+$/1 Ca^{2+} (4:1) stoichiometry was recently proposed (Fujioka et al., 2000; Dong et al., 2002). The data of Kang and Hilgemann (2004) suggest that although 3:1 is the dominant mode of NCX operation, additional modes are possible and account for the reported discrepancies. Because both NCKX and NCX are electrogenic exchangers, i.e., the overall charge associated with Na$^+$ transport exceeds that associated with Ca^{2+} transport, their operation generates membrane potential (E_m) and is affected by the existing E_m.

1.2 The Direction of NCX-Mediated and NCKX-Mediated Ca^{2+} Flow

Whether NCX or NCKX mediate Ca^{2+} efflux (forward mode) or influx (reverse mode) is determined by the difference between E_m and the equilibrium potential of a given exchanger (E_{NCX} or E_{NCKX}). When E_m is lower than E_{NCX} or E_{NCKX}, as under physiological conditions (❍ *Table 12-1*, row 1), the exchangers operate

□ Table 12-1

Equilibrium potentials of NCX (E_{NCX}) and NCKX (E_{NCKX}) under basal conditions and following dissipation of Na$^+$ and K$^+$ concentration gradients

Row number	[Na$^+$]$_c$ (mM)	[Na$^+$]$_o$ (mM)	[K$^+$]$_c$ (mM)	[K$^+$]$_o$ (mM)	[Ca^{2+}]$_c$ (μM)	[Ca^{2+}]$_o$ (μM)	$E_{NCX\ 3:1}$ (mV)	$E_{NCX\ 4:1}$ (mV)	E_{NCKX} (mV)
Basal conditions									
1	4	150	150	5	0.1	1300	+37	+67	+225
Na$^+$ and K$^+$ gradients dissipated									
2	[Na$^+$]$_c$ = [Na$^+$]$_o$		[K$^+$]$_c$ = [K$^+$]$_o$		0.1	1300	−253	−127	−253
3	[Na$^+$]$_c$ = [Na$^+$]$_o$		[K$^+$]$_c$ = [K$^+$]$_o$		0.1	130	−192	−96	−199
4	[Na$^+$]$_c$ = [Na$^+$]$_o$		[K$^+$]$_c$ = [K$^+$]$_o$		1	130	−130	−65	−130
5	[Na$^+$]$_c$ = [Na$^+$]$_o$		[K$^+$]$_c$ = [K$^+$]$_o$		10	130	−69	−34	−69
6	[Na$^+$]$_c$ = [Na$^+$]$_o$		[K$^+$]$_c$ = [K$^+$]$_o$		100	130	−7	−4	−7

The above calculations assume the indicated cytosolic (suffix c) and extracellular (suffix o) concentrations of Na$^+$, K$^+$, and Ca^{2+}, and that stoichiometry of NCX is 3 Na$^+$/1 Ca^{2+} (3:1) or 4 Na$^+$/1 Ca^{2+} (4:1), and that of NCKX is 4 Na$^+$/(1 Ca^{2+} + 1 K$^+$)

$E_{NCX3:1} = 3E_{Na} - 2E_{Ca}$ (Blaustein and Lederer, 1999)

$E_{NCX4:1} = (4E_{Na} - 2E_{Ca})/2$ (Dong et al., 2002)

$E_{NCKX} = 4E_{Na} - 2E_{Ca} - E_K$ (Dong et al., 2001)

where E_{Ca}, E_{Na}, and E_K are equilibrium potentials for Ca^{2+}, Na$^+$, and K$^+$, respectively, calculated for 37°C using the Nernst equation

It should be noted that after dissipation of Na$^+$ and K$^+$ gradients (rows 2–6), the equilibrium potentials of NCX and NCKX are expected to be more negative than the plasma membrane potential. Consequently, NCX and NCKX would operate in the reverse mode and load the cells with Ca^{2+}

in the forward mode and extrude Ca^{2+}. Should Na$^+$ and K$^+$ concentration gradients collapse, yielding E_m close to 0 mV, the equilibrium potentials of NCX and NCKX would be less than −100 (❷ *Table 12-1*, row 2), creating a significant driving force for Ca^{2+} influx via the reversed exchangers. Although this driving force would decrease with the rise of cytosolic [Ca^{2+}] ([Ca^{2+}]$_c$) and drop in external [Ca^{2+}] ([Ca^{2+}]$_o$), the exchangers would continue to mediate Ca^{2+} influx until the Ca^{2+} concentration gradient across the plasma membrane dissipates (❷ *Table 12-1*, rows 2–6). One should note, however, that such a continuous operation of NCX or NCKX in the reverse mode requires that Na$^+$ efflux via the exchangers is matched by Na$^+$ influx via another pathway, for example, via N-methyl-D-aspartate (NMDA) or α-amino-3-hydroxy-5-methyl-4-isoxazolepropionic acid (AMPA)/kainate channel. Should this compensatory Na$^+$ influx be blocked, the reverse NCX or NCKX operation would soon stop due to a decrease in cytosolic [Na$^+$] and a buildup of negative E_m.

1.3 Drugs Interfering with Plasmalemmal Na$^+$/Ca^{2+} Exchange

Presently, no drugs able to inhibit NCKX are available. However, several NCX inhibitors have been developed. The most frequently used inhibitors and their actions are described below.

Amiloride derivatives, of which dichlorobenzamil is the most efficacious, interfere with Na$^+$- and Ca^{2+}-binding sites of the NCX molecule and inhibit both forward and reverse operation of NCX (Slaughter et al., 1988). Bepridil is a diarylaminopropylamine derivative that, unlike amiloride derivatives, only interferes with the Na$^+$-binding site(s) of NCX. Bepridil does not readily cross the plasma membrane and, therefore, preferentially prevents external Na$^+$ binding (Garcia et al., 1988). Consequently, bepridil tends to inhibit the forward rather than reverse mode of NCX (Garcia et al., 1988; Kiedrowski et al., 1994a). Both dichlorobenzamil and bepridil are very unspecific inhibitors of Na$^+$/Ca^{2+} exchange. Bepridil inhibits voltage-gated Na$^+$ and Ca^{2+} channels (Yatani et al., 1986), plasmalemmal Ca^{2+} pump (Raess and Record, 1990), Na$^+$, K$^+$-ATPase (Kovacic et al., 1992), NMDA receptors (Sobolevsky et al., 1997), and interferes with Ca^{2+} transport in isolated mitochondria (Matlib, 1985). Dichlorobenzamil inhibits Ca^{2+} channels, plasmalemmal Ca^{2+} pump, and Na$^+$, K$^+$-ATPase (Kim and Smith, 1986). Therefore, interpreting the effects of these drugs solely in terms of plasmalemmal Na$^+$/Ca^{2+}-exchange inhibition is problematic.

In the search for more specific NCX inhibitors, a benzyloxyphenyl derivative, KB-R7943, has been developed. KB-R7943 preferentially inhibits the reverse mode of NCX (Watano et al., 1996; Iwamoto et al., 1996), although effects on the forward mode have been reported (Kimura et al., 1999). Several unspecific effects of KB-R7943 have also been described. The drug inhibits voltage-gated Ca^{2+} channels (Matsuda et al., 2001; Czyż et al., 2002), nicotinic acetylcholine receptors (Pintado et al., 2000), and NMDA receptors (Sobolevsky and Khodorov, 1999; Czyż et al., 2002; Kiedrowski et al., 2004). The latter effect varies depending on preparation and/or experimental conditions. Sobolevsky and Khodorov (1999) reported that in acutely dissociated hippocampal neurons, 10-μM KB-R7943 inhibits over 50% of the steady-state NMDA receptor-mediated inward current within less than 1 s after its application. By contrast, in cultured forebrain neurons exposed to NMDA, Hoyt et al. (1998) failed to observe any major acute effects of the drug on the NMDA-induced inward current. Although Kiedrowski et al. (2004) showed that KB-R7943 partially inhibits the steady-state NMDA current in forebrain neurons, the inhibitory effect required about 2 min of the drug application in order to fully develop.

Recently, two additional benzyloxyphenyl derivatives, SEA0400 (Matsuda et al., 2001) and SN-6 (Iwamoto et al., 2004b) have been developed. Like KB-R7943, these drugs preferentially inhibit the reverse operation of NCX (Bouchard et al., 2004; Iwamoto et al., 2004a, b). An interesting feature of the benzyloxyphenyl derivatives is their selectivity to certain NCX isoforms. While KB-R7943 shows the highest affinity to NCX3 (Iwamoto et al., 2001), SEA0400 (Iwamoto et al., 2004a) and SN-6 (Iwamoto et al., 2004b) preferentially inhibit NCX1. Although SEA0400 very effectively inhibits NCX1 reversal (IC$_{50}$ = 0.056 μM, Iwamoto et al., 2004a), the drug has some additional effect(s): in heart tubes from fetuses of NCX1 knockout mice, 1-μM SEA0400 inhibits Ca^{2+} transients (Reuter et al., 2002).

Benzothiazepine, CGP-37157, considered to be a specific inhibitor of mitochondrial Na$^+$/Ca^{2+} exchange (Cox et al., 1993) also inhibits plasmalemmal NCX (but not NCKX) in neurons (Czyż and Kiedrowski, 2003) and NCX1-expressing oocytes (Omelchenko et al., 2003).

Finally, inhibition of NCX1 (Li et al., 1991) and NCX2 (Li et al., 1994) can be achieved by intracellular delivery of an exchanger inhibitory peptide (XIP), a homolog of the N-terminal portion (amino acids 219–238) of the cytosolic NCX1 loop. The mechanism of NCX1 inhibition by XIP may involve XIP interaction with a yet undetermined portion of the NCX1 molecule (Ottolia et al., 2001). XIP binds phosphatidylinositol 4,5-bisphosphate (PIP$_2$) (He et al., 2000), and PIP$_2$ strongly stimulates NCX1 (Hilgemann and Ball, 1996). It appears that the PIP$_2$ binding by XIP plays a role in the XIP-mediated inhibition of NCX. However, because of this binding, XIP is not a specific inhibitor of NCX. PIP$_2$ affects plasmalemmal Ca^{2+} pumps, Na$^+$/H$^+$ exchangers, K$^+$ channels, ryanodine-sensitive Ca^{2+} channels, and other mechanisms (reviewed by Hilgemann et al., 2001). Consequently, the exogenous XIP, by binding PIP$_2$, affects many mechanisms.

2 Na$^+$/Ca^{2+} Exchangers, Excitotoxicity, and Ischemic Brain Damage

Large amounts of the excitatory neurotransmitter glutamate are released into the interstitial space during brain ischemia (Benveniste et al., 1984; Hagberg et al., 1985; Globus et al., 1988). Glutamate exerts excitotoxic effects in vivo (Olney, 1969), and ischemic neuronal death has been associated with activation of glutamatergic NMDA (Simon et al., 1984) and AMPA/kainate receptors (Sheardown et al., 1990; Buchan et al., 1991). The prime event unleashed by activation of these receptors, and believed to ultimately lead to neuronal death, is Ca^{2+} overload (for reviews see Lee et al., 1999; Arundine and Tymianski, 2003) that eventually impairs mitochondrial function (most recent review, Nicholls, 2004). Deadly consequences of the excessive Ca^{2+} influx for cellular viability are well recognized (Schanne et al., 1979), and glutamate-induced neuronal death has been linked to Ca^{2+} influx (Choi, 1987; Tymianski et al., 1993).

2.1 Plasmalemmal Na$^+$/Ca^{2+} Exchangers and Glutamate-Induced Excitotoxicity in vitro

Activation of ionotropic glutamate receptors leads to a large increase in cytosolic [Na$^+$] in cultured neurons (Kiedrowski et al., 1994a, b; Pinelis et al., 1994). This increase may contribute to glutamate excitotoxicity by compromising plasmalemmal Na$^+$/Ca^{2+}-exchange operation in the forward mode and/or by reversing the exchange (❷ Table 12-1). Neurons express NCX and NCKX isoforms (Kiedrowski et al., 2002). To determine whether Ca^{2+} influx via reversed NCX and/or NCKX contributes to excitotoxicity, it is necessary to inhibit both NCX and NCKX reversal. Although, as mentioned earlier, no NCKX inhibitors are available, inhibition of both NCX and NCKX is possible in vitro by replacing Na$^+$ with Li$^+$ or Cs$^+$, ions that do not support either NCX or NCKX operation (Blaustein and Lederer, 1999). In depolarized and glucose-deprived cerebellar granule cells (with Na$^+$, K$^+$-ATPase inhibited by ouabain), replacement of Na$^+$ with Li$^+$ or Cs$^+$ robustly reduced NMDA-elicited Ca^{2+} influx and excitotoxicity, suggesting the involvement of plasmalemmal Na$^+$/Ca^{2+} exchange in the NMDA excitotoxicity mechanism (Czyż et al., 2002). To further test whether NCX and NCKX contribute to NMDA excitotoxicity, KB-R7943 was used to inhibit NCX reversal and K$^+$ was removed from the medium to prevent NCKX reversal. This approach revealed that NCX and NCKX contribute about equally to NMDA-induced excitotoxicity in cultured cerebellar granule cells (Czyż and Kiedrowski, 2002), although NCX plays a more important role in forebrain neurons (Kiedrowski et al., 2004).

Plasmalemmal Na$^+$/Ca^{2+} exchangers affect NMDA-induced excitotoxicity differently depending on the status of Na$^+$, K$^+$-ATPase operation. When Na$^+$, K$^+$-ATPase is inhibited, the activation of NMDA receptors leads to plasma membrane depolarization and high elevation in cytosolic [Na$^+$]. As shown in ❷ Figure 12-1a, under such conditions, the exchangers reverse and mediate toxic Ca^{2+} influx (Czyż and Kiedrowski, 2002; Czyż et al., 2002). However, when Na$^+$, K$^+$-ATPase is active and counteracts dissipation of Na$^+$ and K$^+$ concentration gradients (Kiedrowski, 1999; Czyż et al., 2002) (❷ Figure 12-1b), the exchangers operate in the forward mode and promote neuronal survival (Andreeva et al., 1991). KB-R7943, an inhibitor of the NCX reverse mode, fails to protect against NMDA excitotoxicity in neurons with active Na$^+$, K$^+$-ATPase (Hoyt et al., 1998), but plays a protective role in neurons with inhibited Na$^+$, K$^+$-ATPase (Kiedrowski et al., 2004). During brain ischemia Na$^+$, K$^+$-ATPase operation is compromised by ATP depletion, which favors NCX and NCKX reversal.

□ Figure 12-1

The impact of Na$^+$, K$^+$-ATPase activity on the mode of NCX and NCKX operation and glutamate excitotoxicity. (a) When Na$^+$, K$^+$-ATPase activity is compromised, activation of NMDA and AMPA/kainate receptors rapidly dissipates Na$^+$ and K$^+$ concentration gradients across the plasma membrane. Under such conditions, NCX and NCKX reverse and enhance Ca^{2+} accumulation. (b) As long as Na$^+$, K$^+$-ATPase effectively counteracts cytosolic [Na$^+$] increase, NCX and NCKX operate in the forward mode and diminish Ca^{2+} overload

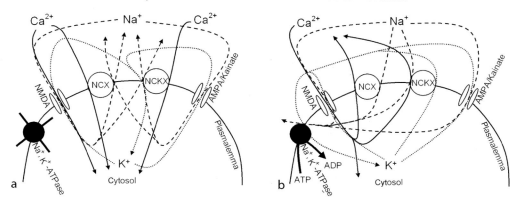

2.2 Plasmalemmal Na^+/Ca^{2+} Exchange Operation During Brain Ischemia

Within the first 2 min of global brain ischemia, anoxic depolarization develops, during which extracellular K^+ ($[K^+]_o$) increases to over 60 mM (Hansen, 1978; Hansen and Zeuthen, 1981; Xie et al., 1994, 1995; Sick et al., 1999), $[Na^+]_o$ drops to about 50 mM (Hansen and Zeuthen, 1981; Xie et al., 1994, 1995; Müller and Somjen, 2000a, b), and $[Ca^{2+}]_o$ decreases about ten times (Hansen and Zeuthen, 1981; Harris et al., 1981; Siemkowicz and Hansen, 1981; Benveniste et al., 1988; Silver and Erecińska, 1990; Xie et al., 1994, 1995). Anoxic depolarization is initiated by Na^+ influx via AMPA/kainate receptors, voltage-gated Na^+ channels (Xie et al., 1994, 1995; Tanaka et al., 1997; Müller and Somjen, 2000a, b), and NMDA receptors (Martin, 1999) and sets the stage for NCX and NCKX reversal (❯ *Table 12-1*).

Neurotoxic effects of global brain ischemia become apparent when ischemia lasts longer than 2 min (Smith et al., 1984; Kato et al., 1991). Because NCX and NCKX may reverse within the first 2 min of ischemia, it is very likely that Ca^{2+} influx via reversed NCX and/or NCKX contributes to ischemic brain damage, as predicted in the late 1980s (Siesjö, 1988; Choi, 1988). Although the role of plasmalemmal Na^+/Ca^{2+} exchange reversal in the ischemic damage of the white matter is well established (for a recent review see Stys, 2004), it has never been adequately tested whether the exchangers also mediate ischemic damage in the gray matter. The progress has been hampered by the lack of specific inhibitors. As mentioned earlier, no inhibitors of NCKX have been developed, whereas NCKX isoforms are expressed in neurons (Kiedrowski et al., 2002), reverse when elevation in cytosolic $[Na^+]$ coincides with plasma membrane depolarization and contribute to NMDA-induced excitotoxicity (Czyż and Kiedrowski, 2002).

Studies using NCX inhibitors, such as amiloride derivatives (Andreeva et al., 1991; Lobner and Lipton, 1993), XIP (Yu and Choi, 1997; Pignataro et al., 2004), KB-R7943 (Hoyt et al., 1998; Schröder et al., 1999; Breder et al., 2000; Aarts et al., 2003), or SEA0400 (Matsuda et al., 2001), and testing the outcome of ischemia or excitotoxicity yielded conflicting results. Neuroprotective effects were observed when inhibitors of NCX reverse mode, KB-R7943 or SEA0400, were used (Schröder et al., 1999; Breder et al., 2000; Matsuda et al., 2001; Czyż and Kiedrowski, 2002; Kiedrowski et al., 2004), whereas amiloride derviatives that inhibit the NCX forward mode enhanced neuronal death (Andreeva et al., 1991). But inhibitors of the NCX reverse mode, such as KB-R7943, were not always neuroprotective (Aarts et al., 2003). It is worth noting, however, that inhibition of NCX reversal alone may be insufficient to reduce Ca^{2+} load below toxic levels. In fact, in primary cultures of cerebellar granule cells that express NCX and NCKX (Kiedrowski et al., 2002), inhibition of NCX reversal (with KB-R7943) and NCKX reversal (by K^+ removal) was necessary to significantly decrease NMDA-induced Ca^{2+} load and excitotoxicity (Czyż and Kiedrowski, 2002).

2.3 High Activity of NCKX in Hippocampal CA1 Neurons

Pyramidal neurons of the hippocampal CA1 region are particularly vulnerable to global brain ischemia (Pulsinelli and Brierley, 1979; Kirino, 1982). They die about 3 days after ischemia in a complex mechanism triggered by an increased expression of the gene silencer REST (Calderone et al., 2003), which suppresses expression of the GluR2 subunit in the CA1 region (Pellegrini-Giampietro et al., 1992, 1997). AMPA channels that lack the GluR2 subunit are Ca-permeable (Hollmann et al., 1991; Hume et al., 1991; Verdoorn et al., 1991), and Ca^{2+} influx via these channels appears to kill CA1 neurons in a mechanism involving cyclin-dependent kinase 5-dependent phosphorylation of NMDA receptors that greatly enhances NMDA receptor activity (Wang et al., 2003; Liu et al., 2004).

Although the events downstream of the REST activation in CA1 neurons have been identified, it remains unclear why the REST expression is specifically enhanced in post-ischemic CA1 neurons, although prior to ischemia this expression is similar in all hippocampal neurons (Calderone et al., 2003). It appears that some ischemic events specific to CA1 neurons trigger REST expression. If NCX or NCKX reversal plays any role in these events, differences in NCX or NCKX activities between CA1 neurons versus other, more resistant, neuronal populations should be evident. Recent data indicate that in cultured CA1 neurons, Ca^{2+} influx via reversed NCKX is several-fold faster than in forebrain neurons or cerebellar granule cells (Kiedrowski, 2004), which lends support for testing the hypothesis that the high activity of reversed NCKX in CA1 neurons may sensitize them to ischemia.

2.4 Dual Role of Plasmalemmal Na$^+$/Ca^{2+} Exchange in Ischemic Brain Damage

The mode of NCX and NCKX operation depends on the degree to which Na$^+$ and K$^+$ concentration gradients are dissipated. The level of this dissipation depends on the degree to which Na$^+$, K$^+$-ATPase operation is compromised by ATP depletion. During focal brain ischemia, ATP depletion is greater in the ischemic core than in the area penumbra (Mies et al., 1991; Hossmann, 1994). Therefore, Na$^+$, K$^+$-ATPase can be operative in the area penumbra and counteract the Na$^+$ and K$^+$ concentration gradient dissipation. As a result, NCX and/or NCKX in the area penumbra may operate in the forward mode and promote neuronal survival (Jeon et al., 2003; Pignataro et al., 2003, 2004). However, the exchangers may reverse transiently when waves of anoxic depolarization, linked to the severity of brain damage, invade the area penumbra (Mies et al., 1993). It is possible that NCX and/or NCKX reverse during each such wave, but otherwise operate in the forward mode. Indeed, inhibition of the NCX reverse mode with the relatively selective drug SEA0400 yielded impressive neuroprotection in focal brain ischemia (Matsuda et al., 2001).

During reperfusion, neuronal [Ca^{2+}]$_c$ returns to low levels (Siemkowicz and Hansen, 1981; Silver and Erecińska, 1992; Tanaka et al., 2002). Very likely, this return involves NCX and/or NCKX operation in the forward mode. Because postischemic restoration of low [Ca^{2+}]$_c$ seems necessary for long-term neuronal survival, plasmalemmal Na$^+$/Ca^{2+} exchangers may play a dual role in ischemia. Their reversal during anoxic depolarization may contribute to ischemic brain damage, but their return to the forward mode during reperfusion may be necessary for neuronal survival.

3   Concluding Remarks

The role of plasmalemmal Na$^+$/Ca^{2+} exchangers in brain ischemia requires further study. Although NCX- and NCKX-mediated Ca^{2+} influx contributes to NMDA-induced excitotoxicity (Czyż and Kiedrowski, 2002), its importance during anoxic depolarization, when pH drops to about 6.6 (Siemkowicz and Hansen, 1981; Kraig et al., 1983; Smith et al., 1986), remains unclear. This low pH not only suppresses NCX (Doering et al., 1996; Linck et al., 1998; Egger and Niggli, 2000) and NCKX activity (Schnetkamp, 1995) but also profoundly inhibits NMDA receptors (Giffard et al., 1990; Tang et al., 1990; Traynelis and Cull-Candy, 1990, 1991). The contribution of NMDA receptors versus reversed NCX and/or NCKX to Ca^{2+} influx in neurons undergoing anoxic depolarization has never been determined.

References

Aarts M, Iihara K, Wei WL, Xiong ZG, Arundine M, et al. 2003. A key role for TRPM7 channels in anoxic neuronal death. Cell 115: 863-877.

Andreeva N, Khodorov B, Stelmashook E, Cragoe E, Victorov I. 1991. Inhibition of Na$^+$/Ca^{2+} exchange enhances delayed neuronal death elicited by glutamate in cerebellar granule cell cultures. Brain Res 548: 322-325.

Arundine M, Tymianski M. 2003. Molecular mechanisms of calcium-dependent neurodegeneration in excitotoxicity. Cell Calcium 34: 325-337.

Benveniste H, Drejer J, Schousboe A, Diemer NH. 1984. Elevation of the extracellular concentrations of glutamate and aspartate in rat hippocampus during transient cerebral ischemia monitored by intracerebral microdialysis. J Neurochem 43: 1369-1374.

Benveniste H, Jorgensen MB, Diemer NH, Hansen AJ. 1988. Calcium accumulation by glutamate receptor activation is involved in hippocampal cell damage after ischemia. Acta Neurol Scand 78: 529-536.

Blaustein MP, Lederer WJ. 1999. Sodium/calcium exchange: Its physiological implications. Physiol Rev 79: 763-854.

Bouchard R, Omelchenko A, Le HD, Choptiany P, Matsuda T, et al. 2004. Effects of SEA0400 on mutant NCX1.1 Na$^+$-Ca^{2+} exchangers with altered ionic regulation. Mol Pharmacol 65: 802-810.

Breder J, Sabelhaus CF, Opitz T, Reymann KG, Schröder UH. 2000. Inhibition of different pathways influencing Na$^+$ homeostasis protects organotypic hippocampal slice cultures from hypoxic/hypoglycemic injury. Neuropharmacology 39: 1779-1787.

Buchan MA, Li H, Cho S, Pulsinelli WA. 1991. Blockade of the AMPA receptor prevents CA1 hippocampal injury following severe but transient forebrain ischemia in adult rats. Neurosci Lett 132: 255-258.

Cai X, Lytton J. 2004. Molecular cloning of a sixth member of the K$^+$-dependent Na$^+$/Ca^{2+} exchanger gene family, NCKX6. J Biol Chem 279: 5867-5876.

Calderone A, Jover T, Noh KM, Tanaka H, Yokota H, et al. 2003. Ischemic insults derepress the gene silencer REST in neurons destined to die. J Neurosci 23: 2112-2121.

Cervetto L, Lagnado L, Perry RJ, Robinson DW, McNaughton PA. 1989. Extrusion of calcium from rod outer segments is driven by both sodium and potassium gradients. Nature 337: 740-743.

Choi DW. 1987. Ionic dependence of glutamate neurotoxicity. J Neurosci 7: 369-379.

Choi DW. 1988. Glutamate neurotoxicity and diseases of the nervous system. Neuron 1: 623-634.

Cox DA, Conforti L, Sperelakis N, Matlib MA. 1993. Selectivity of inhibition on Na$^+$-Ca^{2+} exchange of heart mitochondria by benzothiazepine CGP-37157. J Cardiovasc Pharmacol 21: 595-599.

Czyż A, Kiedrowski L. 2002. In depolarized and glucose-deprived neurons, Na$^+$ influx reverses plasmalemmal K$^+$-dependent and K$^+$-independent Na$^+$/Ca^{2+} exchangers and contributes to NMDA excitotoxicity. J Neurochem 83: 1321-1328.

Czyż A, Kiedrowski L. 2003. Inhibition of plasmalemmal Na$^+$/Ca^{2+} exchange by mitochondrial Na$^+$/Ca^{2+} exchange inhibitor 7-chloro-5-(2-chlorophenyl)-1,5-dihydro-4,1-benzothiazepin-2(3H)-one (CGP-37157) in cerebellar granule cells. Biochem Pharmacol 66: 2409-2411.

Czyż A, Baranauskas G, Kiedrowski L. 2002. Instrumental role of Na$^+$ in NMDA excitotoxicity in glucose-deprived and depolarized cerebellar granule cells. J Neurochem 81: 379-389.

Doering AE, Eisner DA, Lederer WJ. 1996. Cardiac Na-Ca exchange and pH. Ann N Y Acad Sci 779: 182-198.

Dong H, Light PE, French RJ, Lytton J. 2001. Electrophysiological characterization and ionic stoichiometry of the rat brain K$^+$-dependent Na$^+$/Ca^{2+} exchanger, NCKX2. J Biol Chem 276: 25919-25928.

Dong H, Dunn J, Lytton J. 2002. Stoichiometry of the cardiac Na$^+$/Ca^{2+} exchanger NCX1.1 measured in transfected HEK cells. Biophys J 82: 1943-1952.

Egger M, Niggli E. 2000. Paradoxical block of the Na$^+$-Ca^{2+} exchanger by extracellular protons in guinea-pig ventricular myocytes. J Physiol 523: 353-366.

Fujioka Y, Komeda M, Matsuoka S. 2000. Stoichiometry of Na$^+$-Ca^{2+} exchange in inside-out patches excised from guinea-pig ventricular myocytes. J Physiol 523: 339-351.

Garcia ML, Slaughter RS, King F, Kaczorowski GJ. 1988. Inhibition of sodium-calcium exchange in cardiac sarcolemmal membrane vesicles. 1 Mechanism of inhibition by bepridil. Biochemistry 27: 2410-2415.

Giffard RG, Monyer H, Christine CW, Choi DW. 1990. Acidosis reduces NMDA receptor activation, glutamate neurotoxicity, and oxygen-glucose deprivation neuronal injury in cortical cultures. Brain Res 506: 339-342.

Globus MY, Busto R, Dietrich WD, Martinez E, Valdes I, et al. 1988. Effect of ischemia on the in vivo release of striatal dopamine, glutamate, and gamma-aminobutyric acid studied by intracerebral microdialysis. J Neurochem 51: 1455-1464.

Hagberg H, Lehmann A, Sandberg M, Nystrom B, Jacobson I, et al. 1985. Ischemia-induced shift of inhibitory and excitatory amino acids from intra- to extracellular compartments. J Cereb Blood Flow Metab 5: 413-419.

Hansen AJ. 1978. The extracellular potassium concentration in brain cortex following ischemia in hypo- and hyperglycemic rats. Acta Physiol Scand 102: 324-329.

Hansen AJ, Zeuthen T. 1981. Extracellular ion concentrations during spreading depression and ischemia in the rat brain cortex. Acta Physiol Scand 113: 437-445.

Harris RJ, Symon L, Branston NM, Bayhan M. 1981. Changes in extracellular calcium activity in cerebral ischaemia. J Cereb Blood Flow Metab 1: 203-209.

He Z, Feng S, Tong Q, Hilgemann DW, Philipson KD. 2000. Interaction of PIP$_2$ with the XIP region of the cardiac Na/Ca exchanger. Am J Physiol Cell Physiol 278: C661-666.

Hilgemann DW, Ball R. 1996. Regulation of cardiac Na$^+$, Ca^{2+} exchange and K$_{ATP}$ potassium channels by PIP$_2$. Science 273: 956-959.

Hilgemann DW, Feng S, Nasuhoglu C. 2001. The complex and intriguing lives of PIP2 with ion channels and transporters. RE19. Sci STKE.

Hollmann M, Hartley M, Heinemann S. 1991. Ca^{2+} permeability of KA-AMPA-gated glutamate receptor channels depends on subunit composition. Science 252: 851-853.

Hossmann KA. 1994. Viability thresholds and the penumbra of focal ischemia. Ann Neurol 36: 557-565.

Hoyt KR, Arden SR, Aizenman E, Reynolds IJ. 1998. Reverse Na$^+$/Ca^{2+} exchange contributes to glutamate-induced intracellular Ca^{2+} concentration increases in cultured rat forebrain neurons. Mol Pharmacol 53: 742-749.

Hume RI, Dingledine R, Heinemann SF. 1991. Identification of a site in glutamate receptor subunits that controls calcium permeability. Science 253: 1028-1031.

Iwamoto T, Watano T, Shigekawa M. 1996. A novel isothiourea derivative selectively inhibits the reverse mode of Na$^+$/Ca^{2+} exchange in cells expressing NCX1. J Biol Chem 271: 22391-22397.

Iwamoto T, Kita S, Uehara A, Inoue Y, Taniguchi Y, et al. 2001. Structural domains influencing sensitivity to isothiourea derivative inhibitor KB-R7943 in cardiac Na$^+$/Ca^{2+} exchanger. Mol Pharmacol 59: 524-531.

Iwamoto T, Kita S, Uehara A, Imanaga I, Matsuda T, et al. 2004a. Molecular determinants of Na$^+$/Ca^{2+} exchange (NCX1) inhibition by SEA0400. J Biol Chem 279: 7544-7553.

Iwamoto T, Inoue Y, Ito K, Sakaue T, Kita S, et al. 2004b. The exchanger inhibitory peptide region-dependent inhibition of Na$^+$/Ca^{2+} exchange by SN-6 [2-[4-(4-nitrobenzyloxy)benzyl]thiazolidine-4-carboxylic acid ethyl ester], a novel benzyloxyphenyl derivative. Mol Pharmacol 66: 45-55.

Jeon D, Chu K, Kim Y, Yoon B, Shin H. 2003. Na$^+$/Ca^{2+} exchanger2 protects cell death after focal cerebral ischemia. Soc Neurosci [Abstracts 308.310].

Juhaszova M, Church P, Blaustein MP, Stanley EF. 2000. Location of calcium transporters at presynaptic terminals. Eur J Neurosci 12: 839-846.

Kang TM, Hilgemann DW. 2004. Multiple transport modes of the cardiac Na$^+$/Ca^{2+} exchanger. Nature 427: 544-548.

Kato H, Liu Y, Araki T, Kogure K. 1991. Temporal profile of the effects of pretreatment with brief cerebral ischemia on the neuronal damage following secondary ischemic insult in the gerbil: Cumulative damage and protective effects. Brain Res 553: 238-242.

Kiedrowski L. 1999. Elevated extracellular K$^+$ concentrations inhibit N-methyl-D-aspartate-induced Ca^{2+} influx and excitotoxicity. Mol Pharmacol 56: 737-743.

Kiedrowski L. 2004. High activity of plasmalemmal K$^+$-dependent Na$^+$/Ca^{2+} exchangers in hippocampal CA1 neurons. Neuroreport 15: 2113-2116.

Kiedrowski L, Brooker G, Costa E, Wroblewski JT. 1994a. Glutamate impairs neuronal calcium extrusion while reducing sodium gradient. Neuron 12: 295-300.

Kiedrowski L, Wroblewski JT, Costa E. 1994b. Intracellular sodium concentration in cultured cerebellar granule cells challenged with glutamate. Molec Pharmacol 45: 1050-1054.

Kiedrowski L, Czyż A, Li X-F, Lytton J. 2002. Preferential expression of plasmalemmal K-dependent Na$^+$/Ca^{2+} exchangers in neurons versus astrocytes. Neuroreport 13: 1529-1532.

Kiedrowski L, Czyż A, Baranauskas G, Li X-F, Lytton J. 2004. Differential contribution of plasmalemmal Na$^+$/Ca^{2+} exchange isoforms to sodium-dependent calcium influx and NMDA excitotoxicity in depolarized neurons. J Neurochem 90: 117-128.

Kim D, Smith TW. 1986. Inhibition of multiple trans-sarcolemmal cation flux pathways by dichlorobenzamil in cultured chick heart cells. Mol Pharmacol 30: 164-170.

Kim MH, Lee SH, Park KH, Ho WK, Lee SH. 2003. Distribution of K$^+$-dependent Na$^+$/Ca^{2+} exchangers in the rat supraoptic magnocellular neuron is polarized to axon terminals. J Neurosci 23: 11673-11680.

Kimura J, Watano T, Kawahara M, Sakai E, Yatabe J. 1999. Direction-independent block of bi-directional Na$^+$/Ca^{2+} exchange current by KB-R7943 in guinea-pig cardiac myocytes. Br J Pharmacol 128: 969-974.

Kirino T. 1982. Delayed neuronal death in the gerbil hippocampus following ischemia. Brain Res 239: 57-69.

Kofuji P, Hadley RW, Kieval RS, Lederer WJ, Schulze DH. 1992. Expression of the Na-Ca exchanger in diverse tissues—a study using the cloned human cardiac Na-Ca exchanger. Am J Physiol 263: C1241-C1249.

Kovacic H, Gallice P, Crevat A. 1992. Inhibition of sodium pump by bepridil—an invitro and microcalorimetric study. Biochem Pharmacol 44: 1529-1534.

Kraev A, Quednau BD, Leach S, Li XF, Dong H, et al. 2001. Molecular cloning of a third member of the potassium-dependent sodium-calcium exchanger gene family, NCKX3. J Biol Chem 276: 23161-23172.

Kraig RP, Ferreira-Filho CR, Nicholson C. 1983. Alkaline and acid transients in cerebellar microenvironment. J Neurophysiol 49: 831-850.

Lee JM, Zipfel GJ, Choi DW. 1999. The changing landscape of ischaemic brain injury mechanisms. Nature 399: A7-A14.

Li XF, Lytton J. 2002. Differential expression of Na/Ca exchanger and Na/Ca + K exchanger transcripts in rat brain. Ann N Y Acad Sci 976: 64-66.

Li XF, Kraev AS, Lytton J. 2002. Molecular cloning of a fourth member of the potassium-dependent sodium-calcium exchanger gene family, NCKX4. J Biol Chem 277: 48410-48417.

Li Z, Nicoll DA, Collins A, Hilgemann DW, Filoteo AG, et al. 1991. Identification of a peptide inhibitor of the cardiac sarcolemmal Na$^+$-Ca^{2+} exchanger. J Biol Chem 266: 1014-1020.

Li Z, Matsuoka S, Hryshko LV, Nicoll DA, Bersohn MM, et al. 1994. Cloning of the NCX2 isoform of the plasma membrane Na$^+$-Ca^{2+} exchanger. J Biol Chem 269: 17434-17439.

Linck B, Qiu Z, He Z, Tong Q, Hilgemann DW, et al. 1998. Functional comparison of the three isoforms of the Na$^+$/Ca^{2+} exchanger (NCX1, NCX2, NCX3). Am J Physiol 274: C415-423.

Liu S, Lau L, Wei J, Zhu D, Zou S, et al. 2004. Expression of Ca^{2+}-permeable AMPA receptor channels primes cell death in transient forebrain ischemia. Neuron 43: 43-55.

Lobner D, Lipton P. 1993. Intracellular calcium levels and calcium fluxes in the CA1 region of the rat hippocampus slice during in vitro ischemia: Relationship to electrophysiological cell damage. J Neurosci 13: 4861-4871.

Martin RL. 1999. Block of rapid depolarization induced by in vitro energy depletion of rat dorsal vagal motoneurones. J Physiol 519: 131-141.

Matlib MA. 1985. Action of bepridil, a new calcium channel blocker on oxidative phosphorylation, oligomycin-sensitive adenosine triphosphatase activity, swelling, Ca^{++} uptake and Na^+-induced Ca^{++} release processes of rabbit heart mitochondria in vitro. J Pharmacol Exp Ther 233: 376-381.

Matsuda T, Arakawa N, Takuma K, Kishida Y, Kawasaki Y, et al. 2001. SEA0400, a novel and selective inhibitor of the Na^+- Ca^{2+} exchanger, attenuates reperfusion injury in the in vitro and in vivo cerebral ischemic models. J Pharmacol Exp Ther 298: 249-256.

Mies G, Ishimaru S, Xie Y, Seo K, Hossmann KA. 1991. Ischemic thresholds of cerebral protein synthesis and energy state following middle cerebral artery occlusion in rat. J Cereb Blood Flow Metab 11: 753-761.

Mies G, Iijima T, Hossmann KA. 1993. Correlation between peri-infarct DC shifts and ischaemic neuronal damage in rat. Neuroreport 4: 709-711.

Müller M, Somjen GG. 2000a. Na^+ and K^+ concentrations, extra- and intracellular voltages, and the effect of TTX in hypoxic rat hippocampal slices. J Neurophysiol 83: 735-745.

Müller M, Somjen GG. 2000b. Na^+ dependence and the role of glutamate receptors and Na^+ channels in ion fluxes during hypoxia of rat hippocampal slices. J Neurophysiol 84: 1869-1880.

Nicholls DG. 2004. Mitochondrial dysfunction and glutamate excitotoxicity studied in primary neuronal cultures. Curr Mol Med 4: 149-177.

Nicoll DA, Longoni S, Philipson KD. 1990. Molecular cloning and functional expression of the cardiac sarcolemmal Na^+-Ca^{2+} exchanger. Science 250: 562-565.

Nicoll DA, Quednau BD, Qui ZY, Xia YR, Lusis AJ, et al. 1996. Cloning of a third mammalian Na^+-Ca^{2+} exchanger, NCX3. J Biol Chem 271: 24914-24921.

Olney JW. 1969. Brain lesions, obesity, and other disturbances in mice treated with monosodium glutamate. Science 164: 719-721.

Omelchenko A, Bouchard R, Le HD, Choptiany P, Visen N, et al. 2003. Inhibition of canine (NCX1.1) and Drosophila (CALX1.1) Na^+-Ca^{2+} exchangers by 7-chloro-3,5-dihydro-5-phenyl-1H-4,1-benzothiazepine-2-one (CGP-37157). J Pharmacol Exp Ther 306: 1050-1057.

Ottolia M, John S, Qiu Z, Philipson KD. 2001. Split Na^+-Ca^{2+} exchangers Implications for function and expression. J Biol Chem 276: 19603-19609.

Papa M, Canitano A, Boscia F, Castaldo P, Sellitti S, et al. 2003. Differential expression of the Na^+-Ca^{2+} exchanger transcripts and proteins in rat brain regions. J Comp Neurol 461: 31-48.

Pellegrini-Giampietro DE, Zukin RS, Bennett MVL, Cho SH, Pulsinelli WA. 1992. Switch in glutamate receptor subunit gene expression in CA1 subfield of hippocampus following global ischemia in rats. Proc Natl Acad Sci USA 89: 10499-10503.

Pellegrini-Giampietro DE, Gorter JA, Bennett MV, Zukin RS. 1997. The GluR2 (GluR-B) hypothesis: Ca^{2+}-permeable AMPA receptors in neurological disorders. Trends Neurosci 20: 464-470.

Philipson KD, Nicoll DA. 2000. Sodium-calcium exchange: A molecular perspective. Annu Rev Physiol 62: 111-133.

Pignataro G, Castaldo P, Gala R, Cuomo O, Di Renzo GF, 2003. Pattern of expression of Na^+/Ca^{2+} exchanger encoding genes NCX1, NCX2 and NCX3 in focal cerebral ischemia induced by permanent middle cerebral artery occlusion (pMCAO). Soc Neurosci [Abstracts 531.514].

Pignataro G, Tortiglione A, Scorziello A, Giaccio L, Secondo A, et al. 2004. Evidence for a protective role played by the Na^+/Ca^{2+} exchanger in cerebral ischemia induced by middle cerebral artery occlusion in male rats. Neuropharmacology 46: 439-448.

Pinelis VG, Segal M, Greenberger V, Khodorov BI. 1994. Changes in cytosolic sodium caused by a toxic glutamate treatment of cultured hippocampal neurons. Biochem Mol Biol Int 32: 475-482.

Pintado AJ, Herrero CJ, Garcia AG, Montiel C. 2000. The novel Na^+/Ca^{2+} exchange inhibitor KB-R7943 also blocks native and expressed neuronal nicotinic receptors. Br J Pharmacol 130: 1893-1902.

Polumuri SK, Ruknudin A, McCarthy MM, Perrot-Sinal TS, Schulze DH. 2002. Sodium-calcium exchanger NCX1, NCX2, and NCX3 transcripts in developing rat brain. Ann N Y Acad Sci 976: 60-63.

Poon S, Leach S, Li XF, Tucker JE, Schnetkamp PP, et al. 2000. Alternatively spliced isoforms of the rat eye sodium/calcium + potassium exchanger NCKX1. Am J Physiol 278: C651-660.

Prinsen CF, Szerencsei RT, Schnetkamp PP. 2000. Molecular cloning and functional expression of the potassium-dependent sodium-calcium exchanger from human and chicken retinal cone photoreceptors. J Neurosci 20: 1424-1434.

Pulsinelli WA, Brierley JB. 1979. A new model of bilateral hemispheric ischemia in the unanesthetized rat. Stroke 10: 267-272.

Quednau BD, Nicoll DA, Philipson KD. 1997. Tissue specificity and alternative splicing of the Na^+/Ca^{2+} exchanger isoforms NCX1, NCX2, and NCX3 in rat. Am J Physiol 41: C1250-C1261.

Raess BU, Record DM. 1990. Inhibition of erythrocyte Ca^{2+}-pump by Ca^{2+} antagonists. Biochem Pharmacol 40: 2549-2555.

Reiländer H, Achilles A, Friedel U, Maul G, Lottspeich F, et al. 1992. Primary structure and functional expression of the Na/Ca,K-exchanger from bovine rod photoreceptors. EMBO J 11: 1689-1695.

Reuter H, Henderson SA, Han T, Matsuda T, Baba A, et al. 2002. Knockout mice for pharmacological screening:

Testing the specificity of Na$^+$-Ca^{2+} exchange inhibitors. Circ Res 91: 90-92.

Sakaue M, Nakamura H, Kaneko I, Kawasaki Y, Arakawa N, et al. 2000. Na$^+$-Ca^{2+} exchanger isoforms in rat neuronal preparations: Different changes in their expression during postnatal development. Brain Res 881: 212-216.

Schanne FA, Kane AB, Young EE, Farber JL. 1979. Calcium dependence of toxic cell death: A final common pathway. Science 206: 700-702.

Schnetkamp PP. 1995. Chelating properties of the Ca^{2+} transport site of the retinal rod Na-Ca+K exchanger: Evidence for a common Ca^{2+} and Na$^+$ binding site. Biochemistry 34: 7282-7287.

Schnetkamp PP. 2004. The SLC24 Na$^+$/Ca^{2+}-K$^+$ exchanger family: Vision and beyond. Pflugers Arch 447: 683-688.

Schnetkamp PP, Basu DK, Szerencsei RT. 1989. Na$^+$-Ca^{2+} exchange in bovine rod outer segments requires and transports K$^+$. Am J Physiol 257: C153-C157.

Schröder UH, Breder J, Sabelhaus CF, Reymann KG. 1999. The novel Na$^+$/Ca^{2+} exchange inhibitor KB-R7943 protects CA1 neurons in rat hippocampal slices against hypoxic/hypoglycemic injury. Neuropharmacology 38: 319-321.

Sheardown MJ, Nielsen EO, Hansen AJ, Jacobsen P, Honore T. 1990. 2,3-Dihydroxy-6-nitro-7-sulfamoyl-benzo(F)quinoxaline: A neuroprotectant for cerebral ischemia. Science 247: 571-574.

Sick TJ, Tang R, Perez-Pinzon MA. 1999. Cerebral blood flow does not mediate the effect of brain temperature on recovery of extracellular potassium ion activity after transient focal ischemia in the rat. Brain Res 821: 400-406.

Siesjö BK. 1988. Historical overview: Calcium, ischemia and death of brain cells. Ann N Y Acad Sci 522: 638-661.

Siemkowicz E, Hansen AJ. 1981. Brain extracellular ion composition and EEG activity following 10 minutes ischemia in normo- and hyperglycemic rats. Stroke 12: 236-240.

Silver IA, Erecińska M. 1990. Intracellular and extracellular changes of [Ca^{2+}] in hypoxia and ischemia in rat brain in vivo. J Gen Physiol 95: 837-866.

Silver IA, Erecinska M. 1992. Ion homeostasis in rat brain in vivo: Intra-cellular and extracellular [Ca^{2+}] and [H$^+$] in the hippocampus during recovery from short-term, transient ischemia. J Cereb Blood Flow Metab 12: 759-772.

Simon RP, Swan JH, Griffiths T, Meldrum BS. 1984. Blockade of N-methyl-D-aspartate receptors may protect against ischemic damage in the brain. Science 226: 850-852.

Slaughter RS, Garcia ML, Cragoe EJ Jr, Reeves JP, Kaczorowski GJ. 1988. Inhibition of sodium-calcium exchange in cardiac sarcolemmal membrane vesicles. 1 Mechanism of inhibition by amiloride analogues. Biochemistry 27: 2403-2409.

Smith ML, Auer RN, Siesjö BK. 1984. The density and distribution of ischemic brain injury in the rat following 2–10 min of forebrain ischemia. Acta Neuropathol 64: 319-332.

Smith ML, von Hanwehr R, Siesjö BK. 1986. Changes in extra- and intracellular pH in the brain during and following ischemia in hyperglycemic and in moderately hypoglycemic rats. J Cereb Blood Flow Metab 6: 574-583.

Sobolevsky AI, Khodorov BI. 1999. Blockade of NMDA channels in acutely isolated rat hippocampal neurons by the Na$^+$/Ca^{2+} exchange inhibitor KB-R7943. Neuropharmacology 38: 1235-1242.

Sobolevsky A, Koshelev S, Khodorov BI. 1997. Bepridil-induced blockade of NMDA channels in rat hippocampal neurons. Neuropharmacology 36: 319-324.

Stys PK. 2004. White matter injury mechanisms. Curr Mol Med 4: 113-130.

Szerencsei RT, Prinsen CF, Schnetkamp PP. 2001. Stoichiometry of the retinal cone Na/Ca-K exchanger heterologously expressed in insect cells: Comparison with the bovine heart Na/Ca exchanger. Biochemistry 40: 6009-6015.

Tanaka E, Yamamoto S, Kudo Y, Mihara S, Higashi H. 1997. Mechanisms underlying the rapid depolarization produced by deprivation of oxygen and glucose in rat hippocampal CA1 neurons in vitro. J Neurophysiol 78: 891-902.

Tanaka E, Uchikado H, Niiyama S, Uematsu K, Higashi H. 2002. Extrusion of intracellular calcium ion after in vitro ischemia in the rat hippocampal CA1 region. J Neurophysiol 88: 879-887.

Tang C-M, Dichter M, Morad M. 1990. Modulation of the N-methyl-D-aspartate channel by extracellular H$^+$. Proc Natl Acad Sci USA 87: 6445-6449.

Traynelis SF, Cull-Candy SG. 1990. Proton inhibition of N-methyl-D-aspartate receptors in cerebellar neurons. Nature 345: 347-350.

Traynelis SF, Cull-Candy SG. 1991. Pharmacological properties and H$^+$ sensitivity of excitatory amino acid receptor channels in rat cerebellar granule neurons. J Physiol 433: 727-763.

Tsoi M, Rhee KH, Bungard D, Li XF, Lee SL, et al. 1998. Molecular cloning of a novel potassium-dependent sodium-calcium exchanger from rat brain. J Biol Chem 273: 4155-4162.

Tymianski M, Charlton MP, Carlen PL, Tator CH. 1993. Source specificity of early calcium neurotoxicity in cultured embryonic spinal neurons. J Neurosci 13: 2085-2104.

Verdoorn TA, Burnashev N, Monyer H, Seeburg PH, Sakmann B. 1991. Structural determinants of ion flow through recombinant glutamate receptor channels. Science 252: 1715-1718.

Wang J, Liu S, Fu Y, Wang JH, Lu Y. 2003. Cdk5 activation induces hippocampal CA1 cell death by directly phosphorylating NMDA receptors. Nature Neurosci 6: 1039-1047.

Watano T, Kimura J, Morita T, Nakanishi H. 1996. A novel antagonist, No. 7943, of the Na$^+$/Ca^{2+} exchange current in guinea-pig cardiac ventricular cells. Br J Pharmacol 119: 555-563.

Xie Y, Dengler K, Zacharias E, Wilffert B, Tegtmeier F. 1994. Effects of the sodium channel blocker tetrodotoxin (TTX) on cellular ion homeostasis in rat brain subjected to complete ischemia. Brain Res 652: 216-224.

Xie Y, Zacharias E, Hoff P, Tegtmeier F. 1995. Ion channel involvement in anoxic depolarization induced by cardiac arrest in rat brain. J Cereb Blood Flow Metab 15: 587-594.

Yatani A, Brown AM, Schwartz A. 1986. Bepridil block of cardiac calcium and sodium channels. J Pharmacol Exp Ther 237: 9-17.

Yu L, Colvin RA. 1997. Regional differences in expression of transcripts for Na$^+$/Ca^{2+} exchanger isoforms in rat brain. Mol Brain Res 50: 285-292.

Yu SP, Choi DW. 1997. Na$^+$-Ca^{2+} exchange currents in cortical neurons: Concomitant forward and reverse operation and effect of glutamate. Eur J Neurosci 9: 1273-1281.

13 Role and Regulation of Copper and Zinc Transport Proteins in the Central Nervous System

C. W. Levenson · N. M. Tassabehji

Abstract: The trace elements copper and zinc are essential for the molecular and physiological functions of the central nervous system (CNS). These cations act as cofactors for enzymes that regulate every aspect of CNS function, including neuronal development and plasticity, neurotransmitter synthesis and processing, cellular metabolism and energy production, and gene expression. Imbalances in zinc have been associated with a variety of clinical disorders, including Alzheimer's disease (AD) and Parkinson's disease. Zinc has also been implicated in the neuronal damage and death associated with ischemia, seizure disorders, and brain trauma. Genetic disorders characterized by copper toxicity and copper deficiency have severe neurological consequences. Thus, it is important that subcellular copper and zinc balance be maintained precisely. This task is accomplished by several families of metal-specific transport proteins. For each metal, this chapter will begin with a brief introduction to the role of this metal in the CNS. This will be followed by the function and regulation of the known transport proteins involved in cellular uptake, intracellular trafficking, and cellular export in the CNS. There will also be discussions of the clinical implications of zinc and copper transporter abnormalities as well as the possible ways that an understanding of these transporters could lead to the development of new treatments for a variety of neurological disorders.

List of Abbreviations: AD, Alzheimer's disease; AE, acrodermatitis enteropathica; AMPA, alpha-amino-3-hydroxy-5-methyl-4-isoxazolepropionic acid glutamate receptor; ATP7A, Menkes protein, MNK; ATP7B, Wilsons protein, WND; BSE, bovine spongiform encephalopathy; CCK, cholecystokinin; CCO, cytochrome c oxidase; CCS, copper chaperone for SOD; CJD, Creutzfeldt-Jakob disease; CNS, central nervous system; Cp, ceruloplasmin; Cu, copper; DβM, dopamine beta monooxygenase; DMT1, divalent metal transporter-1; FKBP52, FK506-binding protein 52; GABA, gamma-aminobutyric acid; GABA$_A$, GABA$_A$ receptor; Glu, glutamate; GnRH, gonadotropin-releasing hormone; GPI, glycosylphosphatidylinositol; LZT, LIV-1 subfamily of ZIP zinc transporters; MMP, matrix metalloproteinase protein; MNK, Menkes protein, ATP7A; MSH, melanocortin stimulating hormone; MT, metallothionein; NMDA, N-methyl-D-aspartate glutamate receptor; NPY, neuropeptide Y; NRF, nuclear respiratory factor; PAM, peptidylglycine α-amidating monooxygenase; SOD, superoxide dismutase; TGN, *trans*-Golgi network; TRH, thyrotropin-releasing hormone; VGCaC, Voltage-gated calcium channels; VIP, vasoactive intestinal polypeptide; WND, Wilsons disease protein, APT7B; ZIP, Zrt/Irt-like proteins; Zn, zinc; ZnT, zinc transporter

1   Copper

1.1   CNS Functions

The trace element copper is essential for both the development and function of the central nervous system (CNS). Because it is found in both reduced (Cu^+) and oxidized (Cu^{2+}) states and can fluctuate between these two states, it readily serves as an essential cofactor at the catalytic site of many important CNS enzymes. For example, the ability of superoxide dismutase (Cu, Zn-SOD) to convert neurotoxic oxygen free radicals into hydrogen peroxide is dependent on copper (Maier and Chan, 2002). The activity of the catacholaminergic enzyme, dopamine β-monooxygenase (DβM), which converts dopamine into norepinephrine, DβM, requires copper (Hunt and Johnson, 1972), as does the activity of peptidylglycine α-amidating monooxygenase (PAM) that is responsible for the posttranslational modification of dozens of neurohormones and neuropeptides, including neuropeptide Y (NPY), oxytocin, thyrotropin-releasing hormone (TRH), vasoactive intestinal peptide (VIP), gonadotropin-releasing hormone (GnRH), substance P, neurotensin, cholecystokinin (CCK), α-MSH, and galanin (Prigge et al., 2000; Steveson et al., 2003). Copper is needed for normal brain function as an essential cofactor for cytochrome c oxidase, which is an integral part of the electron transport chain (Wikstrom, 2004). The CNS also contains the cuproenzyme ceruloplasmin (Cp) that appears to play an essential role in brain iron metabolism. Cp regulates brain iron concentrations (Patel et al., 2002), particularly, in the astrocytes that line the microvasculature of the CNS and reside between the dopaminergic neurons of the substantia nigra (Klomp and Gitlin, 1996).

In addition to the enzymatic functions of copper, there are also nonenzymatic roles in the CNS. For example, there is evidence that copper may facilitate the formation of bridges between transmitter-containing synaptic vesicles and the plasma membrane in advance of exocytosis (Hoss and Formaniak, 1980). Upon exocytosis, copper is released from the synaptosome into the synaptic cleft (Hartter and Barnea, 1988; Kardos et al., 1989), where it inhibits NMDA (Trombley et al., 1998) and GABA (Trombley et al., 1998; Zhu et al., 2002) receptor-mediated currents. It has also been shown to regulate voltage-gated calcium channels (VGCaC) (Horning and Trombley, 2001; Castelli et al., 2003). Furthermore, metal-lothioneins (MTs) 1, 2, and 3, which bind copper and appear to function as antioxidants and factors that regulate brain development, neuronal growth, differentiation, and survival (Yeiser et al., 1999b; Carrasco et al., 2003; Kohler et al., 2003).

There are also several CNS disease states where copper appears to play a nonenzymatic but important role. For example, alterations in brain copper metabolism and copper-mediated aggregation of amyloid β (Aβ) have been reportedly linked to Alzheimer's disease (AD) (Strausak et al., 2001). Furthermore, while controversial (Amoureux et al., 1997), mutations in the MT3 gene have been linked to AD (Uchida et al., 1991; Yu et al., 2001). Also, the normal isoform of the prion protein, PrpC, is a copper-binding protein. Prion diseases result when this cell surface glycoprotein undergoes a conformational change resulting in the pathological PrP(Sc) isoform responsible for a number of transmissible spongiform encephalopathies such as bovine spongiform encephalopathy (BSE), scrapie, and Creutzfeldt-Jakob disease (CJD). While the role of PrP(C) in CNS copper metabolism, if any, is still being debated (Waggoner et al., 2000; Brown, 2004), there is recent evidence that copper may serve to limit the progression of prion disease (Hijazi et al., 2003).

Copper is not only an essential trace metal but also in high concentrations its redox activity renders it toxic, resulting in neuronal DNA damage and apoptotic cell death. Our lab has published a number of studies examining the molecular mechanisms that are responsible for the induction of apoptosis following abnormal copper accumulation (Narayanan et al., 2001; VanLandingham et al., 2002). For example, we have shown that the tumor suppressor protein p53 is actively involved in copper-induced apoptosis in human neurons (VanLandingham et al., 2002) and may be involved in a wide variety of disorders, including Wilson's disease related dystonia and cognitive impairment, Parkinson's disease, and AD.

Given these roles in the CNS, and the need for cellular copper balance, the copper transport proteins that facilitate copper uptake, export, and intracellular trafficking are clearly important. The identification of mammalian copper transporters is largely the result of initial identifications made in the yeast *Saccharomyces cerevisiae*. This work has been recently reviewed showing not only the isolation of copper transporters in yeast but also describing a great deal of elegant work that has been conducted in this model system to understand the functions and molecular regulation of these transporters (Labbe and Thiele, 1999; Eide, 2000; Van Ho et al., 2002). Thus, this chapter will focus on copper transport and the copper chaperone proteins in the mammalian CNS.

1.2   Cellular Copper Uptake

1.2.1   Ctr1

In the CNS, cellular copper uptake appears to be largely facilitated in an energy-independent fashion by the copper transporter Ctr1 (Lee et al., 2002a). The structure and function of this protein in intestinal transport has recently been reviewed (Sharp, 2003). While three transcripts have been identified (2.0, 5.5, and a much less abundant 8.5 kb transcript), the mature amino acid sequence has been reported to be 190 amino acids forming three transmembrane domains (Zhou and Gitschier, 1997; Klomp et al., 2003a). In the plasma membrane, human Ctr1 exists as highly glycosylated homotrimer (Eisses and Kaplan, 2002) with an extracellular N terminus region that appears to be responsible for both subunit interactions and copper binding (Klomp et al., 2003a).

While the subcellular localization of Ctr1 appears to be cell specific with localization to perinuclear vesicular compartments in some cell types, such as cultured hepatocytes (HepG2), cervical carcinoma (HeLa), and large cell lung cancers (Klomp et al., 2002), the most likely localization for copper transport by Ctr1 in the CNS is the cell membrane. The role of copper in the localization of Ctr1 is, however, being currently debated. Initial work suggested that copper concentration did not alter the subcellular localization of Ctr1 (Klomp et al., 2002), while a more recent report shows that elevations in available copper enhance

Ctr1 endocytosis via clathrin-coated pits (Petris et al., 2003). The copper-stimulated endocytosis was accompanied by a significant increase in Ctr1 degradation, suggesting that cells are using translocation and posttranslational stability, rather than transcriptional regulation (Lee et al., 2000a), to downregulate copper uptake when copper availability is high (❷ *Figure 13-1*).

◻ Figure 13-1

Cellular copper uptake. Normal copper (Cu⁺) uptake is facilitated by the trimer Crt1 located on the plasma membrane (1). Because copper can be highly toxic, under conditions of high copper, Ctr1 undergoes endocytosis (2) via clathrin-coated pits (3), and is then internalized (4), and degraded (5) to limit copper uptake

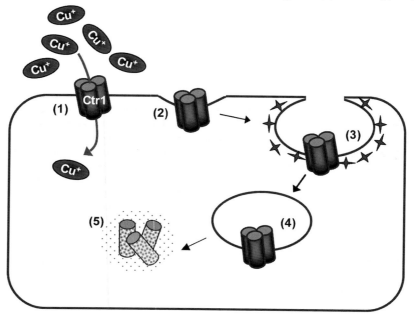

While Ctr1 is ubiquitously expressed, like its subcellular localization, its abundance appears to be cell and organ specific. The highest levels of Ctr1 expression are found in the heart, liver, pancreas and prostate, testes, ovary, and kidney (Zhou and Gitschier, 1997). While whole brain expression is relatively low (Zhou and Gitschier, 1997; Lee et al., 2000b), its importance in this organ should not be underestimated as it has been shown that Ctr1 is highly concentrated in the choroid plexus, suggesting a role for copper uptake into the brain (Nishihara et al., 1998; Kuo et al., 2001). Illustrating the importance of this metal transporter in the brain is the fact that homozygous mutant and null mice lacking functional Ctr1 do not survive beyond embryonic day 9. Furthermore, heterozygotes [Ctr1(+/−)] have significantly reduced brain copper levels (∼50%) and reduced activities of copper dependent enzymes (Kuo et al., 2001; Lee et al., 2001a). It is also worth noting here that while copper uptake is likely to be the primary function of Ctr1, mouse cells deficient in Ctr1 were unable to accumulate the chemotherapeutic agent cisplatin (Ishida et al., 2002). Thus, understanding the regulation of this copper transport protein may permit the design of better chemotherapeutic agents and prevent cisplatin resistance.

1.2.2 Ctr2

Although the data show that Ctr1 is likely the major transporter involved in brain copper uptake, there is also evidence for other transporters that may contribute to brain copper content. Copper uptake into Ctr1 deficient cells, while reduced to 30% of control, was still saturable and exhibited kinetic features that did not resemble the typical pattern of Ctr1-mediated uptake (Lee et al., 2002b). Other work has identified a putative human low-affinity copper transporter known as Ctr2. The ctr2 gene is distinct from ctr1 in that it produces a single transcript with high abundances found in brain, heart, placenta, testes, and leukocytes (Zhou and Gitschier, 1997). The reduced affinity for copper may be the result of differences in the N-terminal region where copper binding was shown to occur (Klomp et al., 2003a).

1.3 Intracellular Copper Trafficking

1.3.1 CCS

The copper chaperone protein CCS (copper chaperone for SOD) was so named because of its essential role in providing copper to Cu, Zn-SOD (Culotta et al., 1997). The subunits of CCS contain three functional domains that alternatively provide the ability of CCS to bind copper (domain I), interact with apo-SOD (domain II), and facilitate the transfer of copper from CCS to SOD (domain III) (Field et al., 2002). This transfer appears to take place largely in the cytosol where Cu, Zn-SOD is found (Culotta et al., 1997). However, a recent publication reported the identification of both CCS and Cu, Zn-SOD in the intermembrane space of the mitochondria, suggesting that this isoform of SOD may provide free radical-scavenging ability between the inner and outer membrane of the mitochondria, while manganese-SOD (Mn-SOD) protects the mitochondrial matrix (Prohaska and Gybina, 2004). The role of CCS in intracellular copper trafficking is illustrated in ❯ *Figure 13-2*.

While the highest concentration of CCS is found in the liver, there is a significant amount of this copper chaperone protein in the CNS (Rothstein et al., 1999). Immunohistochemistry has shown that CCS is

◻ Figure 13-2

Cytosolic and mitochondrial copper trafficking. After entry into the cell via Ctr1, copper (Cu$^+$) is carried by the chaperone proteins CCS and Cox17. CCS is responsible for the delivery of copper to the cytosolic protein superoxide dismutase (Cu, Zn-SOD). Both CCS and Cu, Zn-SOD have also been detected in the inner mitochondrial space. Cox17 is translocated to the inner mitochondrial space, where it has been hypothesized to deliver copper to Cox11 for activation of the copper dependent CCO I. Cox 17 also delivers copper to the Sco2/Sco1 complex for delivery of copper to CCO II

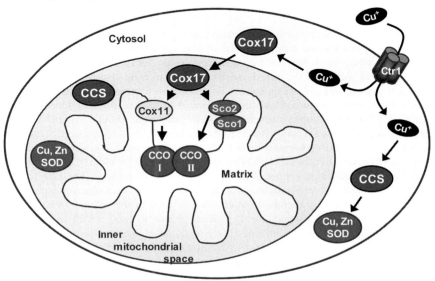

localized primarily to neurons, where it can be seen not only in cell bodies, dendrites, and axonal projections but also in astrocytes. In the spinal cord, CCS is largely confined to motor neurons. In the brain, it is expressed throughout the neuropil, and intense immunoreactivity can be seen in both large and small pyramidal cortical neurons, Purkinjie cells, deep cerebellar neurons. Interestingly, Western analysis suggested that in the cerebellum and kidney there may be two subunits of CCS (Rothstein et al., 1999).

Dietary copper deficiency regulates the abundance of CCS in the brain. Interestingly, unlike most phenotypes associated with copper deficiency, the copper-mediated increases in CCS appear to be dose-dependent. While the initial report of CCS regulation by copper did not show effects in brain (Bertinato et al., 2003), subsequent work used Western analysis to show that dietary copper deficiency produced a 2.8-fold increase in mouse brain CCS and a 2.2-fold increase in rat brain CCS (Gybina and Prohaska, 2003; Prohaska et al., 2003a). No changes in mRNA were detected (Bertinato and L'Abbe, 2003), suggesting that the increases in CCS protein were the result of posttranslational mechanisms. Indeed, it is now known that copper restriction results in a decrease in CCS protein degradation via the 26 S proteosome (Bertinato and L'Abbe, 2003).

The importance of CCS for SOD function in the CNS was shown by the production of CCS null mice [CCS(−/−)]. These mice had brain SOD activity that was as low as 15% of control (Wong et al., 2000). While the fact that there was some preservation of Cu, Zn-SOD activity suggests that there may be other chaperone proteins that can facilitate transfer of copper in the absence of CCS, this hypothesized chaperone clearly lacks the efficiency of CCS. A related study showed that while CCS(−/−) mice had an ~50% decrease in brain SOD activity, there was an even greater reduction in SOD protein levels to 22% of control, which is consistent with the posttranslational regulation of CCS seen in copper deficiency (Prohaska et al., 2003b).

Part of the therapeutic significance of CCS function in SOD activation may lie in the fact that this isoform of SOD is coded for by a gene found on chromosome 21. Patients with trisomy 21, also known as Down's syndrome, have elevated levels of SOD that have been linked to cellular damage (Lee et al., 2001b). Thus, modifications to the ability of CCS to deliver copper may serve as a therapeutic avenue. Furthermore, a number of point mutations in Cu, Zn-SOD have been linked to the development of amyotrophic lateral sclerosis (ALS) (Orrell et al., 1997). Two studies have now shown that CCS interacts with mutant SOD associated with familial ALS (Casareno et al., 1998; Corson et al., 1998), suggesting that CCS may represent a novel approach to the treatment of this disorder as well.

1.3.2 Cox 17

Like the other copper chaperone proteins, Cox 17, also called Cox 17p, was first discovered in yeast (Glerum et al., 1996) enabling the human homolog to be quickly cloned afterward (Amaravadi et al., 1997). Mammalian Cox17, which binds four Cu^+ ions (Palumaa et al., 2004), is responsible for the delivery of copper to the terminal enzyme of the mitochondrial respiratory chain, cytochrome c oxidase (CCO). In yeast, Cox 17 acts downstream of Cox23p, but it is not yet known if there is a human homolog of Cox23p (Barros et al., 2004). After synthesis, Cox17 is translocated to the inner mitochondrial space, where it delivers copper to CCO located on the inner mitochondrial membrane. About 2 of the 13 subunits of CCO require copper. These subunits, alternatively called subunits I and II, or Cox1 and Cox2, contain the copper centers known as CuB and CuA (Hamza and Gitlin, 2002).

As shown in ❷ *Figure 13-2*, the delivery of copper from Cox 17 to subunit II of CCO (CCO II) is facilitated by the initial delivery of copper to the Sco proteins, Sco1 and Sco2. These proteins, which are integral to the inner mitochondrial membrane (Maxfield et al., 2004), are now known to physically interact with each other and exhibit nonredundant but cooperative roles in the delivery of copper to CCO II. Currently, the best model suggests that Cox 17 delivers copper to Sco2, which in turn delivers it to CCO II with the essential cooperation of Sco1 (Leary et al., 2004). There is some evidence that copper can be delivered to CCO II independently of Sco2. Sco2 mutations have been identified in humans resulting in reductions in CCO activity, neurogenic muscular atrophy, and hypertrophic cardioencephalomyopathy (Jaksch et al., 2001; Foltopoulou et al., 2004). Treatment of cultured cells from these patients restored CCO activity from close to normal levels (Salviati et al., 2002). More recently, subcutaneous copper-histidine treatment was used clinically to improve the cardiac function of a patient with mutant Sco2 (Freisinger et al., 2004).

In yeast, the delivery of copper from Cox 17 to CCO subunit I (CCO I) is via the inner mitochondrial membrane protein Cox 11 (Horng et al., 2004). While no human homolog of Cox 11 has been identified to date, it seems reasonable to hypothesize the existence of such an intermediate. Thus, the presence of a putative mammalian homolog of Cox 11 has been included in ❷ *Figure 13-2*.

Because CCO activity is dependent on copper, it is not surprising that Cox 17 null mice [Cox 17($-/-$)] exhibit a severe reduction in CCO activity by embryonic day 6.5 (E6.5) and embryonic lethality between E8.5 and E10 (Takahashi et al., 2002a). Interestingly, Cox 17 heterozygotes [Cox 17($+/-$)] are phenotypically healthy with normal body weight and fertility rates. However, brain CCO activity is ~20% lower than wild-type mice. This reduction did not occur in other tissues, such as kidney or skeletal muscle (Takahashi et al., 2002a), suggesting that the CNS may be more susceptible to reductions in Cox 17 activity. Indeed, Northern analysis has shown that cox 17 gene expression is highest in heart, kidney, and brain (Kako et al., 2000). Recent work has shown that transcription of the cox 17 gene is regulated by Sp1 and the nuclear respiratory factors 1 and 2 (NRF-1, NRF-2) (Takahashi et al., 2002b). NRFs are transcription factors that regulate many of the nuclear encoded mitochondrial proteins such Cox 17 (Scarpulla, 1997).

1.3.3 Atox1

The human and murine forms of the intracellular copper-trafficking protein known as Atox1, or HAH1, were first cloned based on their homology to the yeast copper transport protein ATX1 (Klomp et al., 1997; Hung et al., 1998; Hamza et al., 2000). While its expression is highest in liver, testes, and kidney, it is also expressed in almost every brain region with particularly high levels of expression in the hippocampus, dorsal medial nucleus of the hypothalamus, locus coeruleus, and layers 2, 3, and 5 of the cortex (Naeve et al., 1999). Strikingly, Atox1 was associated primarily with neurons, specifically, in a subset of neurons known to accumulate trace metals such as the pyramidal neurons of the cortex, neurons of the CA3 region of the hippocampus, and those of the locus coeruleus (Naeve et al., 1999; Kelner et al., 2000). In these neurons, it appears that Atox1 may provide protection against oxidant-induced apoptosis and possibly other types of neuronal stress (Kelner et al., 2000).

The mechanism of Atox1 function in neurons appears to be the result of its ability to deliver copper to the P-type ATPases, ATP7A, and ATP7B that are responsible for both copper export and incorporation of copper into copper-dependent enzymes (Hamza et al., 1999; Hamza et al., 2003; Lutsenko et al., 2003) as shown in ❷ *Figure 13-3*. Most Atox1($-/-$) mice do not survive to adulthood and have symptoms associated with inactivity of copper-dependent enzymes, including skin laxity, hypopigmentation, seizures, growth retardation, and congenital malformations (Hamza et al., 2001). The function of these ATPases, also known for the diseases that result from mutations in their associated genes Menkes (MNK) and Wilson (WND), will be discussed in subsequent sections. Interactions between Atox1 and the P-type ATPases appear to involve a direct interaction (Strausak et al., 2003; Walker et al., 2004) and are dependent on the presence of copper (Larin et al., 1999). An analysis of the binding constants suggests that the transfer of copper from Atox1 to the ATPases is under kinetic control (Wernimont et al., 2004).

1.3.4 Menkes Protein

While the disease associated with mutations in the MNK gene, MNK disease, was described many years ago and a link to copper trafficking was suspected (Menkes et al., 1962; Danks et al., 1972), it was not until 1993 that the gene that codes for the P-type ATPase, ATP7A (MNK), was identified and cloned (Chelly et al., 1993; Mercer et al., 1993; Vulpe et al., 1993). The murine homolog, the mottled gene, was quickly cloned thereafter (Levinson et al., 1994). Several splice variants appear to exist (Reddy and Harris, 1998). The

◘ Figure 13-3

Trans-Golgi copper trafficking via MNK. After entry into the cell via Ctr1, copper (Cu⁺) is carried by the chaperone protein Atox1 to the MNK protein on the membrane of the *trans*-Golgi network (TGN). MNK transports copper into the TGN for incorporation into copper dependent proteins such as DβM that is responsible for the conversion of dopamine into norepinephrine in noradrenergic neurons

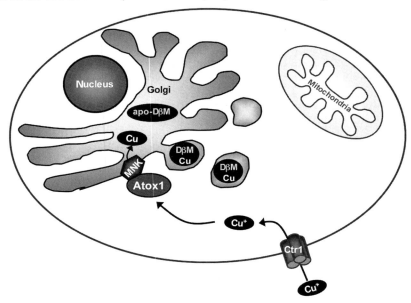

MNK gene is expressed throughout the rat brain, beginning at about day E9, with particularly high expression in the choroid plexus (Kuo et al., 1997).

Clinically, the symptoms of MNK disease are characterized by a disruption in copper-dependent enzyme activity that would be expected in severe copper deficiency, including inadequate thermoregulation, connective tissue defects leading to hyperflexibility of the skin (cutis laxia), hypermobile joints, intestinal diverticula, and torturous, elongated arteries with the presence of aneurysms. There is progressive neurological demyelination and degeneration leading to hypotonia, spasticity, seizures, and profound mental retardation. Hair texture and color abnormalities as well as skin hypopigmentation and pallor are typical. Because of the severity of these symptoms, particularly, the neurological degeneration, infants born with this X-linked disorder exhibit failure to thrive and rarely survive beyond early childhood (Menkes, 1988; Bankier, 1995).

The MNK protein sequence contains an endocytic-targeting motif that appears to target MNK to the final compartment of the Golgi apparatus, the *trans*-Golgi network (TGN) (Francis et al., 1998; Petris et al., 1998). Among the many different types of human MNK mutations that have been identified (Das et al., 1994), at least one results in mistargeting of MNK to the endoplasmic reticulum (Qi and Byers, 1998). Interestingly, this form of MNK that lacks exon 10 results in MNK disease. However, it also appears as a minor splice variant in normal individuals (Francis et al., 1998). As illustrated in ❷ *Figure 13-3*, in its normal *trans*-Golgi location, MNK transports copper to copper-dependent enzymes such as PAM (Steveson et al., 2003), tyrosinase (Petris et al., 2000), and DβM (Kaler et al., 1998). Clearly, the catalytic activity of these enzymes is essential to the normal function of the CNS. In fact, the role of normal MNK in intracellular copper trafficking in the CNS is not confined to neurons. In fact, it has long been recognized that astroglia not only concentrate copper but also play a significant role in the transport and distribution of copper to neurons (Szerdahelyi and Kása, 1986; Kodama, 1993). Thus, it is not surprising that MNK is expressed in both neurons and astrocytes in the rat CNS (Qian et al., 1997).

1.3.5 Wilson Protein

The Wilson P-type ATPase, ATP7B also known as WND, was cloned in 1993 (Bull et al., 1993; Petrukhin et al., 1993; Tanzi et al., 1993). A number of transcript sizes, likely the result of alternate splicing, have been identified (Bull et al., 1993) giving rise to several isoforms, including products of 160 and 140 kDa. In cultured human liver cells, there is also a smaller 16-kDa version that may arise from the proteolytic cleavage of the 160-kDa form to the 140-kDa version, but the function of this fragment, if any, has not been determined (Lutsenko and Cooper, 1998). The 160-kDa WND is localized to the TGN, while the 140-kDa protein is reported in the mitochondria (Lutsenko and Cooper, 1998). There is also evidence that this shorter form may also be present in the cytosol of the brain (Yang et al., 1997) (❯ Figure 13-4).

❑ Figure 13-4

Trans-Golgi copper trafficking via WND. After entry into the cell via Ctr1, copper (Cu⁺) is carried by the chaperone protein Atox1 to the WND protein on the membrane of the TGN. WND transports copper into the TGN for incorporation into copper dependent proteins such as Cp. Holo-Cp (Cu-Cp) is released from the TGN via vesicles that permit targeting of Cp to the plasma membrane, where it functions in iron export from cells of the CNS. Truncated versions of WND have also been localized to the cytosol and mitocondria

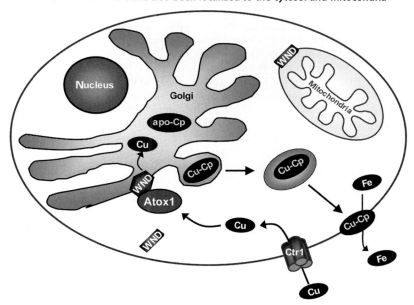

While the gene was only identified and cloned in the past decade, the clinical manifestations of WND mutations and their link to copper metabolism have been known for much longer (Scheinberg and Gitlin, 1952). Mutations in the WND gene, which can occur as a result of nonsense, missense, frameshift, or splice site abnormalities (Shah et al., 1997), produce nonfunctional WND protein or WND that is not localized to the *trans*-Golgi and is subsequently degraded by the proteosomes (Harada et al., 2001). Disruption of the WND gene results in Wilson's disease, which is characterized by copper accumulation in the liver, kidney, brain, and cornea of affected individuals. The symptoms of and current therapies for Wilson's disease are well documented and have been reviewed (Gitlin, 2003; Ferenci, 2004). Briefly, this disorder is most frequently associated with liver disease, including jaundice, hepatitis, cirrhosis, edema, ascites, and if left untreated will lead to fatal liver failure, especially, if accompanied by hemolytic anemia. Serum Cp and billiary copper are decreased, while urinary copper is increased. There may also be copper deposits in the eyes known as Kayser-Fleischer rings and the development of cataracts. Copper accumulation in the kidney results in proximal tubular dysfunction. Patients also experience joint pain, stiffness, paresthesia of the extremities, and loss of bone density and bone lesions.

Interestingly, while all patients appear to have liver involvement, ~20% present first with neurological symptoms. CNS symptoms include spasticity, rigidity, dysarthria, and muscle spasms. Neuropsychiatric symptoms may include depression, memory loss, anxiety, mania, and a variety of schizo-affective type disorders. While the high abundance of WND in the liver and its clear association with liver copper homeostasis has meant that most reviews of WND have focused on the hepatic function (Shim and Harris, 2003; Prohaska and Gybina, 2004), the CNS involvement suggests that WND is important in the brain (Strausak et al., 2001). Indeed, early work showed that WND is expressed in the brain (Bull et al., 1993). It is highly expressed in the pyramidal neurons of the hippocampus (CA1–CA4), the granular cell layer of the dentate gyrus, and the Purkinje cells of the cerebellum (Saito et al., 1999). In the olfactory bulb, WND is highly expressed in the glomerular cell layer. The pontine nuclei and lateral reticular nuclei were also immunoreactive. Lower but still detectable levels of WND were immunolocalized to the caudate putamen and cerebral cortex, where it was localized to neuronal cell bodies (Saito et al., 1999). A novel splice variant of WND has also been identified in the pineal gland and retina. This variant is significantly upregulated during the day (>100-fold compared to expression at night) and suggests a role for copper in the regulation of diurnal rhythms (Borjigin et al., 1999).

It has been known for some time that the WND protein can serve as a functional substitute for MNK and facilitate intracellular copper trafficking at the level of the *trans*-Golgi (Payne et al., 1998). Thus, it is not surprising that the distribution of WND in the CNS is largely similar to that of MNK, the major exception being localization of MNK, but not WND, to glia (Saito et al., 1999). Biochemically, WND also shares several features with MNK. As shown in ❯ *Figure 13-4*, like MNK, WND is located on the membrane of the TGN (Harada et al., 2003; Huster et al., 2003; Cater et al., 2004). In the liver, this localization is responsible for incorporation of copper into apo-ceruloplamin. Holo-Cp is then exported into the serum (Komatsu et al., 2002). In the CNS, it appears that WND can also function to deliver of copper to at least some copper-dependent enzymes as they are synthesized and moved through the *trans*-Golgi. This is likely to include brain Cp. Unlike hepatic Cp, however, in the CNS, Cp is glycosylphosphatidylinositol (GPI)-anchored to the plasma membrane, where it plays an important role in brain iron export (Jeong and David, 2003) (❯ *Figure 13-4*).

1.4 Cellular Copper Export

1.4.1 P-Type ATPases

Under conditions of high-neuronal copper, ATP7A (MNK) is translocated from its normal position in the TGN to the plasma membrane where it facilitates copper efflux (❯ *Figure 13-5*). Atox1 appears to be required for the redistribution of MNK to the plasma membrane because Atox1(−/−) cells are characterized by alterations in ATP7A trafficking and a significant reduction in cellular copper efflux (Hamza et al., 2001, 2003). Neuronal copper balance is maintained by the recycling of MNK from the plasma membrane to TGN once cellular copper levels are restored to normal (Petris et al., 1998).

While ATP7B (WND) is clearly expressed in the CNS, its role in neuronal copper export is less clear. In hepatocytes, WND is found in the TGN when cellular copper levels are low. Increases in copper results in the translocation of WND to vesicles that appear to form the bile canaliculi. Thus, excess copper is excreted into the bile. As seen with MNK, WND is recycled to the *trans*-Golgi following the excretion of excess copper (Schaefer et al., 1999; Roelofsen et al., 2000). In Wilson's disease, WND is unable to translocate from the *trans*-Golgi resulting in copper accumulation (Forbes and Cox, 2000). As discussed previously, Wilson's disease results in the accumulation of copper not only in the liver but also in brain and other tissues where the WND gene is expressed. Thus, it is interesting to speculate, as illustrated in ❯ *Figure 13-5*, that WND may also be part of the export mechanisms that regulate CNS copper levels.

◘ Figure 13-5

Cellular copper export. While WND and MNK are normally located on the membrane of the TGN, under conditions of high copper both WND and MNK are translocated to the plasma membrane and facilitate cellular copper export. The role of WND in copper export may be dependent on an association with the cytosolic protein Murr1. APP and the FKBP52 in association with Atox1 also function in neuronal copper export

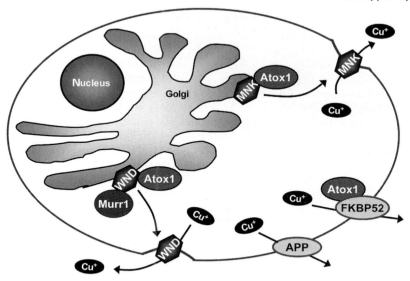

1.4.2 Murr1

Murr1 appears to be a multifunctional protein. It has been shown to inhibit the both cytokine-stimulated and basal activity of nuclear factor-kappaB (NF-κB) (Ganesh et al., 2003) as well as sodium currents (Biasio et al., 2004). Unexpectedly, mutations in the MURR1 gene were shown to cause copper toxicosis in Bedlington terriers characterized by hepatic copper accumulation due to defective billiary copper excretion (Klomp et al., 2003b). Thus, it appears that Murr1 is also involved in hepatic copper export, most likely through its direct association with the WND protein (Tao et al., 2003). The finding that relatively small amounts of Murr1 were associated with vesicular compartments while most Murr1 is in the cytosol (Klomp et al., 2003) is consistent with the known interaction between Murr1 and the amino terminus of WND (Tao et al., 2003). It was recently shown that Murr1 is ubiquitously expressed in the adult murine brain, where it is predominately expressed in neurons. The highest levels were found in hippocampal neurons (Wang et al., 2004b). While it has not been tested directly, these data suggest that in conjunction with WND, Murr1 may play a role in neuronal copper export (❷ *Figure 13-5*).

1.4.3 Other Putative Export Mechanisms

Increases in cellular copper enhance the interaction between domain I of Atox1 and the FK506-binding protein 52 (FKBP52). Overexpression of FKBP52 led to a significant increase in copper efflux. These data suggested that this newly identified protein may function in copper efflux (❷ *Figure 13-5*) and neuroprotection in the presence of high loads of cellular copper (Sanokawa-Akakura et al., 2004).

There is also evidence that amyloid precursor protein (APP) that has been associated with AD may function in neuronal copper export (❷ *Figure 13-5*). Overexpession of APP in transgenic mice resulted in reduced brain copper levels (Maynard et al., 2002; Bayer et al., 2003) and reduced activity of copper-dependent SOD activity (Bayer et al., 2003). APP does not appear to alter cellular copper uptake. Copper uptake was the same in wild-type and APP(−/−) neurons (White et al., 1999). Interestingly, copper depletion has recently been shown to decrease transcription of the APP gene leading to reduced APP protein levels (Bellingham et al., 2004). Together these data suggest a role for APP in the facilitation of neuronal copper export (❷ *Figure 13-5*).

2   Zinc

2.1   CNS Functions

In humans, zinc deficiency has been linked to a variety of behavioral and physiological abnormalities. Dietary zinc deficiency has been reported to cause hypogonadism, geophagia, abnormal taste acuity, immune suppression, and cognitive impairment (Prasad, 2001a, b). Severe zinc deficiency in adults can result in balance and gait disturbances and neuropsychological disorders, including depression, paranoia, and hallucinations (Henkin et al., 1975). Zinc deficiency has also been linked to learning and memory deficits (Tucker and Sandstead, 1984), depression (Maes et al., 1994, 1999), and schizophrenia (Andrews, 1992). However, a recent review of the literature shows that the cognitive and psychological effects of zinc deficiency and zinc supplementation in children and infants are heterogeneous (Black, 2003).

Evidence of the essentiality of the trace element zinc can also be seen in the genetic disorder acrodermatitis enteropathica (AE). AE, which is characterized by a mutation in the Zip4 transporter gene (Wang et al., 2002, 2004c) and the inability to absorb zinc in the gastrointestinal system leading to severe perioral and perianal dermatitis and failure to thrive, is lethal in infancy if left untreated (Perafan-Riveros et al., 2002). To date, 21 different mutations, all leading to AE, have been identified in the Zip4 gene (Kury et al., 2003). Fortunately, this genetic disorder can be successfully treated with life-long, high-dose zinc treatment (Radja and Charles-Holmes, 2002) that bypasses the normal intestinal zinc absorption mechanisms.

2.1.1   Bound Zinc

Given that many of the symptoms associated with zinc deficiency are neurological, it is clear that zinc plays important roles in the CNS. Most zinc in the CNS is bound to proteins, many of which play essential enzymatic roles. In fact, there are at least 80 different mammalian enzymes that require zinc. The catalytic roles of zinc have been recently reviewed (McCall et al., 2000; Tapiero and Tew, 2003). For example, zinc is essential for the activity of DNA and RNA polymerases. Many of the enzymes in intermediary metabolism, including pyruvate carboxylase, fructose 1,6-bis phosphatase, lactate dehydrogenase, and alcohol dehydrogenase, all require zinc. Zinc is also an essential component of the matrix metalloproteinase family of enzymes (MMP) that plays role in the development and plasticity of the CNS (Crocker et al., 2004).

In addition to the enzymatic functions of zinc, zinc is also a structural component of many nonenzymatic proteins. A primary example of this is the binding of zinc to a family of zinc-binding protein known as zinc-finger proteins. These proteins use cysteine and histidine to bind zinc in generally either a Cys_2-His_2 or Cys_2-Cys_2 motif resulting in protein folding consistent with the formation of a "finger-like" domain (Berg and Shi, 1996). Their structure has recently been reviewed (Laity et al., 2001; Zawia, 2003). Hundreds of zinc-finger proteins have been identified to date, with new proteins being identified every year. Many of the members of this family, including Sp1, GATA1, and transcription factor IIIA, act as DNA-binding transcription factors (O'Halloran, 1993; Klug and Schwabe, 1995). They are also highly represented among the steroid-hormone nuclear receptors such as the retinoic acid receptors RXR and RAR, the nuclear vitamin D receptor, glucocorticoid receptor, estrogen receptor, thyroid hormone receptor and the progesterone receptor (Savouret et al., 1994; Brandao-Neto et al., 1995; Haussler et al., 1997; Kroncke and Carlberg, 2000). In addition to these protein–DNA interactions, zinc-finger proteins have also been shown to participate in protein–RNA interactions and form the bridge between DNA–RNA hybrids (Shi and Berg, 1995). Most recently, the thyroid hormone receptor, a key player in brain development and neuronal differentiation, was shown not only to be a DNA-binding nuclear receptor but also to act as a single-stranded RNA-binding protein (Xu and Koenig, 2004). Additionally a number of zinc-finger proteins, particularly, those containing the LIM motif, have been shown to participate in protein–protein interactions between nuclear transcription factors, cytoskeletal proteins, and signaling proteins (Brown et al., 2001). They also interact with lipids (Laity et al., 2001). Because these proteins appear to regulate so many cellular processes, the use of engineered zinc-finger proteins in rational drug design and development is currently being explored (Jamieson et al., 2003).

2.1.2 Free Zinc

Approximately 10% of CNS zinc is not bound to protein or amino acid ligands and is thus known as free, or chelatable, zinc. The identification and function of this neuronal pool of zinc has recently been reviewed (Frederickson et al., 2000; Frederickson and Bush, 2001; Takeda, 2001). In normal neurons, free zinc is predominately localized to the presynaptic vesicles of a subset of glutamatergic neurons (Danscher, 1996; Franco-Pons et al., 2000). Free zinc has also been colocalized with glycine and GABA in the mouse (Kovacs and Larson, 1997). Regions rich in "zincergic" neurons include the mossy fibers of the hippocampus, the amygdala, and the olfactory bulb. Free zinc-containing neurons are also abundant in the cortex (Frederickson et al., 2000). Depolarization and calcium influx result in the exocytotic release of zinc into the synaptic cleft (Assaf and Chung, 1984), where its primary function appears to be the modulation of both ionotropic and metabotropic postsynaptic receptors that have specific zinc-binding sites. For example, zinc inhibits $GABA_A$ receptors, reducing their inhibitory action (Westbrook and Mayer, 1987; Smart et al., 1994). Zinc inhibits the NMDA subtype of the glutamate receptor (Westbrook and Mayer, 1987; Vogt et al., 2000). It also appears that zinc modulates the activity of at least a subset of AMPA receptors, and that this effect may be biphasic and cell type specific (Lin et al., 2001; Zhang et al., 2002; Blakemore and Trombley, 2004). There is also evidence that zinc can potentiate glycine-mediated currents (Trombley and Shepard, 1996), regulate VGCaC (Winegar and Lansman, 1990), as well as potassium, sodium, and chloride channels (Harrison and Gibbons, 1994), and act as an inhibitory neuromodulator of glutamate release (Takeda et al., 2004).

Despite the fact that zinc plays a role in the normal modulation of postsynaptic receptors and other channels, the release of high concentrations of zinc following seizure, ischemia, or traumatic injury have been shown to be neurotoxic (Cuajungco and Lees, 1997). For example, in the rat, ischemia results in the rapid release of zinc from synaptic vesicles so that 7 min after the induction of ischemia by middle cerebral artery occlusion, there were no remaining zinc-positive terminals in neocortical layers II and III. Over the next 24 h there was a progressive decrease in free presynaptic zinc in all ischemic brain areas (Sørensen et al., 1998). The released zinc then accumulates in postsynaptic neurons followed by neuronal death (Tønder et al., 1990; Koh et al., 1996), suggesting that the release of presynaptic vesicular zinc is responsible for the damage and death. Subsequent work has shown that the zinc-mediated neuronal death is the result of a combination of apoptosis and necrosis (Ahn et al., 1998; Kim et al., 1999) that can be prevented by zinc chelation (Koh et al., 1996). There is also evidence that zinc can contribute to neurodegenerative disorders such as Parkinson's disease, some forms of amyolateral lateral sclerosis, and AD (see Cuajungco and Less, 1997 for a recent review).

2.2 Neuronal Zinc Uptake

The structure and function of transporters responsible for the uptake, intracellular trafficking, and export of zinc have recently been reviewed (McMahon and Cousins, 1998; Colvin et al., 2000; Cousins and McMahon, 2000; Takeda, 2000; Kambe et al., 2004; Liuzzi and Cousins, 2004). Most of these reviews have largely dealt with the available information on intestinal and liver transport (where most of the experimental attention has been focused). However, this chapter will examine the recent data on the zinc transport proteins in the CNS. These transport proteins include the ZnT family, the ZIP superfamily, and a variety of postsynaptic receptors that permit the movement of zinc across membranes.

2.2.1 ZIP1

The ZIP (SLC39A) superfamily of transporters (Zrt/Irt-like proteins) has been most closely associated with cellular zinc (Zn^{2+}) uptake. While most of the members of this superfamily have eight membrane-spanning domains, their tissue specificity is rather heterogeneous. For example, ZIP1 and ZIP3 are expressed in the CNS, while ZIP2 and ZIP4 are not. ZIP1 overexpression results in cellular zinc accumulation (Gaither and Eide, 2001). Its abundance in brain is higher than ZIP3, suggesting that ZIP1 is the main facilitator of neuronal zinc uptake discovered to date. Interestingly, neither zinc deficiency nor supplementation appears to alter the expression of ZIP1 (Cousins et al., 2003; Dufner-Beattie et al., 2003). However, decreases in available zinc resulted in an increase in the movement of ZIP1 from intracellular organelles out onto the plasma membrane (Wang et al., 2004a). Thus, it appears that posttranslational regulation of ZIP1 may facilitate neuronal zinc uptake during periods of low-zinc availability.

2.2.2 ZIP3

Overexpression of ZIP3 also led to an increase in cellular zinc accumulation (Dufner-Beattie et al., 2003). Thus, ZIP3, which is expressed in the CNS, is included with ZIP1 in ❯ *Figure 13-6* as a putative neuronal

❏ Figure 13-6

Neuronal zinc uptake and trafficking. Neuronal zinc (Zn) uptake appears to be largely facilitated by the ZIP family proteins, ZIP1 and ZIP3, and LIV-1. ZnT5 may also function in this capacity. Zinc is then translocated into the TGN by the transport protein ZnT4, and possibly ZnT5. There is also evidence of mitochondrial zinc that may play a role in Zn transport. Although the transport mechanisms are not understood, neurons that sequester free zinc in synaptic vesicles must transport zinc down the axon to the synaptic buton

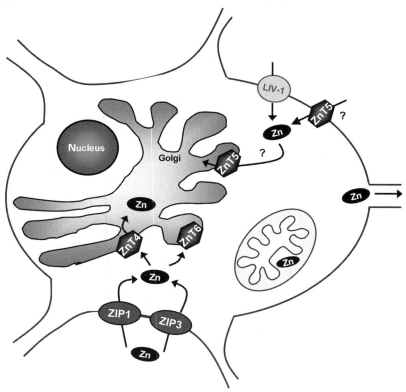

zinc transporter that facilitates zinc uptake. While the effect of zinc availability in ZIP3 expression in the CNS has not been tested directly, zinc deficiency only modestly decreased the expression of ZIP3 in immune cells (Cousins et al., 2003). Even this effect may be tissue specific because ZIP3 was not regulated by zinc in small intestine (Dufner-Beattie et al., 2003). The larger effect of zinc availability is on the posttranslational localization of ZIP3. Similar to the regulation of ZIP1, zinc deficiency increases the amount of ZIP3 that is localized to the plasma membrane to facilitate cellular zinc uptake (Wang et al., 2004a). The ZIP proteins also appear to be responsible for the uptake of oligodendrocyte zinc (Law et al., 2003).

2.2.3 LIV-1

Recently, a new ZIP subfamily was identified and named the LZT family for LIV-1 subfamily of ZIP zinc transporters (Taylor et al., 2003). These proteins, of which ZIP4 is a member, were recently reviewed (Taylor and Nicholson, 2003). The human LZT protein LIV-1 is localized on the plasma membrane (❯ *Figure 13-6*). Consistent with a role in zinc uptake, LIV-1 is expressed in the placenta, prostate, and several cancer cells, including lung cancer and HeLa. In the CNS, LIV-1 is expressed in the cortex, cerebellum, substantia nigra, nucleus accumbens, corpus callosum, amygdala, pituitary, caudate nucleus, medulla, pons, putamen, and spinal cord (Taylor et al., 2003).

2.2.4 Postsynaptic Receptors

Release of zinc from presynaptic neurons, which will be discussed in a subsequent section on neuronal zinc export, results in an increase in free Zn^{2+} in the synaptic cleft. As described previously, this free zinc interacts with and regulates the function of a variety of postsynaptic receptors, including $GABA_A$ receptors, glutamate receptors (NMDA and AMPA receptors), and voltage-gated calcium receptors. However, as shown in ❯ *Figure 13-7*, these receptors also appear to represent a mechanism for the entry of zinc into

❏ Figure 13-7

Transport of vesicular zinc and uptake by postsynaptic neurons. The zinc transporter ZnT3 is localized to presynaptic vesicular membranes by the chaperone protein AP-3. ZnT3 then accepts zinc (Zn^{2+}) from ligands that are likely to include MT3 and sequesters it in glutamate-containing vesicles. Synaptic activity results in exocytosis of zinc and glutamate into the synaptic cleft. Zinc both modifies the synaptic activity of the postsynaptic $GABA_A$ receptors ($GABA_A$), glutamate receptors (NMDA and AMPA), and VGCaC, and uses them as a route of entry into the postsynaptic neuron. Because high concentrations of free zinc are neurotoxic, it is also cleared from the synapse by a Zn^{2+}/H^+ antiporter, and from the postsynaptic neuron by a Na^+/Zn^{2+} exchanger

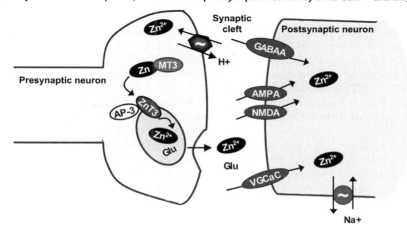

postsynaptic neurons (Sensi et al., 1997; Li et al., 2003). Calcium-permeable AMPA-kainate channel (Ca-A/K) appear to be responsible for most of the postsynaptic Zn^{2+} uptake (Weiss and Sensi, 2000; Martinez-Galan et al., 2003).

2.2.5 Zinc/Proton Antiporter

Reuptake of synaptic zinc into presynaptic terminals is likely to occur by several mechanisms, including ZIP1 and ZIP3 transporters. As illustrated in ❷ *Figure 13-7*, there is also evidence for a zinc/proton (Zn^{2+}/H^+) antiporter that has been hypothesized to function as a mechanism to replenish zinc-containing vesicles (Colvin et al., 2000).

2.2.6 DMT1/DCT1

DMT1 is expressed in hippocampal granular and pyramidal cells, cerebellar granular cells, and pyramidal cells of the piriform cortex and the preoptic nucleus (Gunshin et al., 1997). Because of the ability of zinc to generate inward currents in *Xenopus* oocytes that expressed DMT1, it was hypothesized that this cation transporter was involved in zinc transport (Gunshin et al., 1997). Subsequent work, however, has shown that this member of the Nramp family plays a significant role in iron trafficking but does not transport zinc (Sacher et al., 2001).

2.3 Intracellular Zinc Trafficking

2.3.1 Metallothionein

While there are many different human MT isoforms, it appears that MT1, MT2, and MT3 play the most prominent role in the CNS (Ebadi et al., 1995). Members of the MT family of protein all bind zinc and copper in vivo and reportedly function in the protection against oxidant damage, heavy metal detoxica tion, and possibly protection against injury (Hidalgo et al., 2001). However, the role of MT in zinc metabolism and intracellular zinc trafficking in the CNS is of interest because these proteins also appear to function as storage forms for zinc. This is supported by the fact that the transcription of both MT1 and MT2 (MT1/2) is increased dramatically by zinc. The regulation of MT gene expression has been thoroughly reviewed (Andrews, 1990) and involves the metal-regulated transcription factor MTF-1.

All three isoforms have been shown to donate zinc to apoenzymes (Udom and Brady, 1980; Shi et al., 2002), a process that is facilitated by ATP (Jiang et al., 1998). MT1/2 are expressed in all regions of the CNS as well as other tissues. While the highest abundance in astrocytes, there have been reports of small amounts of MT1/2 and MT1/2 mRNA in neurons (Blaauwgeers et al., 1993). Neither oligodendrocytes nor resting astrocytes appear to express MT1/2. However, there are a number of reports of expression in reactive astrocytes after injury, suggesting a role for MT in buffering zinc levels when high concentrations are released into the synaptic cleft after injury, seizure, or hypoxia-ischemia (Acarin et al., 1999a; Carrasco et al., 2000). Like MT1/2, MT3 is also induced after injury (Yeiser et al., 1999a; Acarin et al., 1999b) and may play a role in intracellular zinc trafficking (Shi et al., 2002). However, it is unique from the predominant MT isoforms in several ways. First, MT3 is almost exclusively expressed in the CNS (Palmiter et al., 1992), where it is found predominately in neurons (Masters et al., 1994). Second, it was first identified as a neuronal growth inhibitory factor (GIF) that, while controversial (Amoureux et al., 1997), was linked to the development of AD (Uchida et al., 1991). MT3 also increases during development (Yeiser et al., 1999b) when it may act to inhibit neurite outgrowth (Chung et al., 2002). Most importantly, for this review, MT3 was localized to neurons that sequester zinc in synaptic vesicles (Masters et al., 1994) and thus has been hypothesized to play a role in the intracellular trafficking of zinc via ZnT3, the transporter that concentrates Zn^{2+} in glutamate-containing synaptic vesicles (❷ *Figure 13-7*).

2.3.2 ZnT4

The structure and function of the ZnT (SLC30) family of zinc transporters have recently been reviewed (Liuzzi and Cousins, 2004; Palmiter and Huang, 2004). These transporters have been associated with the removal of cytosolic zinc either into intracellular compartments, such as vesicles or theTGN, or export from the cell. While nine different mammalian ZnT proteins (ZnT1–ZnT9) have been identified to date, only ZnT1, ZnT3, ZnT4, ZnT5, and ZnT6 have been shown to be expressed in the CNS. Others may follow, but this chapter will focus on the function of the known ZnT family members in the CNS.

The zinc transporter ZnT4 has been identified as the gene that is mutated in the lethal milk mouse (*lm*) (Huang and Gitschier, 1997). Pups born to *lm* dams die of zinc deficiency because of low maternal milk zinc content. Fostering to normal dams prevents the zinc deficiency and permits apparently normal development (Erway and Grider, 1984). However, the finding that in adulthood these pups exhibit zinc deficiency symptoms was the clue that ZnT4 expression is not confined to the mammary tissue. While ZnT4 is indeed highly expressed in mammary tissue, it is also expressed in the brain (Huang and Gitschier, 1997). Other studies have shown that ZnT4 is localized to the *trans*-Golgi (❷ *Figure 13-6*), where it is likely to participate in the movement of zinc across the membrane to supply zinc-dependent enzymes (Palmiter and Huang, 2004). Zinc restriction did not change ZnT4 gene expression in intestine, liver, and kidney (Liuzzi et al., 2001). However, zinc deficiency increases mammary ZnT4 expression (Kelleher and Lönnerdal, 2002). The effect of alterations in neuronal zinc availability on ZnT4 abundance has not been studied.

2.3.3 ZnT5

In mouse tissues, ZnT5 is expressed in kidney>brain>intestine. It is also found in liver, spleen, and mammary tissue (Cragg et al., 2002). The function of this putative transporter in the brain is not understood, and studies in a variety of cell types have been somewhat contradictory. For example, in human cervical cells, ZnT5 is located in Golgi-enriched vesicles. In pancreatic β cells, it was associated with secretory granules (Kambe et al., 2002), but expression in *Xenopus* oocytes and transient expression in human colonic carcinoma cells (Caco-2) suggested that ZnT5 is located at the plasma membrane (Cragg et al., 2002). On the basis of the reported localization and the function of other ZnT family of transporters, it is tempting to hypothesize that ZnT5 functions in some way to reduce cytosolic zinc levels, either by zinc import into intracellular compartments (❷ *Figure 13-6*) or by export from the cell (❷ *Figure 13-8*). However, overexpression studies have also suggested a role for ZnT5 in zinc uptake (Cragg et al., 2002). Thus, we have included it in ❷ *Figure 13-6* depicting possible zinc uptake mechanisms in the CNS.

2.3.4 ZnT6

The transporter ZnT6 is most highly expressed in brain, small intestine, liver, and kidney, where it appears to be largely associated with the TGN (❷ *Figure 13-6*). Like ZnT4 and ZnT5, it appears to transport zinc into the *trans*-Golgi for incorporation into zinc-dependent enzymes (Huang et al., 2002). The next section of this chapter will also show evidence for the role of ZnT6 in cellular zinc export.

2.3.5 Mitochondrial Zinc

There have been a number of studies suggesting the existence of mitochondrial zinc (Colvin et al., 2003). Whether this is Zn^{2+} or MT-bound zinc is currently being debated (Saris and Niva, 1994; Ye et al., 2001). The transport mechanisms into and out of the mitochondria have not been definitively identified, but there is evidence that zinc may be transported into the mitochondria using calcium uptake mechanisms (Saris and Niva, 1994). Clearly more work is needed on the transport and function of zinc in the mitochondria.

■ Figure 13-8

Neuronal export of zinc. The zinc transport protein ZnT1 appears to be the main route of export. Under conditions of high-zinc ZnT4 and ZnT6, which normally reside on membranes of the *trans*-Golgi, are translocated in Golgi-associated vesicles to the plasma membrane where they participate in zinc export. It has also been hypothesized that ZnT5 and the sodium-zinc exchanger, both located on the plasma membrane, may also act to export zinc under conditions of elevated cellular zinc

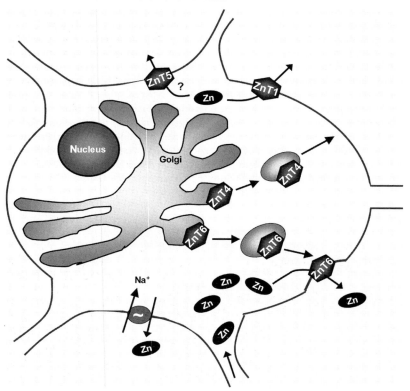

2.4   Neuronal Zinc Export

2.4.1 ZnT1

The ZnT1 protein, with its six transmembrane-spanning domains, was the first reported mammalian zinc transporter. It is localized to the plasma membrane, where it likely forms a multimer that is responsible, at least in part, for the export of cellular zinc (Palmiter and Findley, 1995) (❷ *Figure 13-8*). Overexpression of ZnT1 results in increased cellular zinc export and protection from zinc-mediated neurotoxicity (Kim et al., 2000).

In the brain, ZnT1 expression is developmentally regulated. At birth, ZnT1 expression is low in the cortex, hippocampus, cerebellum, and olfactory bulb. Significant increases are seen by postnatal day 6. ZnT1 expression in the cerebellum is delayed somewhat but is comparable to other areas by postnatal day 9 (Nitzan et al., 2002). In adult mice, ZnT1 is highly expressed in the cortex and cerebellum, with somewhat lower levels in the hippocampus, hypothalamus, and olfactory bulb. Lower but still detectable levels are also seen in the striatum and septum (Sekler et al., 2002).

The regulation of ZnT1 by zinc in cells outside the CNS appears to be tissue specific and has recently been reviewed (Liuzzi and Cousins, 2004). In the brain, there are several lines of evidence suggesting zinc regulation of this important zinc exporter. First, treatment of primary cultures of hippocampal neurons with 150 μM zinc resulted in the rapid induction of ZnT1 mRNA expression that peaked at 2 h after treatment (Tsuda et al., 1997). Second, transient forebrain ischemia, which is known to result in the release of free zinc from synaptic vesicles, produced a significant increase in ZnT1 abundance in the CA1 region of the hippocampus, a region that is particularly high in free zinc (Tsuda et al., 1997). Thus, it is likely that ZnT1 not only participates in export of zinc from neurons under conditions of normal turnover but may also play a role in the protection of neurons from excessive zinc accumulation resulting from release of zinc during pathological conditions such as seizure, ischemia, or trauma (❷ *Figure 13-8*).

2.4.2 ZnT3

Although ZnT1 appears to be the main protein responsible for zinc export, ZnT3 plays an indirect role in zinc export through the sequestration of zinc in vesicles that empty into the synaptic cleft (❷ *Figure 13-7*). ZnT3 is exclusively expressed in the brain and testes. In the brain, it has been localized to the membrane of presynaptic vesicles that contain free zinc and the neurotransmitter glutamate (Palmiter et al., 1996; Wenzel et al., 1997). ZnT3 is translocated to the vesicular membrane with the aid of the chaperone protein AP-3 (Cole et al., 1999). ZnT3 expression appears to be developmentally regulated and has been detected in all regions where free zinc is accumulated in vesicles, including the mossy fibers of the hippocampus, the dentate gyrus, cortex, olfactory bulb, and amygdala (Wenzel et al., 1997; Valente and Auladell, 2002).

ZnT3 null mice that lacked neuronal ZnT3 expression failed to accumulate zinc in synaptic vesicles. Heterozygotes with reduced ZnT3 expression had an intermediate level of free vesicular zinc (Cole et al., 1999), establishing ZnT3 as the sole transporter responsible for the translocation of zinc into synaptic vesicles. Total zinc in the hippocampus and cortex of ZnT3 null mice was reduced by 20% (Cole et al., 1999). Interestingly, the ZnT3 null mouse also showed that vesicular zinc is not the only pool of free zinc in the brain. Injections of kainate are known to cause seizures and the accumulation of free zinc followed by postsynaptic neuronal death. In wild-type mice, this is assumed to be the result of the excessive release of free zinc from presynaptic terminals during seizure activity. However, in ZnT3 null mice that lacked presynaptic zinc, kainite was still able to induce the accumulation of free zinc and neuronal death (Lee et al., 2000a). Thus, while the role of ZnT3 in vesicular zinc accumulation and subsequent exocytotic export from neurons is clear, all of the pools that contribute to free neuronal zinc have not yet been identified.

Finally, it should be pointed out that the function of ZnT3 in vesicular zinc accumulation and presynaptic zinc export may have clinical implications. For example, ZnT3 function has recently been linked to the ageing process. Hippocampal ZnT3 expression is significantly reduced in the mouse model of premature ageing, the senescence-accelerated mouse prone 10 (SAMP10). These mice also exhibited excess glutamate and glycine release as well as an increase in glial fibrillary acidic protein (GFAP), a marker of neuronal injury (Saito et al., 2000). It also appears that ZnT3 activity, probably through the AP-3 protein complex, and vesicular zinc levels are regulated by estrogen. Estrogen replacement in ovariectomized mice lowered free zinc levels in the hippocampus (Lee et al., 2004). Together these data open the door for new work on the role of ZnT3 and free zinc in the ageing process.

2.4.3 Sodium-Zinc Exchanger

Recently Ohana et al. (2004) identified a sodium-zinc (Na^+/Zn^{2+}) exchanger that is distinct from the hypothesized sodium-calcium exchanger that may transport zinc (Sensi et al., 1997). The Na^+/Zn^{2+}s exchanger not only rapidly and actively attenuated the accumulation of zinc following opening of L-type calcium channels, such as those found on the postsynaptic membrane, but also led to neuronal zinc efflux (Ohana et al., 2004). Thus, we have included this possible export mechanism in ❷ *Figures 13-7* and ❷ *13-8*.

2.4.4 ZnT4 and ZnT6

As previously discussed, the transporters ZnT4 and ZnT6 are predominately associated with the *trans*-Golgi function to deliver zinc to zinc-dependent enzymes (❷ *Figure 13-6*). However, initial work in yeast suggested that ZnT6 also transported zinc out of the cytoplasm. While zinc supplementation did not elevate the expression of ZnT6, in mammalian kidney cells subjected to high concentrations of zinc (30–200 µM), both Zn4 and ZnT6 were translocated from the *trans*-Golgi to vesicles and to the plasma membrane. Zinc appears to either leave the cell via the secretory pathway or by ZnT4 and ZnT6 transport at the plasma membrane (Huang et al., 2002). This suggests that in neurons, the translocation of these zinc transporters may participate in zinc export and provide protection from the neurotoxic accumulation of zinc during periods of high-synaptic activity and postsynaptic zinc (❷ *Figure 13-8*).

3 Conclusions

In conclusion, the cellular and molecular roles of zinc and copper in normal CNS function are clear. Imbalances, either deficiency or toxicity, have serious neurological consequences. Furthermore, abnormal intracellular metal trafficking has been associated with a number of disorders of the CNS. The clinical implications of trace metal imbalances and abnormalities in transport can be seen in the toxic accumulation of zinc in postsynaptic neurons following stroke and seizure, the copper-stimulated precipitation of amyloid protein in AD, and the severe neurodegeneration associated with the copper deficiency of MNK disease. While we have only recently begun to characterize the role and regulation of the transport proteins that regulate zinc and copper in the human CNS, these proteins hold a great deal of promise for rationale drug design and the development of future therapies for a host of traumatic and genetic disorders of the CNS.

References

Acarin L, Gonzalez B, Hidalgo J, Castro AJ, Castellano B. 1999a. Primary cortical glial reaction versus secondary thalamic glial response in the excitotoxically injured young brain: Astroglial response and metallothionein expression. Neuroscience 92: 827-839.

Acarin L, Carrasco J, Gonzalez B, Hidalgo J, Castellano B. 1999b. Expression of growth inhibitory factor (metallothionein-III) mRNA and protein following excitotoxic immature brain injury. J Neuropathol Exp Neurol 58: 389-397.

Ahn YH, Kim YH, Hong SH, Koh JY. 1998. Depletion of intracellular zinc induces protein synthesis-dependent neuronal apoptosis in mouse cortical culture. Exp Neurol 154: 47-56.

Amaravadi R, Glerum DM, Tzagoloff A. 1997. Isolation of a cDNA encoding the human homolog of COX17, a yeast gene essential for mitochondrial copper recruitment. Hum Genet 99: 329-333.

Amoureux MC, Gool Van D, Herrero MT, Dom R, Colpaertet FC et al. 1997. Regulation of metallothionein-III (GIF) mRNA in the brain of patients with Alzheimer disease is not impaired. Mol Chem Neuropathol 32: 101-121.

Andrews GK. 1990. Regulation of metallothionein gene expression. Prog Food Nutr Sci 14: 193-258.

Andrews RC. 1992. An update of the zinc deficiency theory of schizophrenia. Identification of the sex determining system as the site of action of reproductive zinc deficiency. Med Hypotheses 38: 284-291.

Assaf SY, Chung SH. 1984. Release of endogenous Zn2+ from brain tissue during activity. Nature 308: 734-736.

Bankier A. 1995. Menkes disease. J Med Genet 32: 213-215.

Barros MH, Johnson A, Tzagoloff A. 2004. COX23, a homologue of COX17, is required for cytochrome oxidase assembly. J Biol Chem 279: 31943-31947.

Bayer TA, Schafer S, Simons A, Kemmling A, Kamer T, et al. 2003. Dietary Cu stabilizes brain superoxide dismutase 1 activity and reduces amyloid Abeta production in APP23 transgenic mice. Proc Natl Acad Sci USA 100: 14187-14192.

Bellingham SA, Lahiri DK, Maloney B, La Fontaine S, Multhaup G, et al. 2004. Copper depletion down-regulates expression of the Alzheimer's disease amyloid-beta precursor protein gene. J Biol Chem 279: 20378-20386.

Berg JM, Shi Y. 1996. The galvanization of biology: A growing appreciation for the roles of zinc. Science 271: 1081-1085.

Bertinato J, L'Abbe MR. 2003. Copper modulates the degradation of copper chaperone for Cu,Zn superoxide dismutase by the 26 S proteosome. J Biol Chem 278: 35071-35078.

Bertinato J, Iskandar M, L'Abbe MR. 2003. Copper deficiency induces the upregulation of the copper chaperone for Cu/Zn superoxide dismutase in weanling male rats. J Nutr 133: 28-31.

Biasio W, Chang T, McIntosh CJ, McDonald FJ. 2004. Identification of Murr1 as a regulator of the human delta epithelial sodium channel. J Biol Chem 279: 5429-5434.

Blaauwgeers HG, Sillevis Smitt PA, De Jong JM, Troost D. 1993. Distribution of metallothionein in the human central nervous system. Glia 8: 62-70.

Black MM. 2003. The evidence linking zinc deficiency with children's cognitive and motor functioning. J Nutr 133: 1473S-1476S.

Blakemore LJ, Trombley PQ. 2004. Diverse modulation of olfactory bulb AMPA receptors by zinc. Neuroreport 15: 919-923.

Borjigin J, Payne AS, Deng J, Li X, Wang MM, et al. 1999. A novel pineal night-specific ATPase encoded by the Wilson disease gene. J Neurosci 19: 1018-1026.

Brandao-Neto J, Madureira G, Mendonca BB, Bloise W, Castro AV. 1995. Endocrine interaction between zinc and prolactin. An interpretative review. Biol Trace Elem Res 49: 139-149.

Brown DR. 2004. Role of the prion protein in copper turnover in astrocytes. Neurobiol Dis 15: 534-543.

Brown S, Coghill ID, McGrath MJ, Robinson PA. 2001. Role of LIM domains in mediating signaling protein interactions. IUBMB Life 51: 359-364.

Bull PC, Thomas GR, Rommens JM, Forbes JR, Cox DW. 1993. The Wilson disease gene is a putative copper transporting P-type ATPase similar to the Menkes gene. Nat Genet 5: 327-337.

Carrasco J, Penkowa M, Hadberg H, Molinero A, Hidalgo J. 2000. Enhanced seizures and hippocampal neurodegeneration following kainic acid-induced seizures in metallothionein-I + II-deficient mice. Eur J Neurosci 12: 2311-2322.

Carrasco J, Penkowa M, Giralt M, Camats J, Molinero A, et al. 2003. Role of metallothionein-III following central nervous system damage. Neurobiol Dis 13: 22-36.

Casareno RL, Waggoner D, Gitlin JD. 1998. The copper chaperone CCS directly interacts with copper/zinc superoxide dismutase. J Biol Chem 273: 23625-23628.

Castelli L, Tanzi F, Taglietti V, Magistretti J. 2003. Cu2+, Co2+, and Mn2+ modify the gating kinetics of high-voltage-activated Ca2+ channels in rat palaeocortical neurons. J Membr Biol 195: 121-136.

Cater MA, Forbes J, La Fontaine S, Cox D, Mercer JF. 2004. Intracellular trafficking of the human Wilson protein: The role of the six N-terminal metal-binding sites. Biochem J 380: 805-813.

Chelly J, Tumer Z, Tonnesen T, Petterson A, Ishikawa-Brush Y, et al. 1993. Isolation of a candidate gene for Menkes disease that encodes a potential heavy metal binding protein. Nat Genet 3: 14-19.

Chung RS, Vickers JC, Chuah MI, Eckhardt BL, West AK. 2002. Metallothionein-III inhibits initial neurite formation in developing neurons as well as postinjury, regenerative neurite sprouting. Exp Neurol 178: 1-12.

Cole TB, Wenzel HJ, Kafer KE, Schwartzkroin PA, Palmiter RD. 1999. Elimination of zinc from synaptic vesicles in the intact mouse brain by disruption of the ZnT3 gene. Proc Natl Acad Sci USA 96: 1716-1721.

Colvin RA, Davis N, Nipper RW, Carter PA. 2000. Evidence for a zinc/proton antiporter in rat brain. Neurochem Int 36: 539-547.

Colvin RA, Fontaine CP, Laskowski M, Thomas D. 2003. Zn2+ transporters and Zn2+ homeostasis in neurons. Eur J Pharmacol 479: 171-185.

Corson LB, Strain JJ, Culotta VC, Cleveland DW. 1998. Chaperone-facilitated copper binding is a property common to several classes of familial amyotrophic lateral sclerosis-linked superoxide dismutase mutants. Proc Natl Acad Sci USA 95: 6361-6366.

Cousins RJ, McMahon RJ. 2000. Integrative aspects of zinc transporters. J Nutr 130: 1384S-1387S.

Cousins RJ, Blanchard RK, Popp MP, Liu L, Cao J, et al. 2003. A global view of the selectivity of zinc deprivation and excess on genes expressed in human THP-1 mononuclear cells. Proc Natl Acad Sci USA 100: 6952-6957.

Cragg RA, Christie GR, Phillips SR, Russi RM, Kury S, et al. 2002. A novel zinc-regulated human zinc transporter, hZTL1, is localized to the enterocyte apical membrane. J Biol Chem 277: 22789-22797.

Crocker SJ, Pagenstecher A, Campbell IL. 2004. The TIMPs tango with MMPs and more in the central nervous system. J Neurosci Res 75: 1-11.

Cuajungco MP, Lees GJ. 1997. Zinc metabolism in the brain: Relevance to human neurodegenerative disorders. Neurobiol Dis 4: 137-169.

Culotta VC, Klomp LW, Strain J, Casareno RL, Krems B, et al. 1997. The copper chaperone for superoxide dismutase. J Biol Chem 272: 23469-23472.

Danks DM, Campell P, Stevens BJ, Howell RR. 1972. Menkes' kinky hair syndrome: An inherited defect of copper absorption with widespread effects. Pediatrics 50: 188-201.

Danscher G. 1996. The autometallographic zinc-sulphide method. A new approach involving in vivo creation of nanometer-sized zinc sulphide crystal lattices in zinc-enriched synaptic and secretory vesicles. Histochem J 28: 361-373.

Das S, Levinson B, Whitney S, Vulpe C, Packman S, et al. 1994. Diverse mutations in patients with Menkes disease often lead to exon skipping. Am J Hum Genet 55: 883-889.

Dufner-Beattie J, Langmade SJ, Wang F, Eide D, Andrews GK. 2003. Structure, function, and regulation of a subfamily of mouse zinc transporter genes. J Biol Chem 278: 50142-50150.

Ebadi M, Iversen PL, Hao R, Cerutis DR, Rojas P, et al. 1995. Expression and regulation of brain metallothionein. Neurochem Int 27: 1-22.

Eide DJ. 2000. Metal ion transport in eukaryotic microorganisms: Insights from Saccharomyces cerevisiae. Adv Microb Physiol 43: 1-38.

Eisses JF, Kaplan JH. 2002. Molecular characterization of hCTR1, the human copper uptake protein. J Biol Chem 277: 29162-29171.

Erway LC, Grider A, Jr. 1984. Zinc metabolism in lethal-milk mice. Otolith, lactation, and aging effects. J Hered 75: 480-484.

Ferenci P. 2004. Review article: Diagnosis and current therapy of Wilson's disease. Aliment Pharmacol Ther 19: 157-165.

Field LS, Luk E, Culotta VC. 2002. Copper chaperones: Personal escorts for metal ions. J Bioenerg Biomembr 34: 373-379.

Foltopoulou PF, Zachariadis GA, Politou AS, Tsiftsoglou AS, Papadopoulou LC. 2004. Human recombinant mutated forms of the mitochondrial COX assembly Sco2 protein differ from wild-type in physical state and copper binding capacity. Mol Genet Metab 81: 225-236.

Forbes JR, Cox DW. 2000. Copper-dependent trafficking of Wilson disease mutant ATP7B proteins. Hum Mol Genet 9: 1927-1935.

Francis MJ, Jones EE, Levy ER, Ponnambalam S, Chelly J, et al. 1998. A Golgi localization signal identified in the Menkes recombinant protein. Hum Mol Genet 7: 1245-1252.

Franco-Pons N, Casanovas-Aguilar C, Arroyo S, Rumia J, Perez-Clausell J, et al. 2000. Zinc-rich synaptic boutons in human temporal cortex biopsies. Neuroscience 98: 429-435.

Frederickson CJ, Bush AI. 2001. Synaptically released zinc: Physiological functions and pathological effects. Biometals 14: 353-366.

Frederickson CJ, Suh SW, Silva D, Frederickson CJ, Thompson RB. 2000. Importance of zinc in the central nervous system: The zinc-containing neuron. J Nutr 130: 1471S-1483S.

Freisinger P, Horvath R, Macmillan C, Peters J, Jaksch M. 2004. Reversion of hypertrophic cardiomyopathy in a patient with deficiency of the mitochondrial copper binding protein Sco2: Is there a potential effect of copper? J Inherit Metab Dis 27: 67-79.

Gaither LA, Eide DJ. 2001. The human ZIP1 transporter mediates zinc uptake in human K562 erythroleukemia cells. J Biol Chem 276: 22258-22264.

Ganesh L, Burstein E, Guha-Niyogi A, Louder MK, Mascola JR, et al. 2003. The gene product Murr1 restricts HIV-1 replication in resting CD4+ lymphocytes. Nature 426: 853-857.

Gitlin JD. 2003. Wilson disease. Gastroenterol 125: 1868-1877.

Glerum DM, Shtanko A, Tzagoloff A. 1996.Characterization of COX17, a yeast gene involved in copper metabolism and assembly of cytochrome oxidase. J Biol Chem 271: 14504-14509.

Gunshin H, Mackenzie B, Berger UV, Gunshin Y, Romero MF, et al. 1997. Cloning and characterization of a mammalian proton-coupled metal-ion transporter. Nature 388: 482-488.

Gybina AA, Prohaska JR. 2003. Increased rat brain cytochrome c correlates with degree of perinatal copper deficiency rather than apoptosis. J Nutr 133: 3361-3368.

Hamza I, Gitlin JD. 2002. Copper chaperones for cytochrome c oxidase and human disease. J Bioenerg Biomembr 34: 381-388.

Hamza I, Schaefer M, Klomp LW, Gitlin JD. 1999. Interaction of the copper chaperone HAH1 with the Wilson disease protein is essential for copper homeostasis. Proc Natl Acad Sci USA 96: 13363-13368.

Hamza I, Klomp LW, Gaedigk R, White RA, Gitlin JD. 2000. Structure, expression, and chromosomal localization of the mouse Atox1 gene. Genomics 63: 294-297.

Hamza I, Faisst A, Prohaska J, Chen J, Gruss P, et al. 2001. The metallochaperone Atox1 plays a critical role in perinatal copper homeostasis. Proc Natl Acad Sci USA 98: 6848-6852.

Hamza I, Prohaska J, Gitlin JD. 2003. Essential role for Atox1 in the copper-mediated intracellular trafficking of the Menkes ATPase. Proc Natl Acad Sci USA 100: 1215-1220.

Harada M, Sakisaka S, Terada K, Kimura R, Kawaguchi T, et al. 2001. A mutation of the Wilson disease protein, ATP7B, is degraded in the proteasomes and forms protein aggregates. Gastroenterol 120: 967-974.

Harada M, Kumemura H, Sakisaka S, Shishido S, Taniguchi E, et al. 2003. Wilson disease protein ATP7B is localized in the late endosomes in a polarized human hepatocyte cell line. Int J Mol Med 11: 293-298.

Harrison NL, Gibbons SJ. 1994. Zn2+: An endogenous modulator of ligand- and voltage-gated ion channels. Neuropharmacology 33: 935-952.

Hartter DE, Barnea A. 1988. Evidence for release of copper in the brain: Depolarization-induced release of newly taken-up 67copper. Synapse 2: 412-415.

Haussler MR, Haussler CA, Jurutka PW, Thompson PD, Hsieh JC, et al. 1997. The vitamin D hormone and its nuclear receptor: Molecular actions and disease states. J Endocrinol 154: S57-S73.

Henkin RI, Patten BM, Re PK, Bronzert DA. 1975. A syndrome of acute zinc loss. Cerebellar dysfunction, mental changes, anorexia, and taste and smell dysfunction. Arch Neurol 32: 745-751.

Hidalgo J, Aschner M, Zatta P, Vasak M. 2001. Roles of the metallothionein family of proteins in the central nervous system. Brain Res Bull 55: 133-145.

Hijazi N, Shaked Y, Rosenmann H, Ben-Hur T, Gabizon R. 2003. Copper binding to PrPC may inhibit prion disease propagation. Brain Res 993: 192-200.

Horng YC, Cobine PA, Maxfield AB, Carr HS, Winge DR. 2004. Specific copper transfer from the cox17 metallochaperone to both sco1 and cox11 in the assembly of yeast cytochrome c oxidase. J Biol Chem 279: 35334-35340.

Horning MS, Trombley PQ. 2001. Zinc and copper influence excitability of rat olfactory bulb neurons by multiple mechanisms. J Neurophysiol 86: 1652-1660.

Hoss W, Formaniak M. 1980. Enhancement of synaptic vesicle attachment to the plasma membrane fraction by copper. Neurochem Res 5: 795-803.

Huang L, Gitschier J. 1997. A novel gene involved in zinc transport is deficient in the lethal milk mouse. Nat Genet 17: 292-297.

Huang L, Kirschke CP, Gitschier J. 2002. Functional characterization of a novel mammalian zinc transporter, ZnT6. J Biol Chem 277: 26389-26395.

Hung IH, Casareno RL, Labesse G, Mathews FS, Gitlin JD. 1998. HAH1 is a copper-binding protein with distinct amino acid residues mediating copper homeostasis and antioxidant defense. J Biol Chem 273: 1749-1754.

Hunt DM, Johnson DR. 1972. An inherited deficiency in noradrenaline biosynthesis in the brindled mouse. J Neurochem 12: 2811-2819.

Huster D, Hoppert M, Lutsenko S, Zinke J, Lehmann C, et al. 2003. Defective cellular localization of mutant ATP7B in Wilson's disease patients and hepatoma cell lines. Gastroenterol 124: 335-345.

Ishida S, Lee J, Thiele DJ, Herskowitz I. 2002. Uptake of the anticancer drug cisplatin mediated by the copper transporter Ctr1 in yeast and mammals. Proc Natl Acad Sci USA 99: 14298-14302.

Jaksch M, Horvath R, Horn N, Auer DP, Macmillan C, et al. 2001. Homozygosity (E140K) in SCO2 causes delayed infantile onset of cardiomyopathy and neuropathy. Neurology 57: 1440-1446.

Jamieson AC, Miller JC, Pabo CO. 2003. Drug discovery with engineered zinc-finger proteins. Nat Rev Drug Discov 2: 361-368.

Jeong SY, David S. 2003. Glycosylphosphatidylinositol-anchored ceruloplasmin is required for iron efflux from cells in the central nervous system. J Biol Chem 278: 27144-27148.

Jiang LJ, Maret W, Vallee BL. 1998. The ATP-metallothionein complex. Proc Natl Acad Sci USA 95: 9146-9149.

Kako K, Tsumori K, Ohmasa Y, Takahashi Y, Munekata E. 2000. The expression of Cox17p in rodent tissues and cells. Eur J Biochem 267: 6699-6707.

Kaler SG, Holmes CS, Goldstein DS. 1998. Dopamine beta-hydroxylase deficiency associated with mutations in a copper transporter gene. Adv Pharmacol 42: 66-68.

Kambe T, Narita H, Yamaguchi-Iwai Y, Hirose J, Amano T, et al. 2002. Cloning and characterization of a novel mammalian zinc transporter, zinc transporter 5, abundantly expressed in pancreatic beta cells. J Biol Chem 277: 19049-19055.

Kambe T, Yamaguchi-Iwai Y, Sasaki R, Nagao M. 2004. Overview of mammalian zinc transporters. Cell Mol Life Sci 61: 49-68.

Kardos J, Kovacs I, Hajos F, Kalman M, Simonyi M. 1989. Nerve endings from rat brain tissue release copper upon depolarization. A possible role in regulating neuronal excitability. Neurosci Lett 103: 139-144.

Kelleher SL, Lönnerdal B. 2002. Zinc transporters in the rat mammary gland respond to marginal zinc and vitamin A intakes during lactation. J Nutr 132: 3280-3285.

Kelner GS, Lee M, Clark ME, Maciejewski D, McGrath D, et al. 2000. The copper transport protein Atox1 promotes neuronal survival. J Biol Chem 275: 580-584.

Kim AH, Sheline CT, Tian M, Higashi T, McMahon RJ, et al. 2000. L-type Ca(2+) channel-mediated Zn(2+) toxicity and modulation by ZnT-1 in PC12 cells. Brain Res 886: 99-107.

Kim YH, Kim EY, Gwag BJ, Sohn S, Koh JY. 1999. Zinc-induced cortical neuronal death with features of apoptosis and necrosis: Mediation by free radicals. Neuroscience 89: 175-182.

Klomp AE, Tops BB, Denberg Van IE, Berger R, Klomp LW. 2002. Biochemical characterization and subcellular localization of human copper transporter 1 (hCTR1). Biochem J 364: 497-505.

Klomp AE, Juijn JA, der Gun van LT, den Berg van IE, Berger R, et al. 2003a. The N-terminus of the human copper transporter 1 (hCTR1) is localized extracellularly, and interacts with itself. Biochem J 370: 881-889.

Klomp AE, de Sluis van B, Klomp LW, Wijmenga C. 2003b. The ubiquitously expressed MURR1 protein is absent in canine copper toxicosis. J Hepatol 39: 703-709.

Klomp LW, Gitlin JD. 1996. Expression of the ceruloplasmin gene in the human retina and brain: Implications for a pathogenic model in aceruloplasminemia. Hum Mol Genet 5: 1989-1996.

Klomp LW, Lin SJ, Yuan DS, Klausner RD, Culotta VC, et al. 1997. Identification and functional expression of HAH1, a novel human gene involved in copper homeostasis. J Biol Chem 272: 9221-9226.

Klug A, Schwabe JW. 1995. Protein motifs 5. Zinc fingers. FASEB J 9: 597-604.

Kodama H. 1993. Recent developments in Menkes disease. J Inherit Metab Dis 16: 791-799.

Koh JY, Suh SW, Gwag BJ, He YY, Hsu CY, et al. 1996. The role of zinc in selective neuronal death after transient global cerebral ischemia. Science 272: 1013-1016.

Kohler LB, Berezin V, Bock E, Penkowa M. 2003. The role of metallothionein II in neuronal differentiation and survival. Brain Res 992: 128-136.

Komatsu Y, Ogra Y, Suzuki KT. 2002. Copper balance and ceruloplasmin in chronic hepatitis in a Wilson disease animal model, LEC rats. Arch Toxicol 76: 502-508.

Kovacs KJ, Larson AA. 1997. Zn2+ inhibition of [3H]MK-801 binding is different in mouse brain and spinal cord: Effect of glycine and glutamate. Eur J Pharmacol 324: 117-123.

Kroncke KD, Carlberg C. 2000. Inactivation of zinc finger transcription factors provides a mechanism for a gene regulator role of nitric oxide. FASEB J 14: 166-173.

Kuo YM, Gitschier J, Packman S. 1997. Developmental expression of the mouse mottled and toxic milk genes suggests distinct functions for the Menkes and Wilson disease copper transporters. Hum Mol Genet 6: 1043-1049.

Kuo YM, Zhou B, Cosco D, Gitschier J. 2001. The copper transporter CTR1 provides an essential function in mammalian embryonic development. Proc Natl Acad Sci USA 98: 6836-6841.

Kury S, Kharfi M, Kamoun R, Taieb A, Mallet E, et al. 2003. Mutation spectrum of human SLC39A4 in a panel of patients with acrodermatitis enteropathica. Hum Mutat 22: 337-338.

Laity JH, Lee BM, Wright PE. 2001. Zinc finger proteins: New insights into structural and functional diversity. Curr Opin Struct Biol 11: 39-46.

Labbe S, Thiele DJ. 1999. Pipes and wiring: The regulation of copper uptake and distribution in yeast. Trends Microbiol 7: 500-505.

Larin D, Mekios C, Das K, Ross B, Yang AS, et al. 1999. Characterization of the interaction between the Wilson and Menkes disease proteins and the cytoplasmic copper chaperone, HAH1p. J Biol Chem 274: 28497-28504.

Law W, Kelland EE, Sharp P, Toms NJ. 2003. Characterisation of zinc uptake into rat cultured cerebrocortical oligodendrocyte progenitor cells. Neurosci Lett 352: 113-116.

Leary SC, Kaufman BA, Pellecchia G, Guercin GH, Mattman A, et al. 2004. Human SCO1 and SCO2 have independent, cooperative functions in copper delivery to cytochrome c oxidase. Hum Mol Genet 13: 1839-1848.

Lee J, Prohaska JR, Dagenais SL, Glover TW, Thiele DJ. 2000b Isolation of a murine copper transporter gene, tissue specific expression and functional complementation of a yeast copper transport mutant. Gene 254: 87-96.

Lee J, Prohaska JR, Thiele DJ. 2001b. Essential role for mammalian copper transporter Ctr1 in copper homeostasis and embryonic development. Proc Natl Acad Sci USA 98 6842-6847.

Lee J, Pena MM, Nose Y, Thiele DJ. 2002a. Biochemical characterization of the human copper transporter Ctr1. J Biol Chem 277: 4380-4387.

Lee J, Petris MJ, Thiele DJ. 2002b. Characterization of mouse embryonic cells deficient in the ctr1 high affinity copper transporter. Identification of a Ctr1-independent copper transport system. J Biol Chem 277: 40253-40259.

Lee JY, Cole TB, Palmiter RD, Koh JY. 2000a. Accumulation of zinc in degenerating hippocampal neurons of ZnT3-null mice after seizures: Evidence against synaptic vesicle origin. J Neurosci 20: RC79.

Lee JY, Kim JH, Hong SH, Lee JY, Cherny RA, et al. 2004. Estrogen decreases zinc transporter 3 expression and synaptic vesicle zinc levels in mouse brain. J Biol Chem 279: 8602-8607.

Lee M, Hyun D, Jenner P, Halliwell B. 2001a. Effect of overexpression of wild-type and mutant Cu/Zn-superoxide dismutases on oxidative damage and antioxidant defences: Relevance to Down's syndrome and familial amyotrophic lateral sclerosis. J Neurochem 76: 957-965.

Levinson B, Vulpe C, Elder B, Martin C, Verley F, et al. 1994. The mottled gene is the mouse homologue of the Menkes disease gene. Nat Genet 6: 369-373.

Li YV, Hough CJ, Sarvey JM. 2003. Do we need zinc to think? Sci STKE 182: pe19.

Lin DD, Cohen AS, Coulter DA. 2001. Zinc-induced augmentation of excitatory synaptic currents and glutamate receptor responses in hippocampal CA3 neurons. J Neurophysiol 85: 1185-1196.

Liuzzi JP, Cousins RJ. 2004. Mammalian zinc transporters. Annu Rev Nutr 24: 151-172.

Liuzzi JP, Blanchard RK, Cousins RJ. 2001. Differential regulation of zinc transporter 1, 2, and 4 mRNA expression by dietary zinc in rats. J Nutr 131: 46-52.

Lutsenko S, Cooper MJ. 1998. Localization of the Wilson's disease protein product to mitochondria. Proc Natl Acad Sci USA 95: 6004-6009.

Lutsenko S, Tsivkovskii R, Walker JM. 2003. Functional properties of the human copper-transporting ATPase ATP7B (the Wilson's disease protein) and regulation by metallochaperone Atox1. Ann N Y Acad Sci 986: 204-211.

Maes M, D'Haese PC, Scharpe S, D'Hondt P, Cosyns P, et al. 1994. Hypozincemia in depression. J Affect Disord 31: 135-140.

Maes M, De Vos N, Demedts P, Wauters A, Neels H. 1999. Lower serum zinc in major depression in relation to changes in serum acute phase proteins. J Affect Disord 56: 189-194.

Maier CM, Chan PH. 2002. Role of superoxide dismutases in oxidative damage and neurodegenerative disorders. Neuroscientist 8: 323-334.

Martinez-Galan JR, Diaz C, Juiz JM. 2003. Histochemical localization of neurons with zinc-permeable AMPA/kainate channels in rat brain slices. Brain Res 963: 156-164.

Masters BA, Quaife CJ, Erickson JC, Kelly EJ, Froelick GJ, et al. 1994. Metallothionein III is expressed in neurons that sequester zinc in synaptic vesicles. J Neurosci 14: 5844-5857.

Maxfield AB, Heaton DN, Winge DR. 2004. Cox17 is functional when tethered to the mitochondrial inner membrane. J Biol Chem 279: 5072-5080.

Maynard CJ, Cappai R, Volitakis I, Cherny RA, White AR, et al. 2002. Overexpression of Alzheimer's disease amyloid-beta opposes the age-dependent elevations of brain copper and iron. J Biol Chem 277: 44670-44676.

McCall KA, Huang C, Fierke CA. 2000. Function and mechanism of zinc metalloenzymes. J Nutr 130: 1437S-1446S.

McMahon RJ, Cousins RJ. 1998. Mammalian zinc transporters. J Nutr 128: 667-670.

Menkes JH. 1988. Kinky hair disease: Twenty-five years later. Brain Dev 10: 77-79.

Menkes JH, Alter M, Steigleder GK, Weakley DR, Sung JH. 1962. A sex-linked recessive disorder with retardation of growth, peculiar hair and focal cerebral and cerebellar degeneration. Pediatrics 29: 764-779.

Mercer JF, Livingston J, Hall B, Paynter JA, Begy C, et al. 1993. Isolation of a partial candidate gene for Menkes disease by positional cloning. Nat Genet 3: 20-25.

Naeve GS, Vana AM, Eggold JR, Kelner GS, Maki R, et al. 1999. Expression profile of the copper homeostasis gene, rAtox1, in the rat brain. Neuroscience 93: 1179-1187.

Narayanan VS, Fitch CA, Levenson CW. 2001. Tumor suppressor protein p53 mRNA and subcellular localization are altered by changes in cellular copper in human Hep G2 cells. J Nutr 131: 1427-1432.

Nishihara E, Furuyama T, Yamashita S, Mori N. 1998. Expression of copper trafficking genes in the mouse brain. Neuroreport 9: 3259-3263.

Nitzan YB, Sekler I, Hershfinkel M, Moran A, Silverman WF. 2002. Postnatal regulation of ZnT-1 expression in the mouse brain. Brain Res Dev Brain Res 137: 149-157.

O'Halloran TV. 1993. Transition metals in control of gene expression. Science 261: 715-725.

Ohana E, Segal D, Palty R, Ton-That D, Moran A, et al. 2004. A sodium zinc exchange mechanism is mediating extrusion of zinc in mammalian cells. J Biol Chem 279: 4278-4284.

Orrell RW, Marklund SL, de Belleroche JS. 1997. Familial ALS is associated with mutations in all exons of SOD1: A novel mutation in exon 3 (Gly72Ser). J Neurol Sci 153: 46-49.

Palmiter RD, Findley SD, Whitmore TE, Durnam DM. 1992. MT-III, a brain-specific member of the metallothionein gene family. Proc Natl Acad Sci USA 89: 6333-6337.

Palmiter RD, Findley SD. 1995. Cloning and functional characterization of a mammalian zinc transporter that confers resistance to zinc. EMBO J 14: 639-649.

Palmiter RD, Cole TB, Quaife CJ, Findley SD. 1996. ZnT-3, a putative transporter of zinc into synaptic vesicles. Proc Natl Acad Sci USA 93: 14934-14939.

Palmiter RD, Huang L. 2004. Efflux and compartmentalization of zinc by members of the SLC30 family of solute carriers. Pflugers Arch 447: 744-751.

Palumaa P, Kangur L, Voronova A, Sillard R. 2004. Metal-binding mechanism of Cox17, a copper chaperone for cytochrome c oxidase. Biochem J 382: 307-314.

Patel BN, Dunn RJ, Jeong SY, Zhu Q, Julien JP, et al. 2002. Ceruloplasmin regulates iron levels in the CNS and prevents free radical injury. J Neurosci 22: 6578-6586.

Payne AS, Kelly EJ, Gitlin JD. 1998. Functional expression of the Wilson disease protein reveals mislocalization and impaired copper-dependent trafficking of the common H1069Q mutation. Proc Natl Acad Sci USA 95: 10854-10859.

Perafan-Riveros C, Franca LF, Alves AC, Sanches JA Jr. 2002. Acrodermatitis enteropathica: Case report and review of the literature. Pediatr Dermatol 19: 426-431.

Petris MJ, Camakaris J, Greenough M, La Fontaine S, Mercer JF. 1998. A C-terminal di-leucine is required for localization of the Menkes protein in the trans-Golgi network. Hum Mol Genet 7: 2063-2071.

Petris MJ, Strausak D, Mercer JF. 2000. The Menkes copper transporter is required for the activation of tyrosinase. Hum Mol Genet 9: 2845-2851.

Petris MJ, Smith K, Lee J, Thiele DJ. 2003. Copper-stimulated endocytosis and degradation of the human copper transporter. J Biol Chem 278: 9639-9646.

Petrukhin K, Pirastu M, Tanzi RE, Chernov I, Devoto M, et al. 1993. Mapping cloning and genetic characterization of the region containing the Wilson disease gene. Nat Gen 5: 338-343.

Prasad AS. 2001a. Discovery of human zinc deficiency: Impact on human health. Nutrition 17: 685-687.

Prasad AS. 2001b. Recognition of zinc-deficiency syndrome. Nutrition 17: 67-69.

Prigge ST, Mains RE, Eipper BA, Amzel LM. 2000. New insights into copper monooxygenases and peptide amidation: Structure, mechanism and function. Cell Mol Life Sci 57: 1236-1259.

Prohaska, JR, Gybina AA. 2004. Intracellular copper transport in mammals. J Nutr 134: 1003-1006.

Prohaska JR, Broderius M, Brokate B. 2003a. Metallochaperone for Cu,Zn-superoxide dismutase (CCS) protein but not mRNA is higher in organs from copper-deficient mice and rats. Arch Biochem Biophys 417: 227-234.

Prohaska JR, Geissler J, Brokate B, Broderius M. 2003b. Copper, zinc-superoxide dismutase protein but not mRNA is lower in copper-deficient mice and mice lacking the copper chaperone for superoxide dismutase. Exp Biol Med 228: 959-966.

Qi M, Byers PH. 1998. Constitutive skipping of alternatively spliced exon 10 in the ATP7A gene abolishes Golgi localization of the menkes protein and produces the occipital horn syndrome. Hum Mol Genet 7: 465-469.

Qian Y, Tiffany-Castiglioni E, Harris ED. 1997. A Menkes P-type ATPase involved in copper homeostasis in the central nervous system of the rat. Brain Res Mol Brain Res 48: 60-66.

Radja N, Charles-Holmes R. 2002. Acrodermatitis enteropathica—lifelong follow-up and zinc monitoring. Clin Exp Dermatol 27: 62-63.

Reddy MC, Harris ED. 1998. Multiple transcripts coding for the menkes gene: Evidence for alternative splicing of Menkes mRNA. Biochem J 334: 71-77.

Roelofsen H, Wolters H, Luyn Van MJ, Miura N, Kuipers F, et al. 2000. Copper-induced apical trafficking of ATP7B in polarized hepatoma cells provides a mechanism for biliary copper excretion. Gastroenterol 119: 782-793.

Rothstein JD, Dykes-Hoberg M, Corson LB, Becker M, Cleveland DW, et al. 1999. The copper chaperone CCS is abundant in neurons and astrocytes in human and rodent brain. J Neurochem 72: 422-429.

Sacher A, Cohen A, Nelson N. 2001. Properties of the mammalian and yeast metal-ion transporters DCT1 and Smf1p expressed in Xenopus laevis oocytes. J Exp Biol 204: 1053-1061.

Saito T, Okabe M, Hosokawa T, Kurasaki M, Hata A, et al. 1999. Immunohistochemical determination of the Wilson Copper-transporting P-type ATPase in the brain tissues of the rat. Neurosci Lett 266: 13-16.

Saito T, Takahashi K, Nakagawa N, Hosokawa T, Kurasaki M, et al. 2000. Deficiencies of hippocampal Zn and ZnT3 accelerate brain aging of Rat. Biochem Biophys Res Commun 279: 505-511.

Salviati L, Hernandez-Rosa E, Walker WF, Sacconi S, Di Mauro S, et al. 2002. Copper supplementation restores cytochrome c oxidase activity in cultured cells from patients with SCO2 mutations. Biochem J 363: 321-327.

Sanokawa-Akakura R, Dai H, Akakura S, Weinstein D, Fajardo JE, et al. 2004. A novel role for the immunophilin FKBP52 in copper transport. J Biol Chem 279: 27845-27848.

Saris NE, Niva K. 1994. Is Zn2+ transported by the mitochondrial calcium uniporter? FEBS Lett 356: 195-198.

Savouret JF, Chauchereau A, Misrahi M, Lescop P, Mantel A, et al. 1994. The progesterone receptor. Biological effects of progestins and antiprogestins. Hum Reprod 9: 7-11.

Scarpulla RC. 1997. Nuclear control of respiratory chain expression in mammalian cells. J Bioenerg Biomembr 29: 109-119.

Schaefer M, Roelofsen H, Wolters H, Hofmann WJ, Muller M, et al. 1999. Localization of the Wilson's disease protein in human liver. Gastroenterology 117: 1380-1385.

Scheinberg IH, Gitlin D. 1952. Deficiency of ceruloplasmin in patients with hepatolenticular degeneration (Wilson's disease). Science 116: 484-485.

Sekler I, Moran A, Hershfinkel M, Dori A, Margulis A, et al. 2002. Distribution of the zinc transporter ZnT-1 in comparison with chelatable zinc in the mouse brain. J Comp Neurol 447: 201-209.

Sensi SL, Canzoniero LM, Yu SP, Ying HS, Koh JY, et al. 1997. Measurement of intracellular free zinc in living cortical neurons: Routes of entry. J Neurosci 17: 9554-9564.

Shah AB, Chernov I, Zhang HT, Ross BM, Das K, et al. 1997. Identification and analysis of mutations in the Wilson disease gene (ATP7B): Population frequencies, genotype-phenotype correlation, and functional analyses. Am J Hum Genet 61: 317-328.

Sharp PA. 2003. Ctr1 and its role in body copper homeostasis. Int J Biochem Cell Biol 35: 288-291.

Shi Y, Berg JM. 1995. Specific DNA-RNA hybrid binding by zinc finger proteins. Science 268: 282-284.

Shi YB, Du L, Zheng WJ, Tang WX. 2002. Isolation of GIF from porcine brain and studies of its zinc transfer kinetics with apo-carbonic anhydrase. Biometals 15: 421-427.

Shim H, Harris ZL. 2003. Genetic defects in copper metabolism. J Nutr 133: 1527S-1531S.

Smart TG, Xie X, Krishek BJ. 1994. Modulation of inhibitory and excitatory amino acid receptor ion channels by zinc. Prog Neurobiol 42: 393-341.

Sørensen JC, Mattsson B, Andreasen A, Johansson BB. 1998. Rapid disappearance of zinc positive terminals in focal brain ischemia. Brain Res 812: 265-269.

Steveson TC, Ciccotosto GD, Ma XM, Mueller GP, Mains RE, et al. 2003. Menkes protein contributes to the function of peptidylglycine alpha-amidating monooxygenase. Endocrinology 144: 188-200.

Strausak D, Mercer JF, Dieter HH, Stremmel W, Multhaup G. 2001. Copper in disorders with neurological symptoms: Alzheimer's, Menkes, and Wilson diseases. Brain Res Bull 55: 175-185.

Strausak D, Howie MK, Firth SD, Schlicksupp A, Pipkorn R, et al. 2003. Kinetic analysis of the interaction of the copper chaperone Atox1 with the metal binding sites of the Menkes protein. J Biol Chem 278: 20821-20827.

Szerdahelyi P, Kasa P. 1986. A highly sensitive method for the histochemical demonstration of copper in normal rat tissues. Histochemistry 85: 349-352.

Takahashi Y, Kako K, Kashiwabara S, Takehara A, Inada Y, et al. 2002a. Mammalian copper chaperone Cox17p has an essential role in activation of cytochrome c oxidase and embryonic development. Mol Cell Biol 22: 7614-7621.

Takahashi Y, Kako K, Arai A, Ohishi T, Inada Y, et al. 2002b. Characterization and identification of promoter elements in the mouse COX17 gene. Biochim Biophys Acta 1574: 359-364.

Takeda A. 2000. Movement of zinc and its functional significance in the brain. Brain Res Rev 34: 137-148.

Takeda A. 2001. Zinc homeostasis and functions of zinc in the brain. Biometals 14: 343-351.

Takeda A, Minami A, Seki Y, Oku N. 2004. Differential effects of zinc on glutamatergic and GABAergic neurotransmitter systems in the hippocampus. J Neurosci Res 75: 225-229.

Tanzi RE, Petrukhin K, Chernov I, Pellequer JL, Wasco W, et al. 1993. The Wilson disease gene is a copper transporting ATPase with homology to the Menkes disease gene. Nat Gen 5: 344-350.

Tao TY, Liu F, Klomp L, Wijmenga C, Gitlin JD. 2003. The copper toxicosis gene product Murr1 directly interacts with the Wilson disease protein. J Biol Chem 278: 41593-41596.

Tapiero H, Tew KD. 2003. Trace elements in human physiology and pathology: Zinc and metallothioneins. Biomed Pharmacother 57: 399-411.

Taylor KM, Nicholson RI. 2003. The LZT proteins; the LIV-1 subfamily of zinc transporters. Biochim Biophys Acta 1611: 16-30.

Taylor KM, Morgan HE, Johnson A, Hadley LJ, Nicholson RI. 2003. Structure-function analysis of LIV-1, the breast cancer-associated protein that belongs to a new subfamily of zinc transporters. Biochem J 375: 51-59.

Tønder N, Johansen FF, Frederickson CJ, Zimmer J, Diemer NH. 1990. Possible role of zinc in the selective degeneration of dentate hilar neurons after cerebral ischemia in the adult rat. Neurosci Lett 109: 247-252.

Trombley PQ, Shepherd GM. 1996. Differential modulation by zinc and copper of amino acid receptors from rat olfactory bulb neurons. J Neurophysiol 76: 2536-2546.

Trombley PQ, Horning MS, Blakemore LJ. 1998. Carnosine modulates zinc and copper effects on amino acid receptors and synaptic transmission. Neuroreport 9: 3503-3507.

Tsuda M, Imaizumi K, Katayama T, Kitagawa K, Wanaka A, et al. 1997. Expression of zinc transporter gene, ZnT-1, is induced after transient forebrain ischemia in the gerbil. J Neurosci 17: 6678-6684.

Tucker DM, Sandstead HH. 1984. Neuropsychological function in experimental zinc deficiency in humans. The Neurobiology of Zinc Part B: Deficiency, Toxicity, and Pathology, Vol 11B. Frederickson CJ, Howell GA, Kasarskis EF, editors. New York: Alan R Liss; pp. 139-152.

Uchida Y, Takio K, Titani K, Ihara Y, Tomonaga M. 1991. The growth inhibitory factor that is deficient in the Alzheimer's disease brain is a 68 amino acid metallothionein-like protein. Neuron 7: 337-347.

Udom AO, Brady FO. 1980. Reactivation in vitro of zinc-requiring apo-enzymes by rat liver zinc-thionein. Biochem J 187: 329-335.

Valente T, Auladell C. 2002. Developmental expression of ZnT3 in mouse brain: Correlation between the vesicular zinc transporter protein and chelatable vesicular zinc (CVZ) cells. Glial and neuronal CVZ cells interact. Mol Cell Neurosci 21: 189-204.

Ho Van A, Ward DM, Kaplan J. 2002. Transition metal transport in yeast. Annu Rev Microbiol 56: 237-261.

Landingham Van JW, Fitch CA, Levenson CW. 2002. Zinc inhibits the nuclear translocation of the tumor suppressor protein p53 and protects cultured human neurons from copper-induced neurotoxicity. Neuromolecular Med 1: 171-182.

Vogt K, Mellor J, Tong G, Nicoll R. 2000. The actions of synaptically released zinc at hippocampal mossy fiber synapses. Neuron 26: 187-196.

Vulpe C, Levinson B, Whitney S, Packman S, Gitschier J. 1993. Isolation of a candidate gene for Menkes disease and evidence that it encodes a copper-transporting ATPase. Nat Genet 3: 7-13.

Waggoner DJ, Drisaldi B, Bartnikas TB, Casareno RL, Prohaska JR, et al. 2000. Brain copper content and cuproenzyme activity do not vary with prion protein expression level. J Biol Chem. 275: 7455-7458.

Walker JM, Huster D, Ralle M, Morgan CT, Blackburn NJ, et al. 2004. The N-terminal metal-binding site 2 of the Wilson's disease protein plays a key role in the transfer of copper from Atox1. J Biol Chem 279: 15376-15384.

Wang A, Dufner-Beattie J, Kim BE, Petris MJ, Andrews G, et al. 2004a. Zinc-stimulated endocytosis controls activity of the mouse ZIP1 and ZIP3 zinc uptake transporters. J Biol Chem 279: 24631-24639.

Wang F, Kim BE, Dufner-Beattie J, Petris MJ, Andrews G, et al. 2004c. Acrodermatitis enteropathica mutations affect transport activity, localization and zinc-responsive trafficking of the mouse ZIP4 zinc transporter. Hum Mol Genet 13: 563-571.

Wang K, Zhou B, Kuo YM, Zemansky J, Gitschier J. 2002. A novel member of a zinc transporter family is defective in acrodermatitis enteropathica. Am J Hum Genet 71: 66-73.

Wang Y, Joh K, Masuko S, Yatsuki H, Soejima H, et al. 2004b. The mouse Murr1 gene is imprinted in the adult brain, presumably due to transcriptional interference by the antisense-oriented U2af1-rs1 gene. Mol Cell Biol 24: 270-279.

Weiss JH, Sensi SL. 2000. Ca2+-Zn2+ permeable AMPA or kainate receptors: Possible key factors in selective neurodegeneration. Trends Neurosci 23: 365-371.

Wenzel HJ, Cole TB, Born DE, Schwartzkroin PA, Palmiter RD. 1997. Ultrastructural localization of zinc transporter-3 (ZnT-3) to synaptic vesicle membranes within mossy fiber boutons in the hippocampus of mouse and monkey. Proc Natl Acad Sci USA 94: 12676-12681.

Wernimont AK, Yatsunyk LA, Rosenzweig AC. 2004. Binding of copper(I) by the Wilson disease protein and its copper chaperone. J Biol Chem 279: 12269-12276.

Westbrook GL, Mayer ML. 1987. Micromolar concentrations of Zn2+ antagonize NMDA and GABA responses of hippocampal neurons. Nature 328: 640-643.

White AR, Multhaup G, Maher F, Bellingham S, Camakaris J, et al. 1999. The Alzheimer's disease amyloid precursor protein modulates copper-induced toxicity and oxidative stress in primary neuronal cultures. J Neurosci 19: 9170-9179.

Wikstrom M. 2004. Cytochrome c oxidase: 25 years of the elusive proton pump. Biochim Biophys Acta 1655: 241-247.

Winegar BD, Lansman JB. 1990. Voltage-dependent block by zinc of single calcium channels in mouse myotubes. J Physiol 425: 563-578.

Wong PC, Waggoner D, Subramaniam JR, Tessarollo L, Bartnikas TB, et al. 2000. Copper chaperone for superoxide dismutase is essential to activate mammalian Cu/Zn superoxide dismutase. Proc Natl Acad Sci USA 97: 2886-2891.

Xu B, Koenig RJ. 2004. An RNA-binding domain in the thyroid hormone receptor enhances transcriptional activation. J Biol Chem 279: 33051-33056.

Yang XL, Miura N, Kawarada Y, Terada K, Petrukhin K, et al. 1997. Two forms of Wilson disease protein produced by alternative splicing are localized in distinct cellular compartments. Biochem J 326: 897-902.

Ye B, Maret W, Vallee BL. 2001. Zinc metallothionein imported into liver mitochondria modulates respiration. Proc Natl Acad Sci USA 98: 2317-2322.

Yeiser EC, Lerant AA, Casto RM, Levenson CW. 1999a. Free zinc increases at the site of injury after cortical stab wound in mature but not immature rat brain. Neurosci Lett 277: 75-78.

Yeiser EC, Fitch CA, Horning MS, Rutkoski N, Levenson CW. 1999b. Regulation of metallothionein-3 mRNA by thyroid hormone in developing rat brain and primary cultures of rat astrocytes and neurons. Brain Res Dev Brain Res 115: 195-200.

Yu WH, Lukiw WJ, Bergeron C, Niznik HB, Fraser PE. 2001. Metallothionein III is reduced in Alzheimer's disease. Brain Res 894: 37-45.

Zawia NH. 2003. Transcriptional involvement in neurotoxicity. Toxicol Appl Pharmacol 190: 177-188.

Zhang DQ, Ribelayga C, Mangel SC, McMahon DG. 2002. Suppression by zinc of AMPA receptor-mediated synaptic transmission in the retina. J Neurophysiol 88: 1245-1251.

Zhou B, Gitschier J. 1997. hCTR1: A human gene for copper uptake identified by complementation in yeast. Proc Natl Acad Sci USA 94: 7481-7486.

Zhu HL, Wang DS, Li JS. 2002. Cu2+ suppresses GABA(A) receptor-mediated responses in rat sacral dorsal commissural neurons. Neurosignals 11: 322-328.

14 Functional and Pharmacological Aspects of GABA Transporters

K. Madsen · H. S. White · R. P. Clausen · B. Frølund · O. M. Larsson ·
P. Krogsgaard-Larsen · A. Schousboe

Abstract: Termination of GABAergic neurotransmission is facilitated via high-affinity GABA transporters (GATs), which use the sodium and chloride gradients to drive the active transport of GABA into both the pre- and post-synaptic neurons and neighboring astroglial cells. The GATs are members of the Solute Carrier 6 (SLC6) transporter family.

Early pharmacological studies revealed a difference between the uptake specificity between neurons and astrocytes. Moreover, glial transport is preferably inhibited since exclusive inhibition of neuronal GABA transports can lead to seizures in-vivo. Twenty-eight years after the discovery of GABA transporters the first GABA transporter designated GAT1 was cloned. Today, five GABA transporters are known, one of them being the vesicular GABA transporter and the other four GAT1, GAT2, GAT3, and GAT4 are associated with the plasma membrane. The GATs have been extensively characterized pharmacologically. The main emphasis has been put on GAT1 which is the most active among the four GATs. Moreover, a large number of studies have been focused on identifying inhibitors which selectively may inhibit astroglial GABA transport. This is related to the proposal that such inhibitors may be effective anticonvulsants.

Subcellular localization studies have shown that the GABA transporters are unevenly distributed within the synapses, GAT1 and GAT4 are primarily located on neurons and astrocytes, respectively and GAT2 and GAT3 are less widely distributed and more diverse. The GAT proteins are composed of 12 transmembrane domains (TMD) and display a high level of homology in their amino acid sequence. Functional analysis has revealed that TMD1, TMD3, Extracellular loop (EL) 2, and EL4 are involved in the binding pocket of GAT1, findings which are confirmed in the bacterial leucine transporter LeuT$_{Aa}$ a transporter which shares 20-25 % sequence homology to the SLC transporter family.

List of Abbreviations: ACHC, *cis*-3-aminocyclohexanecarboxylic acid; BBB, Blood-Brain barrier; BGT, Betaine-GABA transporter; CNS, Central nervous system; DABA, Diaminobutyric acid; DMCM, Methyl-6,7-dimethoxy-4-ethyl-β-carboline-3-carboxylate; EL, Extracellular Loop; GABA, γ-aminobutyric acid; GABA-T, GABA aminotransferase; GAD, Glutamate decarboxylase; GAT, GABA transporter; HEK, Human Embryonic Kidney; IL, Intracellular Loop; LeuT$_{Aa}$, *Aquifix aeolicus* Leucine transporter; MDCK, Madin-Darby canine kidney; PKC, Protein Kinase C; PLP, Pyridoxal 5′-phosphate; SSADH, Succinic semialdehyde dehydrogenase; TCA, Tricarboxylic acid cycle; TMD, Transmembrane domain; VGAT, vesicular GABA transporter

1   GABA: An Introduction

Almost 60 years ago, three research groups independently discovered that GABA is present in the brain (Awapara et al., 1950; Roberts and Frankel, 1950; Udenfriend, 1950). Subsequently, it has been established as the major inhibitory neurotransmitter in the mammalian central nervous system (CNS) (Elliott and van Gelder, 1958; Krnjevic and Schwartz, 1967; Roberts, 1971; Curtis and Johnston, 1974). GABA is estimated to be present in 60–75% of the synapses in the CNS (Durkin et al., 1995), hence it plays a significant role in the maintenance of the normal function in the CNS, which is established in concerted action with the major excitatory neurotransmitter, L-glutamate.

Dysfunction in the CNS neurotransmission, resulting from an imbalance between the inhibitory and excitatory currents, manifests itself in numerous pathological diseases among others, epilepsy. Disinhibition is considered to be the precipitating factor in epilepsy, leading to hyperexcitable neurons which discharge in a highly synchronized manner propagating into a full seizure (Lloyd and Morselli, 1987; De Deyn et al., 1990; Dalby and Mody, 2001). Although this imbalance theory is a gross oversimplification, several experimental results strengthen it; reduced GABA levels in human tissue surgically removed from patients with intractable epilepsy have been found and moreover, the chemoconvulsants pentylenetetrazole (PTZ) and methyl 6,7-dimethoxy-4-ethyl-β-carboline-3-carboxylate (DMCM) reduce the GABA response in a dose-dependent manner (De Deyn et al., 1990). Benzodiazepines and barbiturates enhance the GABA-mediated inhibitory neurotransmission, and tiagabine and vigabatrin increase the synaptic GABA concentration. All of these compounds display an anticonvulsant effect.

2 GABAergic Neurotransmission

GABA is synthesized in neurons by a pathway, often referred to as the "GABA shunt." In short, α-ketoglutarate is funneled out of the tricarboxylic acid cycle and transaminated by GABA transaminase (GABA-T) to L-glutamate which is converted to GABA by glutamate decarboxylase (GAD) (Roberts and Kuriyama, 1968; Balazs et al., 1970). GAD exists in two forms with molecular weights of 67 and 65 kDa referred to as GAD_{67} and GAD_{65}, respectively. GAD_{67} and GAD_{65} differ in subcellular localization; the former being distributed throughout the neuron but primarily in the soma and dendrites, whereas the latter is predominantly located at the nerve endings near the synaptic vesicles. GAD is dependent on its cofactor pyridoxal 5'-phosphate (PLP) for activity. Nearly all GAD_{67} is in the activated holoenzyme form, whereas GAD_{65} is only partly saturated with PLP (Kaufman et al., 1991). Due to the different localizations of GAD_{67} and GAD_{65}, and the fact that GAD_{65} is mainly in the apoenzyme form (inactive, without bound PLP) and readily inducible by neuronal activity, it has been proposed that GAD_{65} is responsible for maintaining adequate amounts of GABA in the nerve terminal during heightened neuronal activity (Erlander and Tobin, 1991; Kaufman et al., 1991).

GABA is predominantly packaged into vesicles by a vesicular GABA transporter (VGAT), which uses the proton gradient to drive the uphill transport, and released into the synaptic cleft in a Ca^{2+}-dependent manner (Nicholls, 1989). However, GABA can also be released into the cleft via reversal of the GABA transporters present on the presynaptic neuron (During et al., 1995).

Upon release to the synaptic cleft, GABA interacts with $GABA_A$, $GABA_C$, and $GABA_B$ receptors; the first two being ionotropic and primarily located postsynaptically and the latter being metabotropic and localized both pre- and postsynaptically (Feldman et al., 1997; Watanabe et al., 2002). The termination of the GABAergic neurotransmission is facilitated via high-affinity transport proteins located in both presynaptic neurons and surrounding glia cells (Iversen and Neal, 1968; Iversen and Kelly, 1975). Upon entry into the presynaptic neuron and glia cells, GABA is degraded by the catabolic enzymes GABA-T and succinate semialdehyde dehydrogenase (SSADH) to succinate, which reenters the TCA cycle (Waagepetersen et al., 2003) and completes the "GABA shunt." It has been estimated that roughly 8–10% of the flux through the TCA cycle in GABAergic neurons is accounted for by the GABA shunt (Balazs et al., 1970).

3 GABA Transporters

With the establishment of GABA as an inhibitory neurotransmitter and the elucidation of its metabolism as described above, a more detailed elaboration on the GABA transporters as pharmacological targets is warranted. Elliott and van Gelder (1958) were among the first to determine that GABA in the incubation medium could accumulate into slices of cerebral cortices. However, it was not until 10 years later that the existence of high-affinity transport proteins for GABA was discovered in both neurons and astrocytes (Iversen and Neal, 1968). Later, it was shown that ^{3}H-GABA in rat cerebellum was predominantly accumulated not only into stellate cells or other interneurons but also into astrocytes (Hösli and Hösli, 1976, 1978). Diaminobutyric acid (DABA) and 3-hydroxy-5-aminovaleric acid have been shown to be selective inhibitors of neuronal GABA transport, whereas β-alanine and β-proline are selective inhibitors of glial GABA transport (Iversen and Kelly, 1975; Schousboe et al., 1979). The neuronal GABA uptake inhibitors DABA and cis-3-aminocyclohexanecarboxylic acid (ACHC) have furthermore been shown to be proconvulsive (Krogsgaard-Larsen, 1981). Taking this into account in combination with the notion that approximately 20% of synaptically released GABA is taken up into astrocytes, where it is subsequently degraded to succinate and lost from the GABA pool, the hypothesis has been proposed that selective inhibition of astrocytic GABA transport would increase the amount of GABA recycled into neurons, enhancing the GABAergic neurotransmission, thereby preventing the generation of seizures (Schousboe et al., 1983; Schousboe, 1990, 2000).

3.1 Cloning of High-Affinity GABA Transporters

In an effort to clone the neuronal and glial GABA transporter further intricacies have been revealed. Radian et al. (1986) were the first to isolate an 80-kDa glycoprotein transporter from rat with a Na^+ and Cl^- dependence for transport and an apparent K_m for GABA of 3 µM. Subsequently, this transporter was cloned and designated GAT-1. It revealed a 67-kDa transporter protein consisting of 599 amino acids with an absolute dependence of Na^+ and Cl^- for transport and a K_m of 7 µM for GABA. Pharmacological characterization of previously established inhibitors of either neuronal or glial GABA transport revealed a pharmacology related to the neuronal subtype (Guastella et al., 1990). The human GAT-1 has also been cloned and consists of 599 amino acids as well (Nelson et al., 1990).

A transport protein capable of transporting both GABA and the osmolyte betaine with an apparent K_m of 93 and 398 µM, respectively, was isolated from rat kidney and named the betaine-GABA transporter 1 (BGT-1). It encodes a 614 amino acid protein also with a dependence on Na^+ and Cl^- for transport. The neuronal GAT inhibitors nipecotic acid and DABA display low affinities for the BGT-1 (Yamauchi et al., 1992). The human BGT-1 has also been cloned and consists of 614 amino acids and is highly dependent on Na^+ and Cl^- for transport. In contrary to rBGT-1, the human clone displays a 25-fold higher affinity for GABA than for betaine. Localization studies in eight brain regions revealed the presence of hBGT-1, but it did not match GABAergic pathways closely; hence, it was concluded that it may not terminate GABA neurotransmission but rather sequester GABA diffused away from the synases (Borden et al., 1995; Rasola et al., 1995).

Two more rat GAT clones designated rGAT-2 and rGAT-3 with a K_m of 8 and 12 µM for GABA, respectively, and an amino acid sequence of 602 and 627, respectively, have also been cloned. Both GAT-2 and GAT-3 display a pharmacological profile different from that of the previously reported clones. β-Alanine has a high affinity toward both clones, whereas nipecotic acid and DABA have low affinities, suggesting a higher resemblance to the glial GABA transporter (Borden et al., 1992). Later, the human GAT-3 clone of 632 amino acids was discovered (Borden et al., 1994).

Four mouse GABA transporters displaying a Na^+ and Cl^- dependence for transport have been cloned and characterized pharmacologically. GAT1, GAT2, GAT3, and GAT4 (without hyphen) are composed of 598, 614, 602, and 627 amino acids, respectively. Interestingly, nipecotic acid, DABA, and guvacine are more potent inhibitors of GAT1, GAT3, and GAT4 than of GAT2. Betaine only inhibits GAT2, whereas β-alanine preferentially inhibits GAT3 and GAT4 (Liu et al., 1993).

The nomenclature of the GATs among species seems rather confusing and therefore some clarification may be warranted. The nomenclature between rat and human clones is the same, but when comparing to the mouse clones problems appear. Consequently, rat GAT-1, BGT-1, GAT-2, and GAT-3 correspond to mouse GAT1, GAT2, GAT3, and GAT4, respectively (see ❷ *Table 14-1* for references). In the following, the nomenclature according to the mouse clones will be used in general terms when referring to homologous

◼ Table 14-1

GABA transporter nomenclature across species

Species	Nomenclature			
Rat	GAT-1[a]	BGT-1[b]	GAT-2[c]	GAT-3[c]
Human	GAT-1[d]	BGT-1[e]	NC	GAT-3[f]
Mouse	GAT1[g]	GAT2[g]	GAT3[g]	GAT4[g]

[a]Guastella et al. (1990)
[b]Yamauchi et al. (1992)
[c]Borden et al. (1992)
[d]Nelson et al. (1990)
[e]Borden et al. (1995)
[f]Borden et al. (1994)
[g]Liu et al. (1992), Liu et al. (1993)
NC not cloned

GABA transporters between species. To characterize these clones, the respective authors listed above expressed the clones in relevant expression systems and tested their pharmacology. However, due to the various compounds tested and the unavailability of all the respective IC_{50} values between their works, the pharmacology of GAT1–4 and neuronal and glial GAT is summarized in ❏ Table 14-2. ❏ Table 14-2 displays the IC_{50} values for the two proposed neuronal inhibitors, namely DABA and ACHC, and the glial inhibitor

❏ Table 14-2

Inhibitory activities of various GABA analogs on cortical neurons and astrocytes, and cloned mouse GAT1–4

Compound	*GABA uptake inhibition IC_{50} or $K_{m/i}$ (μM)					
	Neurons	Astrocytes	GAT1	GAT2	GAT3	GAT4
GABA	8[a]	32[a]	17[a]	51[a]	15[a]	17[a]
Nipecotic acid	12	16	24	>1000	113	159
Guvacine	32	29	39	>1000	228	378
DABA	1000	>5000	128	528[c]	300	710
ACHC	200	700	132	1070[c]	>1000	>10000
β-Alanine	1666[b]	843[b]	2920	1100[c]	66	110
THPO	501[b]	262[b]	1300	3000	800	5000
Exo-THPO	780	250	1000	3000	>3000	>3000
N-Methyl-exo-THPO	405	48	450	>3000	>3000	>3000
N-Ethyl-exo-THPO	390	301	320	>1000	>1000	>1000
N-2-Hydroxyethyl-exo-THPO	300	200	>500	>500	>500	>500
N-4-Phenylbutyl-exo-THPO	100	15	7	>500	>1000	>1000
N-Acetyloxyethyl-exo-THPO	200	18	550	>1000	>1000	>1000
(R/S)-EF1502	2	2	7	26	>300	>300
(R)-EF1502	1.5	0.65	4	22	>150	>150
(S)-EF1502	>100	>100	120	34	>150	>150
N-DPB-THPO	38[b]	26	30	200	>300	>1000
N-DPB-Nipecotic acid	1.3[b]	2.0[b]	0.64	7210[c]	550	4390
N-DPB-guvacine	4.9[b]	4.2[b]	–	–	–	–
N-DPB-exo-THPO	1.4	0.6	6	100	>100	>100
N-DPB-N-Methyl-exo-THPO	5	2	2	200	>100	>100
NNC 05-2090	–	–	19	1.4	41	15
SNAP-5114	–	–	>30	22	20	6.6
NNC-711	1.24	0.64	–	–	–	–
Tiagabine	0.45	0.18	0.11	>100	>100	800

*Data summarized from Bolvig et al. (1999), Borden (1996), Clausen et al. (2005), Falch et al. (1999), Larsson et al. (1981, 1983, 1986, 1988), Sarup et al. (2003a), Schousboe (1979), Suzdak et al. (1992), Thomsen et al. (1997), White et al. (2002)
[a]K_m
[b]K_i
[c]Human BGT-1

β-alanine as well as nipecotic acid, all tested on the mouse clones expressed in HEK-293 cells and on primary cultures of cortical neurons and astrocytes from mice.

In summary, four GABA transporters are expressed on the plasma membrane of neurons and astrocytes. GAT1 represents a pharmacology closely related to neuronal GAT. GAT3 and GAT4, which displayed the highest affinity for β-alanine and lower affinity for nipecotic acid, DABA, and ACHC, were thought to represent the glial GAT. GAT2 is quite distinct from the other GATs, although being a high-affinity GABA transporter; GAT2 is the only GABA transporter capable of transporting the osmolyte betaine. The K_m for betaine is $\sim$398 μM, which is fourfold higher than the K_m for GABA (Yamauchi et al., 1992). However, the above description of the GABA transporter substrate specificity has revealed a much less straightforward relationship between neuronal and glial GATs and the cloned GAT1–4 than would have been expected or hoped. To further emphasize this dilemma, the subcellular localization will briefly be outlined in the following section.

3.2 Subcellular Localization of GABA Transporters

GAT1 is found to be expressed on the apical surface in polarized MDCK cells (Pietrini et al., 1994), which is in agreement with GAT1 being restricted to axonal segments in cultured neurons. Moreover, GAT1 expression closely reflects GABAergic pathways (Radian et al., 1990; Pietrini et al., 1994; Borden, 1996; Conti et al., 1998). Furthermore, the cell body of neurons is devoid of GAT1 (Radian et al., 1990). The distal processes of glial cells are also labeled with GAT1, and they are in close proximity of axons forming symmetric synapses; however, the staining intensity of glial GAT1 is much lower than that seen in neurons (Conti et al., 1998).

GAT2 shows a basolateral targeting in polarized MDCK cells (Pietrini et al., 1994; Ahn et al., 1996) consistent with dendritic and cell body labeling in hippocampal neurons (Zhu and Ong, 2004a). Contrary to GAT1, GAT2 was found not to be located close to GABAergic synapses, rather the dendrites make asymmetric contact with glutamatergic neurons. Moreover, GAT2 was observed to be located in the extrasynaptic region (Borden et al., 1995; Zhu and Ong, 2004a). GAT2 is also found on glia cells and in primary cultures of astrocytes (Zhu and Ong, 2004b; Olsen et al., 2005).

GAT3 is primarily expressed on the basolateral surface of polarized MDCK cells (Ahn et al., 1996), suggesting a dendritic localization on neurons. Furthermore, GAT3 is found on distal astrocytic processes. It is concluded that GAT3 is primarily located in the extrasynaptic region (Conti et al., 1999, 2004). GAT4 is localized to the apical membrane of polarized MDCK cells (Ahn et al., 1996). GAT4 is localized to both neurons and astrocytes; however, it is primarily localized to the latter cell type (Durkin et al., 1995; Minelli et al., 1996).

For a more detailed overview of the GAT localization in different brain regions, the reader is referred to Durkin et al. (1995) which contains a thorough presentation of GAT1, GAT3, and GAT4. For GAT2, the reader is referred to the above-mentioned works of Zhu and Ong (2004a,b). In summary, GAT1 and GAT4 are highly abundant and oppositely distributed within the CNS between neurons and astrocytes, respectively, primarily within the synapses. GAT2 and GAT3 are far less abundant and primarily expressed in the extrasynaptic region; these localizations are summarized in ❷ Figure 14-1.

3.3 Structure

The GABA transporters belong to the SLC6 superfamily of Na^+-dependent transporters that can be divided into four groups: (1) Transporters of the biogenic amines noradrenaline, dopamine, and serotonin; (2) various GABA transporters as well as transporters of taurine and creatine; (3) transporters of proline and glycine; and (4) "orphan" transporters (For revise, see Gether et al., 2006).

Common to all the transporters is the similar secondary structure composed of 12 putative hydrophobic transmembrane domains (TMD) which are connected by intracellular loops (IL) and extracellular loops (EL) (Guastella et al., 1990; Kanner, 1994). Within the SLC6 family, highly conserved regions exist which include TMD1, EL1, part of TMD2, IL2, TMD5, and EL3 (Kanner, 1994); these regions are recognized as gray regions in ❷ Figure 14-2.

The GATs are as previously described dependent on sodium and chloride ions for transport and the stoichiometry for transport is 2–3 sodium ions:1 chloride ion:1 GABA molecule (Keynan and Kanner, 1988). GATs are capable of generating a gradient in the order of 10^5 between the intra- and extracellular GABA concentration (Beleboni et al., 2004). About 30–65% amino acid sequence homology exists between different SLC6 family members. For a more thorough review of the amino acid sequence relationship within the SLC6 transporter superfamily please see Miller et al. (2002).

▣ Figure 14-1

Summary of the subcellular localization of GAT1–4. For convenience, they are represented in the same synapsis, although it is an over simplification. (Madsen et al., 2006—with kind permission of Springer Science and Business Media)

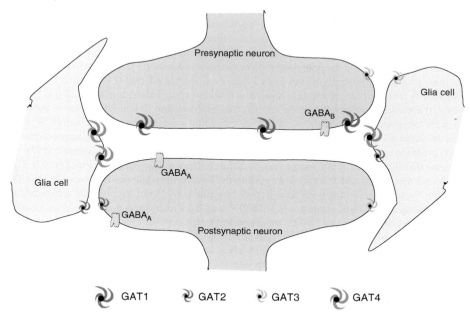

▣ Figure 14-2

Sehematic drawing of the 12-TMD structure of GAT1, showing in gray the conserved domains/loops in the SLC6 transporter family, and a presentation of the discussed amino acids. Furthermore, the three glycosylation sites (Gls) are shown on EL2. Both the N and C terminus are positioned intracellularly

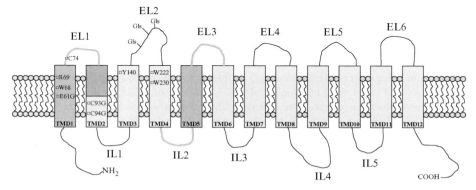

    Several mutation studies have been made in an effort to elucidate specific amino acids involved in the binding of GABA and other substrates and also the regions either TMDs or IL or EL that are involved in lining the GABA binding pocket. Furthermore, several studies address the substrate specificity of GAT1–4 in-between one another. These amino acids/domains are also shown in ❷ *Figure 14-2*.

Arginine R69 that bears a positive charge is essential for transport, since its substitution with other amino acids including charged ones does not recover transport activity. It has been suggested that R69 plays a role in binding of chloride ions (Pantanowitz et al., 1993). Tryptophan W68, W222, and W230 when substituted with either serine or leucine resulted in a 90% reduction in transport activity. It appears that W68 and W222 are required for intrinsic activity. Moreover, W230 has been reported to be involved in plasma membrane targeting (Kleinberger-Doron and Kanner, 1994). Tyrosine Y140 replacement is not tolerated even with the aromatic amino acids phenylalanine or tryptophan. It is speculated that this residue interacts with the amino group of the amino acids and biogenic amines of the SLC6 gene family (Bismuth et al., 1997). Cysteine C74 located in EL1 is also suggested to be involved in the pore formation or GABA translocation (Yu et al., 1998).

The three proposed glycosylation sites in EL2 have been confirmed, and it was found that 40% of the transport activity remained after deletion of these sites. Furthermore, via the introduction of two glycosylation sites in EL3, the transport activity was abolished; hence the glycosylation sites in EL2 appear to be specific and important for transport activity. However, using N-glycosylation a discrepancy in the theoretical transmembrane model occurred since IL1 could be glycosylated in vivo, suggesting an extracellular position of IL1. Moreover, evidence suggests that EL1 actually resides intracellularly (Bennett and Kanner, 1997). Yu et al. (1998) found that the EL1 is located extracellularly quite contrary to Bennett and Kanner (1997). However, they also found that IL1 should be located extracellularly. To accommodate this new topology, the TMD2 is proposed not to span the entire membrane rather to make a reentrant loop which accommodates the extracellular facing of IL1. Furthermore, a new TMD3' is added which is made up of residues toward the N termini of EL2, thereby TMD3 and TMD3' are connected by the new IL1 (Yu et al., 1998). Clark (1997) has proposed a further adaptation of the 12TMD structure of the GABA transporter. Through protease protection studies, they found that EL2 and EL4 are accessible to cytoplasmatic protease activity. This can be explained by EL2 + 4 making a pore loop structure into the membrane and out again. These loops might be involved in the substrate-binding pocket (Clark, 1997). Evidence regarding EL4 involvement in binding and translocation of sodium and GABA has further been established by Zomot and Kanner (2003). Furthermore, TMD1 and TMD3 are found to be in close proximity within the transporter and are involved in the formation of the binding pocket and participate in the translocation pathway, especially the extracellular half of TMD1 that is thought to have a more extended structure than a normal α-helix which would facilitate these actions (Zhou et al., 2004; Zomot et al., 2005). In this context, the recently published crystal structure of a bacterial leucine transporter (Yamashita et al., 2005) homologous to the GABA transporter has provided important structural information (see below), but detailed knowledge about the topology of the bona fide GABA transporters will have to await the availability of crystal structures before precise conclusions can be made.

Mutagenic studies have revealed a functional role for TMD1 + 2 in shaping the substrate-binding pocket of GAT4. The E61G/C93G/C94G mutant shows a 30-fold decrease in K_i for taurine toward the wild-type transporter. The fact that it competitively inhibits GABA transport and that the sizes of the side chains in E61 and C94 are inversely related to the potency of taurine suggests an indirect effect on the GABA binding pocket in GAT4 (Melamed and Kanner, 2004). In another study conducted by Tamura et al. (1995), site-directed mutagenesis was utilized to introduce the EL3 + 5, EL4, and EL6 of GAT3, GAT4, and GAT2, respectively, into GAT1 and the EL5 domain of GAT1 into that of GAT3 to determine the substrate specificity conveyed by these extracellular domains. The introduction of EL3 and EL5 of GAT3 into GAT1 resulted in a significant increase in V_{max} by factors of 2.5 and 4, respectively, but the K_m was not influenced to any significant extent. Furthermore, the EL5 mutant of GAT1 displayed a shift in the β-alanine sensitivity. Moreover, the reverse mutant of GAT3 became less sensitive to β-alanine, suggesting a role of EL5 in the substrate binding of β-alanine. The EL4 GAT1 mutant revealed a fourfold decrease in K_m. The EL6 GAT1 mutant led to a ninefold higher K_m and a twofold increase in V_{max} when compared to the wild-type GAT1. These data suggest that EL4, EL5, and EL6 are involved in the substrate-binding pocket.

The crystal structure of a bacterial homolog of a Na^+/Cl^--dependent transporter (Yamashita et al., 2005), namely the Na^+-dependent leucine transporter from *Aquifex aeolicus* (LeuT$_{Aa}$), reveals interesting structural insight into the SLC6 transporter family. Even though the prokaryotic and eukaryotic only share 20–25% sequence homology in the primary structure within this family, the data still is very relevant. LeuT$_{Aa}$ consists of 12 TMD, and the transporter is shaped like a shallow "shot glass" ~70-Å tall and ~48 Å in diameter. The authors identified a repeat in the first ten TMDs, TMD1–5 and TMD6–10 form a pseudo twofold symmetry along the axis of the membrane, and the two stretches are positioned opposite to one another. A break in the α-helical structure in TM1 and TMD6 from V23-G24 and S256-G260, respectively, exposes the carbonyl oxygen and nitrogen atoms, which are then available for hydrogen bonding and ion coordination in the substrate-binding pocket. Contributing to this effect are TMD3 and TMD8, which display a highly conserved stretch of amino acids surrounding the breaks. These TMDs are thought to represent the core of the transporter. Furthermore, EL2 and EL4, which are juxtaposed across from each other, form the rim of the "shot glass." EL2, TMD9, and TMD12 are also involved in dimerization of the LeuT$_{Aa}$ (Yamashita et al., 2005). The crystal structure of LeuT$_{Aa}$ is shown in ❏ *Figure 14-3*. TMD1, which is

❏ **Figure 14-3**

Crystal structure of LeuT$_{Aa}$. Light gray *triangle represents leucine and the filled circles* represent sodium ions. [Reprinted by permission from Macmillan Publishers Ltd: [Nature] (Yamashita et al., 2005), copyright (2005)]

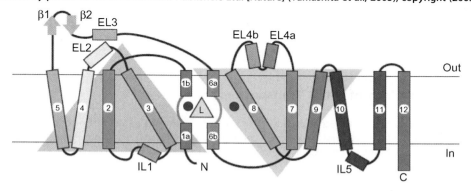

obviously a part of the leucine-binding pocket, and EL2 which forms part of the rim of the transporter along with its involvement in dimerization, present interesting domains in the bacterial LeuT$_{Aa}$, especially because they are highly conserved in the SLC6 transporter family.

The fact that EL2 and EL4 as reported by Clark (1997), and TMD1 and TMD3 as suggested by Zhou et al. (2004) and Zomot et al. (2005) are involved in the binding pocket of GAT draws direct comparison to LeuT$_{Aa}$.

3.4 Trafficking

Studies on the regulation of GAT1 in regard to trafficking have recently been reviewed by Robinson (2002). In the following section, a brief outline of the trafficking behavior of GAT1 will be presented. Activation of protein kinase C (PKC), which can be induced by agonists on different G protein–coupled receptors, results in a decreased cell surface expression of GAT1 in primary cultures of hippocampal neurons (Beckman et al., 1999). Inhibition of tyrosine kinase results in a reduction of the transport activity of GAT1, which correlates with a reduction in V_{max} but not K_m, hence a reduced surface expression of GAT1. These changes are occurring simultaneously with an average reduction of 54% of GAT1 specific tyrosine phosphorylation. Moreover, inhibition of tyrosine phosphatase increases the surface expression of GAT1 and prevents the decrease caused by tyrosine kinase. These data suggest that a balance between tyrosine kinase and phosphatase regulates GAT1 expression. Furthermore, tyrosine kinase/phosphatase and PKC regulation of GAT1 seems to occur through different mechanisms (Law et al., 2000). The regulation of GAT1 also occurs via a transport-mediated process in which GABA and the two substrates nipecotic acid and ACHC cause an upregulation in GAT1 transport activity. This is visualized by an increase in V_{max} and surface expression of GAT1. The nontransportable and competitive inhibitor of GAT1-mediated transport,

SKF89976A (Larsson et al., 1988), shows the exact opposite pattern when compared to GABA. Further-more, intracellular levels of GABA do not regulate GAT1 expression. This suggests that extracellular GABA halts the internalization of GAT1 (Bernstein and Quick, 1999).

GAT1 expressed on the surface is internalized in a clathrin-mediated endocytosis as are synaptic vesicles. Furthermore, GAT1 recycling is regulated in a Ca^{2+}-dependent manner. GAT1-containing vesicles are normally distributed with a diameter of 47 ± 13 nm similar to synaptophysin-containing vesicles. However, they lack synaptophysin and the VGAT, suggesting that they comprise a distinct class of vesicles (Deken et al., 2003). The same research group found that about one third of GAT1 in the cell constitutes the acutely recycling pool, of which one third (about 300 transporters) are expressed on the cell surface in the basal state. Kinetic analysis has revealed the endocytosis and exocytosis time constants of GAT1 to 0.9 and 1.6 min. Furthermore, they investigated three different modulators of GAT1 trafficking, which could be brought about via changes in the acutely recycling pool of GAT1 or on the endocytosis and exocytosis rates. Agonists of PKC were previously found to decrease the surface expression of GAT1, and this was accounted for by increases in endocytosis rate but does not change the acutely recycling pool. Hypertonic concentrations of sucrose were found to inhibit clathrin-dependent internalization not owing the effect to changes in the acutely recycling pool size. Finally, it was shown that Ca^{2+} depletion caused a reduction in GAT1 surface expression due to diminished size of the acutely recycling pool (Wang and Quick, 2005).

4   Pharmacology of GABA Transporters

A number of inhibitors, including substrates, exist that have been key tools in the elucidation of the significance of GABA transport and a brief overview of these compounds will be provided below. As mentioned above, compounds like DABA, ACHC, β-alanine, β-proline, and 3-hydroxy-5-aminovaleric acid have disclosed differ-ences in the transport of GABA into glial and neuronal cells. These compounds are analogs of GABA in which the carbon chain of GABA is modified and/or substituted. Lately, 3-hydroxy-4-N-methylamino-4,5,6,7-tetrahydro-1,2-benzisoxazole (N-Me-exo-THPO) was reported as the most glia-selective inhibitor of GABA uptake yet (White et al., 2002). It was developed from muscimol, a constituent of the fly agaric mushroom *Amanita muscaria*, which can also act as an inhibitor of GABA uptake but has effects on the GABA receptors as well. The activity of muscimol arises from the ability of the 3-hydroxyisoxazole moiety to act as a bioisosteric exchange for the carboxylic acid group in GABA. By using muscimol as lead structure, a series of related compounds was developed and among these THPO, a selective GABA uptake inhibitor was found and this inhibitor enabled the discovery of the potent and selective inhibitors nipecotic acid and guvacine, which are both natural products (Krogsgaard-Larsen and Johnston, 1975; Krogsgaard-Larsen et al., 1975, 2000). These two compounds have not only been valuable pharmacological tools but also very important lead structures for the development of highly potent GABA uptake inhibitors. The breakthrough was the addition of a lipophilic diaromatic side chain (Yunger et al., 1984; Ali et al., 1985), leading to the very potent compounds N-4,4-diphenylbut-3-en-1-yl-nipecotic acid (N-DPB-nipecotic acid/SKF89976A) and N-4,4-diphenylbut-3-en-1-yl-guvacine (N-DPB-guvacine/SKF100330A) that were nonsubstrate inhibitors and able to penetrate the blood–brain barrier (BBB) (Larsson et al., 1988). Following, an impressive number of compounds based on the nipecotic acid and guvacine scaffold with various lipophilic aromatic side chains have been synthesized and characterized (Pavia et al., 1992; Andersen et al., 1993, 1994, 1999, 2001a, b; Dhar et al., 1994; Knutsen et al., 1999). Among these, compounds like (R)-1-[4,4-bis(3-methyl-2-thienyl)-3-butenyl]-3-piperidinecarboxylic acid (tiagabine) and 1-(2-(((diphenylmethylene)amino)oxy)ethyl)-1,2,5,6-tetrahydro-3-pyridinecarboxylic acid (NNC-711) are highly GAT1 selective compounds. Most of the efforts in developing selective GABA uptake inhibitors were performed prior to the cloning of the individual GABA transporters, and highly specific and potent inhibitors are available only at GAT-1. This is probably a consequence of the predominant use of neuronal preparations for the characterization of compounds in which GAT1 is abundantly present as previously mentioned. Very recently, the development of (RS)-4-[N-[1,1-bis(3-methyl-2-thienyl)but-1-en-4-yl]-N-methylamino]-4,5,6,7-tetrahydrobenzo[d]isoxazol-3-ol (EF1502, Clausen et al., 2005) that selectively inhibits GAT1 and GAT2 without affecting GAT3 and

GAT4 was reported, and further in vivo studies disclosed that GAT2 could be an important therapeutic target (White et al., 2005). EF1502 is a structural hybrid of tiagabine and N-Me-exo-THPO. Initially, the exo-THPO series contained small alkyl substituents (Falch et al., 1999), but it was later expanded with lipophilic diaromatic side chains, leading to EF1502. Earlier 1-(3-(9H-carbazol-9-yl)-1-propyl)-4-(2-methoxyphenyl)-4-piperidinol (NNC 05–2090) has been reported as a selective GAT2 inhibitor; however, this compound also affects other transmitter systems (Thomsen et al., 1997). Also GAT3 and GAT4 can be simultaneously targeted with SNAP-5114 (Dhar et al., 1994), but effects at the other GABA transporter subtypes still persist. So whereas GAT1 is well characterized, there is still a need for potent and highly selective inhibitors of the other subtypes. The inhibitory activities of the above-mentioned GABA transport inhibitors are shown in ❷ Table 14-2, and a few important structures of GAT inhibitors are shown in ❷ Figures 14-4 and ❷ 14-5.

❑ **Figure 14-4**
Lead compounds used in the discovery of GABA transport inhibitors

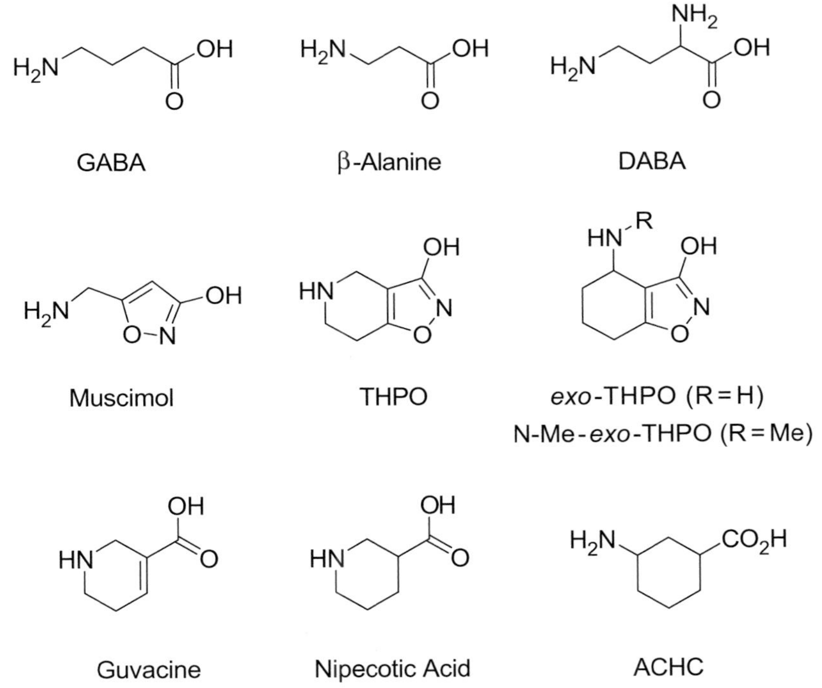

4.1 Anticonvulsant Activity of GABA Transport Inhibitors

Because the structurally restricted GABA analogs originally available (e.g., nipecotic acid, guvacine, and THPO) or later developed (exo-THPO) did not pass the BBB (Schousboe et al., 1986), the general strategy over the years relied on the identification of more lipophilic analogs (Yunger et al., 1984) or prodrugs (Krogsgaard-Larsen, 1981) as described above. N-DPB-nipecotic acid (SKF89976A) and N-DPB-guvacine (SKF100330A) displayed increased potency, the ability to penetrate the BBB, and were orally active when compared to their parent structure (Yunger et al., 1984; Ali et al., 1985). Moreover, they were shown not to be substrates for GABA transporters, although they acted as competitive inhibitors (Larsson et al., 1988). As previously mentioned, tiagabine and NNC-711 were identified from a drug discovery program that targeted

□ Figure 14-5
Structures of more recent GABA transport inhibitors

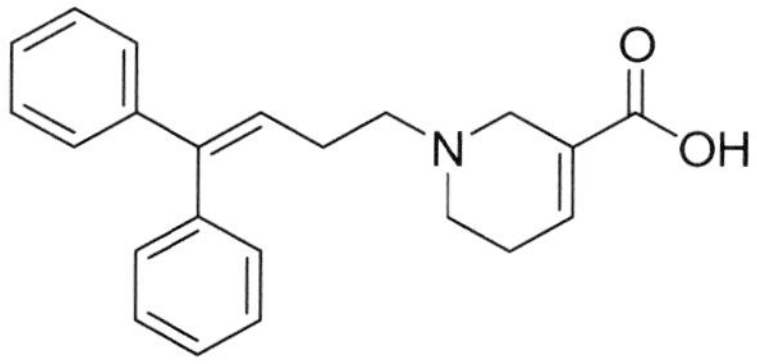

SKF100330A

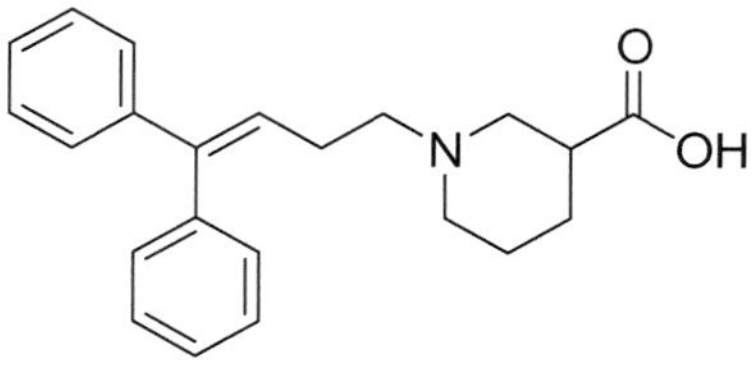

SKF89976A

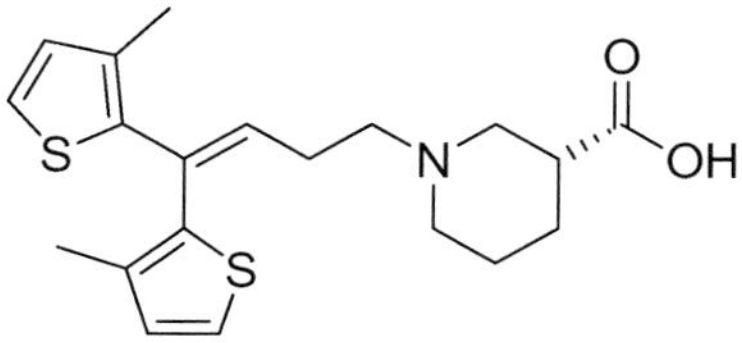

Tiagabine

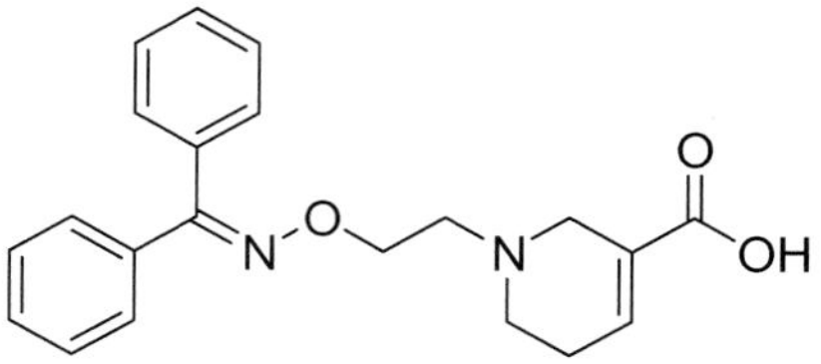

NNC-711

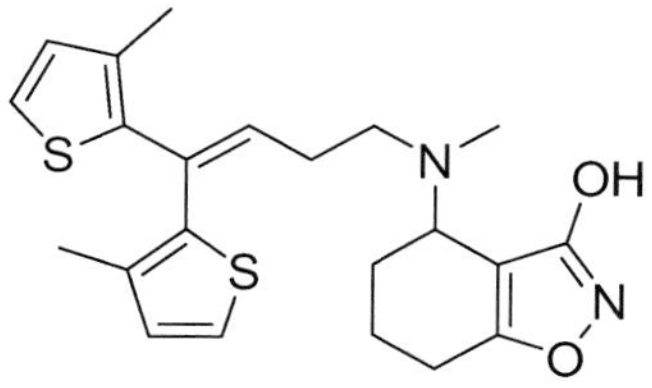

EF 1502

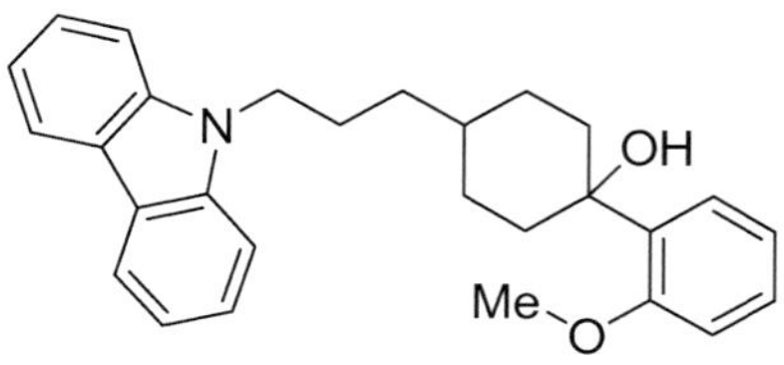

NNC 05-2090

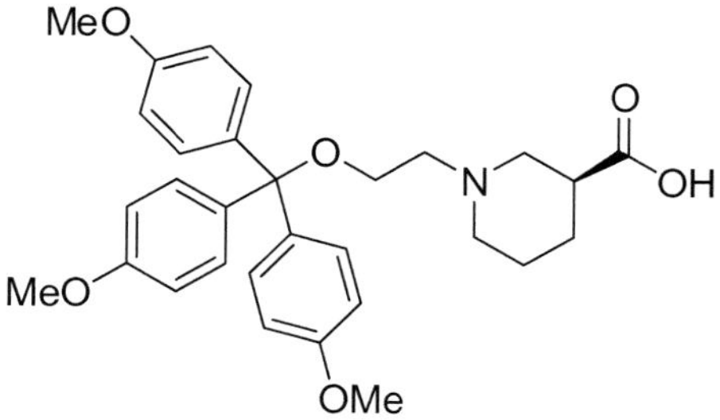

SNAP-5114

modification in the lipophilic aromatic side chain (Braestrup et al., 1990; Suzdak et al., 1992). Tiagabine was subsequently found to be a potent and systemically bioavailable anticonvulsant in rodent seizure and epilepsy models (Suzdak et al., 1992) and was developed and marketed as an add-on treatment for partial epilepsy (Suzdak and Jansen, 1995).

4.2 Glial Versus Neuronal Selective GAT1 Transport Inhibition

The ability of GABA transport inhibitors to prevent audiogenic seizures or chemically induced seizures was demonstrated a quarter of a century ago (Krogsgaard-Larsen, 1981; Croucher et al., 1983; Schousboe et al., 1983; Wood et al., 1983). As shown in ❷ *Table 14-3*, *exo*-THPO and selected *N*-substituted analogs displayed comparable anticonvulsant activity to the clinically active antiepileptic drug tiagabine when

❑ Table 14-3

Anticonvulsant activity of tiagabine, *exo*-THPO and its *N*-substituted analogs

Compound	Anticonvulsant activity (nmol, i.c.v.)	
	ED_{50}	90% CI
Tiagabine	22	11–36
exo-THPO	136	115–155
N-Methyl-*exo*-THPO	59	41–94
N-Ethyl-*exo*-THPO	155	88–255

From White et al. (2002) with permission

injected intracerebroventricularly into the brains of Frings audiogenic seizure-susceptible mice. Given that these compounds are considerably less potent than tiagabine as GABA transport inhibitors, it is somewhat surprising that they proved to be highly efficacious and unexpectedly potent as anticonvulsants when administered intracerebroventricularly (Gonsalves et al., 1989; White et al., 2002). Further pharmacological characterization of the unsubstituted as well as the *N*-methyl and *N*-ethyl substituted compounds disclosed that the anticonvulsive properties of these compounds when injected directly into the brain correlated well with the ability to inhibit glial GABA transport but not the corresponding neuronal transport (White et al., 2002). This finding supports the suggestion put forward two decades ago that inhibition of astrocytic GABA transport would likely lead to an increase in the pool of synaptic GABA and that selective inhibition of this transport system would facilitate reuptake into nerve endings leading to an enhanced GABAergic tone protecting against epileptic seizures (Schousboe et al., 1983). Collectively, these findings demonstrate that if one is able to achieve therapeutic levels of a glial selective GABA transport inhibitor in the brain, it is likely to be as effective as tiagabine as an anticonvulsant.

4.3 Non-GAT1 Transport Inhibitors as Anticonvulsants

As mentioned above, the vast majority of GABA transport inhibitors primarily act on GAT1, which is preferentially located on neuronal elements with less expression on astrocytes. This observation has led to the suggestion that inhibitors of GABA transport mediated by transporters other than GAT1 may be interesting as anticonvulsants, especially those located extrasynaptically (see discussion below) (Dalby, 2003; Sarup et al., 2003b; Schousboe et al., 2004a). Indeed, several nonselective GABA transport inhibitors have been experimentally demonstrated to possess anticonvulsant activity (Dalby et al., 1997; Dalby, 2003; White et al., 2005). In this regard, EF1502 that is substituted with the side chain of tiagabine displays significant inhibitory effects on GAT2, which is notable given the high GAT1 selectivity of tiagabine. Considering that GABA has a lower K_m value at GAT2, EF1502 may be considered equipotent at GAT1 and GAT2.

Not surprisingly, EF1502 was found to possess a reasonably potent and broad-spectrum anticonvulsant profile when tested in a battery of animal seizure and epilepsy models following systemic administration (White et al., 2005). In this regard, EF1502 was found to possess a protective index (i.e., the ratio between median toxic and median effective doses) comparable to that of the selective GAT1 inhibitor tiagabine. Because EF1502 was equally active at both GAT1 and GAT2, isobolographic combination studies with

EF1502, tiagabine, and another liphophilic GAT1-selective GABA-transport inhibitor LU-32–176B (*N*-[4,4-bis(4-fluorophenyl)-butyl]-4-amino-4,5,6,7-tetrahydrobenzo[*d*]isoxazol-3-ol) were conducted to determine to what degree inhibition of GAT2 contributed to the anticonvulsant activity of EF1502. In these studies, EF1502 was found to exert a synergistic anticonvulsant activity when it was administered together with either tiagabine or LU-32–176B (White et al., 2005). More importantly, a less than additive interaction was observed when this combination was evaluated for behavioral toxicity. That the combination of EF1502 with tiagabine did not increase the behavioral toxicity of either drug alone is also of interest because it would suggest that selective inhibitors of the GAT2 transporter may offer some advantage over pure GAT1 selective inhibitors. The demonstration that inhibition of GAT2 by EF1502 likely contributes to its anticonvulsant activity supports the continued identification and development of GAT2-selective GABA transport inhibitors (Schousboe et al., 2004a; Clausen et al., 2005; White et al., 2005). Clearly, the development of a specific GAT2 inhibitor will be required before this hypothesis can be either confirmed or refuted.

5　Concluding Remarks

The GABA system obviously is of fundamental importance for the maintenance of brain function at all levels. Therefore, although the discussions concerning the pharmacology of GABA transporters have been focused on their involvement in the control of seizure activity and epilepsy, it is likely that drugs acting on these transporters may be potential therapeutic candidates for other neurologic and psychiatric conditions believed to be associated with dysfunction of the GABA system, i.e., chronic pain, anxiety, sleep disorders, and others. Actually, several clinically effective drugs used for the treatment of these disorders do in fact act via interactions with entities of the GABA neurotransmission system such as receptor function. In this context, it may be pointed out that for inhibitors of the GABA transporters to have beneficial effects on GABA neurotransmission, their ability to change synaptic GABA levels needs to be translated into signaling through receptor interaction. With regard to the pharmacological interactions, in particular the non-GAT1 active inhibitors, it should be emphasized that since these transporters are located extrasynaptically on both neuronal and glial elements, it is likely that the action may involve extrasynaptic GABA receptors as suggested previously (Schousboe et al., 2004b; White et al., 2005). Of the GABA$_A$ receptor subunits, α6 and α4 associated with δ predominantly constitute the extrasynaptic receptor complexes inside and outside the cerebellum, respectively. It is shown that mice lacking the α6 subunit do not show the tonic component of GABA$_A$ receptor mediated inhibition of cerebellar granula cells (Mody, 2001). The development of the GABAA agonist THIP for the treatment of sleep disorders provides an excellent clinical demonstration supporting the role of extrasynaptic GABA receptors in the control of CNS function (Krogsgaard-Larsen et al., 2004).

Finally, it should be mentioned that in addition to direct interaction with the substrate binding site on GABA transporters, it is possible that modulating the expression of the transporters may represent an alternative therapeutic strategy for controlling CNS excitability. The fact that trafficking of these transporters between the cytoplasm and plasma membrane is rather dynamic (see above) opens the possibility for therapeutic intervention by compounds acting on protein kinases involved in the regulation of this process. However, such manipulation would be expected to be complicated by side effects due to the involvement of such kinases in a multitude of other functions. It may also be noted that endogenous proteins are likely to exist, which may directly regulate surface expression of GABA transporters. One such protein (GABA-CIP) was found to be secreted from cultured neurons (Nissen et al., 1992) and shown to increase the capacity for GABA transport in cerebellar astrocytes. Thus, one possible therapeutic strategy would be the development of molecules that decrease the expression and /or release of GABA-CIP. This would be expected to increase the level of synaptic and extrasynaptic GABA levels.

In summary, it is becoming increasingly clear that the regulation and trafficking of GABA transporters may have important implications for the treatment of a number of neurological disorders and diseases. As such, a greater understanding of the molecular biology, distribution, and factors that regulate their function will be critical for developing a new class of therapeutic agents that target this important regulator of CNS function.

References

Ahn J, Mundigl O, Muth TR, Rudnick G, Caplan MJ. 1996. Polarized expression of GABA transporters in Madin-Darby canine kidney cells and cultured hippocampal neurons. J Biol Chem 271: 6917-6924.

Ali FE, Bondinell WE, Dandridge PA, Frazee JS, Garvey E, et al. 1985. Orally active and potent inhibitors of gamma-aminobutyric acid uptake. J Med Chem 28: 653-660.

Andersen KE, Braestrup C, Grønwald FC, Jørgensen AS, Nielsen EB, et al. 1993. The synthesis of novel GABA uptake inhibitors. 1. Elucidation of the structure-activity studies leading to the choice of (R)-1-[4,4-bis(3-methyl-2-thienyl)-3-butenyl]-3-piperidinecarboxylic acid (tiagabine) as an anticonvulsant drug candidate. J Med Chem 36: 1716-1725.

Andersen KE, Begtrup M, Chorghade MS, Lee EC, Lau J, et al. 1994. The synthesis of novel GABA uptake inhibitors. 2. Synthesis of 5-hydroxytiagabine, a human metabolite of the GABA reuptake inhibitor Tiagabine. Tetrahedron 50: 8699-8710.

Andersen KE, Sørensen JL, Huusfeldt PO, Knutsen LJ, Lau J, et al. 1999. Synthesis of novel GABA uptake inhibitors. 4. Bioisosteric transformation and successive optimization of known GABA uptake inhibitors leading to a series of potent anticonvulsant drug candidates. J Med Chem 42: 4281-4291.

Andersen KE, Lau J, Lundt BF, Petersen H, Huusfeldt PO, et al. 2001a. Synthesis of novel GABA uptake inhibitors. Part 6: Preparation and evaluation of N-Omega asymmetrically substituted nipecotic acid derivatives. Bioorg Med Chem 9: 2773-2785.

Andersen KE, Sørensen JL, Lau J, Lundt BF, Petersen H, et al. 2001b. Synthesis of novel gamma-aminobutyric acid (GABA) uptake inhibitors. 5.(1) Preparation and structure-activity studies of tricyclic analogues of known GABA uptake inhibitors. J Med Chem 44: 2152-2163.

Awapara J, Landua AJ, Fuerst R, Seale B. 1950. Free gamma-aminobutyric acid in brain. J Biol Chem 187: 35-39.

Balazs R, Machiyama Y, Hammond BJ, Julian T, Richter D. 1970. The operation of the gamma-aminobutyrate bypath of the tricarboxylic acid cycle in brain tissue in vitro. Biochem J 116: 445-461.

Beckman ML, Bernstein EM, Quick MW. 1999. Multiple G protein-coupled receptors initiate protein kinase C redistribution of GABA transporters in hippocampal neurons. Protein kinase C regulates the interaction between a GABA transporter and syntaxin 1A. J Neurosci 19: 1-6.

Beleboni RO, Carolino RO, Pizzo AB, Castellan-Baldan L, Coutinho-Netto J, et al. 2004. Pharmacological and biochemical aspects of GABAergic neurotransmission: Pathological and neuropsychobiological relationships. Cell Mol Neurobiol 24: 707-728.

Bennett ER, Kanner BI. 1997. The membrane topology of GAT-1, a (Na$^+$ + Cl$^-$)-coupled gamma-aminobutyric acid transporter from rat brain. J Biol Chem 272: 1203-1210.

Bernstein EM, Quick MW. 1999. Regulation of gamma-aminobutyric acid (GABA) transporters by extracellular GABA. J Biol Chem 274: 889-895.

Bismuth Y, Kavanaugh MP, Kanner BI. 1997. Tyrosine 140 of the gamma-aminobutyric acid transporter GAT-1 plays a critical role in neurotransmitter recognition. J Biol Chem 272: 16096-16102.

Bolvig T, Larsson OM, Pickering DS, Nelson N, Falch E, et al. 1999. Action of bicyclic isoxazole GABA analogues on GABA transporters and its relation to anticonvulsant activity. Eur J Pharmacol 375: 367-374.

Borden LA. 1996. GABA transporter heterogeneity: Pharmacology and cellular localization. Neurochem Int 29: 335-356.

Borden LA, Smith KE, Hartig PR, Branchek TA, Weinshank RL. 1992. Molecular heterogeneity of the gamma-aminobutyric acid (GABA) transport system. Cloning of two novel high affinity GABA transporters from rat brain. J Biol Chem 267: 21098-21104.

Borden LA, Dhar TG, Smith KE, Branchek TA, Gluchowski C, et al. 1994. Cloning of the human homologue of the GABA transporter GAT-3 and identification of a novel inhibitor with selectivity for this site. Receptors Channels 2: 207-213.

Borden LA, Smith KE, Gustafson EL, Branchek TA, Weinshank RL. 1995. Cloning and expression of a betaine/GABA transporter from human brain. J Neurochem 64: 977-984.

Braestrup C, Nielsen EB, Sonnewald U, Knutsen LJ, Andersen KE, et al. 1990. (R)-N-[4,4-bis(3-methyl-2-thienyl)but-3-en-1-yl]nipecotic acid binds with high affinity to the brain gamma-aminobutyric acid uptake carrier. J Neurochem 54: 639-647.

Clark JA. 1997. Analysis of the transmembrane topology and membrane assembly of the GAT-1 gamma-aminobutyric acid transporter. J Biol Chem 272: 14695-14704.

Clausen RP, Moltzen EK, Perregaard J, Lenz SM, Sanchez C, et al. 2005. Selective inhibitors of GABA uptake: Synthesis and molecular pharmacology of 4-N-methylamino-4,5,6,7-tetrahydrobenzo[d]isoxazol-3-ol analogues. Bioorg Med Chem 13: 895-908.

Conti F, Melone M, De Biasi S, Minelli A, Brecha NC, et al. 1998. Neuronal and glial localization of GAT-1, a high-affinity gamma-aminobutyric acid plasma membrane transporter, in human cerebral cortex: With a note on its distribution in monkey cortex. J Comp Neurol 396: 51-63.

Conti F, Zuccarello LV, Barbaresi P, Minelli A, Brecha NC, et al. 1999. Neuronal, glial, and epithelial localization of gamma-aminobutyric acid transporter 2, a high-affinity gamma-aminobutyric acid plasma membrane transporter, in the cerebral cortex and neighboring structures. J Comp Neurol 409: 482-494.

Conti F, Minelli A, Melone M. 2004. GABA transporters in the mammalian cerebral cortex: Localization, development and pathological implications. Brain Res Brain Res Rev 45: 196-212.

Croucher MJ, Meldrum BS, Krogsgaard-Larsen P. 1983. Anticonvulsant activity of GABA uptake inhibitors and their prodrugs following central or systemic administration. Eur J Pharmacol 89: 217-228.

Curtis DR, Johnston GA. 1974. Amino acid transmitters in the mammalian central nervous system. Ergeb Physiol 69: 97-188.

Dalby NO. 2003. Inhibition of gamma-aminobutyric acid uptake: Anatomy, physiology and effects against epileptic seizures. Eur J Pharmacol 479: 127-137.

Dalby NO, Mody I. 2001. The process of epileptogenesis: A pathophysiological approach. Curr Opin Neurol 14: 187-192.

Dalby NO, Thomsen C, Fink-Jensen A, Lundbeck J, Sokilde B, et al. 1997. Anticonvulsant properties of two GABA uptake inhibitors NNC 05–2045 and NNC 05–2090, not acting preferentially on GAT-1. Epilepsy Res 28: 51-61.

De Deyn PP, Marescau B, Mac Donald RL. 1990. Epilepsy and the GABA-hypothesis a brief review and some examples. Acta Neurol Belg 90: 65-81.

Deken SL, Wang D, Quick MW. 2003. Plasma membrane GABA transporters reside on distinct vesicles and undergo rapid regulated recycling. J Neurosci 23: 1563-1568.

Dhar TG, Borden LA, Tyagarajan S, Smith KE, Branchek TA, et al. 1994. Design, synthesis and evaluation of substituted triarylnipecotic acid derivatives as GABA uptake inhibitors: Identification of a ligand with moderate affinity and selectivity for the cloned human GABA transporter GAT-3. J Med Chem 37: 2334-2342.

During MJ, Ryder KM, Spencer DD. 1995. Hippocampal GABA transporter function in temporal-lobe epilepsy. Nature 376: 174-177.

Durkin MM, Smith KE, Borden LA, Weinshank RL, Branchek TA, et al. 1995. Localization of messenger RNAs encoding three GABA transporters in rat brain: An in situ hybridization study. Brain Res Mol Brain Res 33: 7-21.

Elliott KA, van Gelder NM. 1958. Occlusion and metabolism of gamma-aminobutyric acid by brain tissue. J Neurochem 3: 28-40.

Erlander MG, Tobin AJ. 1991. The structural and functional heterogeneity of glutamic acid decarboxylase: A review. Neurochem Res 16: 215-226.

Falch E, Perregaard J, Frølund B, Søkilde B, Buur A, et al. 1999. Selective inhibitors of glial GABA uptake: Synthesis, absolute stereochemistry, and pharmacology of the enantiomers of 3-hydroxy-4-amino-4,5,6,7-tetrahydro-1,2-benzisoxazole (exo-THPO) and analogues. J Med Chem 42: 5402-5414.

Feldman RS, Meyer JS, Quenzer LF. 1997. Amino acid neurotransmitters and histamine. Principles of Neuropsychopharmacology. Farley P, editor. Sunderland: Sinauer Associates; pp. 417-445.

Gether U, Andersen PH, Larsson OH, Schousboe A. 2006. Neuro transmitter transporters: Molecular function of important drug targets. Trends pharmacol Sci 27: 375-383.

Gonsalves SF, Twitchell B, Harbaugh RE, Krogsgaard-Larsen P, Schousboe A. 1989. Anticonvulsant activity of intracerebroventricularly administered glial GABA uptake inhibitors and other GABAmimetics in chemical seizure models. Epilepsy Res 4: 34-41.

Guastella J, Nelson N, Nelson H, Czyzyk L, Keynan S, et al. 1990. Cloning and expression of a rat brain GABA transporter. Science 249: 1303-1306.

Hösli E, Hösli L. 1976. Autoradiographic studies on the uptake of 3H-noradrenaline and 3H-GABA in cultured rat cerebellum. Exp Brain Res 26: 319-324.

Hösli L, Hösli E. 1978. Action and uptake of neurotransmitters in CNS tissue culture. Rev Physiol Biochem Pharmacol 81: 135-188.

Iversen LL, Kelly JS. 1975. Uptake and metabolism of gamma-aminobutyric acid by neurones and glial cells. Biochem Pharmacol 24: 933-938.

Iversen LL, Neal MJ. 1968. The uptake of [3H]GABA by slices of rat cerebral cortex. J Neurochem 15: 1141-1149.

Kanner BI. 1994. Sodium-coupled neurotransmitter transport: Structure, function and regulation. J Exp Biol 196: 237-249.

Kaufman DL, Houser CR, Tobin AJ. 1991. Two forms of the gamma-aminobutyric acid synthetic enzyme glutamate decarboxylase have distinct intraneuronal distributions and cofactor interactions. J Neurochem 56: 720-723.

Keynan S, Kanner BI. 1988. Gamma-aminobutyric acid transport in reconstituted preparations from rat brain: Coupled sodium and chloride fluxes. Biochemistry 27: 12-17.

Kleinberger-Doron N, Kanner BI. 1994. Identification of tryptophan residues critical for the function and targeting of the gamma-aminobutyric acid transporter (subtype A). J Biol Chem 269: 3063-3067.

Knutsen LJ, Andersen KE, Lau J, Lundt BF, Henry RF, et al. 1999. Synthesis of novel GABA uptake inhibitors. 3. Diaryloxime and diarylvinyl ether derivatives of nipecotic acid and guvacine as anticonvulsant agents. J Med Chem 42: 3447-3462.

Krnjevic K, Schwartz S. 1967. The action of gamma-aminobutyric acid on cortical neurones. Exp Brain Res 3: 320-336.

Krogsgaard-Larsen P. 1981. Gamma-aminobutyric acid agonists, antagonists, and uptake inhibitors. Design and therapeutic aspects. J Med Chem 24: 1377-1383.

Krogsgaard-Larsen P, Johnston GA. 1975. Inhibition of GABA uptake in rat brain slices by nipecotic acid, various isoxazoles and related compounds. J Neurochem 25: 797-802.

Krogsgaard-Larsen P, Johnston GA, Curtis DR, Game CJ, McCulloch RM. 1975. Structure and biological activity of a series of conformationally restricted analogues of GABA. J Neurochem 25: 803-809.

Krogsgaard-Larsen P, Frølund B, Frydenvang K. 2000. GABA uptake inhibitors. Design, molecular pharmacology and therapeutic aspects. Curr Pharm Des 6: 1193-1209.

Krogsgaard-Larsen P, Frølund B, Liljefors T, Ebert B. 2004. GABA(A) agonists and partial agonists: THIP (Gaboxadol) as a non-opioid analgesic and a novel type of hypnotic. Biochem Pharmacol 68: 1573-1580.

Larsson OM, Thorbek P, Krogsgaard-Larsen P, Schousboe A. 1981. Effect of homo-beta-proline and other heterocyclic GABA analogues on GABA uptake in neurons and astroglial cells and on GABA receptor binding. J Neurochem 37: 1509-1516.

Larsson OM, Johnston GA, Schousboe A. 1983. Differences in uptake kinetics of cis-3-aminocyclohexane carboxylic acid into neurons and astrocytes in primary cultures. Brain Res 260: 279-285.

Larsson OM, Griffiths R, Allen IC, Schousboe A. 1986. Mutual inhibition kinetic analysis of gamma-aminobutyric acid, taurine, and beta-alanine high-affinity transport into neurons and astrocytes: Evidence for similarity between the taurine and beta-alanine carriers in both cell types. J Neurochem 47: 426-432.

Larsson OM, Falch E, Krogsgaard-Larsen P, Schousboe A. 1988. Kinetic characterization of inhibition of gamma-aminobutyric acid uptake into cultured neurons and astrocytes by 4,4-diphenyl-3-butenyl derivatives of nipecotic acid and guvacine. J Neurochem 50: 818-823.

Law RM, Stafford A, Quick MW. 2000. Functional regulation of gamma-aminobutyric acid transporters by direct tyrosine phosphorylation. J Biol Chem 275: 23986-23991.

Liu QR, Mandiyan S, Nelson H, Nelson N. 1992. A family of genes encoding neurotransmitter transporters. Proc Natl Acad Sci USA 89: 6639-6643.

Liu QR, Lopez-Corcuera B, Mandiyan S, Nelson H, Nelson N. 1993. Molecular characterization of four pharmacologically distinct gamma-aminobutyric acid transporters in mouse brain [corrected]. J Biol Chem 268: 2106-2112.

Lloyd KG, Morselli PL. 1987. Psychopharmacology of GABAergic drugs. Psychopharmacology: The Third Generation of Progress. Meltzer HY, editor. New York: Raven Press; pp. 183-195.

Madsen K, Larsson OM, Schousboe A. 2006. Regulation of excitation by GABA neurotransmission: Focus on metabolism and transport. Inhibitory Regulation of Excitatory Neurotransmission. Darlison MG, editor. London: Springer-Verlag, in press.

Melamed N, Kanner BI. 2004. Transmembrane domains I and II of the gamma-aminobutyric acid transporter GAT-4 contain molecular determinants of substrate specificity. Mol Pharmacol 65: 1452-1461.

Miller JW, Kleven DT, Domin BA, Fremeau RT Jr. 2002. Cloned sodium- (and chloride-) dependent high-affinity transporters for GABA, glycine, proline, betaine, taurine, and creatine. Neurotransmitter Transporters: Structure, Function, and Regulation. Reith MEA, editor. Totowa, New Jersey: Humana Press; pp. 101-150.

Minelli A, De Biasi S, Brecha NC, Zuccarello LV, Conti F. 1996. GAT-3, a high-affinity GABA plasma membrane transporter, is localized to astrocytic processes, and it is not confined to the vicinity of GABAergic synapses in the cerebral cortex. J Neurosci 16: 6255-6264.

Mody I. 2001. Distinguishing between GABA(A) receptors responsible for tonic and phasic conductances. Neurochem Res 26: 907-913.

Nelson H, Mandiyan S, Nelson N. 1990. Cloning of the human brain GABA transporter. FEBS Lett 269: 181-184.

Nicholls DG. 1989. Release of glutamate, aspartate, and gamma-aminobutyric acid from isolated nerve terminals. J Neurochem 52: 331-341.

Nissen J, Schousboe A, Halkier T, Schousboe I. 1992. Purification and characterization of an astrocyte GABA-carrier inducing protein (GABA-CIP) released from cerebellar granule cells in culture. Glia 6: 236-243.

Olsen M, Sarup A, Larsson OM, Schousboe A. 2005. Effect of hyperosmotic conditions on the expression of the betaine-GABA-transporter (BGT-1) in cultured mouse astrocytes. Neurochem Res 30: 855-865.

Pantanowitz S, Bendahan A, Kanner BI. 1993. Only one of the charged amino acids located in the transmembrane alpha-helices of the gamma-aminobutyric acid transporter (subtype A) is essential for its activity. J Biol Chem 268: 3222-3225.

Pavia MR, Lobbestael SJ, Nugiel D, Mayhugh DR, Gregor VE, et al. 1992. Structure-activity studies on benzhydrol-containing nipecotic acid and guvacine derivatives as potent, orally-active inhibitors of GABA uptake. J Med Chem 35: 4238-4248.

Pietrini G, Suh YJ, Edelmann L, Rudnick G, Caplan MJ. 1994. The axonal gamma-aminobutyric acid transporter GAT-1 is sorted to the apical membranes of polarized epithelial cells. J Biol Chem 269: 4668-4674.

Radian R, Bendahan A, Kanner BI. 1986. Purification and identification of the functional sodium- and chloride-coupled gamma-aminobutyric acid transport glycoprotein from rat brain. J Biol Chem 261: 15437-15441.

Radian R, Ottersen OP, Storm-Mathisen J, Castel M, Kanner BI. 1990. Immunocytochemical localization of the GABA transporter in rat brain. J Neurosci 10: 1319-1330.

Rasola A, Galietta LJ, Barone V, Romeo G, Bagnasco S. 1995. Molecular cloning and functional characterization of a GABA/betaine transporter from human kidney. FEBS Lett 373: 229-233.

Roberts E. 1971. The GABA system in brain development. Chemistry and Brain Development. Paoletti R, Davison AN, editors. New York: Plenum Press; pp. 207-214.

Roberts E, Frankel S. 1950. Gamma-aminobutyric acid in brain: Its formation from glutamic acid. J Biol Chem 187: 55-63.

Roberts E, Kuriyama K. 1968. Biochemical-physiological correlations in studies of the gamma-aminobutyric acid system. Brain Res 8: 1-35.

Robinson MB. 2002. Regulated trafficking of neurotransmitter transporters: Common notes but different melodies. J Neurochem 80: 1-11.

Sarup A, Larsson OM, Bolvig T, Frølund B, Krogsgaard-Larsen P, et al. 2003a. Effects of 3-hydroxy-4-amino-4,5,6,7-tetrahydro-1,2-benzisoxazol (exo-THPO) and its N-substituted analogs on GABA transport in cultured neurons and astrocytes and by the four cloned mouse GABA transporters. Neurochem Int 43: 445-451.

Sarup A, Larsson OM, Schousboe A. 2003b. GABA transporters and GABA-transaminase as drug targets. Curr Drug Target CNS Neurol Disord 2: 269-277.

Schousboe A. 1979. Effects of GABA analogues on the high-affinity uptake of GABA in astrocytes in primary cultures. GABA-Biochemistry and CNS Function. Mandel P, De Feudis FV, editors. New York: Plenum Publishing Corp.; pp. 219-237.

Schousboe A. 1990. Neurochemical alterations associated with epilepsy or seizure activity. Comprehensive Epileptology. Dam M, Gram L, editors. New York: Raven Press, Ltd.; pp. 1-16.

Schousboe A. 2000. Pharmacological and functional characterization of astrocytic GABA transport: A short review. Neurochem Res 25: 1241-1244.

Schousboe A, Thorbek P, Hertz L, Krogsgaard-Larsen P. 1979. Effects of GABA analogues of restricted conformation on GABA transport in astrocytes and brain cortex slices and on GABA receptor binding. J Neurochem 33: 181-189.

Schousboe A, Larsson OM, Wood JD, Krogsgaard-Larsen P. 1983. Transport and metabolism of gamma-aminobutyric acid in neurons and glia: Implications for epilepsy. Epilepsia 24: 531-538.

Schousboe A, Larsson OM, Sarup A, White HS. 2004a. Role of the betaine/GABA transporter (BGT-1/GAT2) for the control of epilepsy. Eur J Pharmacol 500: 281-287.

Schousboe A, Sarup A, Larsson OM, White HS. 2004b. GABA transporters as drug targets for modulation of GABAergic activity. Biochem Pharmacol 68: 1557-1563.

Suzdak PD, Jansen JA. 1995. A review of the preclinical pharmacology of tiagabine: A potent and selective anticonvulsant GABA uptake inhibitor. Epilepsia 36: 612-626.

Suzdak PD, Frederiksen K, Andersen KE, Sorensen PO, Knutsen LJ, et al. 1992. NNC-711, a novel potent and selective gamma-aminobutyric acid uptake inhibitor: Pharmacological characterization. Eur J Pharmacol 224: 189-198.

Tamura S, Nelson H, Tamura A, Nelson N. 1995. Short external loops as potential substrate binding site of gamma-aminobutyric acid transporters. J Biol Chem 270: 28712-28715.

Thomsen C, Sorensen PO, Egebjerg J. 1997. 1-(3-(9H-carbazol-9-yl)-1-propyl)-4-(2-methoxyphenyl)-4-piperidinol, a novel subtype selective inhibitor of the mouse type II GABA-transporter. Br J Pharmacol 120: 983-985.

Udenfriend S. 1950. Identification of gamma-aminobutyric acid in brain by the isotope derivative method. J Biol Chem 187: 65-69.

Waagepetersen HS, Sonnewald U, Schousboe A. 2003. Compartmentation of glutamine, glutamate, and GABA metabolism in neurons and astrocytes: Functional implications. Neuroscientist 9: 398-403.

Wang D, Quick MW. 2005. Trafficking of the plasma membrane gamma-aminobutyric acid transporter GAT1. Size and rates of an acutely recycling pool. J Biol Chem 280: 18703-18709.

Watanabe M, Maemura K, Kanbara K, Tamayama T, Hayasaki H. 2002. GABA and GABA receptors in the central nervous system and other organs. A Survey of Cell Biology. Jeon KW, editor. San Diego: Academic Press, Inc.; pp. 1-47.

White HS, Sarup A, Bolvig T, Kristensen AS, Petersen G, et al. 2002. Correlation between anticonvulsant activity and inhibitory action on glial gamma-aminobutyric acid uptake of the highly selective mouse gamma-aminobutyric acid transporter 1 inhibitor 3-hydroxy-4-amino-4,5,6,7-tetrahydro-1,2-benzisoxazole and its N-alkylated analogs. J Pharmacol Exp Ther 302: 636-644.

White HS, Watson WP, Hansen SL, Slough S, Perregaard J, et al. 2005. First demonstration of a functional role for central nervous system betaine/{gamma}-aminobutyric acid transporter (mGAT2) based on synergistic anticonvulsant action among inhibitors of mGAT1 and mGAT2. J Pharmacol Exp Ther 312: 866-874.

Wood JD, Johnson DD, Krogsgaard-Larsen P, Schousboe A. 1983. Anticonvulsant activity of the glial-selective GABA uptake inhibitor, THPO. Neuropharmacology 22: 139-142.

Yamashita A, Singh SK, Kawate T, Jin Y, Gouaux E. 2005. Crystal structure of a bacterial homologue of Na+/Cl− dependent neurotransmitter transporters. Nature 437: 215-223.

Yamauchi A, Uchida S, Kwon HM, Preston AS, Robey RB, et al. 1992. Cloning of a Na(+)- and Cl(−)-dependent betaine transporter that is regulated by hypertonicity. J Biol Chem 267: 649-652.

Yu N, Cao Y, Mager S, Lester HA. 1998. Topological localization of cysteine 74 in the GABA transporter, GAT1, and its importance in ion binding and permeation. FEBS Lett 426: 174-178.

Yunger LM, Fowler PJ, Zarevics P, Setler PE. 1984. Novel inhibitors of gamma-aminobutyric acid (GABA) uptake: Anticonvulsant actions in rats and mice. J Pharmacol Exp Ther 228: 109-115.

Zhou Y, Bennett ER, Kanner BI. 2004. The aqueous accessibility in the external half of transmembrane domain I of the GABA transporter GAT-1 is modulated by its ligands. J Biol Chem 279: 13800-13808.

Zhu XM, Ong WY. 2004a. A light and electron microscopic study of betaine/GABA transporter distribution in the monkey cerebral neocortex and hippocampus. J Neurocytol 33: 233-240.

Zhu XM, Ong WY. 2004b. Changes in GABA transporters in the rat hippocampus after kainate-induced neuronal injury: Decrease in GAT-1 and GAT-3 but upregulation of betaine/GABA transporter BGT-1. J Neurosci Res 77: 402-409.

Zomot E, Kanner BI. 2003. The interaction of the gamma-aminobutyric acid transporter GAT-1 with the neurotransmitter is selectively impaired by sulfhydryl modification of a conformationally sensitive cysteine residue engineered into extracellular loop IV. J Biol Chem 278: 42950-42958.

Zomot E, Zhou Y, Kanner BI. 2005. Proximity of transmembrane domains 1 and 3 of the gamma-aminobutyric acid transporter GAT-1 inferred from paired cysteine mutagenesis. J Biol Chem 280: 25512-25516.

15 Transporters for Excitatory and Neutral Amino Acids

C. P. Landowski · Y. Suzuki · M. A. Hediger

Abstract: The mammalian solute carrier family 1 contains five high affinity, Na$^+$-dependent glutamate transporters and two structurally related Na$^+$-dependent, neutral amino acid transporters. The SLC1 transporters are presumed to be structurally similar given their almost identical hydrophobicity profiles and membrane topologies. Many of the expected features were observed in the crystal structure generated from the glutamate transporter homolog, Glt$_{Ph}$ from *Pyrococcus horikoshii*. The structure features a bowl shaped trimer containing an aqueous basin facing the extracellular solution and extending halfway through the membrane bilayer. Each monomer consists of eight α-helical transmembrane segments and two helical hairpins. While these transporters have similar structural properties, they are functionally distinct. Mammalian glutamate transporters take up 1 L-Glu, L-Asp, or D-Asp molecule along with 3 Na$^+$ and 1 H$^+$ in exchange for 1 K$^+$, whereas the neutral amino acid transporters instead mediate Na$^+$-dependent exchange of small neutral amino acids such as Ala, Ser, Cys and Thr. The regulated action of glutamate transporters permits normal excitatory neurotransmission and protects neurons from overstimulation by glutamate. Excitotoxic damage to neurons has been implicated in neurodegenerative diseases such as amyotrophic lateral sclerosis, Alzheimer's, and Huntington's and ischemia, for example after a stroke or a head injury.

List of Abbreviations: HP, helical hairpin; 3PGDH, 3-phosphoglycerate dehydrogenase; PDC, pyrrolidine dicarboxylate; 4S,5S-POAD, (4S,5S)-2-phenyl-4,5-dihydro-oxazole-4,5-dicarboxylate; SLC, solute carrier; TBOA, β-*threo*-benzyloxyaspartate; T3MG, *threo*-3-methylglutamate; TMOA, *threo*-methoxyaspartate; TMs, transmembrane segments

1   Introduction

The solute carrier family 1 (SLC1) is best known for its high-affinity glutamate transporters. Five high affinity, Na$^+$-dependent glutamate transporters have been identified and characterized: EAAC1 (SLC1A1, EAAT3), GLT1 (SLC1A2/EAAT2), GLAST (SLC1A3/EAAT1), EAAT4 (SLC1A6), and EAAT5 (SLC1A7) (❷ *Table 15-1*). The most well-studied SLC1 members are the high-affinity glutamate transporters EAAC2, GLT1, and GLAST, which play a fundamental role in glutamate uptake in the central nervous system (CNS). As would be expected due to this role, dysfunctions in these transporters lead to neurological diseases. EAAT4 and EAAT5 also have the ability to transport glutamate, but due to their relatively higher chloride conductance they may function like substrate-gated chloride channels and alter neuron excitability. The glutamate transporters exhibit 44–55% amino acid sequence identity with each other and even higher homology in the C-terminal half where the transport function is derived. The SLC1 family also includes two structurally related Na$^+$-dependent, neutral amino acid transporters, ASCT1 (SLC1A4) and ASCT2 (SLC1A5). They share the anion conductance feature with the rest of the family members but do not mediate electrogenic glutamate transport. Instead, these are electroneutral exchangers that mediate neutral amino acid transport. ASCT1 and ASCT2 are 57% identical to each other and show 40–44% sequence identity to glutamate transporters.

In the mammalian CNS, the amino acid L-glutamate is the primary excitatory neurotransmitter (Curtis and Watkins, 1960; Curtis and Johnston, 1974). When glutamate is released into the synaptic cleft, it binds distinct subtypes of ionotropic receptors causing propagation of an action potential, while activation of metabotropic receptors modulates transmission (❷ *Figure 15-1*). After acting upon their receptors, glutamate in the extracellular space must be rapidly cleared so that the receptors are not constantly activated or desensitized, thereby enabling sustained neuronal transmission. Since there are no extracellular enzymes to break down glutamate, this neurotransmitter is removed from the synapse/extracellular space via high-affinity glutamate transporters located predominantly on astrocytic membranes in close proximity to the synapse. The regulated action of these transporters permits normal excitatory neurotransmission, as well as protects neurons from overstimulation by glutamate. Too little glutamate surrounding the receptors can lead to interruption of critical signaling, whereas too much can lead to neuronal death and disease. Excitotoxic damage to neurons has been implicated in neurodegenerative diseases such as amyotrophic lateral sclerosis, Alzheimer's, and Huntington's and ischemia after a stroke or a head injury. On the other

■ Table 15-1
SLC1 family transporters

Gene nomenclature	Gene product	Predominant substrates	Transport type/ coupling ions	Tissue or cellular distribution	Link to disease
SLC1A1	EAAC1/ EAAT3	L-Glu, D,L-Asp	C/Na$^+$, H$^+$, and K$^+$	Brain (neurons), intestine, kidney, lung, heart	Dicarboxylic aminoaciduria
SLC1A2	GLT1/ EAAT2	L-Glu, D,L-Asp	C/Na$^+$, H$^+$, and K$^+$	Brain (astrocytes), retina	Amyotrophic lateral sclerosis
SLC1A3	GLAST1/ EAAT1	L-Glu, D,L-Asp	C/Na$^+$, H$^+$, and K$^+$	Brain (astrocytes), heart, skeletal muscle, retina	
SLC1A4	ASCT1/ SATT	L-Ala, L-Ser, L-Cys, L-Thr	C/Na$^+$, E/amino acid	Brain (astrocytes), ubiquitous	
SLC1A5	ASCT2/ AAAT	L-Ala, L-Ser, L-Cys, L-Thr, L-Gln, L-Asn	C/Na$^+$, E/amino acid	Lung, skeletal muscle, large intestine, kidney, testis, adipose tissue	
SLC1A6	EAAT4	L-Glu, D,L-Asp	C/Na$^+$, H$^+$, and K$^+$	Cerebellum (Purkinje)	
SLC1A7	EAAT5	L-Glu, D,L-Asp	C/Na$^+$, H$^+$, and K$^+$	Retina	

C cotransporter, E exchanger

☐ Figure 15-1

Glutamate transporters and glutamatergic synapses. ʟ-Glutamate is accumulated into synaptic vesicles at presynaptic terminals via vesicular glutamate transporters. The vesicles containing glutamate are released into the synaptic cleft to act upon glutamate receptors. The AMPA receptors mediate fast excitatory postsynaptic potentials, whereas the NMDA receptors possess a cation channel that is permeable to Ca^{2+}. After the receptor activation, the glutamate is removed from the synaptic cleft by high-affinity glutamate transporters using the Na^+ and K^+ ion gradients created by the Na^+/K^+-ATPase. The majority of the glutamate is taken up into glial cells via GLAST or GLT1. The glutamate is converted into glutamine in the glial cell, which is then used to supply the presynaptic nerve terminal with glutamine as a precursor for glutamate synthesis. The glutamine leaves the glial cell via an SLC38 (system N) transporter and enters the neuron via another SLC38 (system A) transporter

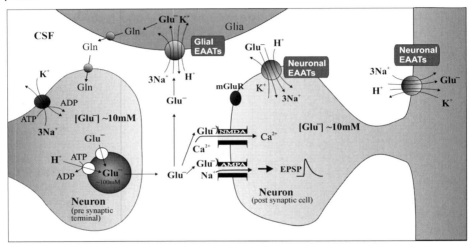

hand, low glutamate levels potentially due to upregulated glutamate uptake has been implicated in the pathogenesis of schizophrenia (Deng et al., 2004; Matute et al., 2005).

Glutamate and aspartate uptake activity were one of the first biochemical indicators for excitatory synapses (Cotman et al., 1981). Two defining properties for glutamate transport in CNS preparations noticed in early studies were that the uptake system had high affinity for the substrate and that it required sodium (Logan and Snyder, 1972). Using pharmacological inhibitors, it became evident that glutamate uptake in CNS occurred through multiple transport systems, depending on the CNS preparation (Balcar and Johnston, 1972; Roberts and Watkins, 1975; Schousboe and Divac, 1979; Robinson et al., 1993). The study of glutamate transport received a tremendous boost in the early 90s when the first three glutamate transporters were cloned and characterized. The identity of these transporters was uncovered when three different high-affinity, sodium-dependent glutamate transporters were reported almost simultaneously: EAAC1 from rabbit intestine (Kanai et al., 1992) and GLAST (Storck et al., 1992) and GLT1 (Pines et al., 1992) from rat brain. The human homologs were isolated from brain a few years after (Arriza et al., 1994). Further screening of cDNA libraries lead to the identification of EAAT4 from human cerebellum (Fairman et al., 1995) and EAAT5 from human retina (Arriza et al., 1997).

Early pharmacology studies designed to distinguish among different excitatory amino acid transporters were performed with radiolabeled substrates (ʟ-glutamate or ʟ-aspartate) in the absence and presence of substrate analogs (Balcar and Johnston, 1972; Logan and Snyder, 1972; Roberts and Watkins, 1975). The structural analogs used in these first structure activity studies varied in stereochemistry, side chain length, and distal acid group make up. While there were some limitations to this approach due to heterogeneous transporter preparations and bias toward competitive inhibition, these experiments provided fundamental insight into the pharmacology of glutamate transport. Compounds that inhibited glutamate or aspartate transport generally were α-amino acids with a carboxylate-like group separated from the α-carboxyl group by two to four carbon atoms. The spacing between the carboxylic groups is limited because long amino acids such as L-α-aminoadipate were ineffective as inhibitors. Generally, modifying the carboxylic acid groups resulted in no inhibition activity; however, the distal carboxylate could be substituted with sulfinic or sulfonic acid groups without affecting the activity. Most of these first generation compounds were competitive substrates, which are not ideal for use as inhibitors. The reason is that these compounds can induce efflux of endogenous glutamate due to transporter-mediated heteroexchange, resulting in an increase in extracellular glutamate (Blitzblau et al., 1996; Koch et al., 1999a, b). Thus, the development of nonsubstrate inhibitors was necessary for characterization of EAAT transporters.

With the availability of individual transporter clones and modern techniques for measuring transport currents, there has been a dramatic increase in excitatory amino acid transporter inhibitor and substrate development in recent years. Most early studies characterizing glutamate transport inhibitors often neglected to consider whether the inhibitors also act as substrates for the transporter. Although this limitation has been overcome by electrophysiology techniques, this remains a significant obstacle in more complex physiological preparations from CNS tissues (e.g., synaptosomes, tissue slices, primary cell culture). Electrophysiological measurements allow transport to be examined in real time and under well-characterized conditions, using such expression systems as *Xenopus laevis* oocytes or mammalian cell lines (e.g., MDCK and HEK-293). The significant advantage of this technique is that it permits the differentiation between substrates and nonsubstrate inhibitors. Utilizing these systems, many nonsubstrate glutamate transporter inhibitors were developed, including the aspartate derivatives β-*threo*-benzyloxyaspartate (TBOA) used for SLC1A1–3 (Shimamoto et al., 2000) and *threo*-methoxyaspartate (TMOA) for both GLT1 and EAAT5 (Shigeri et al., 2001), glutamate derivatives such as *threo*-3-methylglutamate (T3MG) for GLT1 (Vandenberg et al., 1997), and the pyrrolidine dicarboxylates L-*trans*-2,4-PDC used EAAT5 (Bridges et al., 1999) and L-*trans*-2,3-PDC for GLT1 (Willis et al., 1996). Considerable information is available about the localization and density of these transporters, but their relative contribution to the uptake of synaptic glutamate is not completely understood because inhibitors selective for each transporter, with exception of GLT1, have not yet been developed. Therefore, developing subtype selective, nonsubstrate inhibitors is essential for future investigation into their physiological roles and intrinsic properties, as well as use as potential therapeutics.

2 Structural Studies

2.1 Membrane Topology of N-terminal and C-terminal

The membrane topology of the N-terminal half of the glutamate transporter was relatively straightforward to predict. Indeed, the hydropathy plots produced by the three groups who originally cloned EAAC1, GLAST, and GLT1 predicted six transmembrane α-helices at very similar positions (Kanai and Hediger, 1992; Pines et al., 1992; Storck et al., 1992). However, there is much more uncertainty in predicting topology on the carboxyl side, where zero (Storck et al., 1992), two (Pines et al., 1992), and four (Kanai and Hediger, 1992) α-helices have been predicted. Attempts to experimentally determine the glutamate transporter C-terminal topology have suggested that it contains two transmembrane domains (TM7 and TM8), two reentrant loops sinking into each side of the membrane on either side of TM7, and an extracellular hydrophobic linker between the second reentrant loop and TM8 (Grunewald et al., 1998; Slotboom et al., 1999; Grunewald and Kanner, 2000).

2.2 Molecular Architecture of Glutamate Transporters

Biochemical and structural evidence has demonstrated that glutamate transporters, prokaryotic and eukaryotic, exhibit a single oligomeric state formed through assembly of three identical subunits (Yernool et al., 2003, 2004; Gendreau et al., 2004) (❯ *Figure 15-2a*). Many predicted topological features are observed in the recent crystal structure produced from a glutamate transporter homolog, Glt_{Ph} from *Pyrococcus horikoshii*. This structure has revealed the molecular architecture, which appears to be common to all glutamate transporters (Yernool et al., 2004). The bacterial Glt_{Ph} protein shares 37% amino acid identity with excitatory glutamate transporter GLT1 and a relatively high degree of homology with other SLC1 transporters.

◼ Figure 15-2

(a) Top down view of the trimeric structure of Glt_{Ph} from *P. horikoshii* PDB ID 1XFH. The six N-terminal transmembrane domains, shown as a thin wire, form the barrel structure that mediates the interaction between subunits and surrounds the C-terminal domains, shown as thick ribbons. The C-terminal portion contains the glutamate-binding site residues, shown in black. (b) Side view demonstrating the basin-like transporter structure. The glutamate-binding site residues are colored black. (c) Side view showing the six N-terminal domains, thin wire, and the C-terminal helix hairpin (HP) and transmembrane domains, thick ribbon. The HP1 domain toward the bottom, colored dark gray, forms the intracellular gate, while the HP2 domain facing the extracellular basin, colored medium gray, comprises the extracellular gate. Between these HP2 domains are the residues implicated in glutamate binding, shown in black. Glutamate is proposed to enter from the extracellular side while HP2 is open and leave when HP1 opens toward the intracellular space. (d) Close-up view of the proposed binding site residues, in black, the HP1 domain, in dark gray, and HP2 domain, in medium gray

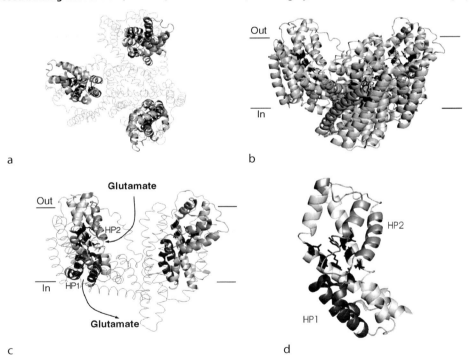

a   b

c   d

2.2.1 3D Structural Data from the Glt_{Ph} Transporter

The insight provided by the Glt_{Ph} structural data demonstrates that glutamate transporters are well adapted for rapid glutamate binding. Perhaps the most striking feature of the structure is bowl-shaped trimer. This trimer structure contains an aqueous basin facing the extracellular solution and extends halfway through the membrane bilayer (❯ *Figure 15-2b*). This feature allows substrates and ions brisk access to the binding sites in the transporters, directly from the bulk solution. Each monomer includes eight α-helical transmembrane segments (TMs) and two helical hairpins (HP) (❯ *Figure 15-3*). The first six transmembrane domains form a distorted N-terminal cylinder, whose outer surface arbitrates the intersubunit

☐ **Figure 15-3**

A transmembrane topology model of Glt$_{Ph}$ from *P. horikoshii*. The filled in circles indicate functionally important residues involved in substrate binding

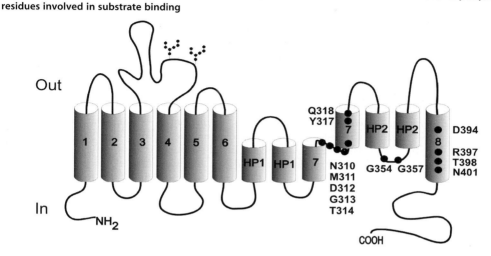

contacts in the trimer (❯ *Figure 15-2a*). The C-terminal portion contains important elements for substrate transport (TM7, TM8, HP1, and HP2 domains) that are contained within the N-terminal cylinder, suggesting that each monomer may function independently. Reaching from opposite sides of the membrane, HP1 and HP2 meet at the bottom of the basin where the glutamate-binding site is proposed to occur (❯ *Figure 15-2c*). A nonprotein electron density, the approximate size of a glutamate molecule, is found near the HP1–HP2 interface, but due to the resolution of the diffraction data it cannot be unmistakably identified (❯ *Figure 15-2d*).

2.3 Experimental Evidence Supporting Substrate-Binding Sites

Experimental evidence to support this proposed binding site comes from the identification of several conserved amino acid residues in this region that are critical to functional activity. There are two conserved serine residues (440 and 443) in GLT1 located in HP2 that are important for the coupling of sodium and glutamate fluxes and are close to the glutamate-binding site (Zhang and Kanner, 1999). Further, when serine 440 is changed to glycine, amino acid transport can be coupled not only to sodium but also to lithium ions. The efficiency of lithium coupled transport is also dependent on the nature of the amino acid at position 443. Interestingly, glycine also occupies the corresponding position Gly 410 in the human glutamate transporter EAAC1, thereby enabling glutamate transport in the sole presence of lithium (Borre and Kanner, 2001). Mutating Gly 410 to Ser causes EAAC1 to lose the ability to couple transport to lithium, but sodium still can drive transport. The corresponding residues in Glt$_{Ph}$, Gly 354 and Gly 357, are near the tip of HP2 and within 5 Å of the substrate-binding site (❯ *Figure 15-3*). In GLT1, two amino acid residues are critical for potassium binding and countertransport. These residues are located in TM7 (Tyr 403 and Glu 404) and close to one of the sodium-binding sites (Kavanaugh et al., 1997; Zhang and Kanner, 1999). Mutations in these two sites can cause transport to be limited to obligatory exchange.

In the Glt$_{Ph}$ structure, the so-called NMDGT motif in TM7 contributes extensively to the substrate-binding site. The conserved residues Asp 394, Arg 397, Thr 398, and Asn 401 are located on the polar side of TM8 and are in positions to interact with the substrate-binding site (❷ *Figure 15-3*). The Arg 397 equivalent in eurkaryotic glutamate homologs provides specificity for substrates containing β- and γ-carboxy groups. This residue is conserved in all dicarboxylic acid transporters in SLC1 but is not present in the small, neutral amino acid transporter, ASCT1 (Arriza et al., 1993; Shafqat et al., 1993), whose substrates have only one carboxyl group. In Glt$_{Ph}$, Arg 397 is in position to interact with the γ-carboxy group of glutamate. In EAAC1, when the conserved residue Arg 447 is converted to a neutral or negatively charged amino acid the glutamate or aspartate transport is abolished, while sodium-dependent, neutral amino acid transport remains intact (Bendahan et al., 2000). Electrophysiological analysis shows that this mutation produces electroneutral transport that no longer countertransports potassium. Therefore, it appears that Arg 447 enables the coupling by sequentially participating in the binding of glutamate and potassium. The two residues that are important for potassium binding and countertransport are in close contact with Arg 447. From the Glt$_{Ph}$ structure, it can be seen that Tyr 317, Gln 318, Arg 397, and the substrate-binding site are close in space (Yernool et al., 2004).

The deep aqueous basin provided by the glutamate transporter allows ion and substrates rapid access to their binding sites in the protein. In an alternative access mechanism model for glutamate transport, the binding site is bordered by two gateway domains that allow the substrate alternating access to the intracellular or extracellular media. Based on the published structural evidence and biochemical data, HP2 is speculated to provide the extracellular gate and HP1 forms the intracellular gate directly under the binding pocket (Yernool et al., 2004). It is known from biochemical studies that residues in HP2 and TM7 undertake conformational changes after binding substrates that make them more solvent exposed (Grunewald et al., 2002; Leighton et al., 2002). More recently, real-time voltage clamp fluorometry measurements on EAAC1 provide evidence for conformational changes in the loop residues that connects HP2 and TM8 in the presence of glutamate or sodium (Larsson et al., 2004).

3 Functional Properties

3.1 Electrogenic Glutamate Transporters, SLC1A1–3 and SLC1A6–7

SLC1A1–3 and SLC1A6–7 are electrogenic, glutamate transporters that can concentrate glutamate into cells against a steep concentration gradient using the electrochemical power from the ion gradients setup by the Na$^+$/K$^+$-ATPase. Glutamate transporters take up 1 glutamate molecule along with 3 Na$^+$ and 1 H$^+$, in exchange for 1 K$^+$, thus resulting in a net translocation of two positive charges per transport cycle (Zerangue and Kavanaugh, 1996b). Based on this coupling stoichiometry, it has been estimated that the glutamate transporters can concentrate glutamate over 10^6 fold. Inside glutamatergic neurons the glutamate concentration can reach ∼10 mM, whereas the extracellular concentration can be reduced to ∼2 nM. Glutamate transport is accompanied by intracellular acidification (Kanai and Hediger, 1992) and driven by the pH gradient (Nelson et al., 1983; Zerangue and Kavanaugh, 1996a). It has been suggested that the cotransported proton binds to the glutamate carrier on a highly conserved glutamate residue Glu 373 in EAAC1 (Grewer et al., 2003).

3.2 Na$^+$/Amino Acid Exchangers, SLC1A4 and SLC1A5

In contrast to the electrogenic glutamate transporters, SLC1A4 (ASCT1) and SLC1A5 (ASCT2) are Na$^+$/amino acid exchangers (Zerangue and Kavanaugh, 1996a; Broer et al., 2000). When Tyr 403 and Glu 404 of GLT1 were mutated the transporter also became a Na$^+$/glutamate exchanger, but lacked the ability for K$^+$-coupling (Kavanaugh et al., 1997; Zhang and Kanner, 1999). These results suggested that K$^+$-coupling was important for the glutamate uptake by the electrogenic glutamate transporters. Moreover, it is likely that this K$^+$-coupled process is rate-limiting step of the transporters in steady state (Grewer and Rauen, 2005).

3.3 Substrate-Gated Anion Conductance

All SLC1 family members demonstrate a substrate-gated anion conductance with characteristics similar to ligand-gated chloride channels (Fairman et al., 1995; Wadiche et al., 1995; Zerangue and Kavanaugh, 1996a; Broer et al., 2000). The observed anion conductance is thermodynamically uncoupled to glutamate transport but is triggered by glutamate and sodium binding only under ionic conditions that promote glutamate translocation (Wadiche et al., 1995; Watzke et al., 2001). The transport-associated conductance is selective for hydrophobic anions showing the following permeability sequence: $SCN^- NO_3^- > I^- > Br^- > Cl^- > F^-$. It appears that glutamate and these anions flow through the transporter via separate routes that can be independently regulated. Site-directed mutagenesis studies have succeeded in eliminating forward and reverse transport without affecting activation of the anion conductance (Seal et al., 2001; Ryan and Vandenberg, 2002). Alternatively, GLAST mutations in the second transmembrane domain change anion permeation characteristics without affecting glutamate transport (Ryan et al., 2004). The residues for glutamate transport are located further toward the C terminus between transmembrane domains 7 and 8 (Yernool et al., 2004). Therefore, these findings demonstrate a structural separation of glutamate transport and the uncoupled anion flux.

Interestingly, those glutamate transporters (i.e., SLC1A1–3) that show the highest glutamate transport rates display the lowest chloride conductance, while EAAT4 and EAAT5 have low glutamate transport rates but high chloride conductance (Picaud et al., 1995; Larsson et al., 1996; Eliasof et al., 1998). These two subgroups of glutamate transporters may have different physiological roles, with one serving classical glutamate uptake and the other functioning as Na^+/glutamate-gated chloride channels. The exact physiological function of the anion current is not known, but it could be used to balance the influx of positive charge (Na^+) during glutamate transport to maintain the resting potential of the cells at a hyperpolarized level (Arriza et al., 1997) or as a mechanism for changing neuronal excitability (Fairman et al., 1995). Associated with the anion conductance, it was recently shown that inward cation current derived from EAAT4 could depolarize the spine membrane in Purkinje cells and that could modify their excitability (Melzer et al., 2005). Moreover, it was revealed that arachidonic acid stimulates an EAAT4-associated proton conductance, which further expands the ligand-gated channel properties of EAAT4 (Fairman et al., 1998).

4 Individual Isoform Descriptions

4.1 SLC1A1

4.1.1 Localization and Function

EAAC1 (EAAT3) was localized on neurons throughout the nervous system and is particularly abundant on postsynaptic membranes (Kanai and Hediger, 1992), as well as on presynaptic GABAergic terminals (Sepkuty et al., 2002). In brain neurons, it is diffusely localized over the processes and cell bodies, most notably in the hippocampus, cerebral cortex, olfactory bulb, striatum, superior colliculus, and thalamus (Rothstein et al., 1994; Kanai et al., 1995; Berger and Hediger, 1998). However, it is not restricted to the CNS tissue, since it is also plentiful in the kidney and intestine where it resides on the apical membrane of epithelial cells (Shayakul et al., 1997). EAAC1 proves to be important in glutamate reabsorption in the kidney because EAAC1 knockout (KO) animals develop dicarboxylic aminoaciduria (Peghini et al., 1997).

In contrast, the function of EAAC1 in the brain has not been clearly established. Early in life, EAAC1 KO mice do not develop remarkable neurological symptoms or neurodegeneration, but they do display reduced spontaneous locomotor activity (Peghini et al., 1997). On the other hand, older KO mice (11 months) showed significant age-dependent morphological abnormalities and associated behavioral changes (Aoyama et al., 2006). The EAAC1 KO mice also had reduced neuronal glutathione content, causing these neurons to be more susceptible to oxidant injury compared to wild-type mice. Moreover, treatment with a membrane-permeable cysteine (*N*-acetylcysteine) reversed this phenotype. The ability of

EAAC1 to transport cysteine and the forementioned observations suggest that EAAC1 provides an important route for neuronal cysteine uptake. Thus, a decrease in EAAC1 activity likely leads to age-dependent neurodegeneration, due to a lack of the antioxidant glutathione. In adult rats, antisense knockdown of EAAC1 disrupted GABA synthesis, since glutamate is a precursor for GABA production. Reduced EAAC1 expression leads to behavioral abnormalities, including staring-freezing episodes, and electrographic seizures (Rothstein et al., 1996; Sepkuty et al., 2002).

4.1.2 Link to Disease and Ischemia

Until recently, no human diseases have been linked to direct defects in EAAC1 function. However, a recent linkage analyses on obsessive-compulsive disorder suggest that EAAC1 mutations are a risk factor for this disease. Some researchers indicated the association between this disease and 9p24, which is in the same region as the SLC1A1 gene (Veenstra-VanderWeele et al., 2001; Hanna et al., 2002; Willour et al., 2004).

While they are not the direct cause, neuronal glutamate transporters, such as EAAC1, are the main contributors to glutamate neurotoxicity in the brain during severe ischemia. Stroke or ischemic conditions lead to ATP depletion causing the loss of the ion gradients necessary for driving sodium-dependent glutamate transport (Rossi et al., 2000). The disruption of these necessary ion gradients results in decreased glutamate uptake or cellular release of glutamate, predominately through neuronal glutamate transporters like EAAC1. The glutamate concentration in the neurons ($\sim$10 mM) is higher compared to that in the glial cells ($\sim$1 mM), where the glutamate concentration is kept low due to conversion to glutamine by glutamine synthetase (Ottersen et al., 1992; Attwell et al., 1993). Therefore, high neuronal glutamate concentrations, as well as the lack of ion gradients, allow for neuronal glutamate transporters to reverse more readily and contribute the most to the extracellular rise in glutamate to neurotoxic levels. Experimentally it has been shown that dihydrokainate, a selective inhibitor for GLT1, used in a hippocampal slice model of ischemia did not have any effect on the observed transporter reversal and accumulation of extracellular glutamate (Rossi et al., 2000). In contrast, a competitive substrate, L-*trans*-pyrrolidine-2,4-dicarboxylate, blocks the reversal of all glutamate transporters and dramatically reduced the amount of glutamate released. Further, hippocampal tissue from GLT1 knockout mice produces the same depolarizing current characteristics as wild-type tissue (Hamann et al., 2002). However, in EAAC1 knockout mice, the time to anoxic depolarization is increased threefold in CA1 pyramidal neurons in the hippocampus (Gebhardt et al., 2002). These studies indicate that the neuronal glutamate transporter EAAC1 causes glutamate neurotoxicity in the brain during ischemia.

4.1.3 Selective Inhibitors

Therefore, developing selective inhibitors for EAAC1 has been a much sought after goal. The design of potent oxazole-based inhibitors represents a recent lead in this effort. One particular compound in this class is (4S,5S)-2-phenyl-4,5-dihydro-oxazole-4,5-dicarboxylate (4S,5S-POAD) which proves to be a nonsubstrate inhibitor, with a K_i value of 15 μM (Campiani et al., 2001). The selectivity has not been demonstrated thus far. The most potent and selective inhibitors for EAAC1 include L-β-*threo*-benzyl-aspartate which shows good selectivity and potency (Esslinger et al., 2005).

4.2 SLC1A2

4.2.1 Localization and Function

GLT1 (EAAT2) is an astroglial subtype expressed abundantly in the forebrain, cerebellum, and spinal cord (Danbolt et al., 1992; Pines et al., 1992). In GLT1 knockout mice, glutamate transport activity in membrane preparations derived from cerebral cortex reduced 94% compared to tissue from wild-type animals (Tanaka et al., 1997). This electrophysiological examination of the CA1 pyramidal neurons from KO mice suggests that this glial glutamate transporter is responsible for the majority of extracellular glutamate clearance in the adult CNS. While GLT1 has been considered a glial transporter, a naturally occurring 3′ splice variant, GLT1b, has been localized to neurons of the central and peripheral nervous system, whereas it was only occasionally detected in astrocytes (Schmitt et al., 2002). In the rat somatosensory cortex, GLT1b was present on the presynaptic terminals and dendritic shafts of neurons (Chen et al., 2002).

The physiological importance of GLT1 has been established using both antisense knockdown and KO mice. GLT1 antisense administration to rats produced progressive hind limb paralysis and motor neuron degeneration (Rothstein et al., 1996). Interestingly, no motor neuron loss is observed in the GLT1 null mice, but they develop hippocampal pathology, lethal spontaneous epileptic seizures, and most mice die within several weeks of birth (Tanaka et al., 1997). It is possible that the GLT1 null mice may not live long enough to display the motor degeneration phenotype. Alternatively, GLAST may be able to compensate during development to prevent the pathology. In retinal tissue, GLT1 is found in the cone and various types of bipolar cells. However, GLT1 null mice show relatively normal electroretinograms and mild increased retinal damage after ischemia, suggesting GLT1 plays a neuroprotective role in the retina (Harada et al., 1998).

4.2.2 ALS and Links to Other Diseases

The important role GLT1 plays in extracellular glutamate clearance in the CNS is critical for maintenance of normal health. Therefore, GLT1 dysfunction can result in several human diseases. Much evidence suggests that glutamate appears to play a neurotoxic role in amyotrophic lateral sclerosis (ALS). The cerebrospinal fluid of many ALS patients (~40%) contains elevated glutamate levels (Rothstein et al., 1990; Spreux-Varoquaux et al., 2002). Additionally, based on the most recent studies, high glutamate concentrations correlated with the spinal onset of the disease, more impaired limb function, and accelerated muscle deterioration. There are several reports indicating that GLT1 expression decreases in the brain of ALS patients and animal models of ALS (Rothstein et al., 1995; Dunlop et al., 2003a; Vanoni et al., 2004). According to Rothstein and colleagues, protein levels in motor cortex decreased 71%, whereas expression in the spinal cord was severely reduced in ALS. In approximately 25% of the ALS motor cortex specimens, the 90% decrease in GLT1 protein was dramatic. It is not certain whether lack of GLT1 is the primary factor driving the development of the motor neuron disease or whether there is a secondary pathophysiological event, but it is important in the propagation of motor neuron loss. A study using transgenic mice overexpressing GLT1, crossed with the ALS model (SOD1-G93A) mice, showed that the double transgenic GLT1/G93A animals display a significant delay in the loss of motor neurons but not in the overall onset of paralysis, body weight decline, or life span compared with their G93A littermates (Guo et al., 2003). The authors suggest that loss of GLT1 may contribute to but does not cause neuronal degeneration in ALS.

Considering its importance in glutamate uptake in the CNS, GLT1 dysfunction is also implicated in several other human diseases. Deficient functioning of glutamate transporters, leading to neurodegeneration, may also contribute to the development of Alzheimer's disease (Li et al., 1997) and Huntington's disease (Behrens et al., 2002). In contrast to the reduced glutamate transport activity seen in ALS, GLT1 mRNA, protein, and function were increased in prefrontal cortex of schizophrenic patients (Matute et al., 2005). Moreover, one report indicates an association between the SLC1A2 gene and schizophrenia (Deng et al., 2004). These findings suggest that SLC1A2 represents at least one susceptibility locus for schizophrenia.

4.2.3 Selective Inhibitors

GLT1 is the most pharmacologically distinct high-affinity glutamate transporter subtype. The vast majority of highly selective subtype-specific inhibitors are limited to GLT1. Due to the long-term use of traditional model systems such as synaptosomes, where GLT1 is highly expressed, a bias for studying this isoform may have influenced the development of inhibitors. This "selection" allowed the GLT1 pharmacology to develop more rapidly in comparison to that of other glutamate transporters. Compounds such as dihydrokainate, L-*trans*-2,3-PDC, TDPA, and WAY-855 are among the most selective for the GLT1 subtype (Arriza et al., 1994; Willis et al., 1996; Brauner-Osborne et al., 2000; Dunlop et al., 2003b).

4.3 SLC1A3

4.3.1 Localization and Function

GLAST (EAAT1) is a glutamate transporter subtype found abundantly distributed on astrocytic plasma membranes associated with excitatory synapses, showing highest density in the Bergmann glia of the cerebellum and less expression in the brain and spinal cord (Storck et al., 1992; Rothstein et al., 1994; Chaudhry et al., 1995).

GLAST knockout mice develop normally and managed simple tasks, such as standing on a stationary or slowly rotating rod, but they showed impaired motor coordination for staying on a more quickly rotating rod (Watase et al., 1998). The cerebellum did not exhibit any visible pathology, and electrophysiology studies in Purkinje cells from cerebellum did not indicate that GLAST plays a role in synaptic clearance of glutamate. However, detailed electrophysiological examination exposed that the Purkinje cells in the knockout animals remained innervated by multiple climbing fibers even in adult tissue, indicating that GLAST plays a role in the cerebellar climbing fiber synapse formation. Knockout mice were more susceptible to cerebellar damage after acute brain injury. The knockout mice also showed more severe pentylenetetrazole-induced seizures, suggesting that GLAST influences seizure susceptibility (Watanabe et al., 1999). In retinal tissue, GLAST is essential for normal signal transmission between photoreceptor and bipolar cells (Harada et al., 1998). Moreover in the peripheral auditory system, the GLAST null mice accumulate higher levels of glutamate in perilymphs after acoustic overstimulation resulting in hastened hearing loss (Hakuba et al., 2000). This suggests that GLAST is important for maintaining glutamate concentration in perilymphs of the inner ear.

4.3.2 Link to Disease

Patients displaying episodic ataxia, hemiplegic migraine, and seizures often have mutations in CACNA1A, neuronal calcium channel, and ATP1A2, ion pump. These conditions are associated with neuronal hyperexcitability; therefore, the gene products of both CACNA1A and ATP1A2 may affect neurotransmission of glutamate. In some patients no mutations in CACNA1A or ATP1A2 were found. Instead, they had a heterozygous mutation of SLC1A3 that codes a dominant-negative GLAST mutant (Jen et al., 2005). This mutant oligomerizes with the wild-type GLAST to exert a dominant-negative effect leading to decreased glutamate uptake, which can contribute to neuronal hyperexcitability that causes seizures, hemiplegia, and episodic ataxia.

4.3.3 Selective Inhibitors

Unlike pharmacologically well-defined GLT1, GLAST lacks selective inhibitors. One of the few inhibitors that shows preference for GLAST over GLT1 is (*R,S*)-2-amino-3-(1-hydroxy-1,2,3-trizol-5-yl)propionate (HTA) that has an IC_{50} value ≈ 100 μM, while its effect on GLT1 (IC_{50} value ≈ 100 μM) and EAAC1 (IC_{50} value $> 1,000$ μM) was much less (Stensbol et al., 2002).

4.4 SLC1A4

4.4.1 Localization and Function

SLC1A4 codes for a Na^+-dependent, small neutral amino acid transporter ASCT1 that accepts L-alanine, L-serine, L-cysteine, and L-threonine (Arriza et al., 1993; Shafqat et al., 1993). Similar to the SLC1 glutamate transporters, ASCT1 mediates an analogous substrate-activated chloride conductance, which is thermodynamically uncoupled from the amino acid flux (Zerangue and Kavanaugh, 1996a). However, unlike the glutamate transporters that complete a transport cycle by potassium countertransport and result in net amino acid flux, ASCT1-mediated transport occurs through potassium-independent electroneutral exchange of neutral amino acids and sodium rather than their net uptake, with the current activated during transport carried by chloride ions (❷ Figure 15-4). Consistent with this mechanism, the amino acid residues (Tyr 403 and Glu 404, in rat GLT1) responsible for K^+-coupling and the relocation step found in glutamate

❑ **Figure 15-4**

Simplified kinetic models of glutamate (*top*) and ASC transporters (*bottom*) (hypothetical). *Top*: under normal conditions, glutamate transport involves loading the empty carrier with glutamate, H^+, and 3 Na^+ (steps 1 and 2), followed by translocation of the fully loaded carrier across the plasma membrane (charge translocation, step 3), and release of the substrates at the intracellular face (steps 4 and 5). Subsequently, K^+ binds to the carrier inside and promotes the relocation of the empty carrier (step 6). Net uptake of glutamate requires completion of this cycle. *Bottom*: when the empty carrier cannot enter the relocation step, the empty carrier binds Na^+ and amino acid substrate again from inside of the cells and translocates back in the reverse direction (steps 5 to 1). In this situation, the transporter behaves like an exchanger. The ASC transporters lack the K^+-coupling step and cannot enter the relocation step, therefore function only in exchange mode

Glutamate transporters

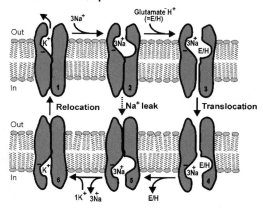

ASC transporters

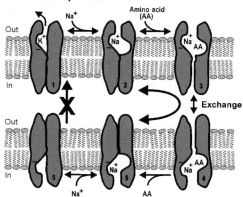

transporters are not conserved in ASC transporters. While system ASC was originally characterized as Na^+ dependent, it does not utilize the Na^+ gradient as a transport-driving force but instead mediates obligatory exchange of substrate amino acids (Arriza et al., 1993; Zerangue and Kavanaugh, 1996a).

In the brain, ASCT1 is found mainly in the radial-astrocyte lineage and olfactory ensheathing glial cells (Sakai et al., 2003). Incidentally, these cells also express the L-serine biosynthetic enzyme 3-phosphoglycerate dehydrogenase (3PGDH) (Yamasaki et al., 2001). Therefore, this suggests that L-serine is synthesized and stored in the glial cells, until it is released to the extracellular space and ultimately to neighboring cells through ASCT1 in exchange for other amino acid substrates. Although L-serine is classified as a nonessential amino acid, it cannot be made in Purkinje neurons because they lack the 3PGDH enzyme required for its synthesis (Furuya et al., 2000). Thus, glial cells appear to be their source of this important amino acid, which is necessary for proper development and function of neurons (Savoca et al., 1995; Mitoma et al., 1998; Furuya et al., 2000).

4.5   SLC1A5

4.5.1   Localization and Function

The ASCT2 transporter is a neutral amino acid transporter that is structurally related to ASCT1 but has different substrate selectivity profile (Kekuda et al., 1996; Utsunomiya-Tate et al., 1996). ASCT2 transporter protein was found to be highly expressed in the brush border membranes of kidney proximal tubule and the intestinal epithelial cells (Avissar et al., 2001). In these tissues, ASCT2 is likely to function in neutral amino acid absorption. In addition to alanine, serine, cysteine, and threonine, ASCT2 also transports glutamine and asparagine with high affinity, as well as methionine, leucine, glycine, valine, and glutamate with lower affinity. In contrast to the SLC1 glutamate transporters, which mediate an electrogenic transport process, ASCT2-mediates Na^+-dependent, electroneutral amino acid exchange. Similar to ASCT1, ASCT2 functions independent of K^+ but cannot undergo a complete transport cycle and therefore is locked into an obligatory homo- or heteroexchange mode (❷ *Figure 15-4*). Benzylserine and benzylcysteine have been shown to competitively inhibit ASCT2 function (Grewer and Grabsch, 2004); however, no specific inhibitors are currently available.

4.6   SLC1A6

4.6.1   Localization and Function

The SLC1A6 encodes a neuronal high-affinity glutamate transporter EAAT4 that is largely limited to cerebellar Purkinje cells on postsynaptic dendritic spines (Fairman et al., 1995; Nagao et al., 1997). EAAT4 is selectively present on this GABAergic cell type and appears to be most concentrated next to excitatory synapses where the glial cell membrane contacts the dendritic spine. Therefore, since EAAT4 is largely located outside the synapse in the perisynaptic membrane and in spine regions, it is positioned to reuptake the glutamate that escapes the synapse to prevent glutamate spillover to neighboring synapses (Takayasu et al., 2005). EAAT4 is poised to be able to indirectly control the amount of glutamate available to activate metabotropic glutamate receptors. Recently, it has been shown that synaptic activation of metabotropic glutamate receptors expressed on Purkinje cells in rat cerebellum is prevented in regions where the glutamate transporter EAAT4 density is high. Thus, regional variations in glutamate transporter abundance are able to affect the amount of metabotropic glutamate receptor activation and therefore regulate synaptic plasticity (Wadiche and Jahr, 2005). In cerebellar Purkinje cells, the analysis of climbing fiber synaptic currents from EAAC1 ($-/-$) mice and EAAT4 ($-/-$) mice revealed that both stoichiometric and anion transporter currents were not present in the EAAT4 ($-/-$) mice, but were observed in EAAC1 ($-/-$) mice. These results suggest that EAAT4 is responsible and thus has a specialized role in clearing glutamate released at climbing fiber–Purkinje cell synapses (Huang et al., 2004).

In addition to glutamate uptake, EAAT4 demonstrates a thermodynamically uncoupled chloride conductance associated with substrate transport that represents over 95% of the steady state current (Fairman et al., 1995). The selectivity of the anion channels associated with the glutamate transporter can be altered from anion selective to partially cation permeable through a voltage- and glutamate-dependent gating process (Melzer et al., 2005). The influx and efflux anion currents are controlled independently, permitting the influx current amplitude to be selectively modified without affecting the efflux current. The gating process results in anion channels that favor cation influx and anion efflux, thus permitting switching between inhibitory currents in resting cells and excitatory currents in electrically active cells. Through this process EAAT4 could modify Purkinje neuron excitability, providing them with a mechanism for adaptation. To date, there are no EAAT4 selective inhibitors; however, the aspartate derivative D,L-*threo*-β-benzyloxyaspartate (TBOA) is a nonsubstrate inhibitor of EAAT4 but also for all the other EAATs (Shimamoto et al., 1998; Shigeri et al., 2001).

4.7 SLC1A7

4.7.1 Localization and Function

EAAT5, encoded by SLC1A7, is a high-affinity glutamate transporter, but the currents elicited by glutamate are largely carried by chloride ions (Arriza et al., 1997). The EAAT5 transporter is primarily expressed in the retina where it is associated with rod photoreceptors and bipolar cells (Pow and Barnett, 2000). Although EAAT5 shares structural homology with the high-affinity glutamate transporters of the SLC1 family, it also features a unique C-terminal motif previously identified in *N*-methyl-D-aspartate receptors and potassium channels. This protein-binding site is intriguing since it confers interactions with a family of synaptic proteins that promote ion channel and receptor clustering (Sheng, 1996). Therefore, EAAT5 may function more like a ligand-gated chloride channel and thus may play a signaling role in photoreceptors.

4.7.2 Nonsubstrate Inhibitors

Interestingly, two aspartate analogs, *threo*-β-hydroxyaspartate and L-*trans*-2,4-PDC, which act as competitive substrates for SLC1A1–3 and SLC1A6 instead are nonsubstrate inhibitors for EAAT5 (Arriza et al., 1997; Bridges et al., 1999). Additionally, the *threo*-methoxyaspartate derivative works as a nonsubstrate inhibitor, but also with GLT1 (Shigeri et al., 2001). While there are several nonsubstrate inhibitors available, thus far none of them are selective for EAAT5.

References

Aoyama K, Suh SW, Hamby AM, Liu J, Chan WY, et al. 2006. Neuronal glutathione deficiency and age-dependent neurodegeneration in the EAAC1 deficient mouse. Nat Neurosci 9: 119-126.

Arriza JL, Kavanaugh MP, Fairman WA, Wu YN, Murdoch GH, et al. 1993. Cloning and expression of a human neutral amino acid transporter with structural similarity to the glutamate transporter gene family. J Biol Chem 268: 15329-15332.

Arriza JL, Fairman WA, Wadiche JI, Murdoch GH, Kavanaugh MP, et al. 1994. Functional comparisons of three glutamate transporter subtypes cloned from human motor cortex. J Neurosci 14: 5559-5569.

Arriza JL, Eliasof S, Kavanaugh MP, Amara SG. 1997. Excitatory amino acid transporter 5, a retinal glutamate transporter coupled to a chloride conductance. Proc Natl Acad Sci USA 94: 4155-4160.

Attwell D, Barbour B, Szatkowski M. 1993. Nonvesicular release of neurotransmitter. Neuron 11: 401-407.

Avissar NE, Ryan CK, Ganapathy V, Sax HC. 2001. Na(+)-dependent neutral amino acid transporter ATB(0) is a rabbit epithelial cell brush-border protein. Am J Physiol Cell Physiol 281: C963-C971.

Balcar VJ, Johnston GA. 1972. The structural specificity of the high affinity uptake of L-glutamate and L-aspartate by rat brain slices. J Neurochem 19: 2657-2666.

Behrens PF, Franz P, Woodman B, Lindenberg KS, Landwehrmeyer GB. 2002. Impaired glutamate transport and glutamate-glutamine cycling: Downstream effects of the Huntington mutation. Brain 125: 1908-1922.

Bendahan A, Armon A, Madani N, Kavanaugh MP, Kanner BI. 2000. Arginine 447 plays a pivotal role in substrate interactions in a neuronal glutamate transporter. J Biol Chem 275: 37436-37442.

Berger UV, Hediger MA. 1998. Comparative analysis of glutamate transporter expression in rat brain using differential double in situ hybridization. Anat Embryol (Berl) 198: 13-30.

Blitzblau R, Gupta S, Djali S, Robinson MB, Rosenberg PA. 1996. The glutamate transport inhibitor L-trans-pyrrolidine-2,4-dicarboxylate indirectly evokes NMDA receptor mediated neurotoxicity in rat cortical cultures. Eur J Neurosci 8: 1840-1852.

Borre L, Kanner BI. 2001. Coupled, but not uncoupled, fluxes in a neuronal glutamate transporter can be activated by lithium ions. J Biol Chem 276: 40396-40401.

Brauner-Osborne H, Hermit MB, Nielsen B, Krogsgaard-Larsen P, Johansen TN. 2000. A new structural class of subtype-selective inhibitor of cloned excitatory amino acid transporter, EAAT2. Eur J Pharmacol 406: 41-44.

Bridges RJ, Kavanaugh MP, Chamberlin AR. 1999. A pharmacological review of competitive inhibitors and substrates of high-affinity, sodium-dependent glutamate transport in the central nervous system. Curr Pharm Des 5: 363-379.

Broer A, Wagner C, Lang F, Broer S. 2000. Neutral amino acid transporter ASCT2 displays substrate-induced Na+ exchange and a substrate-gated anion conductance. Biochem J 346 (Pt. 3): 705-710.

Campiani G, De Angelis M, Armaroli S, Fattorusso C, Catalanotti B, et al. 2001. A rational approach to the design of selective substrates and potent nontransportable inhibitors of the excitatory amino acid transporter EAAC1 (EAAT3). New glutamate and aspartate analogues as potential neuroprotective agents. J Med Chem 44: 2507-2510.

Chaudhry FA, Lehre KP, van Lookeren CM, Ottersen OP, Danbolt NC, et al. 1995. Glutamate transporters in glial plasma membranes: Highly differentiated localizations revealed by quantitative ultrastructural immunocytochemistry. Neuron 15: 711-720.

Chen W, Aoki C, Mahadomrongkul V, Gruber CE, Wang GJ, et al. 2002. Expression of a variant form of the glutamate transporter GLT1 in neuronal cultures and in neurons and astrocytes in the rat brain. J Neurosci 22: 2142-2152.

Cotman CW, Foster A, Lanthorn T. 1981. An overview of glutamate as a neurotransmitter. Adv Biochem Psychopharmacol 27: 1-27.

Curtis DR, Johnston GA. 1974. Amino acid transmitters in the mammalian central nervous system. Ergeb Physiol 69: 97-188.

Curtis DR, Watkins JC. 1960. The excitation and depression of spinal neurones by structurally related amino acids. J Neurochem 6: 117-141.

Danbolt NC, Storm-Mathisen J, Kanner BI. 1992. An [Na+ + K+]coupled L-glutamate transporter purified from rat brain is located in glial cell processes. Neuroscience 51: 295-310.

Deng X, Shibata H, Ninomiya H, Tashiro N, Iwata N, et al. 2004. Association study of polymorphisms in the excitatory amino acid transporter 2 gene (SLC1A2) with schizophrenia. BMC Psychiatry 4: 21.

Dunlop J, Beal MH, She Y, Howland DS. 2003a. Impaired spinal cord glutamate transport capacity and reduced sensitivity to riluzole in a transgenic superoxide dismutase mutant rat model of amyotrophic lateral sclerosis. J Neurosci 23: 1688-1696.

Dunlop J, Eliasof S, Stack G, McIlvain HB, Greenfield A, 2003b. WAY-855 (3-amino-tricyclo[2.2.1.02.6]heptane-1,3-dicarboxylic acid): A novel, EAAT2-preferring, nonsubstrate inhibitor of high-affinity glutamate uptake. Br J Pharmacol 140: 839-846.

Eliasof S, Arriza JL, Leighton BH, Amara SG, Kavanaugh MP. 1998. Localization and function of five glutamate transporters cloned from the salamander retina. Vision Res 38: 1443-1454.

Esslinger CS, Agarwal S, Gerdes J, Wilson PA, Davis ES, et al. 2005. The substituted aspartate analogue L-beta-threo-benzyl-aspartate preferentially inhibits the neuronal excitatory amino acid transporter EAAT3. Neuropharmacology 49: 850-861.

Fairman WA, Vandenberg RJ, Arriza JL, Kavanaugh MP, Amara SG. 1995. An excitatory amino-acid transporter with properties of a ligand-gated chloride channel. Nature 375: 599-603.

Fairman WA, Sonders MS, Murdoch GH, Amara SG. 1998. Arachidonic acid elicits a substrate-gated proton current associated with the glutamate transporter EAAT4. Nat Neurosci 1: 105-113.

Furuya S, Tabata T, Mitoma J, Yamada K, Yamasaki M, et al. 2000. L-serine and glycine serve as major astroglia-derived trophic factors for cerebellar Purkinje neurons. Proc Natl Acad Sci USA 97: 11528-11533.

Gebhardt C, Korner R, Heinemann U. 2002. Delayed anoxic depolarizations in hippocampal neurons of mice lacking the excitatory amino acid carrier 1. J Cereb Blood Flow Metab 22: 569-575.

Gendreau S, Voswinkel S, Torres-Salazar D, Lang N, Heidtmann H, et al. 2004. A trimeric quaternary structure is conserved in bacterial and human glutamate transporters. J Biol Chem 279: 39505-39512.

Grewer C, Grabsch E. 2004. New inhibitors for the neutral amino acid transporter ASCT2 reveal its Na+-dependent anion leak. J Physiol 557: 747-759.

Grewer C, Rauen T. 2005. Electrogenic glutamate transporters in the CNS: Molecular mechanism, pre-steady-state kinetics, and their impact on synaptic signaling. J Membr Biol 203: 1-20.

Grewer C, Watzke N, Rauen T, Bicho A. 2003. Is the glutamate residue Glu-373 the proton acceptor of the excitatory amino acid carrier 1? J Biol Chem 278: 2585-2592.

Grunewald M, Kanner BI. 2000. The accessibility of a novel reentrant loop of the glutamate transporter GLT-1 is restricted by its substrate. J Biol Chem 275: 9684-9689.

Grunewald M, Bendahan A, Kanner BI. 1998. Biotinylation of single cysteine mutants of the glutamate transporter GLT-1 from rat brain reveals its unusual topology. Neuron 21: 623-632.

Grunewald M, Menaker D, Kanner BI. 2002. Cysteine-scanning mutagenesis reveals a conformationally sensitive reentrant pore-loop in the glutamate transporter GLT-1. J Biol Chem 277: 26074-26080.

Guo H, Lai L, Butchbach ME, Stockinger MP, Shan X, et al. 2003. Increased expression of the glial glutamate transporter EAAT2 modulates excitotoxicity and delays the onset but not the outcome of ALS in mice. Hum Mol Genet 12: 2519-2532.

Hakuba N, Koga K, Gyo K, Usami SI, Tanaka K. 2000. Exacerbation of noise-induced hearing loss in mice lacking the glutamate transporter GLAST. J Neurosci 20: 8750-8753.

Hamann M, Rossi DJ, Marie H, Attwell D. 2002. Knocking out the glial glutamate transporter GLT-1 reduces glutamate uptake but does not affect hippocampal glutamate dynamics in early simulated ischaemia. Eur J Neurosci 15: 308-314.

Hanna GL, Veenstra-Vander Weele J, Cox NJ, Boehnke M, Himle JA, et al. 2002. Genome-wide linkage analysis of families with obsessive-compulsive disorder ascertained through pediatric probands. Am J Med Genet 114: 541-552.

Harada T, Harada C, Watanabe M, Inoue Y, Sakagawa T, et al. 1998. Functions of the two glutamate transporters GLAST and GLT-1 in the retina. Proc Natl Acad Sci USA 95: 4663-4666.

Huang YH, Dykes- Hoberg M, Tanaka K, Rothstein JD, Bergles DE. 2004. Climbing fiber activation of EAAT4 transporters and kainate receptors in cerebellar Purkinje cells. J Neurosci 24: 103-111.

Jen JC, Wan J, Palos TP, Howard BD, Baloh RW. 2005. Mutation in the glutamate transporter EAAT1 causes episodic ataxia, hemiplegia, and seizures. Neurology 65: 529-534.

Kanai Y, Hediger MA. 1992. Primary structure and functional characterization of a high-affinity glutamate transporter. Nature 360: 467-471.

Kanai Y, Stelzner MG, Lee WS, Wells RG, Brown D, et al. 1992. Expression of mRNA (D2) encoding a protein involved in amino acid transport in S3 proximal tubule. Am J Physiol 263: F1087-F1092.

Kanai Y, Bhide PG, Di Figlia M, Hediger MA. 1995. Neuronal high-affinity glutamate transport in the rat central nervous system. Neuroreport 6: 2357-2362.

Kavanaugh MP, Bendahan A, Zerangue N, Zhang Y, Kanner BI. 1997. Mutation of an amino acid residue influencing potassium coupling in the glutamate transporter GLT-1 induces obligate exchange. J Biol Chem 272: 1703-1708.

Kekuda R, Prasad PD, Fei YJ, Torres-Zamorano V, Sinha S, et al. 1996. Cloning of the sodium-dependent, broad-scope, neutral amino acid transporter Bo from a human placental choriocarcinoma cell line. J Biol Chem 271: 18657-18661.

Koch HP, Chamberlin AR, Bridges RJ. 1999a. Nontransportable inhibitors attenuate reversal of glutamate uptake in synaptosomes following a metabolic insult. Mol Pharmacol 55: 1044-1048.

Koch HP, Kavanaugh MP, Esslinger CS, Zerangue N, Humphrey JM, et al. 1999b. Differentiation of substrate and nonsubstrate inhibitors of the high-affinity, sodium-dependent glutamate transporters. Mol Pharmacol 56: 1095-1104.

Larsson HP, Picaud SA, Werblin FS, Lecar H. 1996. Noise analysis of the glutamate-activated current in photoreceptors. Biophys J 70: 733-742.

Larsson HP, Tzingounis AV, Koch HP, Kavanaugh MP. 2004. Fluorometric measurements of conformational changes in glutamate transporters. Proc Natl Acad Sci USA 101: 3951-3956.

Leighton BH, Seal RP, Shimamoto K, Amara SG. 2002. A hydrophobic domain in glutamate transporters forms an extracellular helix associated with the permeation pathway for substrates. J Biol Chem 277: 29847-29855.

Li S, Mallory M, Alford M, Tanaka S, Masliah E. 1997. Glutamate transporter alterations in Alzheimer disease are possibly associated with abnormal APP expression. J Neuropathol Exp Neurol 56: 901-911.

Logan WJ, Snyder SH. 1972. High affinity uptake systems for glycine, glutamic and aspaspartic acids in synaptosomes of rat central nervous tissues. Brain Res 42: 413-431.

Matute C, Melone M, Vallejo-Illarramendi A, Conti F. 2005. Increased expression of the astrocytic glutamate transporter GLT-1 in the prefrontal cortex of schizophrenics. Glia 49: 451-455.

Melzer N, Torres-Salazar D, Fahlke C. 2005. A dynamic switch between inhibitory and excitatory currents in a neuronal glutamate transporter. Proc Natl Acad Sci USA 102: 19214-19218.

Mitoma J, Furuya S, Hirabayashi Y. 1998. A novel metabolic communication between neurons and astrocytes: Non-essential amino acid L-serine released from astrocytes is essential for developing hippocampal neurons. Neurosci Res 30: 195-199.

Nagao S, Kwak S, Kanazawa I. 1997. EAAT4, a glutamate transporter with properties of a chloride channel, is predominantly localized in Purkinje cell dendrites, and forms parasagittal compartments in rat cerebellum. Neuroscience 78: 929-933.

Nelson PJ, Dean GE, Aronson PS, Rudnick G. 1983. Hydrogen ion cotransport by the renal brush border glutamate transporter. Biochemistry 22: 5459-5463.

Ottersen OP, Zhang N, Walberg F. 1992. Metabolic compartmentation of glutamate and glutamine: Morphological evidence obtained by quantitative immunocytochemistry in rat cerebellum. Neuroscience 46: 519-534.

Peghini P, Janzen J, Stoffel W. 1997. Glutamate transporter EAAC-1-deficient mice develop dicarboxylic aminoaciduria and behavioral abnormalities but no neurodegeneration. EMBO J 16: 3822-3832.

Picaud SA, Larsson HP, Grant GB, Lecar H, Werblin FS. 1995. Glutamate-gated chloride channel with glutamate-transporter-like properties in cone photoreceptors of the tiger salamander. J Neurophysiol 74: 1760-1771.

Pines G, Danbolt NC, Bjoras M, Zhang Y, Bendahan A, et al. 1992. Cloning and expression of a rat brain L-glutamate transporter. Nature 360: 464-467.

Pow DV, Barnett NL. 2000. Developmental expression of excitatory amino acid transporter 5: A photoreceptor and bipolar cell glutamate transporter in rat retina. Neurosci Lett 280: 21-24.

Roberts PJ, Watkins JC. 1975. Structural requirements for the inhibition for L-glutamate uptake by glia and nerve endings. Brain Res 85: 120-125.

Robinson MB, Sinor JD, Dowd LA, Kerwin JF Jr. 1993. Subtypes of sodium-dependent high-affinity L-[3H]glutamate transport activity: Pharmacologic specificity and regulation by sodium and potassium. J Neurochem 60: 167-179.

Rossi DJ, Oshima T, Attwell D. 2000. Glutamate release in severe brain ischaemia is mainly by reversed uptake. Nature 403: 316-321.

Rothstein JD, Tsai G, Kuncl RW, Clawson L, Cornblath DR, et al. 1990. Abnormal excitatory amino acid metabolism in amyotrophic lateral sclerosis. Ann Neurol 28: 18-25.

Rothstein JD, Martin L, Levey AI, Dykes- Hoberg M, Jin L, et al. 1994. Localization of neuronal and glial glutamate transporters. Neuron 13: 713-725.

Rothstein JD, Van Kammen M, Levey AI, Martin LJ, Kuncl RW. 1995. Selective loss of glial glutamate transporter GLT-1 in amyotrophic lateral sclerosis. Ann Neurol 38: 73-84.

Rothstein JD, Dykes-Hoberg M, Pardo CA, Bristol LA, Jin L, et al. 1996. Knockout of glutamate transporters reveals a major role for astroglial transport in excitotoxicity and clearance of glutamate. Neuron 16: 675-686.

Ryan RM, Vandenberg RJ. 2002. Distinct conformational states mediate the transport and anion channel properties of the glutamate transporter EAAT-1. J Biol Chem 277: 13494-13500.

Ryan RM, Mitrovic AD, Vandenberg RJ. 2004. The chloride permeation pathway of a glutamate transporter and its proximity to the glutamate translocation pathway. J Biol Chem 279: 20742-20751.

Sakai K, Shimizu H, Koike T, Furuya S, Watanabe M. 2003. Neutral amino acid transporter ASCT1 is preferentially expressed in L-Ser-synthetic/storing glial cells in the mouse brain with transient expression in developing capillaries. J Neurosci 23: 550-560.

Savoca R, Ziegler U, Sonderegger P. 1995. Effects of L-serine on neurons in vitro. J Neurosci Methods 61: 159-167.

Schmitt A, Asan E, Lesch KP, Kugler P. 2002. A splice variant of glutamate transporter GLT1/EAAT2 expressed in neurons: Cloning and localization in rat nervous system. Neuroscience 109: 45-61.

Schousboe A, Divac I. 1979. Difference in glutamate uptake in astrocytes cultured from different brain regions. Brain Res 177: 407-409.

Seal RP, Shigeri Y, Eliasof S, Leighton BH, Amara SG. 2001. Sulfhydryl modification of V449C in the glutamate transporter EAAT1 abolishes substrate transport but not the substrate-gated anion conductance. Proc Natl Acad Sci USA 98: 15324-15329.

Sepkuty JP, Cohen AS, Eccles C, Rafiq A, Behar K, et al. 2002. A neuronal glutamate transporter contributes to neurotransmitter GABA synthesis and epilepsy. J Neurosci 22: 6372-6379.

Shafqat S, Tamarappoo BK, Kilberg MS, Puranam RS, McNamara JO, et al. 1993. Cloning and expression of a novel Na($^+$)-dependent neutral amino acid transporter structurally related to mammalian Na$^+$/glutamate cotransporters. J Biol Chem 268: 15351-15355.

Shayakul C, Kanai Y, Lee WS, Brown D, Rothstein JD, et al. 1997. Localization of the high-affinity glutamate transporter EAAC1 in rat kidney. Am J Physiol 273: F1023-F1029.

Sheng M. 1996. PDZs and receptor/channel clustering: Rounding up the latest suspects. Neuron 17: 575-578.

Shigeri Y, Shimamoto K, Yasuda-Kamatani Y, Seal RP, Yumoto N, et al. 2001. Effects of threo-beta-hydroxyaspartate derivatives on excitatory amino acid transporters (EAAT4 and EAAT5). J Neurochem 79: 297-302.

Shimamoto K, Lebrun B, Yasuda-Kamatani Y, Sakaitani M, Shigeri Y, et al. 1998. DL-threo-beta-benzyloxyaspartate, a potent blocker of excitatory amino acid transporters. Mol Pharmacol 53: 195-201.

Shimamoto K, Shigeri Y, Yasuda-Kamatani Y, Lebrun B, Yumoto N, et al. 2000. Syntheses of optically pure beta-hydroxyaspartate derivatives as glutamate transporter blockers. Bioorg Med Chem Lett 10: 2407-2410.

Slotboom DJ, Sobczak I, Konings WN, Lolkema JS. 1999. A conserved serine-rich stretch in the glutamate transporter family forms a substrate-sensitive reentrant loop. Proc Natl Acad Sci USA 96: 14282-14287.

Spreux-Varoquaux O, Bensimon G, Lacomblez L, Salachas F, Pradat PF, et al. 2002. Glutamate levels in cerebrospinal fluid in amyotrophic lateral sclerosis: A reappraisal using a new HPLC method with coulometric detection in a large cohort of patients. J Neurol Sci 193: 73-78.

Stensbol TB, Uhlmann P, Morel S, Eriksen BL, Felding J, et al. 2002. Novel 1-hydroxyazole bioisosteres of glutamic acid.

Synthesis, protolytic properties, and pharmacology. J Med Chem 45: 19-31.

Storck T, Schulte S, Hofmann K, Stoffel W. 1992. Structure, expression, and functional analysis of a Na(+)- dependent glutamate/aspartate transporter from rat brain. Proc Natl Acad Sci USA 89: 10955-10959.

Takayasu Y, Iino M, Kakegawa W, Maeno H, Watase K, et al. 2005. Differential roles of glial and neuronal glutamate transporters in Purkinje cell synapses. J Neurosci 25: 8788-8793.

Tanaka K, Watase K, Manabe T, Yamada K, Watanabe M, et al. 1997. Epilepsy and exacerbation of brain injury in mice lacking the glutamate transporter GLT-1. Science 276: 1699-1702.

Utsunomiya-Tate N, Endou H, Kanai Y. 1996. Cloning and functional characterization of a system ASC-like Na+-dependent neutral amino acid transporter. J Biol Chem 271: 14883-14890.

Vandenberg RJ, Mitrovic AD, Chebib M, Balcar VJ, Johnston GA. 1997. Contrasting modes of action of methylglutamate derivatives on the excitatory amino acid transporters, EAAT1 and EAAT2. Mol Pharmacol 51: 809-815.

Vanoni C, Massari S, Losa M, Carrega P, Perego C, et al. 2004. Increased internalisation and degradation of GLT-1 glial glutamate transporter in a cell model for familial amyotrophic lateral sclerosis (ALS). J Cell Sci 117: 5417-5426.

Veenstra-Vander Weele J, Kim SJ, Gonen D, Hanna GL, Leventhal BL, et al. 2001. Genomic organization of the SLC1A1/EAAC1 gene and mutation screening in early-onset obsessive-compulsive disorder. Mol Psychiatry 6: 160-167.

Wadiche JI, Jahr CE. 2005. Patterned expression of Purkinje cell glutamate transporters controls synaptic plasticity. Nat Neurosci 8: 1329-1334.

Wadiche JI, Amara SG, Kavanaugh MP. 1995. Ion fluxes associated with excitatory amino acid transport. Neuron 15: 721-728.

Watanabe T, Morimoto K, Hirao T, Suwaki H, Watase K, et al. 1999. Amygdala-kindled and pentylenetetrazole-induced seizures in glutamate transporter GLAST-deficient mice. Brain Res 845: 92-96.

Watase K, Hashimoto K, Kano M, Yamada K, Watanabe M, et al. 1998. Motor discoordination and increased susceptibility to cerebellar injury in GLAST mutant mice. Eur J Neurosci 10: 976-988.

Watzke N, Bamberg E, Grewer C. 2001. Early intermediates in the transport cycle of the neuronal excitatory amino acid carrier EAAC1. J Gen Physiol 117: 547-562.

Willis CL, Humphrey JM, Koch HP, Hart JA, Blakely T, et al. 1996. L-trans-2,3-pyrrolidine dicarboxylate: Characterization of a novel excitotoxin. Neuropharmacology 35: 531-539.

Willour VL, Yao SY, Samuels J, Grados M, Cullen B, et al. 2004. Replication study supports evidence for linkage to 9p24 in obsessive-compulsive disorder. Am J Hum Genet 75: 508-513.

Yamasaki M, Yamada K, Furuya S, Mitoma J, Hirabayashi Y, et al. 2001. 3-Phosphoglycerate dehydrogenase, a key enzyme for l-serine biosynthesis, is preferentially expressed in the radial glia/astrocyte lineage and olfactory ensheathing glia in the mouse brain. J Neurosci 21: 7691-7704.

Yernool D, Boudker O, Folta-Stogniew E, Gouaux E. 2003. Trimeric subunit stoichiometry of the glutamate transporters from Bacillus caldotenax and Bacillus stearothermophilus. Biochemistry 42: 12981-12988.

Yernool D, Boudker O, Jin Y, Gouaux E. 2004. Structure of a glutamate transporter homologue from Pyrococcus horikoshii. Nature 431: 811-818.

Zerangue N, Kavanaugh MP. 1996a. ASCT-1 is a neutral amino acid exchanger with chloride channel activity. J Biol Chem 271: 27991-27994.

Zerangue N, Kavanaugh MP. 1996b. Flux coupling in a neuronal glutamate transporter. Nature 383: 634-637.

Zhang Y, Kanner BI. 1999. Two serine residues of the glutamate transporter GLT-1 are crucial for coupling the fluxes of sodium and the neurotransmitter. Proc Natl Acad Sci USA 96: 1710-1715.

Part 3

Neural Membranes and Transport of Neurotransmitters or Other Solutes

16 SLC38 Family of Transporters for Neutral Amino Acids

S. Bröer

Abstract: The solute carrier family 38 (SLC 38) comprises six different Na^+-dependent plasma membrane transporters for neutral amino acids (SNAT1–6). Members of this family have been recognized as molecular correlates of amino acid transport systems A and N. The functional relevance of the SLC 38 family for brain metabolism and function mainly resides in their ability to transport glutamine and the neurotransmitter glycine. As a result, these transporters have been implicated in the glutamate/GABA–glutamine cycle. SNAT1 and 2 are thought to mediate the uptake of glutamine into neurons, whereas SNAT3 is involved in the release of glutamine from astrocytes. The physiological role of the other members in this family remains to be defined.

List of Abbreviations: GABA, Gamma-amino-butyric acid; TCA, Tricarboxylic acid cycle; MeAIB, N-methylaminoisobutyric acid

1   Introduction

The solute carrier family 38 (SLC 38) comprises Na^+-dependent plasma membrane transporters for neutral amino acids (Mackenzie and Erickson, 2004). Members of this family have been recognized as molecular correlates of amino acid transport systems A and N. Traditionally amino acid transport activities in cultured cells have been described as "systems" as long as their molecular identity was unknown (Christensen, 1966). System A is defined as a Na^+-dependent transporter for small neutral amino acids, including alanine, which bestows this system with its acronym "system A". System N has been characterized as a transport system preferring glutamine, asparagine, and histidine. As these amino acids contain an additional nitrogen atom the acronym "system N" was given. The nomenclature of the cloned transporters to some extent followed this scheme but was confusing and inconsistent (❷ *Table 16-1*). To resolve this

❏ Table 16-1
Overview of the SLC38 family

HUGO	System	Name	Alias	Substrates	Mechanism
SLC38A1	A	SNAT1	ATA1, GlnT, SAT1, NAT2, SA2	Q, N, A, C, H, S, M, G, MeAIB	Na^+–AA cotransport
SLC38A2	A	SNAT2	ATA2, SAT2, SA1	A, N, C, Q, G, H, M, P, S, MeAIB	Na^+–AA cotransport
SLC38A3	N	SNAT3	SN1, NAT, g17	Q, N, H	Na^+–AA cotransport H^+-antiport
SLC38A4	A	SNAT4	ATA3, SAT3, NAT3	Q, N, H, S, G, A (K, R, Na^+-independent)	Na^+–AA cotransport
SLC38A5	N	SNAT5	SN2	Q, N, H, S, G, A	Na^+–AA cotransport H^+-antiport
SLC38A6	?	SNAT6	NAT1	Not tested	Not tested

issue, a new nomenclature has recently been introduced, which is used in this chapter (Mackenzie and Erickson, 2004). All members of the SLC 38 family are now named system N/A amino acid transporters (SNAT) and are numbered in the order of their discovery.

The SLC38 family belongs to a larger superfamily of transporters known as the AAAP family of amino acid and auxin permeases (❷ *Figure 16-1*). In mammalians two other solute carrier families belong to this superfamily, namely SLC 32 and SLC 36. Both families are functionally related to SLC 38. The only member of the SLC 32 family is the vesicular GABA transporter. SLC 36 currently comprises four members of proton-coupled amino acid transporters that reside in both the plasma membrane and the lysosomal membrane (Boll et al., 2004).

Hydropathy plotting indicates that all transporters of the SLC38 family most likely have 11 transmembrane helices and an intracellular amino terminus (❷ *Figure 16-2*). However, transmembrane topology

☐ **Figure 16-1**

Sequence similarity between members of the AAAP superfamily of transporters. The sequences of all known human members of solute carrier families 32, 36, and 38 were aligned by using ClustalW software (Thompson et al., 1994). Subsequently, protein distance was calculated by using the Dayhoff PAM matrix (Felsenstein, 1989) and converted into a tree diagram using an additive tree model

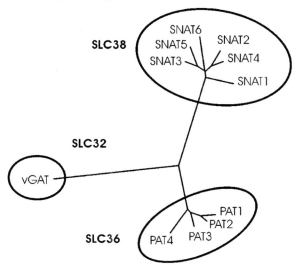

analysis programs consistently bring back SNAT1 with ten transmembrane helices only. Experimental proof for the predicted topology is still lacking. A large loop is predicted between helices five and six, which is predicted to be glycosylated.

Members of this family not only occur in the brain but are also expressed in peripheral tissues. The functional relevance of the SLC 38 family for brain metabolism and function mainly resides in their ability to transport glutamine and the neurotransmitter glycine (Broer and Brookes, 2001; Chaudhry et al., 2002a). As a result these transporters have been proposed to be involved in the glutamate/GABA–glutamine cycle.

It is generally assumed that both GABA and glutamate are recycled in the brain by the glutamate/GABA–glutamine cycle. After being released during neurotransmission, glutamate is taken up largely by astrocytes. There it is converted into glutamine by glutamine synthetase and subsequently released into the extracellular space. Glutamine is then taken up by neurons and converted into glutamate (Shank and Aprison, 1981; Hertz et al., 1999; Daikhin and Yudkoff, 2000). A similar cycle has been proposed for GABA, involving its conversion into glutamine via the tricarboxylic acid cycle and the conversion of glutamate into GABA by glutamate decarboxylase in GABAergic neurons (Shank and Campbell, 1982; Battaglioli and Martin, 1991). Pharmacological studies suggest that a significant proportion of glutamate is recycled by this pathway at least in certain parts of the brain. In the retina, glutamate levels and electrophysiological responses to light were rapidly depleted by inhibiting glial glutamine synthetase with methionine sulfoximine (Pow and Robinson, 1994; Barnett et al., 2000). Similarly, methionine sulfoximine strongly reduced glutamate levels in the neostriatum (Fonnum and Paulsen, 1990) and inhibited recurrent epileptiform activity in the cortex (Bacci et al., 2002). NMR studies in the intact brain (Rothman et al., 2003) and in brain slices (Rae et al., 2003) also demonstrate that glutamate and GABA pools undergo turnover, which in brain slices was inhibited by glutamine transport inhibitors. As will be detailed out in this chapter, there is increasing evidence that members of the SLC 38 family play a vital role in the transfer of glutamine between astrocytes and neurons.

☐ **Figure 16-2**

Topological models of SNAT1 and 3. The peptide sequence of human SNAT1 (a) and human SNAT3 (b) was analyzed by hydropathy plotting using the TMHMM 2.0 program (http://www.cbs.dtu.dk/services/TMHMM-2.0) and the TMpred program (http://www.ch.embnet.org/software/TMPRED_form.html). The structural plots were computed using the transmembrane protein display software (http://www.sacs.ucsf.edu/TOPO/topo.html). Acidic and basic residues in the membrane are shaded. Putative glycosylation sites are shown as boxes

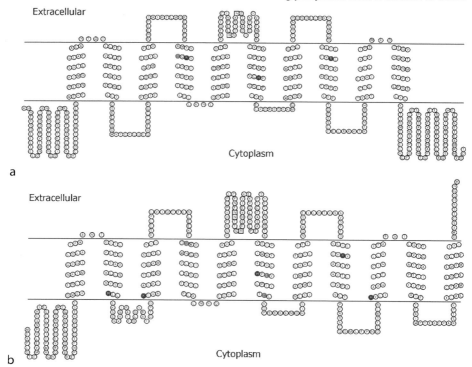

2   Molecular Variants of System A (SNAT1, 2, and 4)

2.1 Molecular Characteristics

Human SNAT1, 2, and 4 are proteins of 527, 506, and 547 amino acids, respectively. SNAT1 and 2 have similar substrate specificity. Both transport most small or hydrophilic neutral amino acids, including glutamine, asparagine, and histidine. By contrast, SNAT4 has a preference for short neutral amino acids, but appears to have a limited capacity to transport glutamine and histidine. In addition it can also transprot cationic amino acids (Hatanaka et al., 2001). Northern-blotting indicates that SNAT4 is a liver-specific transporter and thus will not be further considered in this chapter. SNAT1 shows a preference for glutamine over other amino acids. Interestingly, both SNAT1 and 2 transport serine but not threonine, a hallmark of system A activity. Another hallmark of system A activity is the inhibition by aminomethylated amino acids as exemplified by the nonmetabolizable analog N-methylaminoisobutyric acid (MeAIB). Both SNAT1 and 2 are inhibited by this compound. SNAT1 has a considerable higher affinity for glutamine (K_m of 230 μM) (Albers et al., 2001; Mackenzie et al., 2003) than SNAT2 for which a K_m of 1.65 mM was determined (Yao et al., 2000).

2.2 Localization

The highest expression of SNAT1 is found in the brain (Varoqui et al., 2000). SNAT2, by contrast, is expressed in a wide variety of tissues and appears to be the molecular correlate of the well-characterized system A amino acid transport activity of peripheral cells (Sugawara et al., 2000; Yao et al., 2000). In the rat brain, SNAT1 immunoreactivity is highest in the cerebellum, thalamus, olfactory bulb, and superior colliculus, followed by brainstem and cerebral cortex (Melone et al., 2004). It is found in the membrane of both glutamatergic and GABAergic neurons (Mackenzie et al., 2003; Weiss et al., 2003). A detailed study of its localization in the cerebral cortex showed that 95% of the immunoreactivity was localized in neurons. Double labeling of cells with SNAT1-specific and GABA-specific antibodies indicated its expression in all identified GABAergic neurons (Melone et al., 2004). About 17% of all SNAT1-positive neurons are GABAergic. In cortical neurons, SNAT1 was localized exclusively to the membranes of the cell soma and the dendrites but was notably absent from axon terminals. SNAT2, in agreement with its more widespread distribution, is found in astrocytes and neurons (Reimer et al., 2000). A detailed immunohistochemical analysis of brain tissue has not been reported yet. Both cultured neurons and astrocytes express SNAT1 and 2 but the corresponding transport activity can only be detected in neurons (Heckel et al., 2003).

2.3 Mechanism

Both SNAT1 and 2 cotransport neutral amino acids together with 1 Na^+ ion; (Hatanaka et al., 2000; Yao et al., 2000; Albers et al., 2001; Chaudhry et al., 2002b). Oocytes expressing SNAT1 show increased uptake of Na^+ even in the absence of transporter substrates. The origin of this Na^+ conductance has not been established. Changes of the extracellular Na^+ concentration influence the K_m of glutamine. As a result an ordered binding mechanism, in which Na^+ binds before the substrate to the transporter, has been proposed (Albers et al., 2001; Chaudhry et al., 2002b). Both, SNAT1 and 2 display strong pH dependence, being more active at alkaline pH. The pH dependence is caused by a pH-sensitive modifier site on the transporter (Broer et al., 2002; Chaudhry et al., 2002b). Binding of protons to this site decreases the affinity for Na^+, (Albers et al., 2001) thereby decreasing the transport activity. However, protons cannot replace Na^+ as the cotransported ion.

2.4 Regulation

System A amino acid transporters are tightly regulated and respond to changes of cell growth, cell volume, osmolarity, and amino acid depletion (Shotwell et al., 1983). Most studies have investigated regulation of SNAT2, the molecular correlate of system A activity in many peripheral cells. Alfieri et al. (2001) reported that upregulation of system A activity after hyperosmotic stress in endothelial cells was preceded by a strong upregulation of SNAT2 mRNA. Inhibitors of both transcription and translation inhibited the adaptation to hyperosmotic conditions. A study by Lopez-Fontanals et al. (2003), by contrast, reported that hypertonic incubation of CHO cells did not increase SNAT2 mRNA. In these cells, it was suggested that the response to hyperosmotic medium resulted in an activation of the cyclin-dependent kinase 2 (CDK2)–cyclin A complex. The complex in turn is thought to increase SNAT2 activity via a putative system A activating protein (Ruiz-Montasell et al., 1994). This result suggests a common regulatory pathway involved in cell volume regulation and cell cycle regulation, which is supported by the observation that upregulation of SNAT2 activity during liver regeneration is not accompanied by significant increases of SNAT2 mRNA levels (Freeman and Mailliard, 2000). To some extent protein kinase p38, a component of the mitogen activated protein kinase pathways (MAPK) also appears to be involved in the adaptation to osmotic stress (Lopez-Fontanals et al., 2003).

The mechanism by which SNAT2 activity increases after hypertonic shock has not been established. However, in muscle increased amino acid uptake after stimulation with insulin involves the translocation of

SNAT2 protein from endosomal compartments to the plasma membrane. Similar to the stimulation of insulin-sensitive glucose transport, the signaling pathway was found to involve the insulin receptor and PI-3 kinase (Hyde et al., 2002).

The response to amino acid deprivation apparently uses a different signal transduction pathway. Upregulation of system A activity under these conditions always is accompanied by increased amounts of SNAT2 mRNA (Gazzola et al., 2001; Ling et al., 2001; Lopez-Fontanals et al., 2003; Palii et al., 2004). The adaptive increase of SNAT2 mRNA is prevented by any substrate of SNAT2, including the non-metabolizable amino acid analog MeAIB. However, the immediate sensor of amino acid deprivation remains unknown. Upregulation of SNAT2 transcription under amino acid deprivation is mediated by mitogen activated pathways involving protein kinases ERK1 and 2 or MKK4 and JNK (Franchi-Gazzola et al., 1999; Lopez-Fontanals et al., 2003). Both pathways will result in an increase of transcriptional activity and subsequently in an increase of SNAT2 mRNA and protein levels. Surprisingly, the increase of transcriptional activity is not mediated by amino acid response elements in the promoter of the SNAT2 gene but by elements located in intron 1 (Palii et al., 2004). Mutation of the amino acid response element in intron 1 completely abolished the increase of transcription. This element has enhancer-like properties and confers inducibility at different places and in different orientations. The increase of transport activity after amino acid deprivation is not only mediated by transcriptional regulation but also involves increased forward translocation of transporters from endosomal compartments to the plasma membrane (Ling et al., 2001). Upregulation of SNAT2 mRNA has in addition been observed after treatment of vascular smooth muscle cells with the antigrowth factor TGF-β1. Interestingly, TGF-β1 signaling is thought to involve activation of Smad proteins, which act upon proteins that arrest the cell cycle by blocking cyclin–CDK complexes (Hanahan and Weinberg, 2000). This is an intriguing observation given that upregulation of SNAT2 under hypertonic stress is thought to be caused by an activation of cyclin–CDK complexes but apparently is not associated with increases of SNAT2 mRNA (Lopez-Fontanals et al., 2003).

Much less is known about the regulation of SNAT1. A downregulation of SNAT1 mRNA has been reported after hypoxia in human trophoblasts (Nelson et al., 2003). The signal transduction pathway has not been resolved.

In cultured astrocytes, system A activity can be induced by amino acid depletion of astrocytes or by hyperosmotic shock (Brookes, 1988; Heckel et al., 2003). Furthermore, system A activity mediated by SNAT2 in C6 glioma cells is regulated by changes of transcription and by transporter recruitment to the plasma membrane (Ling et al., 2001). Thus, it appears that similar signal transduction pathways as observed in peripheral cells are functional in the brain.

2.5 Physiological Role

Although both SNAT1 and 2 display system A-like activity, they are likely to play different roles in the brain. It is likely that SNAT2 represents the transport activity that is upregulated whenever amino acids are required for cell growth or increased protein synthesis. SNAT1 on the other hand is expressed at significant levels even in nondividing fully-differentiated GABAergic and glutamatergic neurons. MeAIB, a specific inhibitor of SNAT1 and 2, has been used to investigate the role of these transporters in neurotransmitter metabolism. The results of several studies indicate that saturating concentrations of MeAIB deplete neurotransmitter pools in the hippocampus and in cortical slices (Bacci et al., 2002; Rae et al., 2003). As a result, SNAT1 is thought to mediate uptake of glutamine into neurons after being released from astrocytes (❯ Figure 16-3). Interestingly, Rae et al. (2003) suggested that inhibition of SNAT1 or 2 by the amino acid analog MeAIB mainly affected GABA-labeling in a pool of slow metabolic turnover, most likely cytosolic, but not in the synaptic GABA pool. This notion was subsequently confirmed by the immunolocalization of SNAT1, which is restricted to the soma and dendrites of neurons (Melone et al., 2004). Although this seemingly contradicts the concept of the glutamate/GABA–glutamine cycle, it has to be noted that system A is one of several Na^+-dependent glutamine transport activities in cultured neurons (❯ Figure 16-3).

□ Figure 16-3

Schematic presentation of glutamatergic and GABAergic synapses. The glutamate–glutamine cycle (a) and the glutamate–GABA cycle (b) are depicted with the emphasis on glutamine transporters. Members of the SNAT family are represented by gray shaded circles; the number refers to the numbering of the SNAT family. White circles indicate unidentified transporters. A symbol is included when likely candidates have been proposed (N, system N or N^b, brain-specific system N). Black circles indicate glial glutamate transporters. Other abbreviations: GS, glutamine synthetase and Glnase, glutaminase

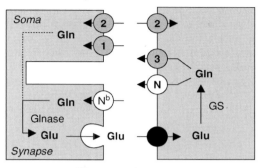

a   Glutamatergic synapse

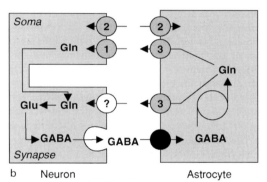

b   Neuron   Astrocyte
GABAergic synapse

Two other transport activities described in cultured neurons that are different from SNAT1 are (1) system N^b, a glutamate-sensitive transporter, which is characterized as a transport system active in the presence of MeAIB, threonine, and histidine (Tamarappoo et al., 1997); and (2) a D-aspartate-sensitive glutamine transporter, which is also resistant to MeAIB but is blocked by threonine and histidine (Heckel et al., 2003). The latter transporter has properties similar to SNAT5 but the corresponding transcript has not been detected in cultured neurons (Heckel et al., 2003).

No attention has yet been paid to the fact that SNAT1 and 2 actively transport glycine. Glycine is a coactivator at NMDA receptors and is found in the extracellular fluid in micromolar concentrations. Because the glial glycine transporter GlyT1b is less able to accumulate glycine than the neuronal GlyT2a, it has been reasoned that reversal of transport in glial cells accounts for nonsynaptic release of glycine (Supplisson and Roux, 2002). The capacity of SNAT1 and 2 to accumulate glycine is in the same order as that of GlyT1b, however they are predominantly expressed in neurons. As a result these transporters constitute a continuous neuronal glycine leak. The functional significance of this putative leak has not been explored.

3   Molecular Variants of System N (SNAT3, 5)

3.1 Molecular Characteristics

SNAT3 was initially cloned from liver and brain tissue (Chaudhry et al., 1999; Gu et al., 2000). Both tissues are known to express system N-like transport activity (Kilberg et al., 1980; Nagaraja and Brookes, 1996). The human SNAT3 cDNA encodes a protein of 504 amino acids (Fei et al., 2000). SNAT3 accepts glutamine, asparagine, and histidine as substrates. Glutamine is transported with an apparent K_m value of 2.4 mM at pH 7.0 (Chaudhry et al., 1999; Broer et al., 2002). Histidine has a similar affinity to the transporter as glutamine. For asparagine a much higher K_m value of 16 mM was reported (Chaudhry et al., 2001).

SNAT5 (472 amino acids) is sequence related to SNAT3 but has a wider substrate specificity than the latter (Nakanishi et al., 2001a, b). SNAT5 transports glycine, asparagine, alanine, serine, glutamine, methionine, and histidine. A K_m value of 4.1 mM for glutamine has been reported for the rat isoform of the transporter (Nakanishi et al., 2001a).

3.2 Localization

SNAT3 is mainly expressed in liver, kidney, and the brain; its distribution in the brain has been studied in some detail (Boulland et al., 2002, 2003). These studies suggest that it is confined to astrocyte processes. Prominent expression was detected in processes adjacent to glutamatergic, GABAergic, and glycinergic synapses. The protein is found in all areas of the brain and shows a relatively even distribution (e.g., less than twofold differences between brain areas). White matter was stained weakly compared to gray matter. In some areas of the brain such as the cerebellum and the hippocampus, SNAT3 was closely positioned to GABAergic synapses but glutamatergic synapses where often not surrounded by SNAT3 containing astrocyte processes. In the cerebellum for example immunoreactivity in the granule cell layer was either associated with GABAergic Golgi-cell terminals or basket-cell terminals. However, Bergmann glia, which express a high density of glutamate transporters were almost devoid of SNAT3 immunoreactivity. This suggests that other release mechanisms might be in place in this cell type. SNAT3 immunoreactivity was also detected in astrocytic perivascular processes and in ependymal cells lining the ventricles. SNAT3 expression increases in the first 2–3 weeks after birth and decreases subsequently to lower levels.

SNAT5 is found in a variety of tissues including the brain. Its cellular distribution in the brain has not been investigated. However, RT-PCR experiments with cultured astrocytes suggest that it is not expressed in astrocytes (Heckel et al., 2003).

3.3 Mechanism

Initial characterization of SNAT3 established and confirmed earlier reports that this transporter is Na^+ dependent (Chaudhry et al., 1999). However, depolarization of cells by addition of KCl had little effect on the transport activity of SNAT3, suggesting that the transporter might not be a simple Na^+–glutamine cotransporter. Expression of the transporter in Na^+/H^+ exchanger-deficient cells revealed that uptake of glutamine caused an alkalinization of the cells. It was concluded that SNAT3 works as a Na^+/H^+ exchanger in which glutamine translocation is coupled to the transport of Na^+ (Chaudhry et al., 1999). Subsequently, it was however reported that transport of glutamine in SNAT3 expressing oocytes was accompanied by inward currents, suggesting that more than one Na^+ was cotransported together with glutamine (Fei et al., 2000). These conflicting data were reconciled by experiments demonstrating that the transporter mediates substrate-induced currents, which are not coupled to substrate translocation (Chaudhry et al., 2001; Broer et al., 2002). Transport of glutamine is energetically coupled to the cotransport of $1Na^+$ and the antiport of $1H^+$. Further experiments revealed that in the transport cycle, substrate binds prior to Na^+ followed by substrate translocation. Return of the substrate-unloaded carrier is facilitated by proton binding. According to the equation $[S]_i/[S]_o = ([Na^+]_o/[Na^+]_i) \times ([H^+]_i/[H^+]_o)$, the transporter will accumulate its substrates [S] inside cells about 20-fold at physiological substrate and ion concentrations.

Small changes of the pH or Na^+ gradient, as a result, can change the prevalent transport direction from influx to efflux (Broer et al., 2002). Accordingly, it has been demonstrated that release of glutamine from astrocytes is reduced when cells are depleted of intracellular Na^+, vice versa efflux increased when the intracellular concentration of Na^+ was raised (Deitmer et al., 2003).

The nature of the glutamine-induced currents observed in SNAT3-expressing *Xenopus laevis* oocytes has not been resolved. Several observations suggest that the current is mediated by the transporter itself and not by oocyte-endogenous ion channels. At 1 mM, for example, currents induced by asparagine and glutamine are similar, although asparagine is transported at a much lower rate than glutamine (Chaudhry et al., 2001). If oocyte endogenous channels were to be activated by alkalinization of the oocyte, smaller currents would be expected for asparagine than for glutamine. It has been suggested that the currents are generated by a H^+ conductance, however, the reversal potential of substrate-induced currents were found to shift with pH in one study but not in another study (Chaudhry et al., 2001; Broer et al., 2002). The amplitude of the currents is strongly Na^+ dependent as is the transport activity, however, their reversal potential is unaffected by changes of the Na^+ concentration suggesting that they are also not mediated by Na^+ ions (Chaudhry et al., 2001; Broer et al., 2002). The substrate-induced currents are rather small, particularly in the case of glutamine, and therefore may not be of physiological relevance.

The transporter has a strong pH dependence being more active at alkaline pH than at acidic pH. The pH dependence is not caused by the proton antiport but is caused by a modifier site (Broer et al., 2002). The pH dependence of the proton antiport function is only observed at pH values >9. Further evidence that the pH sensitivity is conferred by a pH modifier site is provided by the similar pH dependence of the related transporters SNAT1 and 2, both of which do not antiport protons (Albers et al., 2001).

The mechanism of SNAT5 appears to be similar to that of SNAT3. The transporter is Na^+ dependent and substrate-induced inward currents are observed when expressed in oocytes (Nakanishi et al., 2001a). Moreover, substrate uptake is accompanied by intracellular alkalinization, suggesting that it mediates Na^+/H^+ antiport, with Na^+ transport coupled to substrate translocation (Nakanishi et al., 2001a). The Na^+ cotransport stoichiometry has not been established. In analogy to SNAT3, it appears likely that the transport mechanism is electroneutral and substrate-induced currents are generated by a cation conductance.

3.4 Regulation

Regulation of SNAT3 has been studied to a limited extent. In the proximal tubule, SNAT3 mRNA is strongly upregulated in response to chronic metabolic acidosis (Karinch et al., 2002). In the proximal tubule, glutamine is taken up from the blood and subsequently deamidated to synthesize NH_4^+. Ammonium ions are secreted into the urine thereby removing the acid load from the body. In the brain glutamine is used to defuse ammonia followed by secretion of glutamine into the blood. Thus, SNAT3 might play a role in the detoxification of ammonia in the brain, particularly because of its location in perivascular astrocyte processes. However, no regulation of SNAT3 in correspondence to increased levels of ammonia has been reported yet. High levels of SNAT3 mRNA have been reported in brain gliomas, suggesting that SNAT3 may provide glutamine as a nutrient for rapidly growing cells (Sidoryk et al., 2004).

An acute upregulation of SNAT3 activity has been observed after incubation of astrocytes with increased amounts of glutamate (Broer et al., 2004). This action is not mediated by metabotropic glutamate receptors but is caused by elevated intracellular glutamate concentrations. The signal transduction pathway has not been identified but may involve a direct binding of glutamate to the SNAT3 transporter. This regulatory property of SNAT3 explains earlier observations, which indicated an increased release of glutamine after incubation of astrocytes with glutamate (Albrecht, 1989).

Due to its mechanism and the presence of a pH modifier site, SNAT3 is regulated by the intracellular and extracellular Na^+ and H^+ concentration. Under physiological conditions the transporter is close to equilibrium. Small changes of glutamine, Na^+, and H^+ will therefore determine the prevalent direction of substrate transport (Broer et al., 2002).

3.5 Physiological Role

Functional studies in cultured rat astrocytes indicate that SNAT3 activity does not contribute significantly to glutamine uptake (<10% of the uptake activity) (Heckel et al., 2003), which is in agreement with the low affinity of the transporter for its substrates. However, a more prominent system N activity has been reported in mouse astrocytes (Nagaraja and Brookes, 1996). By contrast, 50% of the spontaneous glutamine efflux from astrocytes is mediated by SNAT3 (Deitmer et al., 2003). In the efflux direction, the low affinity is matched by intracellular glutamine concentrations. Moreover, SNAT3 is specific for glutamine and histidine, which prevents interference by other amino acids. The transporter is likely to be important for efflux also in situ (❯ Figure 16-3) (Chaudhry et al., 2002a). Uptake of glutamate or GABA by astrocytes increases intracellular Na^+ concentration, which will foster glutamine efflux. As pointed out earlier, glutamate transporters and SNAT3 are not always colocalized. Bergmann glia cells in the cerebellum, for example express only small amounts of SNAT3 but large amounts of glutamate transporters (Boulland et al., 2002). This result suggests that other routes of glutamine release exist, which is supported by functional studies (Deitmer et al., 2003). These studies indicate that astrocytes express a Na^+-independent glutamine-specific transporter with properties of system N (❯ Figure 16-3). It appears likely that release of glutamine via SNAT3 is more relevant for GABA recycling than for glutamate recycling as suggested by the predominant localization close to GABAergic synapses (❯ Figure 16-3). SNAT3 might also be involved in the release of glutamine into the blood. Immunoreactivity was found both in perivascular astrocyte processes and in ependymal cells, suggesting a role in ammonia detoxification.

The physiological role of SNAT5 remains to be defined. So far no transport activity has been described that matches that of SNAT5. The substrate specificity is quite similar to that of system A or ASC and as a result it may have been characterized as A-like or ASC-like in the past. However, it can be discriminated against the substrate specificity of SNAT1 and 2 by its resistance against MeAIB. The transcript is present in brain (Nakanishi et al., 2001a) and a transport activity similar to SNAT5 has been detected in cultured neurons (Heckel et al., 2003), but the mRNA was notably absent in this preparation.

References

Albers A, Broer A, Wagner CA, Setiawan I, Lang PA, et al. 2001. Na+ transport by the neural glutamine transporter ATA1. Pflugers Arch 443 (1): 92-101.

Albrecht J. 1989. L-Glutamate stimulates the efflux of newly taken up glutamine from astroglia but not from synaptosomes of the rat. Neuropharmacology 28 (8): 885-887.

Alfieri RR, Petronini PG, Bonelli MA, Caccamo AE, Cavazzoni A, et al. 2001. Osmotic regulation of ATA2 mRNA expression and amino acid transport system A activity. Biochem Biophys Res Commun 283 (1): 174-178.

Bacci A, Sancini G, Verderio C, Armano S, Pravettoni E, et al. 2002. Block of glutamate-glutamine cycle between astrocytes and neurons inhibits epileptiform activity in hippocampus. J Neurophysiol 88 (5): 2302-2310.

Barnett NL, Pow DV, Robinson SR. 2000. Inhibition of Muller cell glutamine synthetase rapidly impairs the retinal response to light. Glia 30 (1): 64-73.

Battaglioli G, Martin DL. 1991. GABA synthesis in brain slices is dependent on glutamine produced in astrocytes. Neurochem Res 16 (2): 151-156.

Boll M, Daniel H, Gasnier B. 2004. The SLC36 family: Proton coupled transporters for the absorption of selected amino acids from extracellular and intracellular proteolysis. Pflugers Arch 447 (5): 776-779.

Boulland JL, Osen KK, Levy LM, Danbolt NC, Edwards RH, et al. 2002. Cell-specific expression of the glutamine transporter SN1 suggests differences in dependence on the glutamine cycle. Eur J Neurosci 15 (10): 1615-1631.

Boulland JL, Rafiki A, Levy LM, Storm-Mathisen J, Chaudhry FA. 2003. Highly differential expression of SN1, a bidirectional glutamine transporter, in astroglia and endothelium in the developing rat brain. Glia 41 (3): 260-275.

Broer S, Brookes N. 2001. Transfer of glutamine between astrocytes and neurons. J Neurochem 77 (3): 705-719.

Broer A, Albers A, Setiawan I, Edwards RH, Chaudhry FA, et al. 2002. Regulation of the glutamine transporter SN1 by extracellular pH and intracellular sodium ions. J Physiol 539 (Pt. 1): 3-14.

Broer A, Deitmer JW, Broer S. 2004. Astroglial glutamine transport by system N is upregulated by glutamate. Glia 48: 298-310.

Brookes N. 1988. Neutral amino acid transport in astrocytes: Characterization of Na+-dependent and Na+-independent components of alpha-aminoisobutyric acid uptake. J Neurochem 51 (6): 1913-1918.

Chaudhry FA, Reimer RJ, Krizaj D, Barber D, Storm-Mathisen J, et al. 1999. Molecular analysis of system N suggests novel physiological roles in nitrogen metabolism and synaptic transmission. Cell 99 (7): 769-780.

Chaudhry FA, Krizaj D, Larsson P, Reimer RJ, Wreden C, et al. 2001. Coupled and uncoupled proton movement by amino acid transport system N. EMBO J 20 (24): 7041-7051.

Chaudhry FA, Reimer RJ, Edwards RH. 2002a. The glutamine commute: Take the N line and transfer to the A. J Cell Biol 157 (3): 349-355.

Chaudhry FA, Schmitz D, Reimer RJ, Larsson P, Gray AT, et al. 2002b. Glutamine uptake by neurons: Interaction of protons with system a transporters. J Neurosci 22 (1): 62-72.

Christensen HN. 1966. Methods for distinguishing amino acid transport systems of a given cell or tissue. Fed Proc 25 (3): 850-853.

Daikhin Y, Yudkoff M. 2000. Compartmentation of brain glutamate metabolism in neurons and glia. J Nutr 130 (4S Suppl.): 1026S-1031S.

Deitmer JW, Broer A, Broer S. 2003. Glutamine efflux from astrocytes is mediated by multiple pathways. J Neurochem 87 (1): 127-135.

Fei YJ, Sugawara M, Nakanishi T, Huang W, Wang H, et al. 2000. Primary structure, genomic organization, and functional and electrogenic characteristics of human system N 1, a Na+- and H+-coupled glutamine transporter. J Biol Chem 275 (31): 23707-23717.

Felsenstein J. 1989. PHYLIP—Phylogeny Inference Package (Version 3.2). Cladistics 5: 164-166.

Fonnum F, Paulsen RE. 1990. Comparison of transmitter amino acid levels in rat globus pallidus and neostriatum during hypoglycemia or after treatment with methionine sulfoximine or gamma-vinyl gamma-aminobutyric acid. J Neurochem 54 (4): 1253-1257.

Franchi-Gazzola R, Visigalli R, Bussolati O, Dall' Asta V, Gazzola GC. 1999. Adaptive increase of amino acid transport system A requires ERK1/2 activation. J Biol Chem 274 (41): 28922-28928.

Freeman TL, Mailliard ME. 2000. Posttranscriptional regulation of ATA2 transport during liver regeneration. Biochem Biophys Res Commun 278 (3): 729-732.

Gazzola RF, Sala R, Bussolati O, Visigalli R, Dall' Asta V, et al. 2001. The adaptive regulation of amino acid transport system A is associated to changes in ATA2 expression. FEBS Lett 490 (1–2): 11-14.

Gu S, Roderick HL, Camacho P, Jiang JX. 2000. Identification and characterization of an amino acid transporter expressed differentially in liver. Proc Natl Acad Sci USA 97 (7): 3230-3235.

Hanahan D, Weinberg RA. 2000. The hallmarks of cancer. Cell 100 (1): 57-70.

Hatanaka T, Huang W, Wang H, Sugawara M, Prasad PD, et al. 2000. Primary structure, functional characteristics and tissue expression pattern of human ATA2, a subtype of amino acid transport system A. Biochim Biophys Acta 1467 (1): 1-6.

Hatanaka T, Huang W, Ling R, Prasad PD, Sugawara M, et al. 2001. Evidence for the transport of neutral as well as cationic amino acids by ATA3, a novel and liver-specific subtype of amino acid transport system A. Biochim Biophys Acta 1510 (1–2): 10-17.

Heckel T, Broer A, Wiesinger H, Lang F, Broer S. 2003. Asymmetry of glutamine transporters in cultured neural cells. Neurochem Int 43 (4–5): 289-298.

Hertz L, Dringen R, Schousboe A, Robinson SR. 1999. Astrocytes: Glutamate producers for neurons. J Neurosci Res 57 (4): 417-428.

Hyde R, Peyrollier K, Hundal HS. 2002. Insulin promotes the cell surface recruitment of the SAT2/ATA2 system A amino acid transporter from an endosomal compartment in skeletal muscle cells. J Biol Chem 277 (16): 13628-13634.

Karinch AM, Lin CM, Wolfgang CL, Pan M, Souba WW. 2002. Regulation of expression of the SN1 transporter during renal adaptation to chronic metabolic acidosis in rats. Am J Physiol Renal Physiol 283 (5): F1011-F1019.

Kilberg MS, Handlogten ME, Christensen HN. 1980. Characteristics of an amino acid transport system in rat liver for glutamine, asparagine, histidine, and closely related analogs. J Biol Chem 255 (9): 4011-4019.

Ling R, Bridges CC, Sugawara M, Fujita T, Leibach FH, et al. 2001. Involvement of transporter recruitment as well as gene expression in the substrate-induced adaptive regulation of amino acid transport system A. Biochim Biophys Acta 1512 (1): 15-21.

Lopez-Fontanals M, Rodriguez-Mulero S, Casado FJ, Derijard B, Pastor-Anglada M. 2003. The osmoregulatory and the amino acid-regulated responses of system A are mediated by different signal transduction pathways. J Gen Physiol 122 (1): 5-16.

Mackenzie B, Erickson JD. 2004. Sodium-coupled neutral amino acid (System N/A) transporters of the SLC38 gene family. Pflugers Arch 447 (5): 784-795.

Mackenzie B, Schafer MK, Erickson JD, Hediger MA, Weihe E, et al. 2003. Functional properties and cellular distribution of the system A glutamine transporter SNAT1 support specialized roles in central neurons. J Biol Chem 278 (26): 23720-23730.

Melone M, Quagliano F, Barbaresi P, Varoqui H, Erickson JD, et al. 2004. Localization of the glutamine transporter SNAT1 in rat cerebral cortex and neighboring structures, with a note on its localization in human cortex. Cereb Cortex 14 (5): 562-574.

Nagaraja TN, Brookes N. 1996. Glutamine transport in mouse cerebral astrocytes. J Neurochem 66 (4): 1665-1674.

Nakanishi T, Kekuda R, Fei YJ, Hatanaka T, Sugawara M, et al. 2001a. Cloning and functional characterization of a new subtype of the amino acid transport system N. Am J Physiol Cell Physiol 281 (6): C1757-C1768.

Nakanishi T, Sugawara M, Huang W, Martindale RG, Leibach FH, et al. 2001b. Structure, function, and tissue expression pattern of human SN2, a subtype of the amino acid transport system N. Biochem Biophys Res Commun 281 (5): 1343-1348.

Nelson DM, Smith SD, Furesz TC, Sadovsky Y, Ganapathy V, et al. 2003. Hypoxia reduces expression and function of system A amino acid transporters in cultured term human trophoblasts. Am J Physiol Cell Physiol 284 (2): C310-C315.

Palii SS, Chen H, Kilberg MS. 2004. Transcriptional control of the human sodium-coupled neutral amino acid transporter system A gene by amino acid availability is mediated by an intronic element. J Biol Chem 279 (5): 3463-3471.

Pow DV, Robinson SR. 1994. Glutamate in some retinal neurons is derived solely from glia. Neuroscience 60 (2): 355-366.

Rae C, Hare N, Bubb WA, McEwan SR, Broer A, et al. 2003. Inhibition of glutamine transport depletes glutamate and GABA neurotransmitter pools: Further evidence for metabolic compartmentation. J Neurochem 85 (2): 503-514.

Reimer RJ, Chaudhry FA, Gray AT, Edwards RH. 2000. Amino acid transport system A resembles system N in sequence but differs in mechanism. Proc Natl Acad Sci USA 97 (14): 7715-7720.

Rothman DL, Behar KL, Hyder F, Shulman RG. 2003. In vivo NMR studies of the glutamate neurotransmitter flux and neuroenergetics: Implications for brain function. Annu Rev Physiol 65: 401-427.

Ruiz-Montasell B, Gomez-Angelats M, Casado FJ, Felipe A, McGivan JD, et al. 1994. Evidence for a regulatory protein involved in the increased activity of system A for neutral amino acid transport in osmotically stressed mammalian cells. Proc Natl Acad Sci USA 91 (20): 9569-9573.

Shank RP, Aprison MH. 1981. Present status and significance of the glutamine cycle in neural tissues. Life Sci 28 (8): 837-842.

Shank RP, Campbell GL. 1982. Glutamine and alpha-ketoglutarate uptake and metabolism by nerve terminal enriched material from mouse cerebellum. Neurochem Res 7 (5): 601-616.

Shotwell MA, Kilberg MS, Oxender DL. 1983. The regulation of neutral amino acid transport in mammalian cells. Biochim Biophys Acta 737 (2): 267-284.

Sidoryk M, Matyja E, Dybel A, Zielinska M, Bogucki J, et al. 2004. Increased expression of a glutamine transporter SNAT3 is a marker of malignant gliomas. Neuroreport 15 (4): 575-578.

Sugawara M, Nakanishi T, Fei YJ, Huang W, Ganapathy ME, et al. 2000. Cloning of an amino acid transporter with functional characteristics and tissue expression pattern identical to that of system A. J Biol Chem 275 (22): 16473-16477.

Supplisson S, Roux MJ. 2002. Why glycine transporters have different stoichiometries. FEBS Lett 529 (1): 93-101.

Tamarappoo BK, Raizada MK, Kilberg MS. 1997. Identification of a system N-like Na(+)-dependent glutamine transport activity in rat brain neurons. J Neurochem 68 (3): 954-960.

Thompson JD, Higgins DG, Gibson TJ. 1994. CLUSTAL W: improving the sensitivity of progressive multiple sequence alignment through sequence weighting, position-specific gap penalties and weight matrix choice. Nucleic Acids Res 22 (22): 4673-4680.

Varoqui H, Zhu H, Yao D, Ming H, Erickson JD. 2000. Cloning and functional identification of a neuronal glutamine transporter. J Biol Chem 275 (6): 4049-4054.

Weiss MD, Derazi S, Rossignol C, Varoqui H, Erickson JD, et al. 2003. Ontogeny of the neutral amino acid transporter SAT1/ATA1 in rat brain. Brain Res Dev Brain Res 143 (2): 151-159.

Yao D, Mackenzie B, Ming H, Varoqui H, Zhu H, et al. 2000. A novel system A isoform mediating Na+/neutral amino acid cotransport. J Biol Chem 275 (30): 22790-22797.

17 Monoamine Transporters in the Brain: Structure and Function

H. H. Sitte · M. Freissmuth

Abstract: Monoamine transporters mediate the uptake of serotonin (SERT), norepinephrine (NET), and dopamine (DAT). They are closely related, share many conserved sequence elements and thus overlapping specificities for binding of inhibitors and substrates. The transporter is thought to undergo a conformational cycle that allows for transmembrane translocation of the monoamine substrate and the cosubstrate ions Na^+ and Cl^-. In addition, transporters are known to support currents that are substantially larger than those anticipated from the movement of charges during a translocation cycle. The recently solved structure of the distantly related bacterial leucine transporter ($LeuT_{Aa}$) offers insights that allow to reconcile the channel-like mode in which transporters can operate with the original alternate access model. Access to the substrate and cosubstrate permeation pathway is shielded by juxtamembrane residues, which can operate as gates. When simultaneously open, they allow for large ion fluxes which give rise to excess currents. SERT, NET, and DAT and the other (related) members of the Na^+-dependent neurotransmitter family form constitutive oligomers. Oligomerization is a prerequisite for export of the proteins from the endoplasmic reticulum (ER) because it supports the recruitment of COPII components, most notably Sec24-family members. In addition, the action of amphetamines which induce reverse transport and thus monoamine efflux is proposed to be contingent on the oligomeric assembly of transporters.

List of Abbreviations: COPII, coat protein II; DAT, dopamine transporter; ER, endoplasmic reticulum; ERES, ER exit sites; FRET, Fluorescence resonance energy transfer; GABA, γ-amino butyric acid; GAT1, GABA transporter 1; GEF, guanine nucleotide exchange factor; 5-HT, serotonin; $LeuT_{Aa}$, leucine transporter; MDMA, methylene-dioxymethamphetamine; MTS, methanethiosulfonate; MTSEA, MTS ethylammonium; MTSET, MTS-ethyltrimethylammonium; MTSES, MTS-ethylsulfonate; NET, norepinephrine transporter; PCA, *para*-chloroamphetamine; SERT, serotonin transporter; SNAP25, synaptosomal-associated protein of 25 kDa; TM, transmembrane domain; VAMP, vesicle associated membrane protein

1   Introduction

The term "monoamines" refers to amine neurotransmitters and autacoids, including the classical catecholamines adrenaline, noradrenaline and 1,3-dihydroxy-tryptamine or dopamine (DA), and the indoleamine 5-hydroxytryptamine.

Several Nobel Prizes have been awarded for seminal contributions that paved the way to our current understanding of neurotransmission by monoamines. The most recent was the award in 2000 to Carlsson, Greengard, and Kandel; their discoveries were crucial to our understanding of both, the biochemical and biophysical processes underlying normal brain function and how aberrant signaling can give rise to neurological and psychiatric diseases. The findings of Arvid Carlsson were, in particular, instrumental to linking monoamine deficiency to a state that in experimental animals resembled Parkinson's disease in people (Carlsson, 2001). Oleh Hornykiewicz independently provided the crucial evidence, namely that DA was absent in the basal ganglia of patients with Parkinson's disease (Birkmayer and Hornykiewicz, 1961). Together, these and many additional observations provided the rationale for therapeutic trials with L-dopa. Some 4.5 decades later, it is still safe to claim that no other drug regimen has been as useful in the alleviation of the major symptoms rigor, tremor, and akinesia. Similarly, the groundbreaking work of Axelrod et al. (1971) defined the metabolic pathways by which catecholamines were synthesized and degraded; these insights also defined the site of action of several drugs. If sales figures are used to gauge the impact of scientific discoveries, a top rank is to be reserved to the discovery that antidepressants, cocaine, and amphetamines affect the reuptake of monoamines, for this observation is relevant to the pharmaceutical industry and the illicit drug trade (Axelrod et al., 1961).

In this chapter, we summarize the current knowledge on monoamine transporters from tertiary to quaternary structure and the repercussions that the structural constraints exert on the functional aspects of monoamine transporter physiology.

2   Monoamines

The monoamines comprise the two catecholamines, DA and norepinephrine, which are both derived from the amino acid tyrosine. Serotonin is an indoleamine (5-hydroxytryptamine), which is synthesized from the amino acid tryptophan. The monoaminergic cells produce the monoamines in the periphery, where the complete synthetic machinery resides freely in the cytosol. Newly produced monoamines are packaged into synaptic vesicles and thus made available to exocytotic release. The (presynaptic) depolarization leads to opening of Ca^{2+}-channels. The resulting influx of Ca^{2+} subsequently induces exocytotic release by promoting coupling between the SNARE machinery residing on the vesicle (VAMP) and on the plasma membrane (synaptosomal-associated protein of 25 kDa = SNAP25, syntaxin). During a Rab-dependent process, referred to as nucleation, a temporary fusion event takes place that leads to a brief opening of both the plasma membrane and the vesicular membrane. This establishes an aqueous continuity between vesicle interior and cell exterior and allows densely packed neurotransmitter to exchange between both compartments. The extent to which vesicle and plasma membrane mix varies from a brief interaction, conforming to the model of "kiss-and-run," to a complete fusion of the two membranes. The Ca^{2+} concentration is crucial in specifying the mode of fusion: low Ca^{2+} concentrations lead to a permanent fusion and integration of the vesicle membrane into the plasma membrane while high Ca^{2+} concentrations favor "kiss-and-run" (Harata et al., 2006). The result of both events is a rise in the extracellular concentration of neurotransmitter that stimulates both pre- and postsynaptic receptors to propagate signal, i.e., information. The physiological function of neurotransmitter transporters is to end synaptic transmission: transporters terminate signal transduction by removing one of the main players, the neurotransmitter.

In the axon, the information is encoded in the firing rate, i.e., in a digitized format. This is converted into quantal information transfer, the unit size of which is the vesicular neurotransmitter content. This in turn gives rise to an analog signal on the postsynaptic membrane (because the interaction of neurotransmitter and its cognate receptors is governed by the law of mass action). During this conversion, information is to be lost, if there was no effective means of rapidly resetting the synapse to zero. This is achieved by removing neurotransmitters from the synaptic cleft. Transporters do this very effectively by coupling the translocation of monoamine neurotransmitters to a preexisting gradient of Na^+ and to some extent Cl^- ions.

3   The Therapeutic Efficacy and Abuse Potential of Drugs Acting at Neurotransmitter Transporters

Several distinct classes of drugs target neurotransmitter transporters; some are clinically useful therapeutic agents while others are widely abused because of their psychostimulant actions, which are considered illicit in most—but not all—countries (Iversen, 2000). The therapeutic drugs primarily act by blocking the transporters of serotonin and norepinephrine; this results in elevated concentrations of the neurotransmitter in the synaptic cleft. In the treatment of depression, this is the desired effect which triggers adaptive changes at both the pre- and postsynaptic receptors.

Likewise, drugs of abuse also exert their effects at the level of neurotransmitter transporters; by contrast with antidepressants (which inhibit predominantly either the serotonin transporter (SERT) or the norepinephrine transporter (NET) or both and thus impinge on the serotoninergic and noradrenergic neurons), drugs of abuse activate the dopaminergic rewarding system in the nucleus accumbens (Kuhar et al., 1991). While all drugs of abuse elevate DA in the nucleus accumbens, drugs acting at the dopamine transporter (DAT) can bring about the effect in two different ways: they can either inhibit DA reuptake (Amara and Kuhar, 1993) or induce carrier-mediated release (Levi and Raiteri, 1993). Cocaine is the prototypic inhibitor of the DAT, an action that is also shared by bupropion. This compound is used in many countries to suppress craving during nicotine withdrawal. Amphetamine and a large variety of different congeners induce nonexocytotic release of monoamines by transport reversal.

4   Distribution of Monoamine Transporters in the Brain

According to Sir Henry Dale, the neurochemical identity of a neuron is determined by the nature of the neurotransmitter that is present in its cell soma and its vesicles (Dale, 1935). Sir John Eccles proposed to refer to this concept as Dale's principle; accordingly neurons are referred to as glutamatergic, GABAergic, dopaminergic, etc. (Sulzer and Rayport, 2000). It is worth noting that the discovery of peptides and ATP as cotransmitters has not fundamentally modified this concept because peptide cotransmitters are of modest relevance to rapid neurotransmission and ATP is a ubiquitous cotransmitter; in addition both, peptides and ATP, are degraded by exoenzymes (peptidases and ectonucleotidases) rather than retrieved by specific transporters. Thus, Dale's principle predicts that any given neuron only expresses a single type of neurotransmitter transporter. When analyzed by in situ hybridization, the distribution of neurotransmitter transporters is in line with Dale's principle.

The DAT is expressed in dopaminergic neurons, the bulk of which reside in the substantia nigra and the ventral tegmental area (Hoffman et al., 1998). These neurons also express tyrosine hydroxylase, accordingly the tyrosine hydroxylase promoter can be used to drive the expression of GFP-tagged DAT as a transgene (Zhang et al., 2004). The distribution of the DAT protein is more widespread because it is targeted to the axons and also found in the dendritic compartment: in the mouse and rat brain, immunoreactivity for DAT-like has been described in striatum and in the nucleus accumbens, the olfactory tubercle, the frontal cortex, and cingulate cortex (Ciliax et al., 1995; Freed et al., 1995).

Likewise, the locus coeruleus (and related brain stem nuclei) and the raphe nuclei are the main source of norepinephrine and serotonin, respectively, in the brain. Hence, these neurons are also the main site of synthesis of the norepinephrine transporter (NET) and the SERT. Consistent with the diffuse projection of noradrenergic and serotonergic neurons, immunoreactivity for NET and for SERT is widely distributed in the central nervous system (Qian et al., 1995; Sur et al., 1996; Schroeter et al., 2000). NET colocalizes with synaptic markers such as syntaxin, synaptophysin, and SNAP25 (Schroeter et al., 2000). Immunoelectron microscopy revealed that DAT, NET, and SERT were not directly localized near the synaptic specialization (Nirenberg et al., 1997a, b). This observation is consistent with the concept that the transporters form a metabolic barrier that limits the extrasynaptic action of neurotransmitters. In this work, it was also recognized that the immunoreactivity was not confined to the cell surface but also to intracellular structures; most likely during protein synthesis (see below).

Monoamine neurotransmitter transporters are obviously not confined to the central nervous system; they are also expressed in the periphery (Eisenhofer, 2001): DAT, for instance, is found in the kidney, stomach, and pancreas (Mezey et al., 1998; Sugamori et al., 1999). NET has been detected in peripheral sympathomimetic neurons and ganglia, most prominently in the adrenal gland (Schroeter et al., 1997). SERT was first detected in peripheral blood cells, most importantly in blood platelets. Platelets have served for decades as an easily accessible source of the human transporter (Talvenheimo et al., 1979, 1983); in fact, before the advent of molecular cloning, they were the only readily available source of human SERT. Apart from the blood, SERT has also been detected in placenta (Cool et al., 1991), the mRNA of which originally served as the source for its molecular cloning (Ramamoorthy et al., 1993a).

5   The Tertiary Structure: The Transporter as Folded Membrane Protein

The first transporter for which the cDNA became available was the GABA-transporter (GAT1); this breakthrough was accomplished by the classical tour de force, that is, the protein was purified from brain extracts, subjected to proteolytic digestion, and oligonucleotide probes were designed based on sequence information obtained from Edman degradation of peptide fragments (Guastella et al., 1990). The NET was the first monoamine transporter that was cloned (Pacholczyk et al., 1991) followed by the dopamine and SERTs (Giros et al., 1991; Ramamoorthy et al., 1993a; see ❷ *Figure 17-1*. The primary structure obtained by conceptual translation allowed to generate topological models.

❑ Figure 17-1
Amino acid sequence alignment of monoamine transporters and their published bacterial homologs. Amino acid sequence alignments of monoamine transporters and two bacterial homologs: human DAT, human NET, and human SERT, as well as the leucine transporter (LeuT$_{Aa}$) from *Aquifex aeolicus* and the tryptophan transporter (TnaT) from *Symbiobacterium thermophilum*. The topology of putative transmembrane helices is shown by a surrounding line and indicated by the number of the transmembrane domain (TM); the TMs are shown according to the published high-resolution structure of Yamashita et al. (2005). A block of identical residues is given in white on black background; conservative mutations are printed black highlighted with lightest gray. A block of similar residues is highlighted in darker gray, whereas weakly similar residues are printed in light gray without being highlighted

◘ Figure 17-1 (continued)

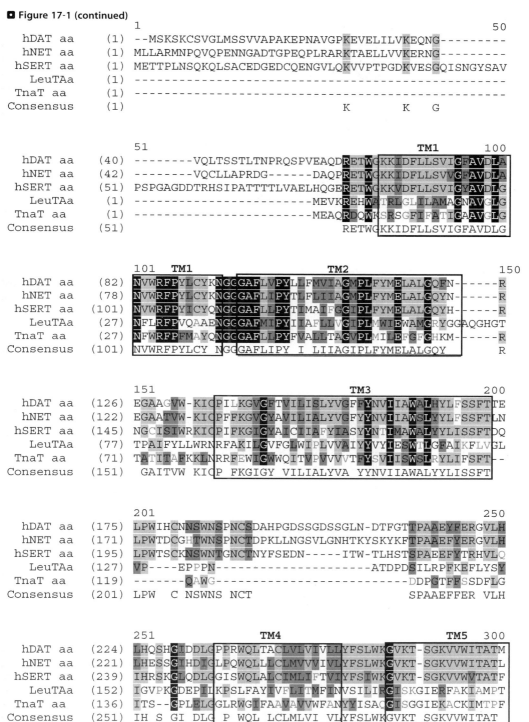

▣ Figure 17-1 (continued)

```
                301    TM5                                        TM6a  350
hDAT aa    (273)  PYVVLTALLIRGVTLPG----AIDGIRAYLSVDFYRLCEAS VWIDAATQV
hNET aa    (270)  PYFVLFVLLVHGVTLPG----ASNGINAYLHIDFYRLKEAT VWIDAATQI
hSERT aa   (288)  PYIILSVLLVRGATLPG----AWRGVLFYLKPNWQKLLETG VWIDAAAQI
LeuTAa     (202)  LFILAVFLVIRVFLLETPNGTAADGLNFLWTPDFEKLKDPG VWIAAVGQI
TnaT aa    (184)  LIVAMLIFVIRGITLPG----ATYGLNYFLNPDFSKIMDPG VWVAAYSQV
Consensus  (301)  PYIVL VLLIRGVTLPG     A  GINFYL PDF KL E GVWIDAATQI


                TM6a/351          TM6b                   TM7               400
hDAT aa    (319)  CFSLGVGFGVLIAFSSYNKFTNNCYRDAIVTTSINSLTSFSSGFVVFSFL
hNET aa    (316)  FFSLGLGAFGVLIAFASYNKFDNNCYRDALLTSSINCITSFVSGFAIFSIL
hSERT aa   (334)  FFSLGPGFGVLLAFASYNKFNNNCYQDALVTSVVNCMTSFVSGFVIFTVL
LeuTAa     (252)  FFILSLGFGAIITYASYVRKDQIIVLSGLTAATLNEKAEVILGGSIS-IP
TnaT aa    (230)  FFSTTLAVGVMIAYASYVPEDSDLANNAFITVFANSSFDFMAGLAVFSTL
Consensus  (351)  FFSLGLGFGVLIAFASYNKFDNNCY DALVTSSIN ITSFVSGFAIFSIL


                401/TM7                                          TM8   450
hDAT aa    (369)  GYMACKHSVPIGDVAKDG-PGLIFIIYPEAIATLP----LSSAWAVVFFI
hNET aa    (366)  GYMAHEHKVNIEDVATEG-AGLVFILYPEAISTLS----GSTFWAVVFFV
hSERT aa   (384)  GYMAEMRNEDVSEVAKDAGPSLLFITYAEAIANMP----ASTFFAIIFFL
LeuTAa     (301)  AAVAFFGVANAVAIAKAGAFNLGFITLPAIFSQTAG----GTFLGFLWFF
TnaT aa    (280)  GYAAVTAGVPFEEMAVAG-PGVAFVAFPKAISMLPGPTWLQSLFGILFFS
Consensus  (401)  GYMA      V I DVAKDG PGLIFI YPEAIS LP    STFFAILFFI


                451      TM8                            TM9     500
hDAT aa    (414)  MLLTLGIDSAMGGMESVITGLIDEFQLLHR-HRELFTLFIVLATFLLSLF
hNET aa    (411)  MLLALGLDSSMGGMEAVITGLADDFQVLKR-HRKLFTFGVTFSTFLLALF
hSERT aa   (430)  MLITLGLDSTFAGLEGVITAVLDEFPHVWAKRRERFVLAVVITCFFGSLV
LeuTAa     (347)  LLFFAGLTSSIAIMQPMIAFLEDELKLSRK----HAVLWTAAIVFFSAHL
TnaT aa    (329)  ALLLAGISSSISQMESFASAVIDRFGVDRK----KLLGWFSLIGFAFSAL
Consensus  (451)  MLL LGLDSSIAGMESVITALIDEF LLRK  R   FVLWV L  F  SLL


                501              TM10                      550
hDAT aa    (463)  CVTNGGIYVFTLLDHFAAGTSILFGVLIEAIGVAWFYGVGQFSDDIQQMT
hNET aa    (460)  CITKGGIYVLTLLDTFAAGTSILFAVLMEAIGVSWFYGVDRFSNDIQQMM
hSERT aa   (480)  TLTFGGAYVVKLLEEYATGPAVLTVALIEAVAVSWFYGITQFCRDVKEML
LeuTAa     (393)  VMFLN--KSLDEMDFWAGTIGVVFFGLTELIIFFWIFGADKAWEEINRGG
TnaT aa    (375)  FATGAGVHILDIVDHFVGSYAIAILGLVEAIVLGYIMGTARIREHVNLTS
Consensus  (501)  IT GGIYVL LLD FAAG AILF GLIEAIGVSWFYGV RF EDIN M


                551                  TM11                 TM12/600
hDAT aa    (513)  GQRPSLYWRLCWKLVSPCFLLFVVVVSIVTFRPPHYGAYIFPDWANALGW
hNET aa    (510)  GFRPGLYWRLCWKFVSPAFLLFVVVVSIINFKPLTYDDYIFPPWANWVGW
hSERT aa   (530)  GFSPGWFWRICWVAISPLFLLFIICSFLMSPPQLRLFQYNYPYWSIILGY
LeuTAa     (441)  IIKVPRIYYYVMRYIPAFLAVLLVVWAREYIPKIMEETHWTVWITRFYI
TnaT aa    (425)  DIRVGMWWDVLVKYVTPVLLGYNILSNFISEFREPYAGYPTGALVLFGWV
Consensus  (551)  G RPGLYWRLCWKYVSP FLLFVIVV IISF P  Y  Y FP WA  LGW
```

□ **Figure 17-1 (continued)**

```
           601/TM12                                                    650
hDAT aa   (563)  VIATSSMAMVPIYAAYK-FCSLPGSFREKLAYAIAPEKDRELVDRGEVRQ
hNET aa   (560)  GIALSSMVLVPIYVIYK-FLSTQGSLWERLAYGITPENEHHLVAQRDIRQ
hSERT aa  (580)  CIGTSSFICIPTYIAYR-LIITPGTFKERIIKSITPETPTEIPCG-DIRL
LeuTAa    (491)  IGLFLFLTFLVFLAERRRNHESAGTLVPR-------------------
TnaT aa   (475)  VAIMFGTSLFMQWRSQQ-LDVTGGEVG---------------------
Consensus (601)  VIA SSM LVP Y AYK    T GSL ERL   I PE    L    DIR
```

```
           651
hDAT aa   (612)  FTLRHWLKV
hNET aa   (609)  FQLQHWLAI
hSERT aa  (628)  NAV------
LeuTAa    (520)  ---------
TnaT aa   (501)  ---------
Consensus (651)    L
```

Hydropathy analyses assigned 12 transmembrane spanning α-helical segments to transporters; On the basis of the analogy with other proteins (e.g., P-glycoprotein, mammalian adenylyl cyclases, etc.), the N and C termini were thought to reside within the cell (Amara and Kuhar, 1993; Chen et al., 1998; Ferrer and Javitch, 1998; Chen and Reith, 2000). Probing with site-specific antibodies confirmed the proposed topology for NET (Bruss et al., 1995) and also for SERT [by use of chemical labeling (Chen et al., 1998)].

There are many different ways to arrange 12 α-helices in the membrane. However, on the basis of the endogenous Zn^{2+}-binding site in the DAT, it is possible to impose reasonably precise distance constraints on any model of monoamine transporters (Norregaard et al., 1998). The Zn^{2+}-binding site in DAT has a tridentate structure: two histidine residues, located in extracellular loop 2 (His193) and the extracellular portion (top) of transmembrane domain 7 (TM7; His375), and a glutamate residue on top of TM8 (Glu396; Norregaard et al., 1998; Loland et al., 1999). The endogenous Zn^{2+}-binding site is unique to DAT, neither the norepinephrine nor the SERTs contain such a high-affinity binding site for Zn^{2+}. The absence of a Zn^{2+}-binding site provided an opportunity to subject the models of helix arrangement to an acid test: if the model is correct, the Zn^{2+}-binding site can be transferred (provided that the amino acid substitutions are tolerated). In the past, this approach had proved useful in defining proximity relationships for instance in G protein-coupled receptors (Elling et al., 1995; Elling and Schwartz, 1996). Indeed, it was possible to engineer a Zn^{2+}-sensitive NET (Norregaard et al., 1998). This was the first characterization of a structural microdomain in a monoamine transporter protein. Importantly, the characterization of endogenous Zn^{2+}-binding sites helped to define the structural features of many other membrane proteins distantly related to the DAT (Gether, 2000; Norregaard et al., 2000; Gether et al., 2001).

Apart from Zn^{2+}, methanethiosulfonate (MTS) reagents have been instrumental to infer the accessibility of distinct amino acid residues within the transmembrane regions: MTS reagents are highly selective for water-accessible ionized cysteines (Karlin and Akabas, 1998). Several different MTS-reagents exist which either permeate across the membrane or are too hydrophilic and thus do not gain access to the lipid phase of the membrane. The hydrophilic MTS reagents (e.g., MTS-ethyltrimethylammonium, MTSET, and MTS-ethylsulfonate, MTSES) and the weak base MTS ethylammonium (MTSEA) represent such a set of reagents; MTSET (or MTDSE) does not permeate across the cell membrane while the weak base MTS ethylammonium (MTSEA) readily diffuses across the membrane in its uncharged form; thus its ability to reach the interior of the cell depends on the pH. If the compounds are used in whole cells and in cell membranes, it is possible to draw conclusions on the extent to which cysteine residues are exposed to the aqueous phase. The analysis is greatly aided by the fact that there are good radioligands that allow to quantitate the extent to which the transporter has been inactivated (Chen et al., 1998; Ferrer and Javitch, 1998; Androutsellis-Theotokis et al., 2001; Kamdar et al., 2001; Reith et al., 2001; Androutsellis-Theotokis and Rudnick, 2002).

The topology of monoamine transporters, which was predicted from hydropathy plots, was probed by using MTS reagents. As predicted from the model, several cysteines located at the extracellular portion of DAT reacted with MTS reagents irrespective of whether tested in a membrane preparation or on whole cells: labeling of Cys90, Cys135, Cys306, and Cys342, located in TM1, TM3, TM6, and TM6, respectively, was consistent with their presence in proximity to the extracellular space (Ferrer and Javitch, 1998). Cys90 on top of TM1 is conserved in all three monoamine transporters; accordingly, Cys109 in SERT is also accessible from the extracellular space (Chen et al., 1997).

However, it is evident that all the approaches outlined above only yield limited structural information. Attempts to obtain high-resolution structures of monoamine transporters have not (yet) been successful. While it has been possible to purify SERT to homogeneity by using either platelets (Launay et al., 1992; Rasmussen et al., 2001; Tate et al., 2003), placenta (Ramamoorthy et al., 1992, 1993b), or brain membranes (Graham et al., 1991, 1992; Habert et al., 1986), further progress has been hampered by the detergent content of the samples. In most instances, digitonin was used to solubilize the transporter and the subsequent purification steps were also done in digitonin-containing solutions; however, the low CMC (critical micellar concentration) of digitonin and the lack of other suitable detergents in which SERT is preserved in active form have proved to be formidable obstacles: digitonin is difficult to remove and protein concentrations required for crystallization cannot be reached without concomitantly concentrating digitonin in parallel. The problem is difficult to remedy. Because thermophilic bacteria—by definition—live at high temperature, their proteins are very resistant to heat denaturation and accordingly substantially more stable than their mammalian counterparts. Hence, the genomes of thermophilic bacteria have been scrutinized for a bacterial homolog of SERT to find a suitable candidate for crystallographic studies; this search has resulted in an interesting candidate, the tryptophan transporter of Symbiophilus thermophilum (Androutsellis-Theotokis et al., 2003).

Most recently, a high-resolution structure has been published for a leucine transporter (LeuT$_{Aa}$) from *Aquifex aeolicus*; this bacterial transporter is distantly related to the mammalian monoamine transporters (Yamashita et al., 2005). The structure obtained for the crystallized LeuT$_{Aa}$ reveals a protein that spans the plasma membrane 12 times thus conforming to the overall topology (see ❷ *Figure 17-2*).

6   A Closer Look at the Transport Cycle

Four decades ago, a model has been put forth that explains the conformational cycle of a transport protein (Jardetzky, 1966), and this "alternating access" model is still considered the working model. The model assumes that the transporter exists in two conformations: first the substrate-binding site of the transporter faces the extracellular milieu; access to the intracellular side is sealed off by the transporter. On binding of the substrate and of the cosubstrates (in monoamine transporters, Na$^+$ and Cl$^-$), a conformational switch is induced, the transporter adopts its inward-facing conformation, whereby the substrate and cosubstrates gain access to the intracellular side, while access to the extracellular side is precluded. The crystal structures of bacterial homologs to both glutamate (Yernool et al., 2004) and monoamine transporters (Yamashita et al., 2005) have been solved at high resolution. The structural details are consistent with many of the implicit predictions of the alternate access model. In fact, LeuT$_{Aa}$ is in a conformation that most likely represents the locked conformation, i.e., the transition state on the reaction trajectory from the outward facing to the inward-facing conformation, where substrate and cosubstrate are accessible neither from the outside nor from the inside.

However, as Gary Rudnick succinctly pointed out in a recent article on the structure–function relationships in SERT: "Many aspects of SERT structure remain unresolved despite the major advance in our understanding provided by the structure of LeuT" (Rudnick, 2006). And this arises from the still unknown mechanistic basis for the movement of single helices during the transport cycle. A rock-and-switch model was proposed based on the structure of two bacterial transporters: both the lactose permease (Abramson et al., 2003) and the glycerol-3-phosphate transporter (Huang et al., 2003) were visualized with a large cavity on the cytoplasmic side, i.e., in the putative inward-facing conformation. In these structures, the transmembrane helices are arranged to form two pseudosymmetric lobes (consisting of transmembrane

◘ Figure 17-2

Putative organization of serotonin transporter threaded onto LeuT$_{Aa}$. *Top* (a) and *side* view (b) of SERT threaded on the backbone of LeuT$_{Aa}$

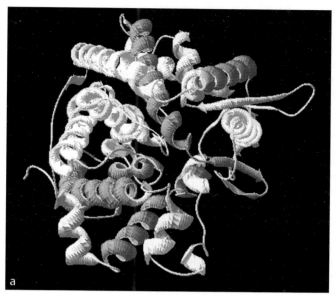

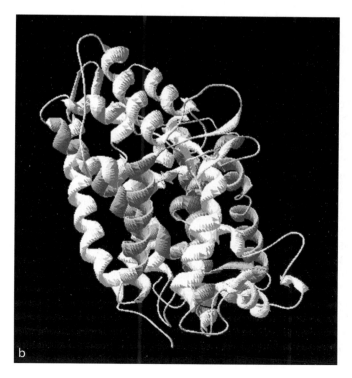

helices 1–6 and 7–12). Binding of substrate may support the movement of the curved helices 1 and 7 by pulling these two helices together (i.e., the helices rock and tilt). The two lobes follow by rigid body movement, which switches the conformation. While the intrinsic beauty of this model is self-evident, its major drawback is the fact that it is most likely not applicable to monoamine transporters. First, there is not any appreciable similarity in primary structure. Second, the intracellular loops of monoamine transporters are far too short to allow for a similar arrangement of the transmembrane helices. Third, a rock-and-switch model is difficult to reconcile with the fact that monoamine transporters can operate in a channel-like mode (see below), i.e., there must be a conformation with a contiguous water-filled channel that spans the lipid phase of the membrane. In fact, the structures of $LeuT_{Aa}$ (Yamashita et al., 2005) and of the bacterial glutamate transporter (Yernool et al., 2004) indicate that there are other solutions to the problem of transmembrane translocation of substrate. These proposals are more compatible with a channel-like mode because they only require modest movements of intramembrane residues that are either close to the extracellular surface or the intracellular portion. By analogy with ion channels, these segments may function as gates; if both are in the position "open," substrate and cosubstrate ions can permeate in a single file mode giving rise to a conducting channel.

Within the family of neurotransmitter:sodium symporters (NSS; Busch and Saier, 2002), the presence of the namesake sodium is an absolute requirement: the action of NSS members is indirectly coupled to the activity of the Na^+/K^+-ATPase by the chemical Na^+-gradient it sustains. Monoamine transport has also been shown to be dependent on the extracellular chloride concentration (Nelson and Rudnick, 1982; Humphreys et al., 1994; Gu et al., 1996b): omission of Cl^- in the extracellular solution results—similar to depletion of Na^+—in profound loss of transport activity (Rudnick and Clark, 1993). DAT and NET fulfill their task by coupling their substrate translocation to the movement of Na^+ and Cl^- across their gradient, as outlined above. In contrast to the two other monoamine transporters, the activity of SERT also depends on K^+. This was already noted in the first studies and the observations were interpreted in a model where SERT-mediated substrate-reuptake was associated with countertransport of K^+ (Nelson and Rudnick, 1979). K^+ serves as the countertransport ion, and this supports the conformational switch of SERT to the outward-facing conformation. However, this view has been challenged recently because there was not any electrophysiological evidence for a movement of K^+ during the transport cycle (Adams and DeFelice, 2002).

Under resting conditions, there is a modest H^+ gradient over the membrane (pH 7.4 and 7.1 on the outside and inside corresponding to ~40 and 80-nM H^+, respectively). The pH has also been claimed to be important for the transport cycle: in experiments directed to elucidate the potential of H^+ to serve as cosubstrate for inwardly directed transport, the authors observed that H^+ can actually substitute for K^+ as ion for the return step (Keyes and Rudnick, 1982). In addition, electrophysiological experiments also revealed the importance of H^+ for carrier-mediated current in SERT (see below; Cao et al., 1997). The physiological relevance of these observations, however, is unclear because other permeating cations (Na^+, K^+) are present at substantially higher (5–6 orders of magnitude) concentrations and the transmembrane gradients are substantially steeper (>tenfold difference in concentration for Na^+ and K^+ as opposed to twofold difference for H^+). Nevertheless, it is interesting that differences in the amino acid composition between the rat and the human SERT affect the ability of the transporter to use H^+ as a cosubstrate (Cao et al., 1998). Finally, the pH is of obvious relevance to defining the concentration of available substrate because only protonated amines can be transported by monoamine transporters (Rudnick et al., 1989; Gu et al., 1996a; Berfield et al., 1999).

Many antidepressant drugs are reuptake inhibitors, i.e., they block SERT and NET. These are widely prescribed drugs, hence there are many compounds and there is a rich pharmacology with extensive studies on structure–activity relations. Thus, the requirement for high-affinity antidepressant binding has been thoroughly studied: similar to binding of the substrate serotonin, binding of inhibitors (tricyclic antidepressants, SSRI = selective serotonin reuptake inhibitors, etc.) also depends on Na^+ and Cl^-. The concentration–response curve for Na^+-dependent stimulation of imipramine binding to SERT was sigmoidal (Talvenheimo et al., 1979). Analogous results have been obtained for NET with its ligand desipramine. This indicates that there is cooperative binding of more than one Na^+ ion. In fact, the structure of $LeuT_{Aa}$ reveals two sodium ions bound simultaneously with the substrate leucine (Yamashita et al., 2005). It has been argued that cosubstrate ion (Na^+ and Cl^-) and substrate or inhibitor bind in random order (Humphreys et al., 1994). Alternatively, binding of inhibitors to transporters can be treated in a manner analogous to the interaction of open channel blockers to ion channels; in this model, the kinetics of binding are compatible with Na^+ triggering the outward-facing conformation, which binds the inhibitor. Thus, binding is sequential, i.e., Na^+-binding precedes inhibitor binding (Korkhov et al., 2006). Binding of substrate and inhibitor is mutually exclusive (Talvenheimo et al., 1979, 1983), it is evident that the binding pocket cannot accommodate the presence of two ligands. The presence of a second binding site has been postulated (Sur et al., 1998) that is claimed to account for the differences between racemic citalopram and the individual *R*- and *S*-isomers thereof (Sanchez et al., 2003; Chen et al., 2005). This is somewhat surprising because one is left to wonder where the second binding site can be accommodated in the structure.

7 Current and Transporters

In the alternating access model of facilitated transport (Jardetzky, 1966), the translocation of substrate is thermodynamically coupled to the movement of cosubstrates along their concentration gradients. These ion gradients are maintained by primary active transporters, i.e., ion pumps like the Na^+/K^+-ATPase or the H^+-ATPase (which is relevant to vesicular transporters). By moving through a fixed cycle of different conformations (Rudnick and Clark, 1993), substrates as well as the cosubstrates are exposed in distinct, sequential manner to the extra- and intracellular sides of the cell. Because the transported molecules are charged, their translocation along with ion cotransport (see below) results in the generation of a charge imbalance; hence, with DAT and NET, a current is to arise over the plasma membrane. SERT, however, does not support a net charge movement and is therefore thought to be electroneutral. By taking into account how rapidly a transport cycle can be performed by monoamine transporters (by using estimates for their turnover number), it is possible to predict the size of putative currents. Hence, the range of possible currents generated by a plasmalemmal transporter would be estimated to be close to nothing in the case of SERT to a few pA for DAT and NET. These estimated values can be shown to be below the detection limit because the signal-to-noise ratio of typical patch-clamp setups does not allow for measurements in this range (see ❷ *Figure 17-3*).

Contrary to these predictions, currents are readily measurable (Lester et al., 1994, 1996; Mager et al., 1994; Galli et al., 1995, 1998; Qian et al., 1997; Sonders et al., 1997; DeFelice and Galli, 1998; Sitte et al., 1998; Hilber et al., 2005). As mentioned above, On the basis of the stoichiometry of the translocation process, currents were to be expected in DAT and NET but not in SERT, for SERT countertransports K^+ from the intracellular side to the extracellular side on return of the unloaded transporter to the outward-facing conformation. As one (positively charged) 5-HT molecule is transported inside plus one Na^+ and one Cl^- and the K^+ ion, there is no net flux over the plasma membrane. Given these considerations, it is ironic that SERT was the first of the three monoamine transporters, which was shown to support a current and this was seen in a serotonergic neuron (from the leech *hirudo medicinalis*), i.e., in a cell where the endogenous transporter was investigated (Bruns et al., 1993). Subsequently, related experiments were done with NET; in these experiments, formal proof was provided that the current was generated by the transporter because it had the appropriate pharmacology (it was blocked by antidepressants in a relevant concentration range) and ionic requirements (Galli et al., 1995). The investigations were extended to show that NET displayed features commonly attributed to ion channels only (Galli et al., 1996). DAT was the last monoamine transporter to be characterized in detail (Sonders et al., 1997); it was also noted to have an uncoupled current, that is, the transport stoichiometry and the current fluxes were not coupled in a fixed stoichiometry (Sonders and Amara, 1996), and this was an additional argument for channel-like properties of DAT. Thus, in summary, channel properties have been observed in all monoamine transporters (DeFelice and Blakely, 1996; Sonders and Amara, 1996).

However, the notion that channel properties might exist in monoamine transporters does not render the alternating access model completely irrelevant. In a recent publication, channel properties have been

□ Figure 17-3

Functional states of the serotonin transporter, prototypical for the monoamine transporters. *Panel a* shows concentration-dependent and saturating uptake of physiological substrate 5-HT. *Panel b* reveals the determination of the SERT density on a plasma membrane preparation of rat SERT expressing cells. *Panel c* shows a current induced by the physiological substrate 5-HT measured in human embryonic kidney cells expressing SERT by the patch-clamp technique in the whole-cell configuration. A typical superfusion experiment is given in *panel d*; concentration-dependent, *para*-chloroamphetamine elicits efflux of preloaded [³H]5-HT (for further details on all the methodology used to reveal the images shown in this figure see Hilber et al., 2005)

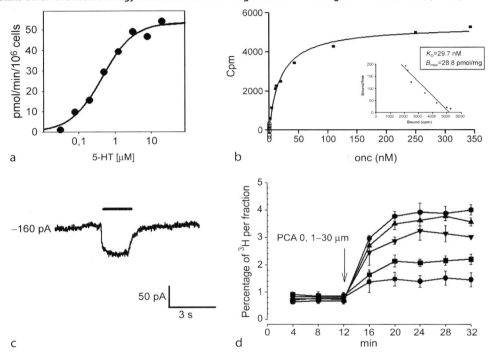

shown to be compatible with alternating access transport mode (Kahlig et al., 2005). Also the possibility was raised that the channel mode represented a side activity during the translocation cycle (Rudnick, 2002). Neurotransmitter transporters are reminiscent of ligand-gated ion channels, both protein families are only "separated by an exceedingly fine line" (Accardi and Miller, 2004). As mentioned earlier, this notion is supported by the recent X-ray crystal structure of bacterial transporters, which are related to the neurotransmitter transporters: in LeuT$_{Aa}$, the substrate leucine and two cosubstrate Na$^+$ ions are locked within the TM. Access to both the extracellular and the intracellular milieu is blocked by amino acid residues above and below the substrate-binding pocket. A gating function can be assigned to these "lid" segments; if they move in a concerted and simultaneous way, a contiguous transmembrane pore is formed and the transporter is converted into a channel. Thus, only subtle structural differences suffice to switch an ion channel to a transporter and vice versa. This concept is reinforced by the observation that the electrophysiological properties of the *Drosophila melanogaster* serotonin (dSERT) differ substantially from that of the mammalian orthologs (Petersen and DeFelice, 1999): during the transport cycle, 5–10 times more charges are moved through dSERT. Thus, the changes in amino acid composition that exist between insect and mammalian SERT affect gating and place dSERT closer to the "true" channels in the continuum of transporters and channels.

Furthermore, Petersen and DeFelice (1999) carried out mole fraction experiments; this and other biophysical analyses demonstrated that substrate permeation at high extracellular substrate concentrations was consistent with a single file model indicative of pore diffusion. This model relies on certain premises: (1) at physiological pH, monoamines are positively charged molecules; therefore, the membrane potential drags them into the cell; (2) vesicular storage of neurotransmitter in vesicles keeps the intracellular concentration of transmitter low; and (3) the pore is also permeable to sodium (and chloride). Accordingly, Na^+ and Cl^- would drive the monoamine through the pore (DeFelice et al., 2001; Adams and DeFelice, 2002, 2003). The single file model shows no well-defined transport cycle and consequently no fixed stoichiometry. In this case, the "stoichiometry of the transport process" reflects a mean value of transported ions per molecule substrate. Permeation in the single file mode is a concept that was originally developed based on electrophysiological and thermodynamic arguments. Recently, it has been directly visualized; the X-ray crystal structure of a K^+ channel shows individual K^+ ions (stripped of their water shell) lined up one after the other within the permeation pathway (MacKinnon, 2003).

Apart from substrate-induced current, there are two distinct other measurable currents: transient and leak currents. Transient current are the result of charge movements, with the capacitance of the membrane serving as temporary storage for charges. When voltage jumps are induced in monoamine transporter expressing cells, additional charge movements in the electrical field of the membrane ensue. These charge movements are referred to as the transient current, which likely reflects the movement of charged residues within the transporter molecule.

In monoamine transporters, there is another current, which is measurable in the absence of voltage jumps or substrate; this is the so-called leak conductance. This state of the transporter reflects a certain leakiness of the pore within the protein. Transporter inhibitors are able to block the leak conductance; by this means, it is possible to estimate the size of the leak. The leak conductance can be regulated by associated proteins: in the case of SERT, syntaxin1a regulates the leak conductance (Beckman and Quick, 2001; Quick, 2003). The physiological relevance of the leak conductance has been questioned because it has so far not been detected in neuronal preparations (Ingram et al., 2002). However, the data obtained in dopaminergic neurons must be interpreted with caution: these neurons display a manifold of different conductances which are large in size and which were therefore blocked to reveal substrate-induced current: hence, the leak might easily have been overseen.

What do all these different transporter-associated currents mean? Is there any physiological role, in particular, for the uncoupled conductances? The uncoupled conductances may influence the membrane potential (Sonders and Amara, 1996; Carvelli et al., 2004): if currents are sustained by Na^+, they can readily depolarize the cell. In DAT, the currents appear to carry mostly Cl^- (Ingram et al., 2002; Meinild et al., 2004). Under these conditions, the membrane potential and the actual reversal potential determine whether the cells can be indeed depolarized by currents through DAT (Sulzer and Galli, 2003). Furthermore, in dopaminergic neurons (i.e., in those cells in which the transporter is expressed under physiological conditions), the activity of DAT impinges on the membrane potential and affects the excitability of the neurons (Falkenburger et al., 2001; Ingram et al., 2002).

8   The Quaternary Structure: Monoamine Transporter Oligomerization

The crystal structure of LeuT$_{Aa}$ by Yamashita and colleagues did not only have implications for models of the tertiary structure of monoamine transporters but also showed that LeuT$_{Aa}$ was a dimer and this is also relevant to monoamine transporters. Monoamine transporters have been repeatedly described to form oligomeric complexes at the plasma membrane of living cells (see ❷ *Figure 17-4*). The structure of LeuT$_{Aa}$ revealed an oligomeric interface predominantly formed by TM9 and TM12. Just et al. (2004) suggested the presence of an oligomeric interface in the region comprising TM11/12 in the human SERT. However, one must bear in mind that the crystals of LeuT$_{Aa}$ have been obtained in detergent solution. Thus, the crystallographic dimer of LeuT$_{Aa}$ may not necessarily represent the quaternary structure adopted by the protein, when residing in the membrane. In recent years, several different interaction domains have been reported to exist in Na^+/Cl^--dependent neurotransmitter transporters (Sitte and Freissmuth, 2003; Sitte et al., 2004).

☐ Figure 17-4

Fluorescence resonance energy transfer (FRET) microscopy image according to Youvan et al. (1997). The image reveals a typical representation of the dopamine transporter at the cell surface in its constitutive oligomerized state. The first image shows cyan fluorescent protein-tagged DAT that has been taken under filter settings for cyan fluorescent protein (excitation 436 nm, emission 488 nm); the second image shows the FRET filter settings (excitation 436 nm, emission 535 nm). The third image represents the ratio or Youvan image. The signal shown here depicts positive resonance energy transfer allowing the conclusion of physical proximity between cyan and yellow fluorescent protein-tagged DAT (for further details see Schmid et al., 2001a, b)

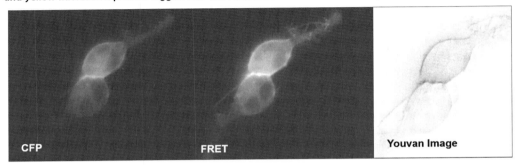

8.1 The Structural Basis of Oligomer Formation

Oligomers of transmembrane proteins may be stabilized by hydrophilic interactions mediated, e.g., by coiled-coils of intracellular segments. Alternatively, the transmembrane segments may pack against each other and these interactions may be stabilized by specific motifs. Two motifs have been recognized that are capable of supporting helix–helix interactions in the lipid milieu of the membrane: the glycophorin A-motif GxxxG (Popot and Engelman, 1990, 2000; MacKenzie and Engelman, 1998; White and Wimley, 1999) and the leucine heptad repeat [LxxxxxxLxxxxxx]$_2$. The latter was originally found in soluble transcription factors (Heldin, 1995). However, a leucine heptad repeat is also present in the transmembrane helix of phospholamban, where it drives the assembly of the pentamere (Reddy et al., 1999; Cornea et al., 2000). The first motif to be investigated was the GxxxG motif in TM6 of the human DAT (Hastrup et al., 2001). On inspection of the serotonin and the norepinephrine, it is evident that this motif is also conserved in these two family members (Sitte et al., 2004).

Likewise, a leucine heptad repeat has been found in the second membrane domain of the human DAT and in the GABA-transporter-1 (GAT1; GABA = γ-amino butyric acid): in both transporters, disruption of this motif disrupts oligomer formation (Scholze et al., 2002; Torres et al., 2003) and correct targeting of the transporters to the plasma membrane. Torres et al. (2003) reported on a second leucine heptad repeat in TM9 of the human DAT; however, this second motif did neither have any impact on the transporters function nor did its deletion affect the targeting of the transporter to the plasma membrane. In the bacterial homologs of the monoamine transporters, it is also readily evident that the motif is conserved, although not to the same extent as in GAT1 (Yamashita et al., 2005).

However, leucine heptad repeats normally do not suffice to sustain a protein–protein interaction in the lipophilic membrane milieu; polar residues must be available to stabilize the leucine zipper by hydrogen bonding and these residues must be sandwiched between the leucine residues, i.e., the hydrogen bond donor must be flanked by a leucine, a helical turn below and above, and presumably for steric reasons, glutamate is the optimal hydrogen bond donor (Zhou et al., 2001). GAT1 contains a glutamate (E[101]) residue in transmembrane helix 2 that fulfills all these criteria; a substitution as subtle as mutation to aspartate suffices to impede oligomer formation (Korkhov et al., 2004). In addition, transmembrane helix 2 also contains a tyrosine residue in position 86 that is required for oligomer formation in GAT1 (Korkhov et al., 2004). In contrast to Glu[101], Tyr[86] does not serve as a hydrogen bond donor. The available evidence indicates that Tyr[86] stabilizes the oligomer by π–π stacking interactions; a substitution by phenylalanine but not by alanine is tolerated.

If the transmembrane helices 2 of the Na^+/Cl^--dependent neurotransmitter transporter family are aligned, it is evident that a canonical leucine heptad repeat is not fully conserved throughout the family: the SERT, for instance, carries an alanine in its amino acid position 125. Therefore, it is somewhat difficult to envisage how TM2 of SERT can form a hydrogen bond-stabilized leucine zipper: when compared to leucine, alanine is far too small to support hydrophobic interactions and helix packing; a cavity is readily evident in a three-dimensional model of the helical dimer. Thus, the three remaining leucines in TM2 of SERT cannot be relevant to oligomerization of the protein. This interpretation is underscored by the fact that mutational exchange of the two crucial leucine residues to alanine does not disrupt oligomer formation in SERT (Just, Sitte, Freissmuth, unpublished observation), while the analogous mutations in GAT1 are detrimental to oligomerization. Therefore, we concluded that oligomer formation in SERT relies on distinct features; notably, this is also supported by the observation that in SERT only a third contact site exists within TM11 and TM12 (Just et al., 2004). By contrast with SERT, the leucine heptad repeats of DAT apparently mediate a homophilic interaction which supports oligomer formation (Torres et al., 2003). This view has been recently challenged by a cross-linking study that was not able to follow this line of argumentation (Sen et al., 2005).

8.2 The Oligomerization Hypothesis

Neurotransmitter transporters reside at the plasma membrane as constitutive oligomers. This notion has been put forth for several neurotransmitter transporters, including transporters for monoamines (Hastrup et al., 2001; Schmid et al., 2001b; Kocabas et al., 2003; Sorkina et al., 2003). It has to be noted that several publications claim the opposite, namely that transporters are exclusively monomers (Hebert and Carruthers, 1992; Lopez-Corcuera et al., 1993; Horiuchi et al., 2001). However, this conclusion is based on experiments in which biochemical approaches were used that may per se disrupt oligomer formation (because of the addition of detergents). As outlined above, oligomers form already at the level of the endoplasmic reticulum (ER; Scholze et al., 2002; Sorkina et al., 2003). On the basis of these observations, we proposed the "oligomerization hypothesis"; the central tenet assumes that (1) oligomer formation is a prerequisite for transporters to exported from ER. This is backed by the observations that mutants exist that disrupt oligomer formation and lead to enhanced ER retention of the transporters (Scholze et al., 2002; Torres et al., 2003). However, these transporters are still fully functional (Scholze et al., 2002). (2) The ER export signal is only present in the oligomer; thus monomers are retained because they lack the appropriate information. Mechanistically, oligomer formation may either lead to complementation of an export signal, which does not work when presented by the monomer, or to masking of a retention signal, which is only accessible in the monomer. Recent evidence—originally obtained with GAT1 (Farhan et al., 2004)—indicates that the C termini of transporters contain an interaction site for COPII components. In GAT1, a segment between L553 and Q572 supports binding of Sec24D. However, the interaction of Sec24D does not rely on oligomerization of the transporter: oligomerization-deficient transporters (GAT1-L2A) are perfectly capable of interacting with Sec24D, as shown by FRET microscopy (Farhan et al., 2004). Nevertheless, GAT1-L2A transporters are not exported from the ER. The assembly of the COPII coat is known to be subject to kinetic proofreading. It has to occur rapidly enough to precede GTP cleavage in Sar1a (Sato and Nakano, 2004, 2005; Forster et al., 2006). Thus, the apparent discrepancy can be rationalized: in our model, the monomeric GAT1-L2A may still bind Sec24D (and the associated Sec23) but a single Sec24D/Sec23 dimer fails to support the efficient assembly of the COPII coat (which requires the rapid recruitment of Sec13–31). (3) The oligomerization hypothesis may be a quaint intellectual exercise, meaningless unless its explanatory power is proved in a disease. This is the case: familial orthostatic intolerance is a disease that is due to a point mutation in NET, NET-A457P. The point mutation prevents the transporter from reaching the cell surface. Phenotypically, the mutation is dominant, mutation in one allele suffice to cause a loss in NET activity of more than 90% (Shannon et al., 2000). A dominant negative effect can only be explained by an action of the mutated transporter on the transporter generated from the healthy allele. In fact, the mutated transporter accumulates in the ER and prevents wild-type NET from reaching the cell surface because wild-type and mutated NET form export-deficient oligomers (Hahn et al., 2003).

Protein export from the ER relies on several mechanisms that also participate in stringent quality control (Ellgaard and Helenius, 2003); in line with this notion, proper oligomer formation of monoamine transporters as well as of other NSS members is a prerequisite for transporters to leave the ER (Sitte et al., 2004). How are transporters targeted to the plasma membrane? This is not clear, but significant progress has been made recently in understanding what happens at the very early steps, that is in the ER. Ribosomal synthesis at the rough ER serves as the starting point of the newly formed membrane protein, which is integrated into ER membranes via the translocon formed by Sec61 channel subunits. While exiting the Sec61 channel, the proteins must undergo rapid folding because improperly folded proteins are directly retrotranslocated and subjected to ER-associated degradation via the proteasome. The content of the ER lumen supports protein maturation by allowing for enzyme-assisted formation of disulfide bonds and by providing several chaperones (e.g., membrane-bound calnexin and soluble calreticulin and BiP/GRP78), which capture and stabilize folding intermediates. The interaction of these chaperons with substrate proteins is, in part, regulated by the glucosylation state of the N-linked glycans. Release from the lectin chaperons is contingent on the trimming of the terminal glucose (Ellgaard and Helenius, 2003).

Typically, there are several ways how membrane proteins can leave the ER: the major route is as cargo of COPII-coated vesicles. To achieve this, the cargo needs to get concentrated at specialized subdomains of the ER that are free of ribosomes: only in these so-called ER exit sites (ERES), budding of vesicles can successfully take place (Orci et al., 1991). Cargo accumulates in these regions and associates with components of the COPII coat. These components include—among others—Sar1, the Sec23–Sec24 complex and the Sec13–Sec31 complex. For recruitment of a COPII coat, and probably initiate assembly, the cargo needs to interact with the Sec23–Sec24 complex; this has been shown for the GABA transporter GAT1 (Farhan et al., 2004); however, we also obtained evidence by Fluorescence resonance energy transfer microscopy that this holds also true for DAT (Stelzeneder and Sitte, unpublished observations).

Assembly of the COPII coat depends on Sar1, which is a small Ras-like GTPase. On activation by its guanine nucleotide exchange factor (GEF) Sec12, Sar1.GTP is recruited to the ER membrane and initiates the recruitment of Sec23–Sec24 dimer to form the so-called prebudding complex. Sec24 mediates the recognition of cargo (Miller et al., 2003; Mossessova et al., 2003). At this stage, cargo and Sec24 interact and initiate formation of the COPII coat, i.e., the additional recruitment of a layer of Sec13–Sec31 dimers (Stagg et al., 2006). The COPII coat is intrinsically unstable, the GTPase of Sar1 is the timer and Sec23 acts as the GTPase activating protein for Sar1, the GAP activity is further enhanced by binding of Sec13/Sec31. Because GTP hydrolysis by Sar1 promotes coat disassembly, budding is presumably disfavored unless the cargo provides an additional interaction site for Sec24 (Forster et al., 2006). From the point of view of quality control, this kinetic proofreading mechanism is likely to prevent erroneous recruitment of proteins for ER export. The final formation of the budding vesicle is driven by the coat lattice which induces and stabilizes the membrane curvature.

We identified a Sec24D interaction motif in the GABA transporter (Farhan et al., 2004), and accordingly, we observed that the C terminus is indispensable for forward trafficking. This is in line with earlier work in which the last 39 amino acids of GAT1 were shown to be required for surface expression (Bendahan and Kanner, 1993). However, both our work and the observations of Kanner and coworkers are difficult to reconcile with a report in which the last 36 amino acids were claimed to be irrelevant to surface expression and trafficking of GAT1 (Perego et al., 1997). In all other instances examined, however, the C terminus was found to specify ER export of monoamine transporters, as shown for DAT (Miranda et al., 2004) and NET (Distelmaier et al., 2004). The homologous position to arginine in position 569 of the rat GABA transporter is lysine 590 in DAT. Mutation of this lysine leads to retention of DAT in the ER. Our (unpublished) observations confirm that DAT requires K^{569} to interact with Sec24D. Finally, it has to be pointed out that there is a nonconcentrative export of membranes and hence proteins residing therein to the cell surface. Thus proteins, which do not contain a specific ER-retrieval or retention motif, are eventually slowly exported to the cell surface. Thus, in experiments which rely on heterologous transfection of mutated transporters, ER-retained versions can in many instances be observed to eventually reach the plasma membrane at some low levels.

8.3 The Importance of Oligomer Formation for the Action of Amphetamine

Amphetamines target monoamine transporters. The family of amphetamine and its congeners includes a large variety of widely abused, psychotropic substances like D-amphetamine (=speed), methamphetamine (=ice) and methylene-dioxymethamphetamine (MDMA; =ecstasy), cathinone (the ingredient of cath) (Seiden et al., 1993; Sulzer et al., 2005). Some compounds are used for therapeutic purposes; the most notable example is methylphenidate (Ritalin) which is used in cases of juvenile attention deficit hyperactivity disorder. The action of methylphenidate is solely accounted for to uptake inhibition (Swanson and Volkow, 2003). Most, if not all, amphetamine-like drugs induce transport reversal (Levi and Raiteri, 1993). Thereby, they elevate extrasynaptic, and synaptic, monoamine concentrations. Amphetamine and its derivatives differ in their affinity for individual monoamine transporters; accordingly, they also elicit distinct pharmacological effects. MDMA targets mainly SERT while D-amphetamine elicits its psychotropic effects at DAT (Seiden et al., 1993).

Amphetamines are to be transported into the cell—i.e., they behave primarily as substrates to monoamine transporters (Trendelenburg et al., 1987; Sitte et al., 1998; Bönisch and Trendelenburg, 1989; Zaczek et al., 1991). The requirements of their uptake are therefore the same as for physiological substrates, this includes cotransport of Na^+ and Cl^- (Sitte et al., 1998). Once inside the cell, amphetamines are taken up into storage vesicles and readily protonated due to the acidic pH value inside these storage vesicles (Sulzer and Rayport, 1990; Sulzer et al., 1995; Pothos and Sulzer, 1998). The acidic pH is needed as energy source for the accumulation of monoamines in a countertransport fashion (Liu et al., 1992). Therefore, a collapse of the proton gradient by amphetamines blunts vesicular uptake of the pertinent monoamine (norepinephrine, serotonin, or DA) and elevates its concentration in the cytosol; this is the mechanistic basis for the weak base hypothesis (Sulzer et al., 1995). Once the concentration of substrate reaches significant amounts in the cytosol, outward transport is initiated. However, certain additional conditions need to be met: (1) outward transport is contingent on a certain level of sodium influx that allows for reverse operation of the transporter (Sulzer et al., 2005). (2) Intracellular kinases need to be activated to promote outward transport.

It is readily evident from the scenario outlined above and has long been known that the first condition, namely increase in intracellular Na^+, is readily achieved by inward transport of amphetamines. However, the role of intracellular kinases has been only appreciated more recently (Gnegy, 2003); both, protein kinase C and Ca^{2+}/calmodulin-dependent protein kinase II are activated during exposure of cells to amphetamine and are required to support transporter-mediated amphetamine induced monoamine efflux (Browman et al., 1998; Kantor and Gnegy, 1998; Kantor et al., 2001; Fog et al., 2006). Truncation of the first 22 N-terminal amino acids removes potential phosphorylation sites and abolishes PKC-dependent phosphorylation. This mutated transporter supports substrate uptake and undergoes regulation of substrate influx by PKC and endocytosis (Granas et al., 2003). However, it fails to support amphetamine-induced substrate efflux (Khoshbouei et al., 2004).

Regardless of whether one tries to understand amphetamine-induced transport reversal by using the alternating excess model or whether one invokes a channel-like mode of substrate entry, the action of amphetamine is difficult to understand, if the transporter is a single entity: the transporter transports amphetamine to the intracellular side and releases it. For reasons that are unclear, it now preferentially binds the monoamine substrate (rather than the amphetamine molecule) and translocates this to the extracellular side. Because there is not any logical argument or experimental evidence for preferential binding of monoamine substrate over that of amphetamine to the inward-facing conformation, we considered an oligomer-based countertransport model. In an oligomer-based countertransport model, substrate is taken up by one moiety and efflux is performed by the counterpart within the oligomer. As the concentration of a releaser (that needs to be taken up) is raised over the concentration, where 50% of the transporters are occupied, the release is actually expected to decline. The reason for this is that the more the single subunits within a transporter oligomer get occupied with substrate being taken up, the less the subunits are available to perform efflux. Therefore, amphetamine-induced efflux is predicted to fade, if its concentrations rise above certain levels. This expectation was fully borne out by a bell-shaped concentration response curve observed with *para*-chloroamphetamine (PCA) and methylene-dioximethamphetamine

(MDMA) in SERT expressing cells (Seidel et al., 2005). We also tested, if the reverse operation of monoamine transporters relied on their oligomeric structure (Seidel et al., 2005). Obviously, it was impossible to use oligomerization deficient transporters since they are retained at the level of the ER (Scholze et al., 2002; Farhan et al., 2004). Thus, we used another approach based on concatemeric fusion of a SERT moiety and a GABA transporter GAT1 moiety. In line with previous work (Horschitz et al., 2003), these transporter subunits were fully functional. Importantly, the GAT1 is resistant to amphetamine, therefore, it is possible to use the GAT1 moiety as a sensor for the efflux-inducing potential of these compounds. The first indication of a functional linkage was obtained in uptake experiments (e.g., using tritiated GABA and unlabeled serotonin or vice versa) in the presence of increasing concentrations of the "countersubstrate" (i.e., serotonin in the case of [³H]GABA uptake). Raising the concentration of the unlabeled countersubstrate inhibited the uptake of the tritiated substrate. This observation can be rationalized in that transport of the unlabeled countersubstrate is also associated with influx of Na⁺, which dissipates the Na⁺ gradient and thus reduces the driving force available for uptake of the radioactive substrate. Thus, Na⁺ influx through one transporter moiety was sensed by the second

□ Figure 17-5

The oligomer-based countertransport model. Low concentrations of *para*-chloroamphetamine (PCA) elicit efflux of intracellular substrate (S): only a fraction of SERT-moieties are occupied by PCA in the oligomeric complex (shown here for the sake of simplicity as a dimer); occupancy by PCA precludes phosphorylation by protein kinase C (PKC; see Ramamoorthy and Blakely, 1999). The other SERT moieties in the oligomeric complex that has not been occupied by PCA are subject to phosphorylation and thereby primed for outward transport of substrate

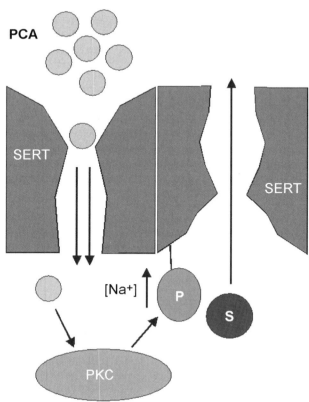

moiety of the concatemer. However, the acid test was to induce GABA release by amphetamine via the SERT-GAT1 concatemer: after preloading a SERT-GAT1-expressing cell line with [^{3}H]GABA, the cells were tested for carrier-mediated release (Sitte et al., 2001) by challenging them with PCA. This caused a tiagabine-sensitive release and provided a formal proof for the model that, during amphetamine-induced monoamine efflux, the transporters operate in a countertransport mode that requires an oligomeric structure (see ❷ *Figure 17-5*).

Acknowledgments

The authors wish to acknowledge support by the following granting institutions: grant P17076 and P18076 (to HHS) from the Austrian Science Foundation/FWF.

References

Abramson J, Smirnova I, Kasho V, Verner G, Kaback HR, et al. 2003. Structure and mechanism of the lactose permease of Escherichia coli. Science 301: 610-615.

Accardi A, Miller C. 2004. Secondary active transport mediated by a prokaryotic homologue of ClC Cl-channels. Nature 427: 803-807.

Adams SV, DeFelice LJ. 2002. Flux coupling in the human serotonin transporter. Biophys J 83: 3268-3282.

Adams SV, DeFelice LJ. 2003. Ionic currents in the human serotonin transporter reveal inconsistencies in the alternating access hypothesis. Biophys J 85: 1548-1559.

Amara SG, Kuhar MJ. 1993. Neurotransmitter transporters: Recent progress. Annu Rev Neurosci 16: 73-93.

Androutsellis-Theotokis A, Ghassemi F, Rudnick G. 2001. A conformationally sensitive residue on the cytoplasmic surface of serotonin transporter. J Biol Chem 276: 45933-45938.

Androutsellis-Theotokis A, Goldberg NR, Ueda K, Beppu T, Beckman ML, et al. 2003. Characterization of a functional bacterial homologue of sodium-dependent neurotransmitter transporters. J Biol Chem 278: 12703-12709.

Androutsellis-Theotokis A, Rudnick G. 2002. Accessibility and conformational coupling in serotonin transporter predicted internal domains. J Neurosci 22: 8370-8378.

Axelrod J. 1971. Noradrenaline: Fate and control of its biosynthesis. Science 173: 598-606.

Axelrod J, Whitby LG, Hertting G. 1961. Effect of psychotropic drugs on the uptake of ^{3}H-norepinephrine by tissues. Science 133: 383-384.

Beckman ML, Quick MW. 2001. Substrates and temperature differentiate ion flux from serotonin flux in a serotonin transporter. Neuropharmacology 40: 526-535.

Bendahan A, Kanner BI. 1993. Identification of domains of a cloned rat brain GABA transporter which are not required for its functional expression. FEBS Lett 318: 41-44.

Berfield JL, Wang LC, Reith ME. 1999. Which form of dopamine is the substrate for the human dopamine transporter: The cationic or the uncharged species? J Biol Chem 274: 4876-4882.

Birkmayer W, Hornykiewicz O. 1961. The ʟ-3,4-dioxyphenylalanine (DOPA)-effect in Parkinson-akinesia. Wien Klin Wochenschr 73: 787-788.

Bönisch H, Trendelenburg U. 1989. The mechanism of action of indirectly acting sympathomimetic amines. Handbook of Experimental Pharmacology: Catecholamines. Trendelenburg U, Weiner N, editors. Berlin, Hamburg, New York: Springer; pp. 247-277.

Browman KE, Kantor L, Richardson S, Badiani A, Robinson TE, et al. 1998. Injection of the protein kinase C inhibitor Ro31–8220 into the nucleus accumbens attenuates the acute response to amphetamine: Tissue and behavioral studies. Brain Res 814: 112-119.

Bruns D, Engert F, Lux H-D. 1993. A fast activating presynaptic reuptake current during serotonergic transmission in identified neurons of Hirudo. Neuron 10: 559-572.

Bruss M, Hammermann R, Brimijoin S, Bonisch H. 1995. Antipeptide antibodies confirm the topology of the human norepinephrine transporter. J Biol Chem 270: 9197-9201.

Busch W, Saier MH Jr. 2002. The transporter classification (TC) system, 2002. Crit Rev Biochem Mol Biol 37: 287-337.

Cao Y, Li M, Mager S, Lester HA. 1998. Amino acid residues that control pH modulation of transport-associated current in mammalian serotonin transporters. J Neurosci 18: 7739-7749.

Cao Y, Mager S, Lester HA. 1997. H$^+$ permeation and pH regulation at a mammalian serotonin transporter. J Neurosci 17: 2257-2266.

Carlsson A. 2001. A half-century of neurotransmitter research: Impact on neurology and psychiatry (Nobel lecture). Chembiochem 2: 484-493.

Carvelli L, McDonald PW, Blakely RD, DeFelice LJ. 2004. Dopamine transporters depolarize neurons by a channel mechanism. Proc Natl Acad Sci USA 101: 16046-16051.

Chen F, Larsen MB, Neubauer HA, Sanchez C, Plenge P, et al. 2005. Characterization of an allosteric citalopram-binding site at the serotonin transporter. J Neurochem 92: 21-28.

Chen JG, Liu CS, Rudnick G. 1997. External cysteine residues in the serotonin transporter. Biochemistry 36: 1479-1486.

Chen JG, Liu CS, Rudnick G. 1998. Determination of external loop topology in the serotonin transporter by site-directed chemical labeling. J Biol Chem 273: 12675-12681.

Chen N, Reith ME. 2000. Structure and function of the dopamine transporter. Eur J Pharmacol 405: 329-339.

Ciliax BJ, Heilman C, Demchyshyn LL, Pristupa ZB, Ince E, et al. 1995. The dopamine transporter: Immunochemical characterization and localization in brain. J Neurosci 15: 1714-1723.

Cool DR, Leibach FH, Bhalla VK, Mahesh VB, Ganapathy V. 1991. Expression and cyclic AMP-dependent regulation of a high affinity serotonin transporter in the human placental choriocarcinoma cell line (JAR). J Biol Chem 266: 15750-15757.

Cornea RL, Autry JM, Chen Z, Jones LR. 2000. Reexamination of the role of the leucine/isoleucine zipper residues of phospholamban in inhibition of the Ca^{2+} pump of cardiac sarcoplasmic reticulum. J Biol Chem 275: 41487-41494.

Dale H. 1935. Reizübertragung durch chemische Mittel im peripheren Nervensystem. Urban & Schwarzenberg. Berlin: Wien; pp. 1-23.

DeFelice LJ, Adams SV, Ypey DL. 2001. Single-file diffusion and neurotransmitter transporters: Hodgkin and Keynes model revisited. Biosystems 62: 57-66.

DeFelice LJ, Blakely RD. 1996. Pore models for transporters? Biophys J 70: 579-580.

DeFelice LJ, Galli A. 1998. Electrophysiological analysis of transporter function. Adv Pharmacol 42: 186-190.

Distelmaier F, Wiedemann P, Bruss M, Bonisch H. 2004. Functional importance of the C-terminus of the human norepinephrine transporter. J Neurochem 91: 537-546.

Eisenhofer G. 2001. The role of neuronal and extraneuronal plasma membrane transporters in the inactivation of peripheral catecholamines. Pharmacol Ther 91: 35-62.

Ellgaard L, Helenius A. 2003. Quality control in the endoplasmic reticulum. Nat Rev Mol Cell Biol 4: 181-191.

Elling CE, Nielsen SM, Schwartz TW. 1995. Conversion of antagonist-binding site to metal-ion site in the tachykinin NK-1 receptor. Nature 374: 74-77.

Elling CE, Schwartz TW. 1996. Connectivity and orientation of the seven helical bundle in the tachykinin NK-1 receptor probed by zinc site engineering. EMBO J 15: 6213-6219.

Falkenburger BH, Barstow KL, Mintz IM. 2001. Dendrodendritic inhibition through reversal of dopamine transport. Science 293: 2465-2470.

Farhan H, Korkhov VM, Paulitschke V, Dorostkar MM, Scholze P, et al. 2004. Two discontinuous segments in the carboxy terminus are required for membrane targeting of the rat GABA transporter-1 (GAT1). J Biol Chem 279: 28553-28563.

Ferrer JV, Javitch JA. 1998. Cocaine alters the accessibility of endogenous cysteines in putative extracellular and intracellular loops of the human dopamine transporter. Proc Natl Acad Sci USA 95: 9238-9243.

Fog JU, Khoshbouei H, Holy M, Owens WA, Vaegter CB, Sen N, Nikandrova Y, Bowton E, McMahon DG, Colbran RJ, Daws LC, Sitte HH, Javitch JA, Galli A, Gether U. 2006. Calmodulin kinase II interacts with the dopamine transporter C terminus to regulate amphetamine-induced reverse transport. Neuron 51: 417-429.

Forster R, Weiss M, Zimmermann T, Reynaud EG, Verissimo F, et al. 2006. Secretory cargo regulates the turnover of COPII subunits at single ER exit sites. Curr Biol 16: 173-179.

Freed C, Revay R, Vaughan RA, Kriek E, Grant S, et al. 1995. Dopamine transporter immunoreactivity in rat brain. J Comp Neurol 359: 340-349.

Galli A, Blakely RD, DeFelice LJ. 1996. Norepinephrine transporters have channel modes of conduction. Proc Natl Acad Sci USA 93: 8671-8676.

Galli A, Blakely RD, DeFelice LJ. 1998. Patch-clamp and amperometric recordings from norepinephrine transporters: Channel activity and voltage-dependent uptake. Proc Natl Acad Sci USA 95: 13260-13265.

Galli A, DeFelice LJ, Duke BJ, Moore KR, Blakely RD. 1995. Sodium-dependent norepinephrine-induced currents in norepinephrine-transporter-transfected HEK-293 cells blocked by cocaine and antidepressants. J Exp Biol 198: 2197-2212.

Gether U. 2000. Uncovering molecular mechanisms involved in activation of G protein-coupled receptors. Endocr Rev 21: 90-113.

Gether U, Norregaard L, Loland CJ. 2001. Delineating structure–function relationships in the dopamine transporter from natural and engineered Zn^{2+} binding sites. Life Sci 68: 2187-2198.

Giros B, el Mestikawy S, Bertrand L, Caron MG. 1991. Cloning and functional characterization of a cocaine-sensitive dopamine transporter. FEBS Lett 295: 149-154.

Gnegy ME. 2003. The effect of phosphorylation on amphetamine-mediated outward transport. Eur J Pharmacol 479: 83-91.

Graham D, Esnaud H, Langer SZ. 1991. Characterization and purification of the neuronal sodium-ion-coupled 5-hydroxytryptamine transporter. Biochem Soc Trans 19: 99-102.

Graham D, Esnaud H, Langer SZ. 1992. Partial purification and characterization of the sodium-ion-coupled 5-hydroxytryptamine transporter of rat cerebral cortex. Biochem J 286 (Pt. 3): 801-805.

Granas C, Ferrer J, Loland CJ, Javitch JA, Gether U. 2003. N-terminal truncation of the dopamine transporter abolishes phorbol ester- and substance P receptor-stimulated phosphorylation without impairing transporter internalization. J Biol Chem 278: 4990-5000.

Gu HH, Ahn J, Caplan MJ, Blakely RD, Levey AI, et al. 1996a. Cell-specific sorting of biogenic amine transporters expressed in epithelial cells. J Biol Chem 271: 18100-18106.

Gu HH, Wall S, Rudnick G. 1996b. Ion coupling stoichiometry for the norepinephrine transporter in membrane vesicles from stably transfected cells. J Biol Chem 271: 6911-6916.

Guastella J, Nelson N, Nelson H, Czyzyk L, Keynan S, et al. 1990. Cloning and expression of a rat brain GABA transporter. Science 249: 1303-1306.

Habert E, Graham D, Langer SZ. 1986. Solubilization and characterization of the 5-hydroxytryptamine transporter complex from rat cerebral cortical membranes. Eur J Pharmacol 122: 197-204.

Hahn MK, Robertson D, Blakely RD. 2003. A mutation in the human norepinephrine transporter gene (SLC6A2) associated with orthostatic intolerance disrupts surface expression of mutant and wild-type transporters. J Neurosci 23: 4470-4478.

Harata NC, Choi S, Pyle JL, Aravanis AM, Tsien RW. 2006. Frequency-dependent kinetics and prevalence of kiss-and-run and reuse at hippocampal synapses studied with novel quenching methods. Neuron 49: 243-256.

Hastrup H, Karlin A, Javitch JA. 2001. Symmetrical dimer of the human dopamine transporter revealed by cross-linking Cys-306 at the extracellular end of the sixth transmembrane segment. Proc Natl Acad Sci USA 98: 10055-10060.

Hebert DN, Carruthers A. 1992. Glucose transporter oligomeric structure determines transporter function. Reversible redox-dependent interconversions of tetrameric and dimeric GLUT1. J Biol Chem 267: 23829-23838.

Heldin CH. 1995. Dimerization of cell surface receptors in signal transduction. Cell 80: 213-223.

Hilber B, Scholze P, Dorostkar MM, Sandtner W, Holy M, Boehm S, Singer EA, Sitte HH. 2005. Serotonin-transporter mediated efflux: A pharmacological analysis of amphetamines and non-amphetamines. Neuropharmacology 49: 811-819.

Hoffman BJ, Palkovits M, Pacak K, Hansson SR, Mezey E. 1998. Regulation of dopamine transporter mRNA levels in the central nervous system. Adv Pharmacol 42: 202-206.

Horiuchi M, Nicke A, Gomeza J, Aschrafi A, Schmalzing G, et al. 2001. Surface-localized glycine transporters 1 and 2 function as monomeric proteins in Xenopus oocytes. Proc Natl Acad Sci USA 98: 1448-1453.

Horschitz S, Hummerich R, Schloss P. 2003. Functional coupling of serotonin and noradrenaline transporters. J Neurochem 86: 958-965.

Huang Y, Lemieux MJ, Song J, Auer M, Wang DN. 2003. Structure and mechanism of the glycerol-3-phosphate transporter from Escherichia coli. Science 301: 616-620.

Humphreys CJ, Wall SC, Rudnick G. 1994. Ligand binding to the serotonin transporter: Equilibria, kinetics, and ion dependence. Biochemistry 33: 9118-9125.

Ingram SL, Prasad BM, Amara SG. 2002. Dopamine transporter-mediated conductances increase excitability of midbrain dopamine neurons. Nat Neurosci 5: 971-978.

Iversen L. 2000. Neurotransmitter transporters: Fruitful targets for CNS drug discovery. Mol Psychiatry 5: 357-362.

Jardetzky O. 1966. Simple allosteric model for membrane pumps. Nature 211: 969-970.

Just H, Sitte HH, Schmid JA, Freissmuth M, Kudlacek O. 2004. Identification of an additional interaction domain in transmembrane domains 11 and 12 that supports oligomer formation in the human serotonin transporter. J Biol Chem 279: 6650-6657.

Kahlig KM, Binda F, Khoshbouei H, Blakely RD, McMahon DG, et al. 2005. Amphetamine induces dopamine efflux through a dopamine transporter channel. Proc Natl Acad Sci USA 102: 3495-3500.

Kamdar G, Penado KM, Rudnick G, Stephan MM. 2001. Functional role of critical stripe residues in transmembrane span 7 of the serotonin transporter. Effects of Na^+, Li^+, and methanethiosulfonate reagents. J Biol Chem 276: 4038-4045.

Kantor L, Gnegy ME. 1998. Protein kinase C inhibitors block amphetamine-mediated dopamine release in rat striatal slices. J Pharmacol Exp Ther 284: 592-598.

Kantor L, Hewlett GH, Park YH, Richardson-Burns SM, Mellon MJ, et al. 2001. Protein kinase C and intracellular calcium are required for amphetamine-mediated dopamine release via the norepinephrine transporter in undifferentiated PC12 cells. J Pharmacol Exp Ther 297: 1016-1024.

Karlin A, Akabas MH. 1998. Substituted-cysteine accessibility method. Methods Enzymol 293: 123-145.

Keyes SR, Rudnick G. 1982. Coupling of transmembrane proton gradients to platelet serotonin transport. J Biol Chem 257: 1172-1176.

Khoshbouei H, Sen N, Guptaroy B, Johnson L, Lund D, et al. 2004. N-terminal phosphorylation of the dopamine transporter is required for amphetamine-induced efflux. PLoS Biol 2: E78.

Kocabas AM, Rudnick G, Kilic F. 2003. Functional consequences of homo- but not hetero-oligomerization between transporters for the biogenic amine neurotransmitters. J Neurochem 85: 1513-1520.

Korkhov VM, Farhan H, Freissmuth M, Sitte HH. 2004. Oligomerization of the {gamma}-aminobutyric acid transporter-1 is driven by an interplay of polar and hydrophobic interactions in transmembrane helix II. J Biol Chem 279: 55728-55736.

Korkhov VM, Holy M, Freissmuth M, Sitte HH. 2006. The conserved glutamate (Glu136) in transmembrane domain 2 of the serotonin transporter is required for the conformational switch in the transport cycle. J Biol Chem 281: 13439-13448.

Kuhar MJ, Ritz MC, Boja JW. 1991. The dopamine hypothesis of the reinforcing properties of cocaine. Trends Neurosci 14: 299-302.

Launay JM, Geoffroy C, Mutel V, Buckle M, Cesura A, et al. 1992. One-step purification of the serotonin transporter located at the human platelet plasma membrane. J Biol Chem 267: 11344-11351.

Lester HA, Cao Y, Mager S. 1996. Listening to neurotransmitter transporters. Neuron 17: 807-810.

Lester HA, Mager S, Quick MW, Corey JL. 1994. Permeation properties of neurotransmitter transporters. Annu Rev Pharmacol Toxicol 34: 219-249.

Levi G, Raiteri M. 1993. Carrier-mediated release of neurotransmitters. Trends Neurosci 16: 415-419.

Liu Y, Peter D, Roghani A, Schuldiner S, Prive GG, et al. 1992. A cDNA that suppresses MPP + toxicity encodes a vesicular amine transporter. Cell 70: 539-551.

Loland CJ, Norregaard L, Gether U. 1999. Defining proximity relationships in the tertiary structure of the dopamine transporter. Identification of a conserved glutamic acid as a third coordinate in the endogenous Zn(2+)-binding site. J Biol Chem 274: 36928-36934.

Lopez-Corcuera B, Alcantara R, Vazquez J, Aragon C. 1993. Hydrodynamic properties and immunological identification of the sodium- and chloride-coupled glycine transporter. J Biol Chem 268: 2239-2243.

MacKenzie KR, Engelman DM. 1998. Structure-based prediction of the stability of transmembrane helix-helix interactions: The sequence dependence of glycophorin A dimerization. Proc Natl Acad Sci USA 95: 3583-3590.

MacKinnon R. 2003. Potassium channels. FEBS Lett 555: 62-65.

Mager S, Min C, Henry DJ, Chavkin C, Hoffman BJ, et al. 1994. Conducting states of a mammalian serotonin transporter. Neuron 12: 845-859.

Meinild AK, Sitte HH, Gether U. 2004. Zinc potentiates an uncoupled anion conductance associated with the dopamine transporter. J Biol Chem 279: 49671-49679.

Mezey E, Eisenhofer G, Hansson S, Hunyady B, Hoffman BJ. 1998. Dopamine produced by the stomach may act as a paracrine/autocrine hormone in the rat. Neuroendocrinology 67: 336-348.

Miller EA, Beilharz TH, Malkus PN, Lee MC, Hamamoto S, et al. 2003. Multiple cargo binding sites on the COPII subunit Sec24p ensure capture of diverse membrane proteins into transport vesicles. Cell 114: 497-509.

Miranda M, Sorkina T, Grammatopoulos TN, Zawada WM, Sorkin A. 2004. Multiple molecular determinants in the carboxyl terminus regulate dopamine transporter export from endoplasmic reticulum. J Biol Chem 279: 30760-30770.

Mossessova E, Bickford LC, Goldberg J. 2003. SNARE selectivity of the COPII coat. Cell 114: 483-495.

Nelson PJ, Rudnick G. 1979. Coupling between platelet 5-hydroxytryptamine and potassium transport. J Biol Chem 254: 10084-10089.

Nelson PJ, Rudnick G. 1982. The role of chloride ion in platelet serotonin transport. J Biol Chem 257: 6151-6155.

Nirenberg MJ, Chan J, Pohorille A, Vaughan RA, Uhl GR, et al. 1997a. The dopamine transporter: Comparative ultrastructure of dopaminergic axons in limbic and motor compartments of the nucleus accumbens. J Neurosci 17: 6899-6907.

Nirenberg MJ, Chan J, Vaughan RA, Uhl GR, Kuhar MJ, et al. 1997b. Immunogold localization of the dopamine transporter: An ultrastructural study of the rat ventral tegmental area. J Neurosci 17: 5255-5262.

Norregaard L, Frederiksen D, Nielsen EO, Gether U. 1998. Delineation of an endogenous zinc-binding site in the human dopamine transporter. EMBO J 17: 4266-4273.

Norregaard L, Visiers I, Loland CJ, Ballesteros J, Weinstein H, et al. 2000. Structural probing of a microdomain in the dopamine transporter by engineering of artificial Zn^{2+} binding sites. Biochemistry 39: 15836-15846.

Orci L, Ravazzola M, Meda P, Holcomb C, Moore HP, et al. 1991. Mammalian Sec23p homologue is restricted to the endoplasmic reticulum transitional cytoplasm. Proc Natl Acad Sci USA 88: 8611-8615.

Pacholczyk T, Blakely RD, Amara SG. 1991. Expression cloning of a cocaine- and antidepressant-sensitive human noradrenaline transporter. Nature 350: 350-354.

Perego C, Bulbarelli A, Longhi R, Caimi M, Villa A, et al. 1997. Sorting of two polytopic proteins, the gamma-aminobutyric acid and betaine transporters, in polarized epithelial cells. J Biol Chem 272: 6584-6592.

Petersen CI, DeFelice LJ. 1999. Ionic interactions in the Drosophila serotonin transporter identify it as a serotonin channel. Nat Neurosci 2: 605-610.

Popot JL, Engelman DM. 1990. Membrane protein folding and oligomerization: The two-stage model. Biochemistry 29: 4031-4037.

Popot JL, Engelman DM. 2000. Helical membrane protein folding, stability, and evolution. Annu Rev Biochem 69: 881-922.

Pothos EN, Sulzer D. 1998. Modulation of quantal dopamine release by psychostimulants. Adv Pharmacol 42: 198-202.

Qian Y, Galli A, Ramamoorthy S, Risso S, DeFelice LJ, et al. 1997. Protein kinase C activation regulates human serotonin transporters in HEK-293 cells via altered cell surface expression. J Neurosci 17: 45-57.

Qian Y, Melikian HE, Rye DB, Levey AI, Blakely RD. 1995. Identification and characterization of antidepressant-sensitive serotonin transporter proteins using site-specific antibodies. J Neurosci 15: 1261-1274.

Quick MW. 2003. Regulating the conducting states of a mammalian serotonin transporter. Neuron 40: 537-549.

Ramamoorthy S, Blakely RD. 1999. Phosphorylation and sequestration of serotonin transporters differentially modulated by psychostimulants. Science 285: 763-766.

Ramamoorthy S, Bauman AL, Moore KR, Han H, Yang FT, et al. 1993a. Antidepressant- and cocaine-sensitive human serotonin transporter: Molecular cloning, expression, and chromosomal localization. Proc Natl Acad Sci USA 90: 2542-2546.

Ramamoorthy S, Cool DR, Leibach FH, Mahesh VB, Ganapathy V. 1992. Reconstitution of the human placental 5-hydroxytryptamine transporter in a catalytically active form after detergent solubilization. Biochem J 286 (Pt. 1): 89-95.

Ramamoorthy S, Leibach FH, Mahesh VB, Ganapathy V. 1993b. Partial purification and characterization of the human placental serotonin transporter. Placenta 14: 449-461.

Rasmussen SG, Carroll FI, Maresch MJ, Jensen AD, Tate CG, et al. 2001. Biophysical characterization of the cocaine binding pocket in the serotonin transporter using a fluorescent cocaine analogue as a molecular reporter. J Biol Chem 276: 4717-4723.

Reddy LG, Jones LR, Thomas DD. 1999. Depolymerization of phospholamban in the presence of calcium pump: A fluorescence energy transfer study. Biochemistry 38: 3954-3962.

Reith ME, Berfield JL, Wang LC, Ferrer JV, Javitch JA. 2001. The uptake inhibitors cocaine and benztropine differentially alter the conformation of the human dopamine transporter. J Biol Chem 276: 29012-29018.

Rudnick G. 2002. Mechanism of biogenic amine neurotransmitter transporters. Neurotransmitter Transporters: Structure, Function, and Regulation. Reith MEA, editor. Totowa, NJ: Humana Press Inc.; pp. 25-52.

Rudnick G. 2006. Structure/function relationship in serotonin transporter. Neurotransmitter Transporters. Sitte HH, Freissmuth M, editors. Berlin, Heidelberg: Springer-Verlag; pp. 59-73.

Rudnick G, Clark J. 1993. From synapse to vesicle: The reuptake and storage of biogenic amine neurotransmitters. Biochim Biophys Acta 1144: 249-263.

Rudnick G, Kirk KL, Fishkes H, Schuldiner S. 1989. Zwitterionic and anionic forms of a serotonin analog as transport substrates. J Biol Chem 264: 14865-14868.

Sanchez C, Bergqvist PB, Brennum LT, Gupta S, Hogg S, et al. 2003. Escitalopram, the S-(+)-enantiomer of citalopram, is a selective serotonin reuptake inhibitor with potent effects in animal models predictive of antidepressant and anxiolytic activities. Psychopharmacology (Berl) 167: 353-362.

Sato K, Nakano A. 2004. Reconstitution of coat protein complex II (COPII) vesicle formation from cargo-reconstituted proteoliposomes reveals the potential role of GTP hydrolysis by Sar1p in protein sorting. J Biol Chem 279: 1330-1335.

Sato K, Nakano A. 2005. Dissection of COPII subunit-cargo assembly and disassembly kinetics during Sar1p-GTP hydrolysis. Nat Struct Mol Biol 12: 167-174.

Schmid JA, Just H, Sitte HH. 2001a. Impact of oligomerization on the function of the human serotonin transporter. Biochem Soc Trans 29: 732-736.

Schmid JA, Scholze P, Kudlacek O, Freissmuth M, Singer EA, et al. 2001b. Oligomerization of the human serotonin transporter and of the rat GABA transporter 1 visualized by fluorescence resonance energy transfer microscopy in living cells. J Biol Chem 276: 3805-3810.

Scholze P, Freissmuth M, Sitte HH. 2002. Mutations within an intramembrane leucine heptad repeat disrupt oligomer formation of the rat GABA transporter 1. J Biol Chem 277: 43682-43690.

Schroeter S, Apparsundaram S, Wiley RG, Miner LH, Sesack SR., et al. 2000. Immunolocalization of the cocaine- and antidepressant-sensitive l-norepinephrine transporter. J Comp Neurol 420: 211-232.

Schroeter S, Levey AI, Blakely RD. 1997. Polarized expression of the antidepressant-sensitive serotonin transporter in epinephrine-synthesizing chromaffin cells of the rat adrenal gland. Mol Cell Neurosci 9: 170-184.

Seidel S, Singer EA, Just H, Farhan H, Scholze P, et al. 2005. Amphetamines take two to tango: An oligomer-based counter-transport model of neurotransmitter transport explores the amphetamine action. Mol Pharmacol 67: 140-151.

Seiden LS, Sabol KE, Ricaurte GA. 1993. Amphetamine: Effects on catecholamine systems and behavior. Annu Rev Pharmacol Toxicol 33: 639-677.

Sen N, Shi L, Beuming T, Weinstein H, Javitch JA. 2005. A pincer-like configuration of TM2 in the human dopamine transporter is responsible for indirect effects on cocaine binding. Neuropharmacology 49: 780-790.

Shannon JR, Flattem NL, Jordan J, Jacob G, Black BK, et al. 2000. Orthostatic intolerance and tachycardia associated with norepinephrine-transporter deficiency. N Engl J Med 342: 541-549.

Sitte HH, Farhan H, Javitch JA. 2004. Sodium-dependent neurotransmitter transporters: Oligomerization as a determinant of transporter function and trafficking. Mol Intervent 4: 38-47.

Sitte HH, Freissmuth M. 2003. Oligomer formation by Na+Cl–coupled neurotransmitter transporters. Eur J Pharmacol 479: 229-236.

Sitte HH, Hiptmair B, Zwach J, Pifl C, Singer EA, et al. 2001. Quantitative analysis of inward and outward transport rates in cells stably expressing the cloned human serotonin transporter: Inconsistencies with the hypothesis of facilitated exchange diffusion. Mol Pharmacol 59: 1129-1137.

Sitte HH, Huck S, Reither H, Boehm S, Singer EA, et al. 1998. Carrier-mediated release, transport rates, and charge transfer induced by amphetamine, tyramine, and dopamine in mammalian cells transfected with the human dopamine transporter. J Neurochem 71: 1289-1297.

Sonders MS, Amara SG. 1996. Channels in transporters. Curr Opin Neurobiol 6: 294-302.

Sonders MS, Zhu SJ, Zahniser NR, Kavanaugh MP, Amara SG. 1997. Multiple ionic conductances of the human dopamine transporter: The actions of dopamine and psychostimulants. J Neurosci 17: 960-974.

Sorkina T, Doolen S, Galperin E, Zahniser NR, Sorkin A. 2003. Oligomerization of dopamine transporters visualized in living cells by FRET microscopy. J Biol Chem 278: 28274-28283.

Stagg SM, Gurkan C, Fowler DM, LaPointe P, Foss TR, et al. 2006. Structure of the Sec13/31 COPII coat cage. Nature 439: 234-238.

Sugamori KS, Lee FJ, Pristupa ZB, Niznik HB. 1999. A cognate dopamine transporter-like activity endogenously expressed in a COS-7 kidney-derived cell line. FEBS Lett 451: 169-174.

Sulzer D, Chen TK, Lau YY, Kristensen H, Rayport S, et al. 1995. Amphetamine redistributes dopamine from synaptic vesicles to the cytosol and promotes reverse transport. J Neurosci 15: 4102-4108.

Sulzer D, Galli A. 2003. Dopamine transport currents are promoted from curiosity to physiology. Trends Neurosci 26: 173-176.

Sulzer D, Rayport S. 1990. Amphetamine and other psychostimulants reduce pH gradients in midbrain dopaminergic neurons and chromaffin granules: A mechanism of action. Neuron 5: 797-808.

Sulzer D, Rayport S. 2000. Dale's principle and glutamate corelease from ventral midbrain dopamine neurons. Amino Acids 19: 45-52.

Sulzer D, Sonders MS, Poulsen NW, Galli A. 2005. Mechanisms of neurotransmitter release by amphetamines: A review. Prog Neurobiol 75: 406-433.

Sur C, Betz H, Schloss P. 1996. Immunocytochemical detection of the serotonin transporter in rat brain. Neuroscience 73: 217-231.

Sur C, Betz H, Schloss P. 1998. Distinct effects of imipramine on 5-hydroxytryptamine uptake mediated by the recombinant rat serotonin transporter SERT1. J Neurochem 70: 2545-2553.

Swanson JM, Volkow ND. 2003. Serum and brain concentrations of methylphenidate: Implications for use and abuse. Neurosci Biobehav Rev 27: 615-621.

Talvenheimo J, Fishkes H, Nelson PJ, Rudnick G. 1983. The serotonin transporter-imipramine "receptor". J Biol Chem 258: 6115-6119.

Talvenheimo J, Nelson PJ, Rudnick G. 1979. Mechanism of imipramine inhibition of platelet 5-hydroxytryptamine transport. J Biol Chem 254: 4631-4635.

Tate CG, Haase J, Baker C, Boorsma M, Magnani F, et al. 2003. Comparison of seven different heterologous protein expression systems for the production of the serotonin transporter. Biochim Biophys Acta 1610: 141-153.

Torres GE, Carneiro A, Seamans K, Fiorentini C, Sweeney A, et al. 2003. Oligomerization and trafficking of the human dopamine transporter. Mutational analysis identifies critical domains important for the functional expression of the transporter. J Biol Chem 278: 2731-2739.

Trendelenburg U, Langeloh A, Bönisch H. 1987. Mechanism of action of indirectly acting sympathomimetic amines. Blood Vessels 24: 261-270.

White SH, Wimley WC. 1999. Membrane protein folding and stability: Physical principles. Annu Rev Biophys Biomol Struct 28: 319-365.

Yamashita A, Singh SK, Kawate T, Jin Y, Gouaux E. 2005. Crystal structure of a bacterial homologue of Na+/Cl–dependent neurotransmitter transporters. Nature 437: 215-223.

Yernool D, Boudker O, Jin Y, Gouaux E. 2004. Structure of a glutamate transporter homologue from *Pyrococcus horikoshii*. Nature 431: 811-818.

Youvan DC, Silva CM, Bylina EJ, Coleman WJ, Dilworth MR, et al. 1997. Calibration of fluorescence resonance energy transfer in microscopy using genetically engineered GFP derivatives on nickel chelating beads. Biotechnology et alia 3: 1-18.

Zaczek R, Culp S, De SE. 1991. Interactions of [3H]amphetamine with rat brain synaptosomes. II. Active transport. J Pharmacol Exp Ther 257: 830-835.

Zhang DQ, Stone JF, Zhou T, Ohta H, McMahon DG. 2004. Characterization of genetically labeled catecholamine neurons in the mouse retina. Neuroreport 15: 1761-1765.

Zhou FX, Merianos HJ, Brunger AT, Engelman DM. 2001. Polar residues drive association of polyleucine transmembrane helices. Proc Natl Acad Sci USA 98: 2250-2255.

18 Regulation of Biogenic Amine Transporters

L. D. Jayanthi · D. J. Samuvel · E. R. Buck · M. E. A. Reith · S. Ramamoorthy

Abstract: The uptake of dopamine, serotonin, and norepinephrine following release into nerve terminals through monoamine transporters is the principal process for termination of monoaminergic transmission. This chapter focuses on the monoamine transporter for dopamine (DAT), serotonin (SERT), and norepinephrine (NET). As these transporters are additionally the high-affinity targets for various therapeutic agents and substances of abuse, knowledge regarding their structure, function, and regulation is of obvious importance. The role of each transporter in monoaminergic transmission is reviewed, followed by a description of long- and short-term regulation of transporter activity. The latter includes trafficking-dependent and –independent regulation, phosphorylation, and protein-protein interactions. The impact of substrates and blockers on transporter regulation is discussed, as well as dysregulation of monoamine transporters in human diseases, and, finally, the central role of monoamine transporters in the action of drugs of abuse. The critical role of monoamine transporters in brain function is underscored by the wide range of drugs that target monoamine transporters, including medications for depression, attention-deficit disorder, smoking, addiction, obsessive-compulsive disorder, and sleep disorders.

List of Abbreviations: 5-HT, serotonin; ADHD, attention deficit hyperactivity disorder; BDNF, brain-derived growth factor; CaMKII, calcium/calmodulin-dependent kinase II; CNS, central nervous system; DA, dopamine; DAT, dopamine transporter; EBV, Epstein–Barr virus; hNET, human NET; IBS, irritable bowel syndrome; MAP kinase, mitogen-activated protein kinase; NE, norepinephrine; NET, norepinephrine transporter; NGF, nerve growth factor; OK, okadaic acid; PICK, protein-1 that interacts with C-kinase; PKA, protein kinase A; PKC, protein kinase C; PNS, peripheral nervous system; PPH, primary pulmonary hypertension; SERT, serotonin transporter; SIDS, sudden infant death syndrome; SP, substance P; SSRIs, selective serotonin reuptake inhibitors; VMATs, vesicular monoamine transporters

1   Introduction

Effective neuronal communication in the brain requires precise and dynamic regulation of neurotransmitter concentrations. The monoamines, dopamine (DA), norepinephrine (NE), and serotonin (5-HT), act as neurotransmitters in peripheral and central nervous systems (PNS and CNS) in a variety of physiological (cognitive, autonomic, reward-reinforced learning, and emotional) functions (Bunney et al., 1987; Nicoll et al., 1987; Fozzard, 1989; Jacobs and Fornal, 1991; Jacobs and Azmitia, 1992; Goldstein, 1995). At the molecular level, monoamine signaling is dynamically regulated by a diverse set of macromolecules including biosynthetic enzymes, secretory proteins, ion channels, pre- and postsynaptic receptors, and transporters.

2   Structure, Function, and Pharmacology of Monoamine Transporters

The uptake of DA, 5-HT, and NE following release into the nerve terminals through monoamine transporters is the principal process for termination of respective monoaminergic (dopaminergic, serotonergic, and noradrenergic) neurotransmission. The high-affinity plasma membrane dopamine transporter (DAT), norepinephrine transporter (NET), and serotonin transporter (SERT) dictate the concentration, duration, and magnitude of postsynaptic responses. Several different types of cell-surface receptors exist to confer the specific actions of DA, 5-HT, and NE on target cells (Glennon and Dukat, 1995). However, the extracellular clearance of DA, 5-HT, or NE is carried out by only one form (Ramamoorthy et al., 1993) of DAT, SERT, or NET, respectively, in the brain and periphery (Blakely et al., 1991; Hoffman et al., 1991; Lesch et al., 1993). Monoamine transporters belong to the Na^+/Cl^--dependent γ-aminobutyric acid (GABA)/norepinephrine transporter (GAT1/NET) gene family (Amara and Kuhan, 1993; Miller et al., 1997; Povlock and Amara, 1997). The amino acid sequence predicts the presence of 12 hydrophobic transmembrane domains with cytoplasmic NH_2 and COOH termini. Also, the amino acid sequence reveals several potential phosphorylation sites for multiple kinases in the cytoplasmic domains (Ramamoorthy et al., 1993). The translocation of amines by amine transporter requires Na^+ and Cl^- in the external medium. Monoamine transporters are the high-affinity targets for various therapeutic agents and substances of abuse (Ramamoorthy et al., 1993). The critical role of monoamine transporters for normal brain function is underscored by the wide range of drugs that target monoamine transporters, including medications for depression, attention deficit hyperactivity disorder (ADHD), smoking, addiction, obsessive–compulsive disorder, and sleep disorders. The majority of these drugs interfere with the transporter-mediated clearance of extracellular biogenic amine neurotransmitters. An ensuing surge of extracellular monoamines activates monoamine receptors and triggers a cascade of molecular and cellular events to produce therapeutic benefit.

3   The Serotonin Transporter

The monoamine neurotransmitter serotonin (5-hydroxytryptamine, 5-HT) plays an important role as a neuromodulator in adult central and peripheral nervous system regulating a variety of different physiological processes including mood, sleep, sexual drive, appetite, memory, thyroid function, gastrointestinal motility, vasoconstriction, and addiction (Fozzard, 1989; Jacobs and Azmitia, 1992). The uptake of synaptic 5-HT through Na^+/Cl^--dependent SERT is the principal process of terminating serotonergic neurotransmission. Though more than 15 different types of cell-surface receptors exist to confer the specific actions of 5-HT on target cells (Glennon and Dukat, 1995), a single gene (Ramamoorthy et al., 1993) encoding the SERT appears to be responsible for extracellular 5-HT clearance in the brain and periphery. SERT is mapped to chromosome 17 at 17q11.1–17q12 (Blakely et al., 1991; Hoffman et al., 1991; Lesch et al., 1993). In addition to serotonergic neurons, SERTs are also expressed in platelets (Rudnick, 1977; Lesch et al., 1993), placenta (Balkovetz et al., 1989), intestinal crypt epithelia (Wade et al., 1996), adrenal chromaffin cells (Tecott et al., 1995; Schroeter et al., 1997), mast cells (Hoffman et al., 1991; Miller and Hoffman, 1994), medullary thyroid carcinoma cells (Clark et al., 1995), thyroid follicular cells (Tamir et al., 1996), and lymphocytes (Lesch et al., 1996; Faraj et al., 1997). While clearance of synaptic and extrasynaptic 5-HT appears to be the principal function of SERTs, certain cells, notably platelets, utilize SERTs to acquire 5-HT from the extracellular environment for subsequent release, involved in the process of platelet activation (Cirillo et al., 1999; Musselman et al., 2002). Platelets and 5-HT neurons share many common properties, including vesicular monoamine transporters (VMATs), 5-HT release, biochemistry, identical SERT sequences, and 5-HT receptors (Owens and Nemeroff, 1994). Therefore, platelets have been widely used as a peripheral indicator of central 5-HT metabolism and SERT function in psychiatric disorders and vascular diseases in which 5-HT has been implicated (Meltzer et al., 1981; Wirz-Justice, 1988). In the lung, SERTs efficiently clear plasma-borne 5-HT and regulate blood 5-HT levels with the help of platelets.

Altered serotonergic neurotransmission and 5-HT have long been associated with psychiatric disorders, including depression, suicide, impulsive violence, and alcoholism (Heinz et al., 2001; Hahn and Blakely, 2002a). Reduced binding of SERT ligands imipramine and paroxetine to brain and platelet SERTs in patients with depression and suicide victims indicate that altered SERT function might contribute to aberrant behaviors. All SERT antagonists have been shown to be effective antidepressants. Drugs that block SERT, including tricyclic antidepressants such as imipramine, and selective serotonin reuptake inhibitors (SSRIs) like fluoxetine (Prozac), paroxetine (Paxil), sertraline (Zoloft), and citalopram (*Celexa*), are successfully used in the treatment of depression. SSRIs rapidly inhibit the uptake of 5-HT. However, the therapeutic efficacy of antidepressants develops slowly during several weeks of continuous treatment. The therapeutic efficacies of antidepressant drugs have been realized for years; however, current knowledge regarding their mechanisms of action remains incomplete. Because it has been well recognized that treatment response to antidepressants generally requires two or more weeks, studies on long-term adaptive changes have been focused on regulation of receptors, transcription factors, and kinases. SERT antagonists, including antidepressants and cocaine, limit clearance of neuronally released 5-HT and elevate available 5-HT to receptors. These observations suggest that the elevation of extraneuronal 5-HT induces alterations in compensatory or intracellular regulatory pathways impacted by 5-HT signaling, and hence neural plasticity. Therefore, changes in SERT kinetics and number will strongly influence the efficacy of antidepressants in the treatment of depression.

Receptors that are known to influence amine transporter function have been implicated in depression as well as in animal models (Langer, 1987, 1997; Stockmeier et al., 1998; Maes et al., 1999; Murphy et al., 1999; Stockmeier et al., 2002). Altered receptor expression, and sensitivity to receptor ligands, and changes in downstream signaling cascades have been demonstrated in antidepressant drug-treated animals. Chronic antidepressant administrations alter activity and expression of second messenger-regulated protein kinases such as protein kinase C (PKC), calcium/calmodulin-dependent kinase II (CaMKII), protein kinase A (PKA), mitogen-activated protein kinase (MAP kinase) as well as expression of cAMP-specific phosphodi-esterase 4A and 4B isoforms and CREB protein (Popoli et al., 1995, 1997, 2000; Tadokoro et al., 1998; Battersby et al., 1999; Takahashi et al., 1999; Consogno et al., 2000). These neuronal adaptations could serve as molecular switches for amine clearance in vivo by changing the degree of receptor sensitivity, and thus signals linked to SERT regulation. Some examples below describe how receptor-linked regulation of SERT may play a role in depression and antidepressant treatments and vice versa.

Presynaptic inhibitory α_2-adrenoceptors are present on serotonergic nerve endings, and endogenous NE is able to control the release and uptake of 5-HT (Ansah et al., 2000). Decreased platelet α_2-adrenoceptor density and dysregulation of nerve terminal α_2-adrenoceptor density and sensitivity have been shown in depressed patients (Maes et al., 1999). Genetic deletion of the α_2-adrenoceptor in mice renders animals to behave depressed, suggesting a role for α_2-adrenoceptor in the modulation of depression and anxiety (Schramm et al., 2001). Receptors for α_2-adrenoceptor, adenosine, histamine, and 5-HT also regulate 5-HT uptake (Launay et al., 1994; Miller and Hoffman, 1994; Ansah et al., 2000). Chronic antidepressant treatment increases expression of brain-derived growth factor (BDNF), BDNF receptor, and TrkB receptor function (Morinobu et al., 1995; Nibuya et al., 1995; Russo-Neustadt et al., 2000). BDNF produces antidepressant-like behavioral effects and increases serotonergic neurotransmission (Celada et al., 1996; Altar, 1999; Shirayama et al., 2002). BDNF, but not nerve growth factor (NGF), has been shown to regulate SERT expression in B lymphoblasts, suggesting the role of BDNF in functional SERT expression (Mossner et al., 2000). Evidence shows that BDNF and activation of TrkB receptors are required for antidepressant-induced behavioral effects. In vivo activation of 5-HT$_{1B}$ receptors increases 5-HT clearance by increasing SERT activity in the rat hippocampus (Daws et al., 1999, 2000). Mice lacking SERT have altered expression and function of 5-HT$_{1A}$ and 5-HT$_{1B}$ receptors (Fabre et al., 2000). On the other hand, mice lacking the 5-HT$_{1A}$ and 5-HT$_{1B}$ receptors show altered expression of SERT (Ase et al., 2001). Thus, elevated extraneuronal 5-HT could influence 5-HT$_{1A}$ and 5-HT$_{1B}$ receptor signals, and hence SERT activity. Substance P (SP) and substance P receptor (NK1) have been implicated in the pathophysiology of depression (Rupniak and Kramer, 1999; Lieb et al., 2002). Furthermore, genetic deletion and pharmaco-logical blockade of NK1 receptor decrease depressive behaviors and increase serotonergic activity (Rupniak et al., 2001; Bilkei-Gorzo et al., 2002), suggesting the serotonergic system as a potential target for effects of SP on depression-related behaviors (Haddjeri and Blier, 2001; Rupniak et al., 2001; Santarelli et al., 2001). Reduction of SP in the rat brain after chronic antidepressant treatment (Shirayama et al., 1996, 2002) raises the possibility that the degree of NK1 receptor regulating SERT function may be altered after chronic exposure of antidepressants.

4   The Norepinephrine Transporter

The noradrenergic system modulates attention, alertness, arousal, and vigilance. Noradrenergic signaling is intimately linked with behavioral arousal (Astier et al., 1990) and is affected in stress-related paradigms linked to depression (Pavcovich et al., 1990). NE is an important chemical messenger in the nervous system and regulates affective states, learning and memory, and endocrine and autonomic functions. It has been implicated in depression, aggression, addiction, and cardiac and thermal regulation. NE acutely inhibits nociceptive transmission mediated by substance P (NK1), potentiates opioid analgesia, and underlies part of the antinociceptive effects of tricyclic antidepressants (Holden and Naleway, 2001; Jasmin et al., 2002). NE transporter regulates noradrenergic signaling in the CNS and PNS by mediating the clearance of NE and is an important target for antidepressants and psychostimulants (Axelrod and Kopin, 1969; Iversen, 1978; Pacholczyk et al., 1991; Amara and Arriza, 1993). The importance of NET to NE homeostasis suggests a role for NET in disorders of both central and autonomic nervous systems. Involvement of noradrenergic systems in mood disorders is suggested by the evidence that depression is accompanied by altered indices of noradrenergic function and that effective antidepressants enhance extracellular NE levels (Ressler and Nemeroff, 1999, 2001). Furthermore, NET-binding sites are decreased in brains of patients with major depression (Klimek et al., 1997). The activation and sensitization of NE systems in response to stress suggest that NE may play a role in disorders triggered by early life trauma, including depression and posttraumatic stress disorder (Heim and Nemeroff, 2001). NE also plays an important role in attention, vigilance, learning, and memory and is hypothesized to contribute to ADHD (Biederman and Spencer, 1999). Stimulant drugs used to treat ADHD act on both the NET and the DAT, and atomoxetine, which selectively targets NET, is also effective in treating ADHD (Biederman and Spencer, 1999). The activity of NET at postganglionic sympathetic nerve terminals, especially in the heart, is impacted in diseases of the cardiovascular system (Blakely, 2001; Robertson et al., 2001). Diminished NE uptake sites and activity have been observed in hypertension, diabetes, cardiomyopathy, and heart failure, and ischemia-induced efflux of nonvesicular, cytoplasmic NE via NET may also contribute to fatal arrhythmias (Hahn and Blakely, 2002). NETs are also expressed in peripheral tissues like adrenal glands, vas deferens, and placenta. NET is the only catecholamine transporter present in the placenta and is thought to shield the fetus from fluctuating catecholamine levels in the maternal circulation. Analogous to the brain, blockade of placental NET by cocaine may result in elevated catecholamines in the maternal circulation. It is likely that pregnancy complications like preterm birth, spontaneous abortion, and abruptio placentae associated with maternal cocaine abuse relate to changes in the placental vascular physiology resulting from altered catecholamine signaling. DA affinity for NET is higher compared with its affinity for DAT, and NET density in the prefrontal cortex of the brain is higher than DAT density (Horn, 1973; Giros et al., 1994; Eshleman et al., 1999; Moron et al., 2002). NET-knockout (K/O) mice do not effectively clear DA in the frontal cortex, underscoring the NET as a DA carrier in the frontal cortex (Moron et al., 2002), and amphetamine reportedly releases DA from noradrenergic neurons in the prefrontal cortex (Shoblock et al., 2004). NET is poorly expressed in the striatum and robustly expressed in the frontal cortex. Therefore, selective NET inhibitors can raise DA levels in the frontal cortex, but not in the striatum. Thus, DAT/NET ratios in discrete brain regions are likely to govern selective catecholamine transport as well as selective drug effects on catecholamine transport. The behavioral outcome depends on the test used. In studies on locomotion in NET K/O mice, it has been suggested (Mead et al., 2002) that differences in baseline locomotion should be taken into account in interpreting the observed psychostimulant supersensitivity (Xu et al., 2000) and reduced cocaine sensitivity (Mead et al., 2002). While these studies indicate a role for the NET in the acute drug effect, the NET is not a prerequisite for the locomotor effect as opposed to the DAT that is critical as shown by the lack of effect of cocaine or amphetamine in DAT K/O mice (Giros et al., 1996; Mead et al., 2002). In contrast, in cocaine self-administration studies, likely measuring cocaine's reinforcing effect, NET becomes a major contributor in the absence of DAT. Thus, while cocaine self-administration in DAT K/O mice is intact (Rocha et al., 1998), DA is cleared by NET in DAT K/O animals (Moron et al., 2002). In support of this notion, cocaine and amphetamine increased dialysate DA in the nucleus accumbens of DAT K/O mice as did the specific NET blocker reboxetine; selective blockade of DAT by GBR 12909 in DAT K/Os had no effect on nucleus accumbens DA (Carboni et al., 2001). It appears therefore that cocaine or amphetamine can act at the NET, which takes over the clearance of DA in the nucleus accumbens when DAT is absent in DAT K/Os. However, more information is needed to fully understand the mechanism as desipramine did not enhance DA uptake measured in vitro by voltammetry in the nucleus accumbens of DAT K/Os (Budygin et al., 2002).

5 The Dopamine Transporter

DA signaling regulates many crucial functions such as movement, emotion, and cognition (Carlsson et al., 2001; Greengard, 2001). DAT terminates dopaminergic neurotransmission by re-uptake of DA in presynaptic neurons and plays a key role in DA recycling. DAT can also provide reverse transport of DA under certain circumstances. Psychostimulants such as cocaine and amphetamine and drugs used for ADHD such as methylphenidate exert their actions via DAT (Sulzer et al., 1995; Sora et al., 1998). Recent molecular and pharmacological analyses using monoamine transport-K/O mice have confirmed the physiological importance and requirement of presynaptic amine transporter expression for normal transmitter clearance, presynaptic transmitter homeostasis, postsynaptic action, and drug responses (Rioux et al., 1999; Xu et al., 2000; Carboni et al., 2001). In particular, functional loss of DAT either through pharmacological inhibition (Kula and Baldessarini, 1991; Giros et al., 1992) or through gene knockout (Giros et al., 1996) results in profound physical, physiological, and behavioral changes.

DAT not only functions as a carrier for DA but also mediates other processes, adding another level of complexity to its potential role in neuropsychiatric diseases. In the substantia nigra, DAT can regulate DA release, previously thought to be the domain of D_2 DA autoreceptors. Originally discovered in DAT-expressing cells, DAT produces at least three types of ion channel-like conductances (Sonders et al., 1997; Ingram et al., 2002). In the substantia nigra, substrate transport by the DAT initiates an excitatory DAT-mediated current, cell depolarization, and consequent augmentation of somatodendritic DA release (Falkenburger et al., 2001; Ingram et al., 2002). DAT-mediated regulation of DA release differs from the D_2 autoreceptor control of release. In the presence of DA, DAT promotes DA release, whereas D_2 autoreceptor attenuates release. DAT-mediated DA release is triggered at relatively low DA levels, whereas D_2 autoreceptor control of DA release requires significantly higher DA concentrations (Ingram et al., 2002). Finally, DAT substrate clearance (and associated ion conductances) results in DA-neuron depolarization and increased neuronal firing rate, even if D_2 receptors are blocked (Mortensen and Amara, 2003). DAT control of DA release is region specific. In the striatum, DA clearance is a primary function of the DAT, whereas in the substantia nigra the DAT regulates extracellular DA levels by controlling both clearance and release. In DA terminal regions, D_2 receptor activation has been reported to enhance DAT function, adding another autoreceptor-mediated mechanism in regulating extraneuronal DA levels (see Gulley and Zahniser, 2003; Wu et al., 2002). Evidence for the critical and brain region-specific role of the DAT in regulating DA neurotransmission and presynaptic homeostasis comes from targeted deletion of the DAT gene in mice. In comparison with wild-type controls, DAT mutant mice exhibit significant phenotypic transformations, including hyperactivity, small size, skeletal abnormalities, pituitary hypoplasia, impaired care by females for their offspring, cognitive and sensorimotor gating deficits, and sleep dysregulation. The striatum of the mutant mice adapts by reducing the DA-synthesizing enzyme tyrosine hydroxylase, vesicular DA stores, stimulated DA release, and D_1 and D_2 (but not D_3) receptor densities and function (for review, see Gainetdinov and Caron, 2003). The extreme changes in DA-signaling systems of the striatum are not replicated in the frontal cortex, and indeed, this brain region retains normal dopaminergic systems. Because DAT density in the frontal cortex is low and DA uptake proceeds normally in the frontal cortex of DAT-K/O mice, it is unlikely that drug-induced blockade of the DAT is a significant contributor to elevated DA levels in the prefrontal cortex (see ❷ Sect. 4 for a role for NET when DAT density is low). In the normal brain, the frontal cortex expresses much lower levels of the DAT and DA autoreceptors, stores less DA, and relies more on DA synthesis than on vesicular recycling for DA release. These contrasting cortical and striatal DA regulatory processes have implications for ADHD.

6   Monoamine Transporters and Their Functional Regulation

Monoamine transporters, in general, function by sequestering monoamines from specific nerve terminals. However, in several brain regions and under certain conditions, monoamine transporter functions can overlap (Cases et al., 1998; Pan et al., 2001; Moron et al., 2002). Pharmacological and behavioral studies in genetic animal models with targeted disruption of monoamine transporters suggest functional overlap between these transporters. Consequently, pharmacological and physiological characterizations to distinguish their role in psychiatric illnesses and drug abuse require proper understanding of the mechanisms regulating monoamine transporter function.

A range of physiologic, pharmacologic, and activity-dependent mechanisms can regulate monoamine transporters acutely. Changes in the transporter activity or expression will have a significant impact on the duration and concentration of monoamines present in and outside the synaptic cleft. These changes resulting in the regulation of transport function, in turn, would influence pre- and postsynaptic responses to released monoamines. Several studies suggest the presence of endogenous regulatory mechanisms that influence transporter expression and function at the level of gene transcription and translation (long-term or chronic regulation requiring hours or days) or posttranslational protein modifications (short-term or acute regulation requiring seconds to minutes) (❷ *Figure 18-1*) (Blakely et al., 1997; Ramamoorthy, 2002; Jayanthi and Ramamoorthy, 2005).

6.1   Long-Term Regulation of Amine Transporters at the Gene Level

Structural analysis of transporter gene promoter regions reveals a number of canonical transcription-binding sites that may be important in controlling the responses of the transporter genes to regulatory factors (Lesch et al., 1994; Kawarai et al., 1997; Fritz et al., 1998; Flattem and Blakely, 2000; Murphy et al., 2004; Kelada et al., 2005; Marziniak et al., 2005). Relevant investigations performed on JAR cells have shown that activation of cAMP-dependent (mimicked by cholera toxin, forskolin, dibutryl cAMP) and -independent pathways (mimicked by staurosporine, interleukin-1β) increases 5-HT uptake. Increases in 5-HT uptake require prolonged stimulation as well as messenger RNA and protein synthesis (Ramamoorthy et al., 1995b, c). Similarly, angiotensin II increases NET activity at the level of regulating NET gene transcription (Lu et al., 1996).

6.2   Short-Term Regulation of Amine Transporters

Amino acid sequence analysis of SERT, DAT, and NET proteins reveal numerous consensus sites for protein kinases as well as putative interactive motifs in cytoplasmic domains suggesting that second messengers are able to play a role in posttranslational regulation of monoamine transporters. Before the cloning of monoamine transporters, evidence suggested a pivotal role for second messenger-linked pathways in the acute modulation of neurotransmitter uptake (Ramamoorthy, 2002). Potential pathways linked to second messenger-linked pathways might regulate transporter function acutely. Multiple reports have demonstrated a capacity of native and heterologously expressed amine transporters to be regulated rapidly following acute elevation/depletion of intracellular Ca^{2+}, treatment with calmodulin inhibitors, or via activation of PKC, NOS/cGMP, and MAPK pathways. Since the second messenger-linked pathways noted above can be linked to presynaptic receptors, these pathways may provide positive/negative feedback mechanisms in control of amine clearance in vivo (Blakely et al., 1998, 2005; Ramamoorthy, 2002; Melikian, 2004; Zahniser and Sorkin, 2004; Jayanthi and Ramamoorthy, 2005).

6.2.1   Mechanisms of Short-Term Monoamine Transporter Regulation

Regulation of transport function can occur directly by phosphorylation of transporter protein. Phosphorylation of transporter protein might in turn change its intrinsic transport activity, turnover rate, plasma membrane insertion by modulating exocytic fusion, or sequestration from the plasma membrane by modulating endocytic machinery. Alternatively, transporters can be regulated through their association with other interacting proteins by phosphorylation-dependent or -independent pathways. Substrate or antagonist binding may also modulate transport activity via its influence on transporter phosphorylation, trafficking, and interaction with transporter-interacting proteins. Posttranslational modifications such as glycosylation, phosphorylation, and ubiquitination regulate monoamine transporter function and expression levels (Vaughan et al., 1997; Ramamoorthy et al., 1998; Jayanthi et al., 2004; Jiang et al., 2004; Li et al., 2004; Miranda et al., 2005). In addition, variations in monoamine transporter gene sequences known as polymorphisms may also alter transporter expression levels, activity and/or regulation. Recent studies demonstrate that the activity and expression of monoamine transporters are regulated by phosphorylation

■ Figure 18-1

Regulated life cycle of the monoamine amine transporters. Since transporter activity is a property of the protein at the cell surface, the entire picture of "how" and "where" transporter proteins become modified during the course of normal biosynthesis or as a result of regulatory events is important. ❷ *Figure 18-1* illustrates a general hypothetical model that currently accounts for the known data on the regulation of monoamine transporters. Expression of transporter is regulated at the level of gene transcription and transporter protein expression. At the gene level, transporters are regulated by many cellular signals that control SERT gene transcription factors. At the protein level, monoamine transporters may be organized as a complex in the plasma membrane that can be regulated by several cellular mechanisms, such as phosphorylation, protein–protein interactions, and ubiquitination. Phosphorylated transporter enters into a regulated endocytosis pathway. Transporters may enter into a regulated endocytic pathway, and internalized transporters may be subjected to degradation or recycling depending on the signals and cell system. Internalized transporters could be dephosphorylated by associated protein phosphatase, allowing the return of nonphosphorylated transporters to the cell surface. In certain cases, transporter substrates may increase the plasma membrane residency time of the transporter. This may serve as a built-in "feedback" mechanism to autoregulate the transporter and suppress the influence of a specific stimulus. Thus, cocaine and other transporter ligands such as antidepressants can have effects on these regulatory mechanisms by themselves or via altered monoamine levels. Dysregulation of these normal, regulated life cycle of monoamine transporters may lead to altered synaptic monoamines and altered behaviors linked to psychiatric diseases and addiction. T, transporters; TAP, transporter-associated proteins; PP2A, protein phosphatase 2A; P, phosphorylation; ER, endoplasmic reticulum

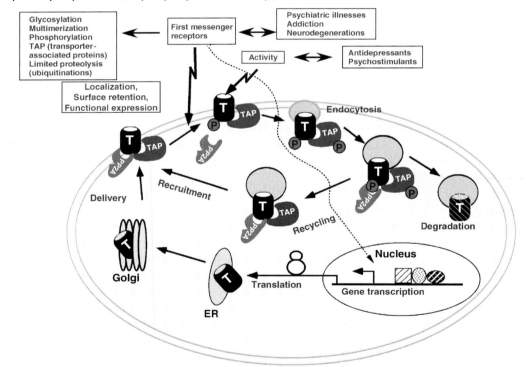

and dephosphorylation of the transporter proteins. Thus, monoamine transporters are dynamically regulated by intracellular and extracellular regulation of phosphorylation state, which in turn significantly impacts the duration and concentration of monoamines present in and outside the synaptic cleft (❷ *Figure 18-1*).

6.2.2 Trafficking-Dependent and Trafficking-Independent Regulation of Monoamine Transporters

Among various stimuli that acutely regulate monoamine transporters, the majority regulates transport function by altering transporter surface expression. Activation of PKC pathways by phorbol esters reduces 5-HT, NE, and DA transport capacity and the number of binding sites on the cell surface (for reviews, see Gulley and Zahniser, 2003; Mortensen and Amara, 2003). Presynaptic receptor activation such as NK1 activation leads to activation of PKC, and subsequently downregulation of DAT and NET. DA itself regulates the DAT, directly by downregulating surface expression, or indirectly by upregulating the DAT via D_2 autoreceptors (for review, see Gulley and Zahniser, 2003; Wu et al., 2002). Using PKC isoform-specific inhibitors as well as coexpression studies reveals the involvement of classical PKCβII in DAT downregulation. DAT function is also regulated by arachidonic acid, ethanol, tyrosine kinase activator/inhibitors, and nitric oxide (Lonart and Johnson, 1994; Zhang and Reith, 1996; Mayfield and Zahniser, 2001). Analogous PKC-mediated transporter redistribution has been detected for NET and SERT (Kitayama et al., 1994; Zhang et al., 1997; Apparsundaram et al., 1998a; 1998b; Jayanthi et al., 2004). In the transformed cell line SK-N-SH cells, where NET is expressed endogenously, activation of muscarinic acetylcholine receptors also results in NET downregulation. Moreover, inhibition of PKC by antagonists abolishes PKC-mediated effects but produces only partial blockade of methacholine-mediated effect. PKC activation and pathways dependent on mobilization of Ca^{2+} stores are involved in muscarinic receptor-mediated NET regulation (Apparsundaram et al., 1998a). Thus, studies show the existence of PKC-independent regulatory pathways supporting NET surface expression and/or intrinsic transporter catalytic activity.

Downregulation of transporters by PKC may be present but could occur across a different time frame. Indeed, recent studies using natively expressed SERT in platelets show diminished catalytic activity before an enhancement of SERT endocytic rate that ultimately reduces cell-surface SERT expression. Thus, these findings suggest that PKC activation regulates SERT in a biphasic manner, where the initial phase of inhibition occurs independent of trafficking and the later phase characterized by an enhanced endocytosis.

Hormones and trophic factors acting through tyrosine kinase-linked receptors have also been implicated in monoamine transport regulation. Insulin regulates NE transport (Boyd et al., 1985, 1986; Figlewicz et al., 1993, 1994, 1999). Recent work also shows regulation of DAT function by insulin, presumably through PI3-kinase (which is activated by the insulin receptor) (Carvelli et al., 2002), and downstream Akt (Garcia et al., 2005); this presumably plays a role in effects of food restriction on psychostimulant reinforcement. In the case of NET, MAPKs are involved, differentially regulating NET function by trafficking-dependent and -independent mechanisms (Apparsundaram et al., 2001).

Not only NET (Apparsundaram et al., 2001) but also DAT (Carvelli et al., 2002; Moron et al., 2003) and SERT (Zhu et al., 2004; Samuvel et al., 2005) are regulated by MAPKs. While studies on DAT (Moron et al., 2003) and SERT (Samuvel et al., 2005) implicate MAPK effects on transporter trafficking, other studies on NET and SERT indicate modulation of transporter catalytic activity. p38 MAPK-mediated SERT redistribution involves enhanced plasma membrane insertion of the transporter (Samuvel et al., 2005). Numerous studies have indicated alterations in 5-HT levels, SERT-binding sites, and serotonergic neuronal firing in response to numerous stressors (Chaouloff et al., 1999). Thus, the regulation of SERT by p38 MAPK, a stress-induced kinase, may provide a novel presynaptic mechanism in maintaining appropriate synaptic 5-HT levels during stressful conditions. Several studies indicate that SERT is upregulated by a cGMP/PKG-mediated pathway through altered surface expression (Miller and Hoffman, 1994; Kilic et al., 2003; Zhu et al., 2004). Interestingly, MAPK effects on SERT intrinsic activity are also sensitive to PKG activity (Zhu et al., 2004). Thus, monoamine transporters are subjected to multiple, interacting modes of kinase-dependent modulation via trafficking-dependent and -independent mechanisms.

6.3 Internalization Pathways

6.3.1 Clathrin-Dependent DAT Internalization

Monoamine transporters are internalized via clathrin-dependent and -independent pathways. Dominant-negative mutants of dynamin-1, which is shown to block clathrin-mediated endocytosis, are able to block

PKC-dependent DAT internalization (Daniels and Amara, 1999). These observations suggest that PKC regulates DAT internalization by clathrin-mediated and dynamin-dependent cellular mechanisms. They also provide evidence that internalized DAT is targeted to endosomal/lysosomal pathways for degradation. However, other studies show that internalized DAT is directed to the recycling pool (Melikian and Buckley, 1999), and plasma membrane DAT sequestration can occur due to a combination of accelerated internalization or reduced recycling (Loder and Melikian, 2003). However, the molecular mechanisms responsible for different PKC-dependent DAT internalization pathways (recycling endosomes versus degradative lysosomes) between these studies are unknown. Recently, clathrin-dependent mechanisms have been demonstrated for both constitutive and PKC-mediated DAT internalization (Sorkina et al., 2005). Nonclassical, distinct endocytic signals drive constitutive and PKC-regulated DAT internalization (Holton et al., 2005). The DAT internalization signal is conserved across SLC6 neurotransmitter carriers and is functional in the homologous NET. Together, the above studies suggest the involvement of unconventional mechanisms in DAT and NET internalization.

6.3.2 Caveolae/Lipid Raft-Mediated NET and SERT Internalization

Recent studies provided evidence for lipid raft localization and raft-mediated internalization of NET and SERT (Jayanthi et al., 2004; Samuvel et al., 2005). SERT and NET are also expressed in nonneuronal tissues such as placenta and intestinal epithelial cells (Ramamoorthy et al., 1993, 1995a; Jayanthi et al., 1993). PKC activation stimulates lipid raft-mediated internalization of native NETs expressed in placental trophoblasts (Jayanthi et al., 2004). Interestingly, PKC- but not p38 MAPK-mediated SERT regulation in the rat brain involves raft-mediated distribution (Samuvel et al., 2005). The presence of NET and SERT in lipid rafts suggests that signaling machinery specific to lipid rafts may be linked to PKC-mediated transporter downregulation. Raft-associated sorting has been proposed to underlie several cellular processes including signal transduction, protein sorting, and membrane trafficking (Chamberlain and Gould, 2002). Receptors such as NK1R, 5-HT$_3$, and TrkB, several channel proteins, many components of GPCR signal transduction proteins such as adenylyl cyclase, Akt1, PLC, activated PKC, PP2Ac, nonreceptor tyrosine kinases, and other signaling molecules such as syntaxin 1A (a SNARE protein), α-synuclein, and the PKC-binding protein PICK1 have been shown to be associated with lipid rafts (Simons and Toomre, 2000; Chamberlain and Gould, 2002). The localization of receptors such as NK1R that regulate monoamine transporter function and potential transporter-interacting proteins (syntaxin 1A, PP2Ac, PKC), as well as transporters in lipid raft microdomains, raises the possibility that lipid rafts may act as morphological "conveners" of signal transduction by placing various signal transduction molecules near the transporter molecule. For example, transporter-interacting proteins may "guide" targeting the transporter to lipid rafts, and phosphorylation of a "motif/site" within the transporter may act as a "signal" for fostering protein–protein interactions and redistribution. Thus, protein redistribution from plasma membrane microdomains may be one of the several mechanisms by which synaptic plasticity and neurotransmitter homeostasis are maintained (Simons and Ikonen, 1997; Parton and Richards, 2003). More interestingly, antidepressants and antipsychotic drugs are found to be colocalized in raft-like domains suggesting that lipid raft-localized amine transporters SERT and NET as well as 5-HT$_3$ receptors functionally interact with antidepressants and antipsychotic drugs in lipid rafts, and this interaction may play a role in the effect of these drugs in behavioral responses (Eisensamer et al., 2005).

6.4 Altered Transporter Phosphorylation

Recent studies on monoamine transporters reveal that changes in activity and expression are regulated by transporter phosphorylation and dephosphorylation. Thus, the transporters are dynamically regulated by intracellular and extracellular regulation of phosphorylation state, which in turn should have a significant impact on the duration and concentration of monoamines present extraneuronally. DAT, SERT, and

NET proteins are phosphorylated in response to PKC activation (Vaughan et al., 1997; Ramamoorthy et al., 1998; Jayanthi et al., 2004). SERTs are phosphorylated following PKC and PKA activation and protein phosphatase 2A (PP2A) inhibition. DAT proteins are also phosphorylated in transfected cells and synaptosomal preparations following treatment with PKC activators and PP2A inhibitors (Huff et al., 1997; Vaughan et al., 1997). The PKC-dependent phosphorylation shows a close temporal correlation with reduction in transport capacity (Ramamoorthy et al., 1998; Ramamoorthy and Blakely, 1999). SERT substrates and antagonists influence PKC-dependent SERT phosphorylation and surface redistribution (Ramamoorthy and Blakely, 1999). Recent studies indicate that while PKC activation increases SERT basal phosphorylation, p38 MAPK inhibition decreases SERT basal phosphorylation indicating a role for p38 MAPK-induced phosphorylation in constitutive SERT expression (Samuvel et al., 2005). More recently, investigations from Ramamoorthy's laboratory identified a previously unidentified biphasic regulation of endogenous SERTs expressed in platelets (Jayanthi et al., 2005). The findings from this study suggest that PKC activation regulates SERT in a biphasic manner, where the initial phase of inhibition occurs independent of trafficking and the later phase is characterized by an enhanced endocytosis. The biphasic inhibition of SERT is accompanied by a sequential phosphorylation of plasma membrane-resident SERT initially on serine residue(s) and then on threonine residue(s), suggesting that the initial phosphorylation on serine residues might be responsible for changes in the intrinsic properties and/or silencing of SERT and that the phosphorylation on threonine residues later on might trigger internalization of phosphorylated SERT.

DAT is phosphorylated on N-terminal serine residues (Foster et al., 2002). The PKC-mediated internalization of monoamine transporters occurs in parallel to an enhanced phosphorylation of the transporter. Although the transporters undergo phosphorylation in response to PKC activation or PP1/2A inhibition, it is not known whether phosphorylation of the transporter leads to its internalization. However, recent studies using phospho-site mutants of transporters provided positive as well as negative correlations between phosphorylation and transporter functional regulation (Bonisch et al., 1998; Whitworth and Quick, 2001b; Granas et al., 2003; Lin et al., 2003). Studies demonstrate that tyrosine kinase activity is also critical in maintaining NET (Apparsundaram et al., 2001), DAT (Doolen and Zahniser, 2001), and GAT (Law et al., 2000; Whitworth and Quick, 2001a) cell-surface levels. Phosphorylation of Y107 and Y317 on GAT1 is required for tyrosine kinase-mediated GABA transport regulation (Whitworth and Quick, 2001). Interestingly, the reciprocal relationship between PKC- and tyrosine kinase-mediated GAT1 phosphorylation suggests that a balance between these two states of phosphorylation may dictate relative abundance of GAT1 on the cell surface (Quick et al., 2004).

While a part of N-terminal domain appears to interact with syntaxin 1A involved in PKC-mediated regulation (Sung et al., 2003), determinants within the C terminus of human NET (hNET) dictate NET trafficking, stability, and activity (Bauman and Blakely, 2002). Interestingly, nonclassical endocytic signals dictate constitutive and PKC-regulated internalization of DAT (Holton et al., 2005; Sorkina et al., 2005). These signals are conserved in NET. However, it is not known whether there is a relationship between NET phosphorylation and PKC-induced transporter regulation. NET protein contains multiple consensus sites for several kinases including PKC that are distinct from those present in DAT or SERT, and therefore, NET may be regulated by mechanisms that are different than those of DAT and SERT. Recent work by Jayanthi's laboratory (Jayanthi et al., 2006) demonstrates that a PKC-site mutant of hNET is resistant to PKC-mediated downregulation and phosphorylation. This study provides the first evidence that phosphorylation of a PKC motif on a monoamine transporter is linked to transporter internalization. In addition, this PKC-site mutant of hNET exhibits altered transport properties such as increased affinity for NE and substrate-like ligand D-amphetamine and decreased affinity for inhibitory ligands like cocaine, desipramine, and nisoxetine. Phospho-site mutations could contribute to altered NE transport process due to physical conformational changes occurring as the result of mutation or the altered phosphorylation state itself. Such changes can result in altered binding or recognition of the ligands. Recent studies on DAT harboring mutations in the second intracellular loop reported altered ligand-binding properties attributed to structural changes in the physical conformation of DAT protein (Uhl and Lin, 2003; Goldberg et al., 2003; Loland et al., 2004; Fornes et al., 2004). Such investigations would prove useful in developing antidepressant drugs with higher efficacy and reduced potential side effects.

6.5 Regulated Protein–Protein Interactions

Monoamine transporters can act as a single unit, self-associate, or bind to other proteins. As described earlier, agents that maintain the phosphorylated state modulate amine transporter activity. For example, inhibition of PP1/PP2A by okadaic acid (OK) downregulates SERT, DAT, and NET activity. Phosphorylation state and regulation of amine transporter is a balance between the actions and localization of protein kinases and protein phosphatases. The pronounced effect of PP1/PP2A inhibition on amine uptake and amine transporter phosphorylation suggests the possible physical association of PP1/PP2A as a regulatory complex with amine transporter proteins. Indeed, physical complexes containing biogenic amine transporter and PP2Ac protein were recently demonstrated (Bauman et al., 2000). The SERT/PP2A complex is disrupted by PP1/PP2A inhibitors as well as PKC activators and can be stabilized by the SERT substrate 5-HT, suggesting that modulation of SERT/phosphatase association is involved in regulated transporter phosphorylation and trafficking. Similar transporter and PP2Ac associations were found for DAT and NET proteins. Analogous to findings in SERT studies, PP2Ac association with NET in vas deferens was also decreased by PKC activation and PP1/PP2A inhibition.

While direct phosphorylation and/or dephosphorylation of transporters by cellular protein kinases and phosphatases is involved in the dynamic regulation and expression of transporters, other integral membrane proteins also appear to play an important role in trafficking and catalytic function of transporters. The first evidence for the physical association of GAT1 GABA transporter with (t)-SNARE protein syntaxin-1A as a complex comes from studies by Quick and his coworkers (Deken et al., 2000; Horton and Quick, 2001). DAT, SERT, and NET are also physically associated with syntaxin-1A (Haase et al., 2001; Sung et al., 2003; Lee et al., 2004; Samuvel et al., 2005). Using noradrenergic tissues such as vas deferens and transfected cell lines, Sung and coworkers (2003) reported that syntaxin-1A is found in NET immunoprecipitates. Activation of PKC or phosphatase inhibition decreases syntaxin-1A level with NET. Altering intracellular Ca^{2+} also regulates syntaxin-1A/NET interaction. p38 MAPK inhibition and PKC activation decreases SERT and syntaxin-1A interactions in rat brain synaptosomes (Samuvel et al., 2005). Together these findings suggest an important role for syntaxin-1A in neurotransmission by regulating both transmitter release and reuptake.

DAT interacts with several regulatory proteins, including α-synuclein, syntaxin-1A, and PICK. Monoamine transporters also exist in oligomeric forms, but their functional significance is not known (Schmid et al., 2001; Norgaard-Nielsen et al., 2002; Torres et al., 2003) (also see reviews by Schmid et al., 2001; Sitte et al., 2004). Certain intracellular proteins such as PICK1 (protein-1 that interacts with C-kinase) and α-synuclein also interact with the DAT to stabilize its cell-surface expression (Torres et al., 2001; Sidhu et al., 2004). Signals following presynaptic receptor stimulation may influence transporter function and expression by regulating the stability of transporter heteromeric complexes. Studies show interaction of PDZ domain-containing protein PICK1 with C-terminal cytoplasmic domains of DAT and NET (Torres et al., 2001). Coexpression of DAT and PICK1 enhances DAT activity and PICK1 co-immunoprecipitates with DAT. Confocal microscopy analysis reveals colocalization of both DAT and PICK1 in heterologous systems and in dissociated dopaminergic neurons. Since PICK1 is a PKC-binding protein, it is possible that PICK1 acts like an adaptor to bring PKC near DAT proteins, which in turn could regulate PKC-evoked DAT phosphorylation, trafficking, and function. Such DAT and PKCβII interactions have been recently demonstrated (Johnson et al., 2005). α-Synuclein is enriched in dopaminergic nerve terminals and has been implicated in Parkinson's and other neurodegenerative disorders (Polymeropoulos et al., 1997). α-Synuclein binds directly to the C-terminal region of DAT and facilitates plasma membrane clustering and increase in DAT activity (Lee et al., 2001; Wersinger et al., 2004). This study suggests that the α-synuclein/DAT complex regulates normal dopaminergic neurotransmission and altered interactions may result in abnormal DAT function causing dopaminergic neurodegeneration seen in Parkinson's disease. DAT also interacts with LIM domain-containing adapter protein, Hic-5 (Carneiro et al., 2002). Hic-5 is known to interact with signaling molecules such as nonreceptor protein tyrosine kinases FAK and FYN. This raises the possibility that Hic-5 may be involved in tyrosine kinase-mediated DAT regulation. Together, these studies indicate that protein–protein interactions play an important role in influencing transporter phosphorylation, trafficking, and intrinsic activity.

6.6 Influence of Substrates and Antagonists on Monoamine Transport Regulation

Amine transporter substrates and antagonists are known to regulate transporter function and expression (Bernstein and Quick, 1999; Munir et al., 2000; Quick, 2002; Samuvel et al., 2005). Since transporters are subjected to phosphorylation by multiple kinase-dependent modulations, it is possible that substrates may also influence transporter surface expression by regulating kinase-mediated transporter phosphorylation. For example, SERT substrates such as 5-HT, amphetamines, and fenfluramine and antagonists such as antidepressants and cocaine control PKC-dependent SERT phosphorylation and surface redistribution (Ramamoorthy and Blakely, 1999). SERT-transporting substrates, 5-HT, amphetamine, and fenfluramine, protect SERT from PKC-linked phosphorylation and sequestration. The effect of 5-HT is SERT dependent but not 5-HT receptor-dependent, and the nontransported ligands such as cocaine and antidepressants block the effect of 5-HT. Interestingly, amphetamines substitute for substrates in suppressing PKC-mediated SERT phosphorylation. Such action could override homeostatic transporter sequestration processes and provide for psychostimulant sensitization by increasing the number of psychostimulant targets available to a subsequent stimulus. On the other hand, nonpermeant SERT ligands including SSRIs and cocaine that prevent 5-HT permeation block the effect of 5-HT, thus SSRIs may have therapeutic utility in disease states, not only by preventing 5-HT uptake but also by shifting the cellular distribution of SERT. D-Amphetamine, which is also a substrate for SERT, increases SERT basal phosphorylation that is sensitive to p38 MAPK inhibition suggesting that p38 MAPK may govern substrate-mediated effects on SERT basal phosphorylation (Samuvel et al., 2005).

NET proteins are downregulated following chronic treatment (3 days) with the NET substrate NE, amphetamine, and antagonist desipramine, perhaps through changes in protein expression and/or NET turnover (Zhu and Ordway, 1997; Zhu et al., 2000; Ordway et al., 2005).

DAT antagonists and substrates differentially modulate basal and PKC-mediated DAT phosphorylation in rat brain synaptosomes and DAT-expressing cell lines. Acute exposure to transporter substrates reduces DAT membrane expression, while brief treatment with transporter blockers increases DAT cell-surface expression. In addition, the regulation of DAT trafficking has been shown to tightly correlate with the functional regulation of DA transport capacity. Amphetamines trigger DAT internalization (Saunders et al., 2000), and while acute cocaine exposure increases DAT surface levels (Daws et al., 2002; Little et al., 2002), amphetamine-induced DAT internalization is blocked by cocaine (Saunders et al., 2000). This inverse relationship between antagonist binding and substrate translocation suggests that various transporter conformational states may promote or preclude their engagement with cellular endocytic machinery, dictating transporter surface levels.

Substrate translocation or ligand occupancy may influence the equilibrium of protein conformation required for transporter phosphorylation or transporter association with other regulators. Thus, a feedback loop may exist providing a mechanism by which changes in extracellular neurotransmitter concentrations could rapidly modulate neurotransmitter transport capacity. This way, the control of transporter cell-surface expression by its substrates or ligands would provide a novel homeostatic mechanism in the neuron to fine-tune transport capacity to match demands imposed by fluctuating levels of the neurotransmitter. Signaling pathways linked to presynaptic auto- and heteroreceptors could provide a positive/negative feedback control and provide a mechanism by which changes in extraneuronal neurotransmitters could rapidly modulate transport capacity of the transporter. Altered or inappropriate regulatory mechanisms may contribute to transporter dysregulation described in psychiatric and other disorders. Any disturbance in this homeostatic regulatory mechanism, for example by antidepressants or psychostimulants, would be predicted to alter the normative physiological regulation of 5-HT levels and potentially produce pathological or therapeutic effects. Determining the mechanism by which transporter substrates and blockers affect transporter cell-surface expression is certain to be important for the development of new therapies for the treatment of psychiatric illnesses, drug abuse, as well as other disease states such as ADHD and Parkinson's disease.

6.7   Dysregulation of Amine Transporters in Human Diseases

Biogenic amines 5-HT, DA, and NE control many behavioral and physiological functions in the CNS and PNS. Altered amines as well as amine transporters have been implicated in several psychiatric, neurodegenerative, and addictive disorders. Several other diseases and neuropsychiatric disorders are also likely to have genetic contributions from SERT, NET, and DAT. These include developmental disorders such as ADHD, autism, sudden infant death syndrome (SIDS), and Tourette's syndrome as well as equally complex disorders such as polysubstance abuse, irritable bowel syndrome (IBS), primary pulmonary hypertension (PPH), and myocardial infarction.

Two polymorphic regions, the long (*l*) and short (*s*) have been identified in the SERT promoter. The long (*l*) variant is associated with increased 5-HT uptake, and the short (*s*) with low 5-HT uptake. The "*s*" variant plays a functional dominance over the long allele. SERT-linked promoter regions have been implicated in anxiety, mood disorders, alcohol abuse, and other neuropsychiatric disorders. The degree to which SERT-linked promoter variants influence SERT expression in vivo is controversial, with both supportive and contradictory evidence (Flattem and Blakely, 2000; McCauley et al., 2004). A recent search for sequence variants in the SLC6A4 gene, encoding SERT, uncovered 15 variants in genomic DNA from a population of 450 individuals in the DNA Polymorphism Discovery Resource (Ozaki et al., 2003). Of these, six were synonymous and the remaining nine resulted in an amino acid change (Thr4Ala, Gly56Ala, Leu255Met, Ser293Phe, Pro339Leu, Leu362Met, Ile425Val, Lys605Asn, and Pro621Ser. Dennis Murphy of the NIMH reported that two unrelated probands and their family members with OCD contained the Ile425Val coding variant carried on the 5-HTTLPR/1/1 background (Ozaki et al., 2003). In functional studies, this variant has been found to exhibit elevated 5-HT uptake activity without any changes in SERT surface expression and insensitive to stimulation by nitric oxide donors in transfected cells (Kilic et al., 2003). Recently, Blakely's group identified several other human variants that are linked to autistic disorder (Prasad et al., 2005; Sutcliffe et al., 2005). Human SERT variants, T4A and G56A, failed to show 5-HT uptake stimulation when tested with 8-Br-cGMP and anisomycin, typical of wild-type hSERT. Importantly, in a physiologically relevant human cell model, such as Epstein–Barr virus (EBV)-transformed lymphocyte natively expressing the most common of these variants (Gly56Ala), a loss of 5-HT uptake stimulation by PKG and p38 MAPK activators was observed. Furthermore, HeLa cells transfected with the Gly56Ala variant exhibited elevated basal phosphorylation and, unlike wild-type hSERT, could not be further phosphorylated after 8-Br-cGMP treatment (Prasad et al., 2005). On the basis of these findings, it is hypothesized that OCD and autistic subjects carrying mutant SERT show elevated levels of SERT expression as if they were being stimulated constitutively through a cGMP-linked pathway.

The hNET gene is a single-copy gene (SLC6A2) located on chromosome 16 and containing 16 exons (Hahn and Blakely, 2002b). A number of hNET promoter, intron, and coding region polymorphisms have been identified through both discovery-oriented studies of hNET in various clinical populations or during the course of genome sequencing efforts (Hahn and Blakely, 2002). To date, approximately 20 nonsynonymous single nucleotide polymorphisms (SNPs), which result in amino acid substitutions, have been reported in hNET. Many of these variants were derived from psychiatric and cardiovascular phenotypes, yet only a limited number has been examined for alterations in expression or function (Halushka et al., 1999; Runkel et al., 2000; Stober et al., 2000; Iwasa et al., 2001). In a familial form of orthostatic intolerance, Blakely's laboratory identified a nonsynonymous hNET SNP that produces the protein variant, A457P, a loss of function, dominant-negative transporter that contributes to increased heart rate, high plasma NE levels, and reduced systemic NE clearance (Shannon et al., 2000; Hahn et al., 2003). This study demonstrates the impact of the hNET coding variant on NE clearance contributing to a human disease condition. Another recent study from Blakely's laboratory revealed striking effects of these naturally occurring SNPs on transporter protein expression, substrate transport, antagonist interaction, and regulation by kinase-mediated signaling pathways. Of particular interest are hNET F528C and hNET R121Q variants identified in some cardiovascular phenotypes that showed altered regulation by the PKC-mediated pathway. While F528C was insensitive, R121Q was more sensitive to PKC-dependent regulation suggesting that similar mechanisms may underlie differences observed in both basal and regulated transport (Hahn et al., 2005). These findings signify the search for underlying mechanisms of transporter regulation by signaling pathways in normal physiology and pathophysiology.

Altered DAT function or density has been implicated in various types of psychopathology, including depression, suicide, anxiety, aggression, and schizophrenia (Eichelman, 1990; Carlsson et al., 2001; Comings, 2001; Meyer et al., 2002). Associations between DAT gene polymorphisms and human disorders with possible links to the DA system, including ADHD and consequences of cocaine and alcohol abuse, have been reported (Miller et al., 2001; Hahn and Blakely, 2002a). Although the coding region of the human DAT gene contains very limited genetic variation, variants of the DAT gene may exist, and possibly arise from RNA editing or via other mechanisms (Miller et al., 2001). A repeat sequence in the 39-untranslated region (39-UTR) of the human DAT is associated with ADHD (Cook et al., 1995). A thorough examination of potential coding sequence polymorphisms in the human DAT failed to identify any common DAT sequence variants in more than 150 unrelated individuals free of neuropsychiatric disease, or with Tourette's syndrome, a diagnosis of ethanol dependence, or ADHD (Vandenbergh et al., 2000). The study did reveal a low frequency of two naturally occurring human DAT variants, i.e., V55A and V382A (Vandenbergh et al., 2000). In a subsequent report on COS cells expressing these variants, V55A was shown to display a lower K_m for DA uptake compared with wild type, and V382 a lower V_{max} (a dominant effect on expression observed also in the presence of wild type) as well as lower affinity of DA for DAT as measured by inhibition of cocaine analog binding (Lin and Uhl, 2003). In a separate study of 91 healthy controls or subjects with bipolar disease, Grunhage and coworkers (2000) detected two rare missense substitutions and three silent mutations in the whole coding region of the DAT. Altered transport properties associated with some of the coding variants of DAT suggest that individuals with these DAT variants could experience functional changes in their DA system (Lin and Uhl, 2002, 2003).

6.8 Monoamine Transporters in Addiction

Monoamine transporters are also of particular interest in the field of addiction because they constitute high-affinity molecular targets mediating the cellular and behavioral effects of psychostimulants such as amphetamine and cocaine (Reith et al., 1986; Seiden et al., 1993). Repeated use of certain transport inhibitors, such as cocaine, can eventually result in compulsive drug-seeking behavior. Given the importance of monoamine transmission in various aspects of addiction, and the profound influence that monoamine transport has on the extracellular levels of monoamines, as well as intracellular monoamine homeostasis, long-term changes in transporter level, kinetics, or regulation would be expected to greatly influence spontaneous and drug-induced behaviors. This possibility is clearly evidenced by the large effects on drug-induced behaviors, as well as on neurotransmitter synthesis, storage, and release by removing monoamine transporter genes in mutant mice (Giros et al., 1996; Bengel et al., 1998; Rocha et al., 1998; Sora et al., 1998). Receptors that are known to influence amine transporter functions, such as 5-HT$_{1B}$ (SERT), and D$_2$, opioid, or mGluR5 (DAT) have been implicated in cocaine sensitization (Nestler and Aghajanian, 1997; Pierce and Kalivas, 1997; Thompson et al., 2000; Page et al., 2001). Such changes in receptor-linked signaling cascades could influence phosphorylation of transporters or associated proteins, and thereby transport activity.

Since the second messenger-linked pathways can be linked to presynaptic receptors, these pathways may provide positive/negative feedback mechanisms in control of DA, 5-HT, and NE clearance in vivo.

Acknowledgments

The support from the National Institutes of Health, (DA016753 to LDJ), (MH062612, PO1AG023630-01A20004 and P50DA015369 to SR), and (DA 11978 to MEAR), is greatly acknowledged.

References

Altar CA. 1999. Neurotrophins and depression. Trends Pharmacol Sci 20: 59-61.

Amara SG, Arriza JL. 1993. Neurotransmitter transporters: Three distinct gene families. Curr Opin Neurobiol 3: 337-344.

Amara SG, Kuhan MJ. 1993. Neurotransmitter transporters: Recent progress. Annu Rev Neurosci 16: 73-93.

Ansah TA, Ramamoorthy S, Blakely RD. 2000. Elucidation of α_2-adrenergic receptor-mediated regulation of serotonin transport. Society for Neuroscience. New Orleans. 17.16.

Apparsundaram S, Galli A, De Felice LJ, Hartzell HC, Blakely RD. 1998a. Acute regulation of norepinephrine transport: I. PKC-linked muscarinic receptors influence transport capacity and transporter density in SK-N-SH cells. J Pharmacol Exp Ther 287: 733-743.

Apparsundaram S, Schroeter S, Blakely RD. 1998b. Acute regulation of norepinephrine transport. II. PKC-modulated surface expression of human norepinephrine transporter proteins. J Pharmacol Exp Ther 287: 744-751.

Apparsundaram S, Sung U, Price RD, Blakely RD. 2001. Trafficking-dependent and -independent pathways of neurotransmitter transporter regulation differentially involving p38 mitogen-activated protein kinase revealed in studies of insulin modulation of norepinephrine transport in SK-N-SH cells. J Pharmacol Exp Ther 299: 666-677.

Ase AR, Reader TA, Hen R, Riad M, Descarries L. 2001. Regional changes in density of serotonin transporter in the brain of 5-HT$_{1A}$ and 5-HT$_{1B}$ knockout mice, and of serotonin innervation in the 5-HT$_{1B}$ knockout. J Neurochem 78: 619-630.

Astier B, Van Bockstaele EJ, Aston-Jones G, Pieribone VA. 1990. Anatomical evidence for multiple pathways leading from the rostral ventrolateral medulla (nucleus paragigantocellularis) to the locus coeruleus in rat. Neurosci Lett 118: 141-146.

Axelrod J, Kopin IJ. 1969. The uptake, storage, release, and metabolism of noradrenaline in sympathetic nerves. Prog Brain Res 31: 21-32.

Balkovetz DF, Tiruppathi C, Leibach FH, Mahesh VB, Ganapathy V. 1989. Evidence for an imipramine-sensitive serotonin transporter in human placental brush-border membranes. J Biol Chem 264: 2195-2198.

Battersby S, Ogilvie AD, Blackwood DH, Shen S, Muqit MM, et al. 1999. Presence of multiple functional polyadenylation signals and a single nucleotide polymorphism in the $3'$ untranslated region of the human serotonin transporter gene. J Neurochem 72: 1384-1388.

Bauman AL, Apparsundaram S, Ramamoorthy S, Wadzinski BE, Vaughan RA, et al. 2000. Cocaine and antidepressant-sensitive biogenic amine transporters exist in regulated

complexes with protein phosphatase 2A. J Neurosci 20: 7571-7578.

Bauman PA, Blakely RD. 2002. Determinants within the C-terminus of the human norepinephrine transporter dictate transporter trafficking, stability, and activity. Arch Biochem Biophys 404: 80-91.

Bengel D, Murphy DL, Andrews AM, Wichems CH, Feltner D, et al. 1998. Altered brain serotonin homeostasis and locomotor insensitivity to 3,4-methylenedioxymetamphetamine ("ecstasy") in serotonin transporter-deficient mice. Mol Pharmacol 53: 649-655.

Bernstein EM, Quick MW. 1999. Regulation of γ-aminobutyric acid (GABA) transporters by extracellular GABA. J Biol Chem 274: 889-895.

Biederman J, Spencer T. 1999. Attention-deficit/hyperactivity disorder (ADHD) as a noradrenergic disorder. Biol Psychiatry 46: 1234-1242.

Bilkei-Gorzo A, Racz I, Michel K, Zimmer A. 2002. Diminished anxiety- and depression-related behaviors in mice with selective deletion of the Tac1 gene. J Neurosci 22: 10046-10052.

Blakely RD. 2001. Physiological genomics of antidepressant targets: Keeping the periphery in mind. J Neurosci 21: 8319-8323.

Blakely RD, Berson HE, Fremeau RT Jr, Caron MG, Peek MM, et al. 1991. Cloning and expression of a functional serotonin transporter from rat brain. Nature 354: 66-70.

Blakely RD, Defelice LJ, Galli A. 2005. Biogenic amine neurotransmitter transporters: Just when you thought you knew them. Physiology (Bethesda) 20: 225-231.

Blakely RD, Ramamoorthy S, Qian Y, Schroeter S, Bradley C. 1997. Regulation of antidepressant-sensitive serotonin transporters. Neurotransmitter Transporters: Structure, Function, and Regulation. Reith MEA, editor. Totowa, NJ: Humana Press; pp. 29-72.

Blakely RD, Ramamoorthy S, Schroeter S, Qian Y, Apparsundaram S, et al. 1998. Regulated phosphorylation and trafficking of antidepressant-sensitive serotonin transporter proteins. Biol Psychiatry 44: 169-178.

Bonisch H, Hammermann R, Bruss M. 1998. Role of protein kinase C and second messengers in regulation of the norepinephrine transporter. Adv Pharmacol 42: 183-186.

Boyd FT Jr, Clarke DW, Muther TF, Raizada MK. 1985. Insulin receptors and insulin modulation of norepinephrine uptake in neuronal cultures from rat brain. J Biol Chem 260: 15880-15884.

Boyd FT Jr, Clarke DW, Raizada MK. 1986. Insulin inhibits specific norepinephrine uptake in neuronal cultures from rat brain. Brain Res 398: 1-5.

Budygin EA, John CE, Mateo Y, Jones SR. 2002. Lack of cocaine effect on dopamine clearance in the core and shell of the nucleus accumbens of dopamine transporter knock-out mice. J Neurosci 22: RC222.

Bunney BS, Sesack SR, Silva NL. 1987. Midbrain dopaminergic systems: Neurophysiology and electrophysiological pharmacology. Melter HY, editor. Psychopharmacology: The Third Generation of Progress. Raven Press; New York: pp. 1113-1139.

Carboni E, Spielewoy C, Vacca C, Nosten-Bertrand M, Giros B, et al. 2001. Cocaine and amphetamine increase extracellular dopamine in the nucleus accumbens of mice lacking the dopamine transporter gene. J Neurosci 21: RC141: 141-144.

Carlsson A, Waters N, Holm-Waters S, Tedroff J, Nilsson M, et al. 2001. Interactions between monoamines, glutamate, and GABA in schizophrenia: New evidence. Ann Rev Pharmacol Toxicol 41: 237-260.

Carneiro AM, Ingram SL, Beaulieu JM, Sweeney A, Amara SG, et al. 2002. The multiple LIM domain-containing adaptor protein Hic-5 synaptically colocalizes and interacts with the dopamine transporter. J Neurosci 22: 7045-7054.

Carvelli L, Moron JA, Kahlig KM, Ferrer JV, Sen N, et al. 2002. PI-3-kinase regulation of dopamine uptake. J Neurochem 81: 859-869.

Cases O, Lebrand C, Giros B, Vitalis T, De Maeyer E, et al. 1998. Plasma membrane transporters of serotonin, dopamine, and norepinephrine mediate serotonin accumulation in atypical locations in the developing brain of monoamine oxidase A knock-outs. J Neurosci 18: 6914-6927.

Celada P, Siuciak JA, Tran TM, Altar CA, Tepper JM. 1996. Local infusion of brain-derived neurotrophic factor modifies the firing pattern of dorsal raphe serotonergic neurons. Brain Res 712: 293-298.

Chamberlain LH, Gould GW. 2002. The vesicle- and target-SNARE proteins that mediate Glut4 vesicle fusion are localized in detergent-insoluble lipid rafts present on distinct intracellular membranes. J Biol Chem 277: 49750-49754.

Chaouloff F, Berton O, Mormede P. 1999. Serotonin and stress. Neuropsychopharmacology 21: 28S-32S.

Cirillo P, Golino P, Ragni M, Battaglia C, Pacifico F, et al. 1999. Activated platelets and leucocytes cooperatively stimulate smooth muscle cell proliferation and proto-oncogene expression via release of soluble growth factors. Cardiovascular Res 43: 210-218.

Clark MS, Lanigan TM, Page NM, Russo AF. 1995. Induction of a serotonergic and neuronal phenotype in thyroid C-cells. J Neurosci 15: 6167-6178.

Comings DE. 2001. Clinical and molecular genetics of ADHD and Tourette syndrome. Two related polygenic disorders. Ann N Y Acad Sci 931: 50-83.

Consogno E, Dorigo C, Racagni G, Popoli M. 2000. Modification of presynaptic CaM kinase II affinity for ATP in hippocampus after long term blockade of serotonin reuptake. Life Sci 67: 1959-1967.

Cook EH, Stein MA, Krasowski MD, Cox NJ, Olkon DM, et al. 1995. Association of attention-deficit disorder and the dopamine transporter gene. Am J Med Genet 56: 993-998.

Daniels GM, Amara SG. 1999. Regulated trafficking of the human dopamine transporter. Clathrin-mediated internalization and lysosomal degradation in response to phorbol esters. J Biol Chem 274: 35794-35801.

Daws LC, Callaghan PD, Moron JA, Kahlig KM, Shippenberg TS, et al. 2002. Cocaine increases dopamine uptake and cell surface expression of dopamine transporters. Biochem Biophys Res Commun 290: 1545-1550.

Daws LC, Gerhardt GA, Frazer A. 1999. 5-HT$_{1B}$ antagonists modulate clearance of extracellular serotonin in rat hippocampus. Neurosci Lett 266: 165-168.

Daws LC, Gould GG, Teicher SD, Gerhardt GA, Frazer A. 2000. 5-HT$_{1B}$ receptor-mediated regulation of serotonin clearance in rat hippocampus in vivo. J Neurochem 75: 2113-2122.

Deken SL, Beckman ML, Boos L, Quick MW. 2000. Transport rates of GABA transporters: Regulation by the N-terminal domain and syntaxin 1A. Nat Neurosci 3: 998-1003.

Doolen S, Zahniser NR. 2001. Protein tyrosine kinase inhibitors alter human dopamine transporter activity in Xenopus oocytes. J Pharmacol Exp Ther 296: 931-938.

Eichelman BS. 1990. Neurochemical and psychopharmacologic aspects of aggressive behavior. Annu Rev Med 41: 149-158.

Eisensamer B, Uhr M, Meyr S, Gimpl G, Deiml T, et al. 2005. Antidepressants and antipsychotic drugs colocalize with 5-HT$_3$ receptors in raft-like domains. J Neurosci 25: 10198-10206.

Eshleman AJ, Carmolli M, Cumbay M, Martens CR, Neve KA, et al. 1999. Characteristics of drug interactions with recombinant biogenic amine transporters expressed in the same cell type. J Pharmacol Exp Ther 289: 877-885.

Fabre V, Beaufour C, Evrard A, Rioux A, Hanoun N, et al. 2000. Altered expression and functions of serotonin 5-HT$_{1A}$ and 5-HT$_{1B}$ receptors in knock-out mice lacking the 5-HT transporter. Eur J Neurosci 12: 2299-2310.

Falkenburger BH, Barstow KL, Mintz IM. 2001. Dendrodendritic inhibition through reversal of dopamine transport. Science 293: 2465-2470.

Faraj BA, Olkowski ZL, Jackson RT. 1997. Prevalence of high serotonin uptake in lymphocytes of abstinent alcoholics. Biochem Pharmacol 53: 53-57.

Figlewicz DP, Patterson TA, Zavosh A, Brot MD, Roitman M, et al. 1999. Neurotransmitter transporters: Target for endocrine regulation. Hormone Metab Res 31: 335-339.

Figlewicz DP, Szot P, Chavez M, Woods SC, Veith RC. 1994. Intraventricular insulin increases dopamine transporter mRNA in rat VTA/substantia nigra. Brain Res 644: 331-334.

Figlewicz DP, Szot P, Israel PA, Payne C, Dorsa DM. 1993. Insulin reduces norepinephrine transporter mRNA in vivo in rat locus coeruleus. Brain Res 602: 161-164.

Flattem NL, Blakely RD. 2000. Modified structure of the human serotonin transporter promoter. Mol Psychiatry 5: 110-115.

Fornes A, Nunez E, Aragon C, Lopez-Corcuera B. 2004. The second intracellular loop of the glycine transporter 2 contains crucial residues for glycine transport and phorbol ester-induced regulation. J Biol Chem 279: 22934-22943.

Foster JD, Pananusorn B, Vaughan RA. 2002. Dopamine transporters are phosphorylated on N-terminal serines in rat striatum. J Biol Chem 277: 25178-25186.

Fozzard J. 1989. Peripheral actions of 5-hydroxytryptamine. New York: Oxford University Press.

Fritz JD, Jayanthi LD, Thoreson MA, Blakely RD. 1998. Cloning and chromosomal mapping of the murine norepinephrine transporter. J Neurochem 70: 2241-2251.

Gainetdinov RR, Caron MG. 2003. Monoamine transporters: From genes to behavior. Annu Rev Pharmacol Toxicol 43: 261-284.

Garcia BG, Wei Y, Moron JA, Lin RZ, Javitch JA, et al. 2005. Akt is essential for insulin modulation of amphetamine-induced human dopamine transporter cell-surface redistribution. Mol Pharmacol 68: 102-109.

Giros B, El Mestikawy S, Godinot N, Zheng K, Han H, et al. 1992. Cloning, pharmacological characterization, and chromosome assignment of the human dopamine transporter. Mol Pharmacol 42: 383-390.

Giros B, Jaber M, Jones SR, Wightman RM, Caron MG. 1996. Hyperlocomotion and indifference to cocaine and amphetamine in mice lacking the dopamine transporter. Nature 379: 606-612.

Giros B, Wang YM, Suter S, McLeskey SB, Pifl C, et al. 1994. Delineation of discrete domains for substrate, cocaine, and tricyclic antidepressant interactions using chimeric dopamine-norepinephrine transporters. J Biol Chem 269: 15985-15988.

Glennon RA, Dukat M. 1995. Serotonin receptor subtypes. Psychopharmacology: The Fourth Generation of Progress. Bloom FE, Kupfer DJ, editors. New York: Raven Press; pp. 415-429.

Goldberg NR, Beuming T, Soyer OS, Goldstein RA, Weinstein H, et al. 2003. Probing conformational changes in neurotransmitter transporters: A structural context. Eur J Pharmacol 479: 3-12.

Goldstein DS. 1995. Stress, catecholamines, and cardiovascular disease. New York: Oxford University Press; pp. 280-286.

Granas C, Ferrer J, Loland CJ, Javitch JA, Gether U. 2003. N-terminal truncation of the dopamine transporter abolishes phorbol ester- and substance P receptor-stimulated phosphorylation without impairing transporter internalization. J Biol Chem 278: 4990-5000.

Greengard P. 2001. The neurobiology of slow synaptic transmission. Science 294: 1024-1030.

Grunhage F, Schulze TG, Muller DJ, Lanczik M, Franzek E, et al. 2000. Systematic screening for DNA sequence variation in the coding region of the human dopamine transporter gene (DAT1). Mol Psychiatry 5: 275-282.

Gulley JM, Zahniser NR. 2003. Rapid regulation of dopamine transporter function by substrates, blockers and presynaptic receptor ligands. Eur J Pharmacol 479: 139-152.

Haase J, Killian AM, Magnani F, Williams C. 2001. Regulation of the serotonin transporter by interacting proteins. Biochem Soc Transm 29: 722-728.

Haddjeri N, Blier P. 2001. Sustained blockade of neurokinin-1 receptors enhances serotonin neurotransmission. Biol Psychiatry 50: 191-199.

Hahn MK, Blakely RD. 2002a. Monoamine transporter gene structure and polymorphisms in relation to psychiatric and other complex disorders. Pharmacogenomics J 2: 217-235.

Hahn M, Blakely RD. 2002b. Gene organization and polymorphisms of monoamine transporters. Relationship to psychiatric and other complex diseases. Totowa: Humana Press; pp. 111-169.

Hahn MK, Robertson D, Blakely RD. 2003. A mutation in the human norepinephrine transporter gene (SLC6A2) associated with orthostatic intolerance disrupts surface expression of mutant and wild-type transporters. J Neurosci 23: 4470-4478.

Hahn MK, Mazei-Robison MS, Blakely RD. 2005. Single nucleotide polymorphisms in the human norepinephrine transporter gene affect expression, trafficking, antidepressant interaction, and protein kinase C regulation. Mol Pharmacol 68: 457-466.

Halushka MK, Fan JB, Bentley K, Hsie L, Shen N, et al. 1999. Patterns of single-nucleotide polymorphisms in candidate genes for blood-pressure homeostasis. Nat Genet 22: 239-247.

Heim C, Nemeroff CB. 2001. The role of childhood trauma in the neurobiology of mood and anxiety disorders: Preclinical and clinical studies. Biol Psychiatry 49: 1023-1039.

Heinz A, Mann K, Weinberger DR, Goldman D. 2001. Serotonergic dysfunction, negative mood states, and response to alcohol. Alcohol Clin Exp Res 25: 487-495.

Hoffman BJ, Mezey E, Brownstein MJ. 1991. Cloning of a serotonin transporter affected by antidepressants. Science 254: 579-580.

Holden JE, Naleway E. 2001. Microinjection of carbachol in the lateral hypothalamus produces opposing actions on nociception mediated by α_1- and α_2-adrenoceptors. Brain Res 911: 27-36.

Holton KL, Loder MK, Melikian HE. 2005. Nonclassical, distinct endocytic signals dictate constitutive and PKC-regulated neurotransmitter transporter internalization. Nat Neurosci 8: 881-888.

Horn AS. 1973. Structure-activity relations for the inhibition of catecholamine uptake into synaptosomes from noradrenaline and dopaminergic neurones in rat brain homogenates. Br J Pharmacol 47: 332-338.

Horton N, Quick MW. 2001. Syntaxin 1A up-regulates GABA transporter expression by subcellular redistribution. Mol Membr Biol 18: 39-44.

Huff RA, Vaughan RA, Kuhar MJ, Uhl GR. 1997. Phorbol esters increase dopamine transporter phosphorylation and decrease transport V_{max}. J Neurochem 68: 225-232.

Ingram SL, Prasad BM, Amara SG. 2002. Dopamine transporter-mediated conductances increase excitability of midbrain dopamine neurons. Nat Neurosci 5: 971-978.

Iversen LL. 1978. Uptake processes for biogenic amines. Handbook of Psychopharmacology. Iversen I, editor. New York: Plenum Press; pp. 381-442.

Iwasa H, Kurabayashi M, Nagai R, Nakamura Y, Tanaka T. 2001. Genetic variations in five genes involved in the excitement of cardiomyocytes. J Hum Genet 46: 549-552.

Jacobs B, Azmitia EC. 1992. Structure and function of the brain serotonin system. Physiol Rev 72: 165-229.

Jacobs BL, Fornal CA. 1991. Activity of brain serotonergic neurons in the behaving animal. Pharmacol Rev 43: 563-578.

Jasmin L, Tien D, Weinshenker D, Palmiter RD, Green PG, et al. 2002. The NK1 receptor mediates both the hyperalgesia and the resistance to morphine in mice lacking noradrenaline. Proc Natl Acad Sci USA 99: 1029-1034.

Jayanthi LD, Ramamoorthy S. 2005. Regulation of monoamine transporters: Influence of psychostimulants and therapeutic antidepressants. AAPS J 7: E728-E738.

Jayanthi LD, Balasubramaniam A, Samuvel DJ, Gether U, Ramamoorthy S. 2006. Phosphorylation of the norepinephrine transporter at threonine 258 and serine 259 is linked to protein kinase C-mediated transporter internalization. J Biol Chem 281: 23326-23340.

Jayanthi LD, Prasad PD, Ramamoorthy S, Mahesh VB, Leibach FH, et al. 1993. Sodium- and chloride-dependent, cocaine-sensitive, high-affinity binding of nisoxetine to the human placental norepinephrine transporter. Biochemistry 32: 12178-12185.

Jayanthi LD, Samuvel DJ, Blakely RD, Ramamoorthy S. 2005. Evidence for biphasic effects of protein kinase C on serotonin transporter function, endocytosis, and phosphorylation. Mol Pharmacol 67: 2077-2087.

Jayanthi LD, Samuvel DJ, Ramamoorthy S. 2004. Regulated internalization and phosphorylation of the native

norepinephrine transporter in response to phorbol esters: Evidence for localization in lipid rafts and lipid raft mediated internalization. J Biol Chem 279: 19315-19326.

Jiang H, Jiang Q, Feng J. 2004. Parkin increases dopamine uptake by enhancing the cell surface expression of dopamine transporter. J Biol Chem 279: 54380-54386.

Johnson LA, Guptaroy B, Lund D, Shamban S, Gnegy ME. 2005. Regulation of amphetamine-stimulated dopamine efflux by protein kinase C β. J Biol Chem 280: 10914-10919.

Kawarai T, Kawakami H, Yamamura Y, Nakamura S. 1997. Structure and organization of the gene encoding human dopamine transporter. Gene 195: 11-18.

Kelada SN, Costa-Mallen P, Checkoway H, Carlson CS, Weller TS, et al. 2005. Dopamine transporter (SLC6A3) 5′ region haplotypes significantly affect transcriptional activity in vitro but are not associated with Parkinson's disease. Pharmacogenet Genomics 15: 659-668.

Kilic F, Murphy DL, Rudnick G. 2003. A human serotonin transporter mutation causes constitutive activation of transport activity. Mol Pharmacol 64: 440-446.

Kitayama S, Dohi T, Uhl G. 1994. Phorbol esters alter functions of the expressed dopamine transporter. Eur J Pharmacol Molecular Pharmacology Section 268: 115-119.

Klimek V, Stockmeier C, Overholser J, Meltzer HY, Kalka S, et al. 1997. Reduced levels of norepinephrine transporters in the locus coeruleus in major depression. J Neurosci 17: 8451-8458.

Kula NS, Baldessarini RJ. 1991. Lack of increase in dopamine transporter binding or functions in rat brain tissue after treatment with blockers of neuronal uptake of dopamine. Neuropharmacology 30: 89-92.

Langer SZ. 1987. Presynaptic Regulation of Monoaminergic Neurons. Psychopharmacology: The Third Generation of Progress. Meltzer HY, editor. New York: Raven Press; pp. 151-157.

Langer SZ. 1997. 25 years since the discovery of presynaptic receptors: Present knowledge and future perspectives. Trends Pharmacol Sci 18: 95-99.

Launay J, Bondoux D, Oset-Gasque M, Emami S, Mutel V, et al. 1994. Increase of human platelet serotonin uptake by atypical histamine receptors. Am J Physiol 266: 526-536.

Law RM, Stafford A, Quick MW. 2000. Functional regulation of γ-aminobutyric acid transporters by direct tyrosine phosphorylation. J Biol Chem 275: 23986-23991.

Lee FJ, Liu F, Pristupa ZB, Niznik HB. 2001. Direct binding and functional coupling of α-synuclein to the dopamine transporters accelerate dopamine-induced apoptosis. FASEB J 15: 916-926.

Lee KH, Kim MY, Kim DH, Lee YS. 2004. Syntaxin 1A and receptor for activated C kinase interact with the N-terminal region of human dopamine transporter. Neurochem Res 29: 1405-1409.

Lesch KP, Balling U, Gross J, Strass K, Wolozin BL, et al. 1994. Organization of the human serotonin transporter gene. J Neural Transm 95: 157-162.

Lesch KP, Bengel D, Heils A, Sabol SZ, Greenberg BD, et al. 1996. Association of anxiety-related traits with a polymorphism in the serotonin transporter gene regulatory region. Science 274: 1527-1531.

Lesch KP, Wolozin BL, Murphy DL, Riederer P. 1993. Primary structure of the human platelet serotonin uptake site: Identity with the brain serotonin transporter. J Neurochem 60: 2319-2322.

Lieb K, Ahlvers K, Dancker K, Strohbusch S, Reincke M, et al. 2002. Effects of the neuropeptide substance P on sleep, mood, and neuroendocrine measures in healthy young men. Neuropsychopharmacology 27: 1041-1049.

Lin Z, Uhl GR. 2002. Dopamine transporter mutants with cocaine resistance and normal dopamine uptake provide targets for cocaine antagonism. Mol Pharmacol 61: 885-891.

Lin Z, Uhl GR. 2003. Human dopamine transporter gene variation: Effects of protein coding variants V55A and V382A on expression and uptake activities. Pharmacogenomics J 3: 159-168.

Lin Z, Zhang PW, Zhu X, Melgari JM, Huff R, et al. 2003. Phosphatidylinositol-3-kinase, protein kinase C, MEK1/2 kinase regulation of dopamine transporters (DAT) require N-terminal DAT phospho acceptor sites. J Biol Chem 278: 20162-20170.

Little KY, Elmer LW, Zhong H, Scheys JO, Zhang L. 2002. Cocaine induction of dopamine transporter trafficking to the plasma membrane. Mol Pharmacol 61: 436-445.

Loder MK, Melikian HE. 2003. The dopamine transporter constitutively internalizes and recycles in a protein kinase C-regulated manner in stably transfected PC12 cell lines. J Biol Chem 278: 22168-22174.

Loland CJ, Granas C, Javitch JA, Gether U. 2004. Identification of intracellular residues in the dopamine transporter critical for regulation of transporter conformation and cocaine binding. J Biol Chem 279: 3228-3238.

Lonart G, Johnson KM. 1994. Inhibitory effects of nitric oxide on the uptake of [^{3}H]dopamine and [^{3}H]glutamate by striatal synaptosomes. J Neurochem 63: 2108-2117.

Lu D, Yu K, Paddy MR, Rowland NE, Raizada MK. 1996. Regulation of norepinephrine transport system by angiotensin II in neuronal cultures of normotensive and spontaneously hypertensive rat brains. Endocrinology 137: 763-772.

Li LB, Chen N, Ramamoorthy S, Chi L, Cui XN, et al. 2004. The role of N-glycosylation in function and surface trafficking of the human dopamine transporter. J Biol Chem 279: 21012-21020.

Maes M, Van Gastel A, Delmeire L, Meltzer HY. 1999. Decreased platelet α_2-adrenoceptor density in major depression: Effects of tricyclic antidepressants and fluoxetine. Biol Psychiatry 45: 278-284.

Marziniak M, Mossner R, Schmitt A, Lesch KP, Sommer C. 2005. A functional serotonin transporter gene polymorphism is associated with migraine with aura. Neurology 64: 157-159.

Mayfield RD, Zahniser NR. 2001. Dopamine D_2 receptor regulation of the dopamine transporter expressed in Xenopus laevis oocytes is voltage-independent. Mol Pharmacol 59: 113-121.

McCauley JL, Olson LM, Dowd M, Amin T, Steele A, et al. 2004. Linkage and association analysis at the serotonin transporter (SLC6A4) locus in a rigid-compulsive subset of autism. Am J Med Genet 127B: 104-112.

Mead AN, Rocha BA, Donovan DM, Katz JL. 2002. Intravenous cocaine induced-activity and behavioural sensitization in norepinephrine-, but not dopamine-transporter knockout mice. Eur J Neurosci 16: 514-520.

Melikian HE. 2004. Neurotransmitter transporter trafficking: Endocytosis, recycling, and regulation. Pharmacol Therap 104: 17-27.

Melikian HE, Buckley KM. 1999. Membrane trafficking regulates the activity of the human dopamine transporter. J Neurosci 19: 7699-7710.

Meltzer HY, Arora RC, Baber R, Tricou BJ. 1981. Serotonin uptake in blood platelets of psychiatric patients. Arch Gen Psychiatry 38: 1322-1326.

Meyer JH, Goulding VS, Wilson AA, Hussey D, Christensen BK, et al. 2002. Bupropion occupancy of the dopamine transporter is low during clinical treatment. Psychopharmacology (Berl) 163: 102-105.

Miller GM, De La Garza RD, 2nd, Novak MA, Madras BK. 2001. Single nucleotide polymorphisms distinguish multiple dopamine transporter alleles in primates: Implications for association with attention deficit hyperactivity disorder and other neuropsychiatric disorders. Mol Psychiatry 6: 50-58.

Miller JW, Kleven DT, Domin BA, Fremeau RT Jr. 1997. Cloned sodium- (and chloride-) dependent high-affinity transporters for GABA, glycine, proline, betaine, taurine, and creatine. Neurotransmitter Transporters: Structure, Function, and Regulation. Reith MEA, editor. Totowa, NJ: Humana Press; pp. 101-150.

Miller KJ, Hoffman BJ. 1994. Adenosine A_3 receptors regulate serotonin transport via nitric oxide and cGMP. J Biol Chem 269: 27351-27356.

Miranda M, Wu CC, Sorkina T, Korstjens DR, Sorkin A. 2005. Enhanced ubiquitylation and accelerated degradation of the dopamine transporter mediated by protein kinase C. J Biol Chem 280: 35617-35624.

Morinobu S, Nibuya M, Duman RS. 1995. Chronic antidepressant treatment down-regulates the induction of c-fos mRNA in response to acute stress in rat frontal cortex. Neuropsychopharmacology 12: 221-228.

Moron JA, Brockington A, Wise RA, Rocha BA, Hope BT. 2002. Dopamine uptake through the norepinephrine transporter in brain regions with low levels of the dopamine transporter: Evidence from knock-out mouse lines. J Neurosci 22: 389-395.

Moron JA, Zakharova I, Ferrer JV, Merrill GA, Hope B, et al. 2003. Mitogen-activated protein kinase regulates dopamine transporter surface expression and dopamine transport capacity. J Neurosci 23: 8480-8488.

Mortensen OV, Amara SG. 2003. Dynamic regulation of the dopamine transporter. Eur J Pharmacol 479: 159-170.

Mossner R, Daniel S, Albert D, Heils A, Okladnova O, et al. 2000. Serotonin transporter function is modulated by brain-derived neurotrophic factor (BDNF) but not nerve growth factor (NGF). Neurochem Int 36: 197-202.

Munir M, Correale DM, Robinson MB. 2000. Substrate-induced up-regulation of Na^+-dependent glutamate transport activity. Neurochem Int 37: 147-162.

Murphy DL, Lerner A, Rudnick G, Lesch KP. 2004. Serotonin transporter: Gene, genetic disorders, and pharmacogenetics. Mol Interv 4: 109-123.

Murphy DL, Wichems C, Li Q, Heils A. 1999. Molecular manipulations as tools for enhancing our understanding of 5-HT neurotransmission. Trends Pharmacol Sci 20: 246-252.

Musselman DL, Marzec U, Davidoff M, Manatunga AK, Gao F, et al. 2002. Platelet activation and secretion in patients with major depression, thoracic aortic atherosclerosis, or renal dialysis treatment. Depress Anxiety 15: 91-101.

Nestler EJ, Aghajanian GK. 1997. Molecular and cellular basis of addiction. Science 278: 58-63.

Nibuya M, Morinobu S, Duman RS. 1995. Regulation of BDNF and trkB mRNA in rat brain by chronic electroconvulsive seizure and antidepressant drug treatments. J Neurosci 15: 7539-7547.

Nicoll RA, Madison DV, Lancaster B. 1987. Noradrenergic modulation of neuronal excitability in mammalian hippocampus. Psychopharmacology: The Third Generation of Progress. Meltzer HY, editor. New York: Raven Press; pp. 105-112.

Norgaard-Nielsen K, Norregaard L, Hastrup H, Javitch JA, Gether U. 2002. Zn^{2+} site engineering at the oligomeric interface of the dopamine transporter. FEBS Lett 524: 87-91.

Ordway GA, Jia W, Li J, Zhu MY, Mandela P, et al. 2005. Norepinephrine transporter function and desipramine: Residual drug effects versus short-term regulation. Neurosci Methods 143: 217-225.

Owens MJ, Nemeroff CB. 1994. Role of serotonin in the pathophysiology of depression: Focus on the serotonin transporter. Clin Chem 40: 288-295.

Ozaki N, Goldman D, Kaye WH, Plotnicov K, Greenberg BD, et al. 2003. Serotonin transporter missense mutation associated with a complex neuropsychiatric phenotype. Mol Psychiatry 8: 895, 933-936.

Pacholczyk T, Blakely RD, Amara SG. 1991. Expression cloning of a cocaine- and antidepressant-sensitive human noradrenaline transporter. Nature 350: 350-354.

Page G, Peeters M, Najimi M, Maloteaux JM, Hermans E. 2001. Modulation of the neuronal dopamine transporter activity by the metabotropic glutamate receptor mGluR5 in rat striatal synaptosomes through phosphorylation-mediated processes. J Neurochem 76: 1282-1290.

Pan Y, Gembom E, Peng W, Lesch KP, Mossner R, et al. 2001. Plasticity in serotonin uptake in primary neuronal cultures of serotonin transporter knockout mice. Brain Res Dev Brain Res 126: 125-129.

Parton RG, Richards AA. 2003. Lipid rafts and caveolae as portals for endocytosis: New insights and common mechanisms. Traffic 4: 724-738.

Pavcovich LA, Cancela LM, Volosin M, Molina VA, Ramirez OA. 1990. Chronic stress-induced changes in locus coeruleus neuronal activity. Brain Res Bulletin 24: 293-296.

Pierce RC, Kalivas PW. 1997. Repeated cocaine modifies the mechanism by which amphetamine releases dopamine. J Neurosci 17: 3254-3261.

Polymeropoulos MH, Lavedan C, Leroy E, et al. 1997. Mutation in the α-synuclein gene identified in families with Parkinson's disease. Science 276: 2045-2047.

Popoli M, Brunello N, Perez J, Racagni G. 2000. Second messenger-regulated protein kinases in the Brain: Their functional role and the action of antidepressant drugs. J Neurochem 74: 21-33.

Popoli M, Venegoni A, Vocaturo C, Buffa L, Perez J, et al. 1997. Long term blockade of serotonin reuptake affects synaptotagmin phosphorylation in the hippocampus. Mol Pharmacol 51: 19-26.

Popoli M, Vocaturo C, Perez J, Smeraldi E, Racagni G. 1995. Presynaptic Ca^{2+}/calmodulin-dependent protein kinase II: Autophosphorylation and activity increase in the hippocampus after long-term blockade of serotonin reuptake. Mol Pharmacol 48: 623-629.

Povlock SL, Amara SG. 1997. The structure and function of norepinephrine, dopamine, and serotonin transporters. Neurotransmitter Transporters: Structure, Function, and Regulation. Reith MEA, editor. Totowa, NJ: Humana Press; pp. 1-28.

Prasad HC, Zhu CB, McCauley JL, Samuvel DJ, Ramamoorthy S, et al. 2005. Human serotonin transporter variants display altered sensitivity to protein kinase G and p38 mitogen-activated protein kinase. Proc Natl Acad Sci USA 102: 11545-11550.

Quick MW. 2002. Substrates regulate γ-aminobutyric acid transporters in a syntaxin 1A-dependent manner. Proc Natl Acad Sci USA 99: 5686-5691.

Quick MW, Hu J, Wang D, Zhang HY. 2004. Regulation of a γ-aminobutyric acid transporter by reciprocal tyrosine and serine phosphorylation. J Biol Chem 279: 15961-15967.

Ramamoorthy JD, Ramamoorthy S, Leibach FH, Ganapathy V. 1995a. Human placental monoamine transporters as targets for amphetamines. Am J Obstet Gynecol 173: 1782-1787.

Ramamoorthy JD, Ramamoorthy S, Papapetropoulos A, Catravas JD, Leibach FH, et al. 1995b. Cyclic AMP-independent up-regulation of the human serotonin transporter by staurosporine in choriocarcinoma cells. J Biol Chem 270: 17189-17195.

Ramamoorthy S, Ramamoorthy JD, Prasad P, Bhat GK, Mahesh VB, et al. 1995c. Regulation of the human serotonin transporter by interleukin-1β. Biochem Biophys Res Commun 216: 560-567.

Ramamoorthy S. 2002. Regulation of monoamine transporters: Regulated phosphorylation, dephosphorylation, and trafficking. Totowa, NJ: Humana Press Inc.; pp. 1-23.

Ramamoorthy S, Blakely RD. 1999. Phosphorylation and sequestration of serotonin transporters differentially modulated by psychostimulants. Science 285: 763-766.

Ramamoorthy S, Bauman AL, Moore KR, Han H, Yang-Feng T, et al. 1993. Antidepressant- and cocaine-sensitive human serotonin transporter: Molecular cloning, expression, and chromosomal localization. Proc Natl Acad Sci USA 90: 2542-2546.

Ramamoorthy S, Giovanetti E, Qian Y, Blakely RD. 1998. Phosphorylation and regulation of antidepressant-sensitive serotonin transporters. J Biol Chem 273: 2458-2466.

Ramamoorthy S, Prasad PD, Kulanthaivel P, Leibach FH, Blakely RD, et al. 1993. Expression of a cocaine-sensitive norepinephrine transporter in the human placental syncitiotrophoblast. Biochemistry 32: 1346-1353.

Reith MEA, Meisler BE, Sershen H, Lajtha A. 1986. Structural requirements for cocaine congeners to interact with dopamine and serotonin uptake sites in mouse brain and to induce stereotyped behavior. Biochem Pharmacol 35: 1123-1129.

Ressler KJ, Nemeroff CB. 1999. Role of norepinephrine in the pathophysiology and treatment of mood disorders. Biol Psychiatry 46: 1219-1233.

Ressler KJ, Nemeroff CB. 2001. Role of norepinephrine in the pathophysiology of neuropsychiatric disorders. CNS Spectra 6: 663-666, 670.

Rioux A, Fabre V, Lesch KP, Moessner R, Murphy DL, et al. 1999. Adaptive changes of serotonin 5-HT$_{2A}$ receptors in mice lacking the serotonin transporter. Neurosci Lett 262: 113-116.

Robertson D, Flattem N, Tellioglu T, Carson R, Garland E, et al. 2001. Familial orthostatic tachycardia due to norepinephrine transporter deficiency. Ann N Y Acad Sci 940: 527-543.

Rocha BA, Fumagalli F, Gainetdinov RR, Jones SR, Ator R, et al. 1998. Cocaine self-administration in dopamine-transporter knockout mice. Nat Neurosci 1: 132-137.

Rudnick G. 1977. Active transport of 5-hydroxytryptamine by plasma membrane vesicles isolated from human blood platelets. J Biol Chem 252: 2170-2174.

Runkel F, Bruss M, Nothen MM, Stober G, Propping P, et al. 2000. Pharmacological properties of naturally occurring variants of the human norepinephrine transporter. Pharmacogenetics 10: 397-405.

Rupniak NM, Kramer MS. 1999. Discovery of the antidepressant and anti-emetic efficacy of substance P receptor (NK1) antagonists. Trends Pharmacol Sci 20: 485-490.

Rupniak NM, Carlson EJ, Webb JK, Harrison T, Porsolt RD, et al. 2001. Comparison of the phenotype of NK1R−/−mice with pharmacological blockade of the substance P (NK1) receptor in assays for antidepressant and anxiolytic drugs. Behav Pharmacol 12: 497-508.

Russo-Neustadt AA, Beard RC, Huang YM, Cotman CW. 2000. Physical activity and antidepressant treatment potentiate the expression of specific brain-derived neurotrophic factor transcripts in the rat hippocampus. Neuroscience 101: 305-312.

Samuvel DJ, Jayanthi LD, Bhat NR, Ramamoorthy S. 2005. A role for p38 mitogen-activated protein kinase in the regulation of the serotonin transporter: Evidence for distinct cellular mechanisms involved in transporter surface expression. J Neurosci 25: 29-41.

Santarelli L, Gobbi G, Debs PC, Sibille ET, Blier P, et al. 2001. Genetic and pharmacological disruption of neurokinin 1 receptor function decreases anxiety-related behaviors and increases serotonergic function. Proc Natl Acad Sci USA 98: 1912-1917.

Saunders C, Ferrer JV, Shi L, Chen J, Merrill G, et al. 2000. Amphetamine-induced loss of human dopamine transporter activity: An internalization-dependent and cocaine-sensitive mechanism. Proc Natl Acad Sci USA 97: 6850-6855.

Schmid JA, Just H, Sitte HH. 2001. Impact of oligomerization on the function of the human serotonin transporter. Biochem Soc Transm 29: 732-736.

Schmid JA, Scholze P, Kudlacek O, Freissmuth M, Singer EA, et al. 2001. Oligomerization of the human serotonin transporter and of the rat GABA transporter 1 visualized by fluorescence resonance energy transfer microscopy in living cells. J Biol Chem 276: 3805-3810.

Schramm NL, McDonald MP, Limbird LE. 2001. The α$_{2a}$-adrenergic receptor plays a protective role in mouse behavioral models of depression and anxiety. J Neurosci 21: 4875-4882.

Schroeter S, Levey AI, Blakely RD. 1997. Polarized expression of the antidepressant-sensitive serotonin transporter in epinephrine-synthesizing chromaffin cells of the rat adrenal gland. Mol Cell Neurosci 9: 170-184.

Seiden LS, Sabol KE, Ricaurte GA. 1993. Amphetamine: Effects on catecholamine systems and behavior. Ann Rev Pharmacol Toxicol 32: 639-677.

Shannon JR, Flattem NL, Jordan J, Jacob G, Black BK, et al. 2000. Orthostatic intolerance and tachycardia associated with norepinephrine-transporter deficiency. N Engl J Med 342: 541-549.

Shirayama Y, Chen AC, Nakagawa S, Russell DS, Duman RS. 2002. Brain-derived neurotrophic factor produces antidepressant effects in behavioral models of depression. J Neurosci 22: 3251-3261.

Shirayama Y, Mitsushio H, Takashima M, Ichikawa H, Takahashi K. 1996. Reduction of substance P after chronic antidepressants treatment in the striatum, substantia nigra and amygdala of the rat. Brain Res 739: 70-78.

Shoblock JR, Maisonneuve IM, Glick SD. 2004. Differential interactions of desipramine with amphetamine and methamphetamine: Evidence that amphetamine releases dopamine from noradrenergic neurons in the medial prefrontal cortex. Neurochem Res 29: 1437-1442.

Sidhu A, Wersinger C, Vernier P. 2004. α-Synuclein regulation of the dopaminergic transporter: A possible role in the pathogenesis of Parkinson's disease. FEBS Lett 565: 1-5.

Simons K, Ikonen E. 1997. Functional rafts in cell membranes. Nature 387: 569-572.

Simons K, Toomre D. 2000. Lipid rafts and signal transduction. Nat Rev Mol Cell Biol 1: 31-39.

Sitte HH, Farhan H, Javitch JA. 2004. Sodium-dependent neurotransmitter transporters: Oligomerization as a determinant of transporter function and trafficking. Mol Interv 4: 38-47.

Sonders MS, Zhu SJ, Zahniser NR, Kavanauch MP, Amara SG. 1997. Multiple ionic conductances of the human dopamine transporter: The actions of dopamine and psychostimulants. J Neurosci 17: 960-974.

Sora I, Wichems C, Takahashi N, Li XF, Zeng Z, et al. 1998. Cocaine reward models: Conditioned place preference can be established in dopamine- and in serotonin-transporter knockout mice. Proc Natl Acad Sci USA 95: 7699-7704.

Sorkina T, Hoover BR, Zahniser NR, Sorkin A. 2005. Constitutive and protein kinase C-induced internalization of the dopamine transporter is mediated by a clathrin-dependent mechanism. Traffic 6: 157-170.

Stober G, Meyer J, Nanda I, Wienker TF, Saar K, et al. 2000. Linkage and family-based association study of schizophrenia and the synapsin III locus that maps to chromosome 22q13. Am J Med Genet 96: 392-397.

Stockmeier CA, Shapiro LA, Dilley GE, Kolli TN, Friedman L, et al. 1998. Increase in serotonin-1A autoreceptors in the

midbrain of suicide victims with major depression—postmortem evidence for decreased serotonin activity. J Neurosci 18: 7394-7401.

Stockmeier CA, Shi X, Konick L, Overholser JC, Jurjus G, et al. 2002. Neurokinin-1 receptors are decreased in major depressive disorder. Neuroreport 13: 1223-1227.

Sulzer D, Chen TK, Lau YY, Kristensen H, Rayport S, et al. 1995. Amphetamine redistributes dopamine from synaptic vesicles to the cytosol and promotes reverse transport. J Neurosci 15: 4102-4108.

Sung U, Apparsundaram S, Galli A, Kahlig KM, Savchenko V, et al. 2003. A regulated interaction of syntaxin 1A with the antidepressant-sensitive norepinephrine transporter establishes catecholamine clearance capacity. J Neurosci 23: 1697-1709.

Sutcliffe JS, Delahanty RJ, Prasad HC, McCauley JL, Han Q, et al. 2005. Allelic heterogeneity at the serotonin transporter locus (SLC6A4) confers susceptibility to autism and rigid-compulsive behaviors. Am J Hum Genet 77: 265-279.

Tadokoro C, Kiuchi Y, Yamazaki Y, Oguchi K, Kamijima K. 1998. Effects of imipramine and sertraline on protein kinase activity in rat frontal cortex. Eur J Pharmacol 342: 51-54.

Takahashi M, Terwilliger R, Lane C, Mezes PS, Conti M, et al. 1999. Chronic antidepressant administration increases the expression of cAMP-specific phosphodiesterase 4A and 4B isoforms. J Neurosci 19: 610-618.

Tamir H, Hsiung SC, Liu KP, Blakely RD, Russo AF, et al. 1996. Expression and development of a functional plasmalemmal 5-hydroxytryptamine transporter by thyroid follicular cells. Endocrinology 137: 4475-4485.

Tecott L, Shtrom S, Julius D. 1995. Expression of a serotonin-gated ion channel in embryonic neural and nonneural tissues. Mol Cell Neurosci 6: 43-55.

Thompson AC, Zapata A, Justice JB, Vaughan RA, Sharpe LG, et al. 2000. κ-opioid receptor activation modifies dopamine uptake in the nucleus accumbens and opposes the effects of cocaine. J Neurosci 20: 9333-9340.

Torres GE, Carneiro A, Seamans K, Fiorentini C, Sweeney A, et al. 2003. Oligomerization and trafficking of the human dopamine transporter. Mutational analysis identifies critical domains important for the functional expression of the transporter. J Biol Chem 278: 2731-2739.

Torres GE, Yao WD, Mohn AR, Quan H, Kim KM, et al. 2001. Functional interaction between monoamine plasma membrane transporters and the synaptic PDZ domain-containing protein PICK1. Neuron 30: 121-134.

Uhl GR, Lin Z. 2003. The top 20 dopamine transporter mutants: Structure-function relationships and cocaine actions. Eur J Pharmacol 479: 71-82.

Vandenbergh DJ, Thompson MD, Cook EH, Bendahhou E, Nguyen T, et al. 2000. Human dopamine transporter gene: Coding region conservation among normal, Tourette's disorder, alcohol dependence and attention-deficit hyperactivity disorder populations. Mol Psychiatry 5: 283-292.

Vaughan RA, Huff RA, Uhl GR, Kuhar MJ. 1997. Protein kinase C-mediated phosphorylation and functional regulation of dopamine transporters in striatal synaptosomes. J Biol Chem 272 (24): 15541-15546.

Wade PR, Chen J, Jaffe B, Kassem IS, Blakely RD, et al. 1996. Localization and function of a 5-HT transporter in crypt epithelia of the gastrointestinal tract. J Neurosci 16: 2352-2364.

Wersinger C, Vernier P, Sidhu A. 2004. Trypsin disrupts the trafficking of the human dopamine transporter by α-synuclein and its A30P mutant. Biochemistry 43: 1242-1253.

Whitworth TL, Quick MW. 2001a. Substrate-induced regulation of γ-aminobutyric acid transporter trafficking requires tyrosine phosphorylation. J Biol Chem 276: 42932-42937.

Whitworth TL, Quick MW. 2001b. Upregulation of γ-aminobutyric acid transporter expression: Role of alkylated γ-aminobutyric acid derivatives. Biochem Soc Transm 29: 736-741.

Wirz-Justice A. 1988. Platelet research in psychiatry. Experientia 44: 145-152.

Wu Q, Reith ME, Walker QD, Kuhn CM, Carroll FI, et al. 2002. Concurrent autoreceptor-mediated control of dopamine release and uptake during neurotransmission: An in vivo voltammetric study. J Neurosci 22: 6272-6281.

Xu F, Gainetdinov RR, Wetsel WC, Jones SR, Bohn LM, et al. 2000. Mice lacking the norepinephrine transporter are supersensitive to psychostimulants. Nat Neurosci 3: 465-471.

Zahniser NR, Sorkin A. 2004. Rapid regulation of the dopamine transporter: Role in stimulant addiction? Neuropharmacology 47 (Suppl. 1): 80-91.

Zhang L, Reith ME. 1996. Regulation of the functional activity of the human dopamine transporter by the arachidonic acid pathway. Eur J Pharmacol 315: 345-354.

Zhang L, Coffey LL, Reith, MEA. 1997. Regulation of the functional activity of the human dopamine transporter by protein kinase C. Biochem Pharmacol 53: 677-688.

Zhu CB, Hewlett WA, Feoktistov I, Biaggioni I, Blakely RD. 2004. Adenosine receptor, protein kinase G, and p38 mitogen-activated protein kinase-dependent up-regulation of serotonin transporters involves both transporter trafficking and activation. Mol Pharmacol 65: 1462-1474.

Zhu MY, Ordway GA. 1997. Down-regulation of norepinephrine transporters on PC12 cells by transporter inhibitors. J Neurochem 68: 134-141.

Zhu MY, Shamburger S, Li J, Ordway GA. 2000. Regulation of the human norepinephrine transporter by cocaine and amphetamine. J Pharmacol Exp Ther 295: 951-959.

19 Expression and Functional Activities of Glucose Transporters in the Central Nervous System

G. G. Piroli · C. A. Grillo · L. R. Reznikov · L. P. Reagan

Abstract: The family of facilitative glucose transporter (GLUT) proteins is responsible for the entry of glucose into cells throughout the periphery and the brain. The expression, regulation and activity of glucose transporters play an essential role in neuronal homeostasis, since glucose represents the primary energy source for the brain. Brain GLUTs exhibit both cell type and region specific localizations suggesting that the transport and utilization of glucose in the CNS is tightly regulated and compartmentalized. Brain GLUTs also exhibit discrete localizations, as well as unique subcellular localizations, indicating that GLUTs may be involved in highly specialized activities in the CNS such as glucose sensing. Insulin sensitive GLUTs are expressed in the brain suggesting that GLUTs may participate in the central actions of insulin, including cognitive function and homeostatic control of food intake. These results illustrate that the expression, regulation and trafficking of brain GLUTs are critically involved in maintaining neuronal homeostasis and responsiveness.

List of Abbreviations: AD, Alzheimer's disease; ANLSH, astrocyte-neuron lactate shuttle hypothesis; BBB, blood–brain barrier; CNS, central nervous system; CORT, corticosterone; EM, electron microscopic; GC, glucocorticoid; GE, glucose-excited; GFAP, glial fibrillary acidic protein; GI, glucose-inhibited; GLUT, glucose transporter; GLUT1DS, GLUT1 deficiency syndrome; HDM, high-density microsomal; LDM, low-density microsomal; MCI, mild cognitive impairment; MCT, monocarboxylate transporter; NG, nonglucosensing; SUR1, sulfonylurea receptor; VMN, ventromedial nucleus of the hypothalamus

1   Introduction

The family of facilitative glucose transporter (GLUT) proteins is responsible for the entry of glucose into cells throughout the periphery and the brain (Maher et al., 1994; Vannucci et al., 1997; Shepherd and Kahn, 1999). The expression, regulation, and activity of GLUTs play an essential role in neuronal homeostasis since glucose represents the primary energy source for the brain (Lund-Anderen, 1979; Pardridge, 1983). The expanding GLUT gene family has recently added several novel members, which required reclassification of GLUT nomenclature into three different classes based upon their sequence similarities (Joost et al., 2002). The brain GLUTs are represented in Class I (GLUTs 1–4), Class II (GLUT5), and Class III (GLUT8). Brain GLUTs exhibit both cell type and region specific localizations, suggesting that the transport and utilization of glucose in the central nervous system (CNS) is tightly regulated and compartmentalized. The 55-kDa isoform of GLUT1 expressed in microvessels, the 45-kDa isoform of GLUT1 expressed in glia, and neuronal expression of GLUT3 are proposed to be responsible for the majority of glucose uptake and utilization in the brain (Duelli and Kuschinsky, 2001). Other GLUTs exhibit more discrete localizations (GLUTs 2 and 4), as well as unique subcellular localizations (GLUT8), indicating that these GLUTs may be involved in highly specialized activities in the CNS (❷ *Figure 19-1*). Insulin sensitive GLUTs are expressed in the brain (GLUTs 4 and 8), suggesting that GLUTs may participate in the central actions of insulin, including cognitive function (Park, 2001) and homeostatic control of food intake (Schwartz et al., 1992). The aim of this chapter will be to discuss the localization of GLUTs expressed in the CNS, with a special emphasis on the functional roles that GLUTs play in maintaining neuronal homeostasis and responsiveness.

2   Expression and Localization of Brain Glucose Transporters

2.1 GLUT1

GLUT1, also referred to as the erythrocyte glucose transporter, is expressed both in the brain and the periphery. In the brain, GLUT1 is involved in both the passage of glucose into the brain through the BBB and the uptake of glucose by astrocytes (Giaume et al., 1997) and was originally identified as a 55-kDa protein (Dick et al., 1984). This highly glycosylated isoform of GLUT1 was localized to microvessels of the blood–brain barrier by cytochalasin B binding and was identified as GLUT1 by immunoblotting using

☐ Figure 19-1

Localization of GLUT isoforms in the CNS. Shown in green is the 55-kDa isoform of GLUT1 expressed in endothelial cells. Shown in light blue is the 45-kDa isoform of GLUT1 expressed in astrocytes. Neuropil expression of GLUT3 is depicted in yellow. Illustrated in dark blue is the somatodendritic labeling of GLUT4. Potential overlap of GLUTs 3 and 4 distribution in some neurons of the brain is shown as yellow and dark blue-hatched areas. Shown in brown is GLUT5 expressed in microglia. Illustrated as red dots is the intracellular and somatodendritic localization of GLUT8. Not shown is the astrocytic and neuronal localization of GLUT2. Reprinted from McEwen and Reagan (2004), with permission from Elsevier

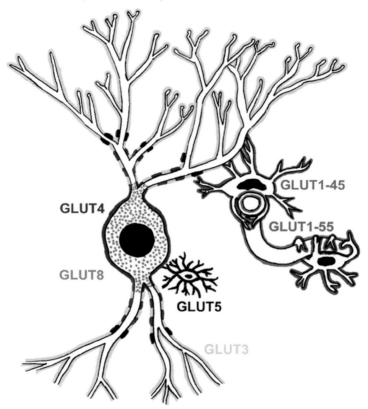

antisera raised against the human erythrocyte GLUT (Dick et al., 1984). These early findings were confirmed by cloning of GLUT1 from a rat brain cDNA library (Birnbaum et al., 1986). While a widespread distribution of GLUT1 in the rat brain was observed (Brant et al., 1993; Rayner et al., 1994), the cells expressing the transporter were more selectively identified as endothelial cells of cerebral microvessels (Kasanicki et al., 1987; Boado and Pardridge, 1990). Immunohistochemical staining showed that GLUT1 was present in the luminal and abluminal surfaces of cerebral microvessels. Interestingly, abluminal levels of GLUT1 are higher than luminal expression, an asymmetric distribution that would direct the glucose flux toward the brain parenchyma (Gerhart et al., 1989; Kasanicki et al., 1989; Farrell and Pardridge, 1991). Additional observations (Boado and Pardridge, 1990; Pardridge et al., 1990; Farrell et al., 1992) also suggested that GLUT1 was associated exclusively with endothelial cells and was not expressed in other cells in the brain. However, the existence of a 45-kDa isoform of GLUT1 was identified by analysis of microvessel-free brain preparations (Maher et al., 1994; Vannucci, 1994), rat brain synaptosomes (Bhattacharyya and

Brodsky, 1988), and crude brain homogenates (Morgello et al., 1995). Additional studies revealed an association of GLUT1 with astrocytes surrounding cerebral microvessels as well as astrocytic cell bodies and processes (Morgello et al., 1995; Leino et al., 1997). Colocalization of GLUT1 with the astrocytic marker glial fibrillary acidic protein (GFAP) further supported astrocytic expression of GLUT1 (Yu and Ding, 1998). In summary, these studies demonstrate that GLUT1 exists as two isoforms transcribed from the same gene in the brain: a more heavily glycosylated 55-kDa isoform expressed in endothelial cells and a less glycosylated 45-kDa isoform localized to astrocytes.

GLUT1 partial deficiency syndrome (GLUT1DS) illustrates the importance of this transporter in brain metabolism (De Vivo et al., 1991). While GLUT1 complete deficiency is lethal in knockout mice (Heilig et al., 2003), reduced expression of GLUT1 as observed in GLUT1DS decreases glucose uptake, which in turn leads to lower glucose and lactate concentrations in the cerebrospinal fluid (CSF) of GLUT1DS patients (Pascual et al., 2004). Developmental encephalopathy is observed in these patients, along with cognitive impairment, microcephaly, and seizures. A variety of mutations of the GLUT1 gene were identified in GLUT1DS (Wang et al., 2005) and are believed to contribute to these clinical manifestations. Seizures usually do not respond or even worsen with the use of classic antiepileptic drugs, probably due to the inhibitory effect on glucose transport exerted by these compounds (Pascual et al., 2004). On the other hand, seizures disappear under ketogenic diet; ketone bodies are taken by the brain through the monocarboxylate transporter (MCT), and completely oxidized in the mitochondria, providing the brain the energy to drive different processes in replacement of glucose (Klepper et al., 2004).

2.2 GLUT2

GLUT2 was first described in the periphery as part of the glucosensor mechanism present in pancreatic β-cells and liver, functional activities that include the enzyme glucokinase. Both GLUT2 and glucokinase show high K_m values for glucose transport and phosphorylation, respectively, and are fully active at high glucose concentrations. Pancreatic β-cells also express ATP-sensitive K^+-channels consisting of the Kir6.2 subunit and sulfonylurea receptors (SUR1). As a consequence of glucose metabolism in β-cells, ATP levels increase and ATP-sensitive K^+-channels close leading to depolarization that increases Ca^{2+} levels and stimulation of insulin release. In the brain, glucosensing neurons expressed in the hypothalamic ventromedial nucleus (VMN) are proposed to be activated in a similar manner (Levin et al., 2001). In this regard, colocalization studies identified GLUT2, glucokinase, and SUR1 in several brain areas including the hypothalamus (Li et al., 2003; Roncero et al., 2004). Central administration of GLUT2 antisense oligonucleotides decreased cumulative food intake and body weight, and also attenuated glucoprivic feeding in rats (LeLoup et al., 1998; Wan et al., 1998), further supporting an important functional role for GLUT2 in the hypothalamus. Histological studies showed that the localization of GLUT2 is limited to certain brain areas, including the hypothalamus, amygdala, and cortex, with scattered expression in the rest of the brain (LeLoup et al., 1994; Arluison et al., 2004a). Other studies revealed a widespread distribution of GLUT2 in the brain (Brant et al., 1993) or failed to detect GLUT2 protein (Rayner et al., 1994). The cellular type expressing GLUT2 is also equivocal, with reports showing localization in astrocytes (LeLoup et al., 1994; Arluison et al., 2004b; Young and McKenzie, 2004), tanycytes (Garcia et al., 2003; Young and McKenzie, 2004), and neurons (Arluison et al., 2004b). Given the recent molecular characterization of glucosensing neurons in the VMN (see in a later section; Kang et al., 2004), additional investigations of GLUT2 are required to clarify the expression and functional role of this transporter in the brain.

2.3 GLUT3

GLUT3, referred to as the neuron specific glucose transporter, was first cloned from a human fetal muscle cDNA library and was found to be widely expressed in human tissues, including the brain (Kayano et al., 1988). Further reports observed a more restricted expression of GLUT3 in human tissues, with predominance in brain, testis, and spermatozoa (Haber et al., 1993). The distribution of GLUT3 mRNA and protein is even more restricted in rodents, being observed only in the brain (Yano et al., 1991; Maher et al., 1992; Nagamatsu et al., 1992). Several studies localized GLUT3 to neurons by in situ hybridization histochemistry (Nagamatsu et al., 1993) and immunohistochemistry (McCall et al., 1994; Gerhart et al., 1995). In the rat brain, GLUT3 was localized to the neuropil; this is most evident in the hippocampus where mossy fibers showed a strong immunopositive signal for GLUT3, while pyramidal cell and granule cell bodies displayed little GLUT3-positive labeling (McCall et al., 1994; Gerhart et al., 1995). Electron microscopic (EM) studies provided additional support for a neuropil localization of GLUT3, and also confirmed that GLUT3 immunoreactivity was not associated with nonneuronal cell types (Leino et al., 1997). In the mouse brain, GLUT3 immunoreactivity is observed but not limited to the neuropil since lower levels of GLUT3 expression are also observed in neuronal cell bodies (Choeiri et al., 2002). Regional distribution within the brain showed high expression of GLUT3 mRNA in the cerebellum, striatum, cortex, and hippocampus (Nagamatsu et al., 1993), whereas GLUT3 protein was detected throughout the rat CNS as a 45-kDa band by immunoblot analysis (Nagamatsu et al., 1993; Maher et al., 1994). Radioimmunocytochemistry, a technique in which immunoreactivity is detected using radiolabeled secondary antisera, showed similar profiles for GLUT3 protein expression (Zeller et al., 1995; Reagan et al., 1999). Since local cerebral glucose utilization is relatively similar for neuronal cell body layers when compared with the neuropil (Zeller et al., 1995; Duelli et al., 1999), the absence of expression of GLUT3 in cell bodies in the rat brain suggests that other GLUT isoforms may be expressed in the soma to fulfill the metabolic demands of neuronal cell bodies (see later).

2.4 GLUT4

It is well established that glucose transport in adipocytes and muscle is rapidly induced by insulin, suggesting that redistribution of a putative insulin-sensitive transporter from intracellular organelles to the plasma membrane occurs following insulin receptor activation. This transporter, GLUT4, was first cloned from a rat skeletal muscle cDNA library, and its expression was localized to insulin respon- sive tissues such as skeletal muscle, adipose tissue and heart as well as kidney (Birnbaum, 1989; Charron et al., 1989). Western blot experiments showed that GLUT4 was present not only in the plasma membrane but also in low-density microsomes and that insulin elicited trafficking of GLUT4 from the microsomal fraction to the plasma membrane (Birnbaum, 1989). This mechanism is the basis for insulin-induced glucose uptake and has been confirmed by many other techniques (for review see Saltiel and Pessin, 2002). More recently, GLUT4 expression in the brain was identified in the hypothalamus (LeLoup et al., 1996), cerebellum (Brant et al., 1993; Rayner et al., 1994; Kobayashi et al., 1996; Vannucci et al., 1998b), cortex, and hippocampus (Messari et al., 1998; Vannucci et al., 1998b; Reagan, 2002; McEwen and Reagan, 2004). Immunohistochemical detection of GLUT4 at light and EM levels showed a neuronal somatodendritic labeling (Messari et al., 1998; McEwen and Reagan, 2004), with absence of expression in nonneural cells except for endothelial vascular cells (Ngarmukos et al., 2001). Furthermore, GLUT4 expression was present in a subset of GLUT3 expressing neurons in the rat brain, cells that were also positive for parvalbumin or choline acetyltransferase (Aplet et al., 1999). Interestingly, the insulin receptor and GLUT4 exhibit overlapping distributions in the brain, including the cerebellum, hypothalamus, and hippocampus (Marks et al., 1991; Doré et al., 1997), suggesting that insulin may elicit GLUT4 translocation from internal pools to the plasma membrane in the CNS as it does in the periphery. In support of this hypothesis, GLUT4 immunoreactivity is associated not only with the plasma membrane but also with the cytoplasm (Messari et al., 1998), and in animal models of diabetes, impaired trafficking of GLUT4 has been described in cortex, cerebellum (Vannucci et al., 1998b), and hippocampus (Reagan, 2002). Moreover, glucose-induced increases in plasma insulin levels stimulates GLUT4 translocation to the plasma membrane in the hippocampus (McEwen and Reagan, 2004). These results support the hypothesis that insulin stimulates GLUT4 translocation in the brain and suggests that GLUT4 could be a mediator of central effects of insulin. However, it is important to note that the magnitude of these insulin stimulated events are greater in peripheral tissues, such as muscle, when compared to the hippocampus, and GLUT4 may therefore not make significant contributions to neuronal glucose utilization. Nonetheless, insulin-stimulated translocation of GLUT4 to the plasma membrane in the hippocampus may serve additional functional roles, perhaps acting as a metabolic sensor that serves to monitor the preexisting neuronal milieu (see later).

2.5 GLUT5

GLUT5 was first cloned from a cDNA library of human small intestine and subsequently described in human kidney (Kayano et al., 1990) and spermatozoa (Burant et al., 1992). This pattern of distribution of GLUT5 is consistent with its selectivity for fructose transport (Burant et al., 1992), considering the high concentration of fructose in those tissues. Further studies showed that GLUT5 was also present in fat, muscle, and brain, and that GLUT5 was not insulin responsive (Shepherd et al., 1992). In the rat, GLUT5 localization is restricted to intestine, kidney, and brain (Rand et al., 1993). Immunoblot analysis of human brain determined that GLUT5 antisera recognized a protein of similar molecular weights in human brain and cultured peripheral macrophages (Maher et al., 1994). Immunohistochemical studies revealed the expression of GLUT5 in microglial cells in the normal brain (Payne et al., 1997) and also in brain tumors (Sasaki et al., 2004). A recent study revealed that GLUT5 expression is present only in the microglia among cells of the mononuclear phagocyte system and is absent in monocyte-derived cells that infiltrate lesions in brain infarcts (Sasaki et al., 2003). Since fructose levels in brain are low and GLUT5 transporter activity for glucose is much lower than for fructose (Burant et al., 1992), the physiological role of GLUT5 in microglia remains to be determined.

2.6 GLUT8

Whereas most tissues express GLUTs 1–5, other tissues express low levels of these "classic" GLUTs (Marger and Saier, 1993). In addition, GLUT4 knockout mice exhibit an unexpected phenotype with almost normal glucose transport in muscle in the absence of compensatory overexpression of GLUT1 or 3 (Katz et al., 1995). These intriguing observations, along with the possibility of searching databases for sequence similarities with GLUTs 1–5, stimulated cloning of new GLUTs. Among these newly identified GLUTs was GLUT8 (previously referred to as GLUTx1), which exhibits only 20–30% identity with GLUTs 1–5, depending on the species (Carayannopoulos et al., 2000; Doege et al., 2000; Ibberson et al., 2000). These first studies revealed the presence of GLUT8 mRNA in several tissues, including the testis, adrenal gland, liver, spleen, adipose tissue, and brain (Ibberson et al., 2000); GLUT8 was also identified in blastocysts (Carayannopoulos et al., 2000). In the brain, our previous studies provided the first description of GLUT8 mRNA and protein expression in the hippocampus (Reagan et al., 2001). Unlike GLUT3, GLUT8 is expressed primarily in neuronal cell bodies and the most proximal apical dendrites (Reagan et al., 2001, 2002). The expression of GLUT8 protein in the rat brain appears to be widespread, as shown by immunofluorescence in the cortex, cerebellum, the paraventricular hypothalamic nucleus, the amygdala, and the supraoptic nucleus (McEwen and Reagan, 2004). Other studies showed similar localization of GLUT8 (Ibberson et al., 2002; Sankar et al., 2002). In addition, our studies also illustrated that GLUT8 was not colocalized with the astroglia marker GFAP or the microglia marker OX-42, suggesting that GLUT8 was selectively expressed in neurons (Reagan et al., 2002). This exclusive neuronal expression of GLUT8 was further supported by our immunogold EM studies in the hippocampus of the rat (Piroli et al., 2002).

Functionally, initial experiments showed that expression of GLUT8 in *Xenopus* oocytes did not increase 2-deoxyglucose uptake (Ibberson et al., 2000). The presence of a dileucine motif at the amino terminus of GLUT8 may serve as an internalization signal that prevents sufficient plasma membrane expression of the transporter, thereby preventing glucose transport in transfected cells (Ibberson et al., 2000). Mutagenesis or disruption of intracellular trafficking mechanisms promotes GLUT8 association with the plasma membrane and stimulates cytochalasin-B sensitive 2-deoxy-D-glucose uptake (Ibberson et al., 2000; Lisinski et al., 2001). In the in vivo setting, GLUT8 is not associated with the plasma membrane under physiological settings or in experimental models of type 1 diabetes in the CNS (Reagan et al., 2001). Alternatively, GLUT8 was immunodetected in high-density microsomal (HDM) and low-density microsomal (LDM) fractions, but not in plasma membranes in the hippocampus (Reagan et al., 2001). Furthermore, EM analyses revealed that GLUT8 was associated with the endoplasmic reticulum and the cytosol of the rat hippocampus but not with the plasma membrane (Piroli et al., 2002). GLUT8 exhibits a similar ultrastructural profile in the rat cortex (❷ *Figure 19-2*), suggesting that GLUT8 transport activity resides in the rough endoplasmic reticulum (Piroli et al., 2002). We have previously hypothesized that GLUT8 transports the glucose molecules released during protein glycosylation events that occur in the endoplasmic reticulum lumen into the cytoplasm, and in this manner GLUT8 plays a key role in maintaining neuronal glucose homeostasis.

◻ Figure 19-2

Ultrastructural localization of GLUT8 in neurons of normal rat cortex. GLUT8 immunoreactivity (ir) as demonstrated by immunogold labeling (black particles) is found in the cytosolic compartment as well as near and abutting the membranes of the endoplasmic reticulum (ER; indicated by *arrowheads*). GLUT8 immunogold particles are usually not associated with the plasma membrane (PM), the nucleus (N), or the mitochondria (m). Scale bar = 0.5 μm

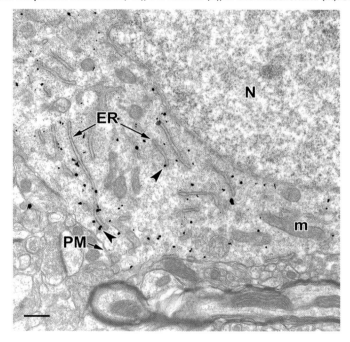

Considering that glucose utilization in neuronal cell bodies is similar to that of the neuropil in the hippocampus (Zeller et al., 1995; Duelli et al., 1999), it is therefore possible that the somatodendritic expression of GLUT8, as well as GLUT4, supports the metabolic requirements of neuronal cell bodies. Interestingly, the trafficking of these somatodendritic GLUT isoforms appears to be insulin sensitive, as will be discussed later.

3 GLUT Regulation in the CNS: Transient Trafficking Versus Maintained Modifications

Brain GLUT isoforms respond to a variety of physiological and pathophysiological stimuli, resulting in alterations in transcription, translation, and trafficking. The developing and emerging hypotheses regarding the role of GLUTs in glucose sensing, energy utilization, and cognitive function have provided a more dynamic description of the functional activities of these proteins in the CNS. Some of these responses of GLUTs may be rapid, transient, and involve trafficking or translocation events, while other GLUT responses may develop more slowly, requiring transcriptional and translational events. Such differences emphasize the multileveled regulation of GLUT expression and activity and the essential role that GLUTs perform in maintaining neuronal and nonneuronal homeostasis.

3.1 Rapid, Insulin-Stimulated GLUT Trafficking in the CNS

The insulin-stimulated translocation of GLUT4 is well characterized in peripheral tissues (Pessin et al., 1999) and more recent investigations revealed that GLUT4 trafficking may also be insulin-sensitive in the brain. In support of this hypothesis and similar to observations in peripheral tissues (Garvey et al., 1993; Kainulainen et al., 1994; Marcus et al., 1994; Smith et al., 1999; Li and McNeill, 2001), plasma membrane association of GLUT4 is modulated in the cerebellum, cortex (Vannucci et al., 1998b), and hippocampus (Reagan, 2002) in rodent models of type 1 and type 2 diabetes. Similarly, GLUT8 association with the HDM fraction, and presumably the endoplasmic reticulum, is reduced in experimental models of type 1 diabetes (Piroli et al., 2002, 2004). However, these observations cannot exclusively identify a role for insulin in these trafficking events due to the variety of pathophysiological alterations associated with diabetes phenotypes (McCall, 1992; Gispen and Biessels, 2000). Our more recent studies examined the ability of physiologically relevant stimuli to elicit GLUTs 4 and 8 trafficking in the hippocampus. For example, peripheral administration of glucose, which increases plasma insulin levels, rapidly stimulates GLUT4 translocation to the plasma membrane and GLUT8 trafficking to the endoplasmic reticulum in the rat hippocampus (Piroli et al., 2002; McEwen and Reagan, 2004). In view of the important relationships between glucose, insulin, and cognition (Park, 2001; Messier, 2004), the enhanced trafficking of GLUTs 4 and 8 in the hippocampus may represent a fundamental cellular mechanism associated with cognitive function.

While these studies provide provocative data to support the hypothesis that insulin stimulates GLUTs 4 and 8 trafficking in the CNS, it is important to note that diabetes phenotypes and glucose administration are associated with changes in plasma glucose and plasma insulin levels. Therefore, GLUTs 4 and 8 translocation under these conditions may not be stimulated by increases in insulin but rather by increases in central concentrations of glucose. An experimental approach that would allow for the more selective analysis of GLUT trafficking would be to examine the actions of insulin using in vitro approaches. Cell culture techniques have provided invaluable insight into the trafficking mechanisms responsible for insulin-stimulated translocation events in peripheral tissues (Saltiel and Pessin, 2002). Moreover, use of cloned neuronal cells offers distinct advantages, particularly, when examining signal transduction cascades employed by neurons since these measures are often difficult to ascertain using in vivo approaches. In this regard, Devaskar and coworkers have utilized N2A neuroblastoma cells to examine the GLUT8 trafficking mechanisms utilized by neurons (Shin et al., 2004). While GLUT8 was localized to the intracellular compartment in N2A cells, insulin administration did not alter HDM and LDM levels of GLUT8, suggesting that GLUT8 trafficking is not insulin sensitive. However, it is important to note that these authors did not demonstrate that the N2A cells were insulin responsive, which could account for the lack of insulin-stimulated GLUT8 trafficking. Most recently, we have examined insulin activity in several cloned neuronal cell lines, namely N1E-115 cells and NG108-15 cells. We have previously demonstrated that these cells may be differentiated to a neuronal phenotype (Reagan et al., 1990), thereby providing a model system with which to examine the insulin-signaling mechanisms activated by neuronal insulin receptors. For example, incubation of differentiated N1E-115 cells with 1 μM insulin rapidly stimulates the phosphorylation of Akt without altering total Akt levels (❷ Figure 19-3). Moreover, incubation of N1E-115 cells with 1 μM insulin elicits a greater than two-fold increase in GLUT8 trafficking to the HDM fraction (❷ Figure 19-3). Similarly, insulin stimulates phosphorylation of Akt and increases plasma membrane association of GLUT4 in NG108-15 cells (❷ Figure 19-4). These results using cloned neuronal cells support

◻ Figure 19-3

Insulin stimulates phosphorylation of Akt and translocation of GLUT8 in N1E-115 cells. To determine insulin-stimulated GLUT8 trafficking mechanisms in neurons, immunoblot analysis was performed on HDM fractions isolated from N1E-115 neuroblastoma cells incubated with 1 μM insulin. Insulin-treated N1E-115 cells exhibited robust increases in Akt phosphorylation (pAkt) without modulating total Akt levels. In addition, insulin stimulated GLUT8 translocation to the HDM fraction in differentiated N1E-115 cells, suggesting that phosphorylation of Akt serves as an intermediate in GLUT8 trafficking in neurons

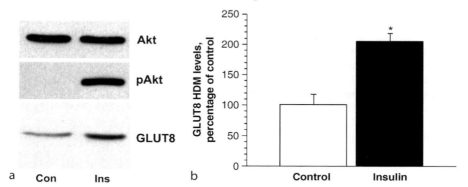

◻ Figure 19-4

Insulin stimulates phosphorylation of Akt and translocation of GLUT4 in NG108-15 cells. Activation of PI-3 kinase and subsequent phosphorylation of Akt are essential intermediates in insulin signal transduction events leading to GLUT4 trafficking in peripheral tissues. In an attempt to determine if neurons utilize similar mechanisms, NG108-15 cells differentiated to a neuronal phenotype were incubated in the presence and absence of 1 μM insulin. While total Akt levels were unaffected, insulin-treatment stimulated a robust increase in the phosphorylation of Akt (pAkt). In addition, insulin stimulated GLUT4 translocation to the plasma membrane fraction in differentiated NG-108 cells. These results suggest that insulin-stimulated translocation of GLUT4 to the plasma membrane may occur through similar pathways in neurons as has been described for peripheral tissues

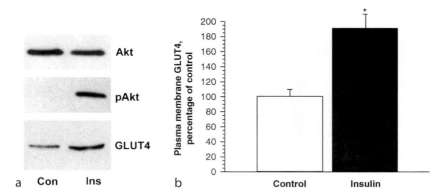

our earlier in vivo findings suggesting that insulin stimulates the translocation of GLUTs 8 and 4 in the hippocampus. Nonetheless, additional studies will be required to fully elucidate the role of insulin and insulin receptor-signaling cascades in neuronal GLUTs 4 and 8 trafficking as well as the physiological and functional consequences of these insulin mediated events.

3.2 Maintained Modification of GLUT Expression: Changes in Glycemic Conditions

Unlike the rapid redistribution of a readily mobilizable pool of GLUTs described above, CNS GLUT regulation may also include modulation of transcription and translation in response to acute and/or chronic homeostatic changes. One area of intense research has been the regulation of GLUT isoforms in experimental models of diabetes and how changes in GLUT expression may modulate brain glucose uptake and utilization. The effects of acute and chronic hyperglycemia have been shown to modulate brain GLUT mRNA and protein expression, trafficking of GLUT4 to the plasma membrane, as well as brain glucose uptake and utilization. However, these studies have failed to reach a consensus, which may be related to region specific, as well as time-dependent effects of hyperglycemia upon brain GLUT expression and activity (for recent reviews see Vannucci et al., 1998b; Duelli and Kuschinsky, 2001; Reagan, 2002). For example, GLUT3 levels are decreased in the hippocampus of aged Akita diabetic mice but not in the cerebellum (Choeiri et al., 2005a). Conversely, while our previous studies demonstrated that 1 week of STZ-induced diabetes does not modulate GLUT3 protein expression (Reagan et al., 1999), 5 weeks of hyperglycemia significantly increased GLUT3 expression in the CA3 region of the rat hippocampus but not in other hippocampal neuronal populations (❷ Figure 19-5). Since chronic hyperglycemia is associated with

❑ Figure 19-5

Chronic streptozotocin (STZ)-induced hyperglycemia produces region-specific increases in GLUT3 expression in the rat hippocampus. Radioimmunocytochemical analysis for GLUT3 was performed in the hippocampus of rats subjected to 5 weeks of STZ-induced hyperglycemia and euglycemic control rats. Autoradiographic analysis revealed that STZ diabetes increased GLUT3 expression in the CA3 region of the hippocampus when compared with euglycemic control rats, increases not observed in other hippocampal neuronal populations. Data expressed as percentage of values obtained in vehicle-treated controls; $*p \leq 0.001$

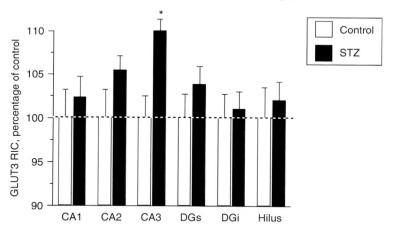

dendritic remodeling and synaptogenesis in the CA3 region (Grillo et al., 2005), increases in GLUT3 protein expression may assist in the increased metabolic demands that would accompany these morphological changes in the hippocampus.

As described for studies that examined the effects of hyperglycemia upon GLUT expression, the effects of hypoglycemia upon brain GLUTs 1 and 3 expression have yielded dissimilar results (Kumagai et al., 1995; Uehara et al., 1997; Duelli et al., 1999; Simpson et al., 1999), discrepancies that may be related to differences in experimental designs as well as region-specific alterations in GLUT expression. An additional caveat to these studies is the hypoglycemia-induced alterations in the relative distributions of brain GLUTs. In this regard, Simpson et al. (1999) demonstrated that chronic hypoglycemia increases GLUT1 mRNA as well as total and luminal GLUT1 protein levels, suggesting that hypoglycemia-induced increases in GLUT1 transcription and translation will lead to the preferential trafficking of GLUT1 to microvessel luminal membranes (Simpson et al., 1999). Collectively, these results suggest that hyperglycemic and hypoglycemic conditions can modulate transcription, translation, trafficking, and distribution of CNS GLUT isoforms.

3.3 Maintained Modification of GLUT Expression: Role of Stress Hormones

Experimental or pathophysiological increases in plasma glucocorticoid (GC) levels are associated with increases in plasma glucose and insulin levels as well as insulin resistance (Stojanovska et al., 1990; Rosmond et al., 1998; Severino et al., 2002) and impairment of GLUT4 expression and translocation in peripheral tissues (for review see Kahn and Flier, 1990; also see Weinstein et al., 1998). In the CNS, stress or exposure to stress levels of GCs produces a wide variety of molecular, cellular, electrophysiological, morphological, and behavioral changes (for review see McEwen, 1999). However, few studies have examined the effects of stress or stress hormones upon GLUT expression and activity, in spite of the well-described effects of GCs upon neuronal function, plasticity, and cognition. McCall and coworkers previously examined the effects of short-term administration of the synthetic GC dexamethasone upon GLUT1 expression in isolated rat brain microvessels (Chipkin et al., 1998). Dexamethasone administration produced the expected hyperglycemia and hyperinsulinemia; dexamethosone also increased GLUT1 protein levels, increases that were associated with increased glucose uptake in isolated cerebral microvessels. Unlike these increases in GLUT1 expression, our previous studies revealed that short-term exposure to stress levels of GCs does not modulate GLUT3 mRNA or protein expression (Reagan et al., 1999) and total GLUT8 expression in the rat hippocampus (Piroli et al., 2004). However, short-term stress stimulates GLUT8 trafficking from the LDM fraction to the HDM fraction in the rat hippocampus, an effect that may be mediated in part by stress-induced increases in plasma insulin levels (Piroli et al., 2004).

More recently, our laboratory has examined the effects of 5-week administration of corticosterone (CORT) upon GLUT expression and trafficking in the rat hippocampus. Chronic exposure to stress levels of CORT is associated with a variety of changes in hippocampal synaptic plasticity, including alterations in long-term potentiation (Pavlides et al., 1993), decreases in cell proliferation (Gould et al., 1992, 1997), dendritic remodeling (Woolley et al., 1990), and decreased performance of hippocampal-dependent behaviors (Conrad et al., 1997). Five-week CORT administration produced the expected increases in plasma glucose levels (vehicle: 115.6 ± 3.1 mg/dL; CORT: 138.8 ± 4.0 mg/dL) and plasma insulin levels (vehicle: 0.676 ± 0.12 ng/mL; CORT: 4.65 ± 0.62 ng/mL). In addition, chronic CORT administration significantly increased plasma membrane GLUT4 levels (❷ Figure 19-6) and HDM GLUT8 levels (❷ Figure 19-7). However, unlike peripheral tissues that exhibit insulin resistance in response to GC exposure, insulin-stimulated trafficking of GLUTs 4 and 8 was significantly enhanced in the hippocampus of chronic CORT treated rats. Specifically, while glucose administration produced the expected increases in GLUT4 translocation in vehicle-treated rats, CORT-treated rats exhibited nearly an eightfold increase in plasma membrane GLUT4 levels (❷ Figure 19-6). CORT administration also maximally stimulated hippocampal GLUT8 trafficking to the HDM fraction compared to vehicle-treated rats (❷ Figure 19-7). Since GC exposure is associated with insulin resistance and decreases in insulin-stimulated trafficking of GLUT4 in peripheral tissues (Weinstein et al., 1998), these results suggest that chronic exposure to stress levels of GCs may enhance insulin sensitivity and responsiveness in the rat hippocampus.

Collectively, these data demonstrate that among the hippocampal responses to chronic exposure to stress levels of GCs are increases in hippocampal insulin sensitivity as measured by enhanced trafficking GLUTs 4 and 8, adaptive responses that may increase neuronal responsiveness during stress or periods of increased neuronal allostatic load (McEwen, 1998). In spite of these observations, additional investigations will be required to more fully elucidate the expression and functional roles of CNS GLUT isoforms in response to GC exposure, especially, in view of the important role of stress and stress hormones in normal brain physiology as well as in disease states such as diabetes, depressive illness, posttraumatic stress disorder, and Alzheimer's disease (AD) (McEwen, 1998, 2003; Sheline et al., 1999; Reagan, 2002).

◘ Figure 19-6

Chronic CORT administration enhances insulin-stimulated GLUT4 trafficking in the rat hippocampus. Hippo campal plasma membrane fractions were isolated 2 hours following an intraperitoneal (i.p.) injection of either saline or glucose in rats treated for 5 weeks with either CORT or vehicle (Veh). Glucose stimulated increases in plasma insulin levels produced the expected translocation of GLUT4 to the plasma membrane in vehicle treated rats [Veh (+)]. CORT administration increased plasma membrane levels of GLUT4 [CORT (−)], increases that were potentiated by glucose administration [CORT (+)]. Data expressed as percentage of values obtained in vehicle-treated controls given saline; *$p \leq 0.05$ compared to same treatment in absence of glucose challenge #$p \leq 0.05$ compared to Veh treatment

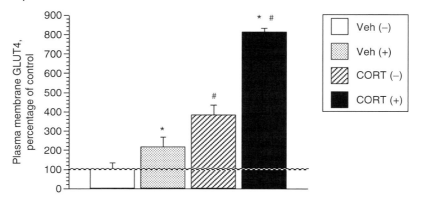

◘ Figure 19-7

Chronic CORT administration enhances insulin-stimulated GLUT8 trafficking in the rat hippocampus. Hippo campal HDM fractions were isolated 2 hours following an i.p. injection of either saline or glucose in rats treated for 5 weeks with either CORT or vehicle (Veh). Western blotting analysis revealed that glucose stimulated increases in plasma insulin levels lead to a significant increase in GLUT8 levels in the HDM fraction. CORT administration maximally stimulated GLUT8 translocation to the HDM fraction of the hippocampus irrespective of glucose treatment. Data expressed as percentage of values obtained in vehicle-treated controls given saline *$p \leq 0.01$ compared to Veh-saline group

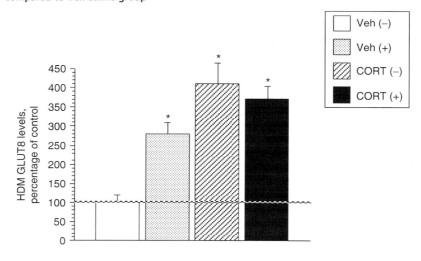

4   Future Perspectives: Brain GLUTs in Specialized Functional Activities

As detailed earlier, the regulation of brain GLUT expression, trafficking, and activity plays a critical role in maintaining metabolic homeostasis in the CNS. In addition, there is emerging evidence for more specialized roles for GLUTs in the CNS. For example, the astrocyte-neuron lactate shuttle hypothesis (ANLSH) proposes that lactate produced by astrocytes serves as a metabolic fuel for neurons (Magistretti et al., 1999; Pellerin and Magistretti, 2004). According to the ANLSH, most of the glucose that enters the brain through the BBB is transported into astrocytes and converted to glycogen or transformed into lactate, which in turn is shuttled to neurons (Shulman et al., 2001; Pellerin and Magistretti, 2004). The entry of glucose to the astrocyte is mediated by GLUT1, whereas the shuttling of lactate out of astrocytes to neurons is mediated by the MCTs (Pierre et al., 2000). The developmental profiles of the MCTs further support this hypothesis, since MCT levels are similar to if not greater than GLUTs 3 and 1 levels in many brain regions in the adult CNS (Vannucci and Simpson, 2003). Accordingly, the functional interactions between brain MCTs and GLUTs in relation to the maintenance of neuronal metabolic homeostasis represents an important and fascinating avenue for future analyses.

The role of brain GLUTs in the activity of glucosensing neurons in the hypothalamus has also come under greater scrutiny. Glucosensing neurons may be classified based upon their electrophysiological responses to changes in glucose levels. Glucose-excited (GE) neurons increase their firing rate as ambient glucose levels rise; glucose-inhibited (GI) neurons exhibit decreased firing rates under these conditions (Levin et al., 2004). While phenotypic characterization has revealed that 40–60% of GE and GI neurons express glucokinase and most GE neurons express the ATP-dependent K^+ channels (K_{ATP}), the brain GLUT that participates in the functional activity of these neurons remains elusive (Levin et al., 2001). More recently, Levin and coworkers performed molecular characterizations of glucosensing neurons using single-cell RT-PCR analysis in ventromedial hypothalamic nucleus (VMN) neurons (Kang et al., 2004). These studies revealed that GLUT3 is ubiquitously expressed in GE and GI neurons as well as in nonglucosensing (NG) neurons. Although GLUT2 has been suggested as a component in the functional activity of glucosensing neurons, GLUT2 was expressed in only a small percentage of VMN neurons and its expression did not correlate with the glucosensing capacity of a given neuron. Therefore, these studies suggest that while neuronal GLUTs may play a facilitory role, the specific GLUT isoform expressed in these neurons may be less important than the expression of glucokinase, which appears to be the major regulator of the activity of glucosensing neurons (Levin BE, personal communication; see also Kang et al., 2004; Levin et al., 2004).

Additional functional roles of GLUTs in the CNS await identification and characterization, including the role of GLUTs in cognitive performance. As described previously, such studies are particularly relevant in view of the association between glucose, insulin, and cognition (for review see Park, 2001; Messier, 2004). Decreases in GLUT expression and trafficking may contribute to cognitive impairment since brain glucose transport and utilization are impaired in elderly patients with mild cognitive impairment (MCI) (De Santi et al., 2001) as well as in AD (Benson et al., 1983; Duara et al., 1986; Friedland et al., 1989; Harr et al., 1995; Piert et al., 1996; De Santi et al., 2001). For example, postmortem studies of AD patients revealed that GLUTs 1 and 3 expression are decreased in several brain regions, including the hippocampus, supporting the hypothesis that decreases in GLUT expression may contribute to impairments in glucose utilization in these patient populations (Kalaria and Harik, 1989; Simpson et al., 1994; Harr et al., 1995; Mooradian et al., 1997; Vannucci et al., 1998a). Conversely, insulin-stimulated GLUTs 4 and 8 trafficking (see earlier) and modulation of GLUT expression represent examples of synaptic plasticity that may contribute to learning and memory formation. In this regard, recent investigations by Messier and colleagues demonstrated that performance of hippocampal-dependent tasks is associated with transient increases in GLUT1 expression in the rat hippocampus (Choeiri et al., 2005b), increases that may be required during increased metabolic demand associated with task learning.

As this section demonstrates, the long-term challenge facing investigators will be to more accurately define the role of brain GLUTs in neuronal homeostasis under "resting" conditions or during periods of increased metabolic demand. Gaining insight into the physiology and function of brain GLUTs in physiological settings would provide invaluable information regarding how GLUT expression and activities may be compromised under pathological conditions, thereby facilitating the development of novel therapeutic interventions in the treatment of a variety of CNS disorders associated with impaired glucoregulation, including MCI, AD, and diabetes.

Acknowledgments

The authors' work is supported in part by the Juvenile Diabetes Research Foundation and The University of South Carolina Research Foundation (LPR); CONICET and the University of Buenos Aires (GGP). The authors would like to acknowledge the efforts of their collaborators, including Dr. Bruce McEwen and Dr. Keith Akama (The Rockefeller University); Dr. Teresa Milner and Nora Tabori (Weill Medical College of Cornell University); and Dr. Maureen Charron (Albert Einstein College of Medicine). The authors would also like to thank Dr. Claude Messier (University of Ottawa), Dr. Cosette Choieri (University of Ottawa), Dr. Barry Levin (Department of Veterans Affairs New Jersey Health Care System), and Dr. Anthony McCall (University of Virginia) for helpful discussions and comments.

References

Aplet J, Melhorn G, Schliebs R. 1999. Insulin-sensitive GLUT4 glucose transporters are colocalized with GLUT3-expressing cells and demonstrate a chemically distinct neuron-specific localization in rat brain. J Neurosci Res 57: 693-705.

Arluison M, Quignon M, Nguyen P, Thorens B, LeLoup C, et al. 2004a. Distribution and anatomical localization of the glucose transporter 2 (GLUT2) in the adult rat brain—an immunohistochemical study. J Chem Neuroanat 28: 117-136.

Arluison M, Quignon M, Thorens B, LeLoup C, Penicaud L. 2004b. Immunocytochemical localization of the glucose transporter 2 (GLUT2) in the adult rat brain. II. Electron microscopic study. J Chem Neuroanat 28: 137-146.

Benson DF, Kuhl DE, Hawkins RA, Phelps ME, Cummings JL, et al. 1983. The fluorodeoxyglucose 18F scan in Alzheimer's disease and multi-infarct dementia. Arch Neurol 40: 711-714.

Bhattacharyya MV, Brodsky JL. 1988. Characterization of the glucose transporter from rat brain synaptosomes. Biochem Biophys Res Commun 155: 685-691.

Birnbaum MJ. 1989. Identification of a novel gene encoding an insulin-responsive glucose transporter protein. Cell 57: 305-315.

Birnbaum MJ, Haspel HC, Rosen OM. 1986. Cloning and characterization of a cDNA encoding the rat brain glucose-transporter protein. Proc Natl Acad Sci USA 83: 5784-5788.

Boado RJ, Pardridge WM. 1990. The brain-type glucose transporter mRNA is specifically expressed at the blood-brain barrier. Biochem Biophys Res Commun 166: 174-179.

Brant AM, Jess TJ, Milligan G, Brown CM, Gould GW. 1993. Immunological analysis of glucose transporters expressed in different regions of the rat brain and central nervous system. Biochem Biophys Res Commun 192: 1297-1302.

Burant CF, Takeda J, Brot-Laroche E, Bell GI, Davidson NO. 1992. Fructose transporter in human spermatozoa and small intestine is GLUT5. J Biol Chem 267: 14523-14526.

Carayannopoulos MO, Chi MMY, Cui Y, Pingsterhaus JM, McKnight RA, et al. 2000. GLUT8 is a glucose transporter responsible for insulin-stimulated glucose uptake in the blastocyst. Proc Natl Acad Sci USA 97: 7313-7318.

Charron MJ, Brosius FC III, Alper SL, Lodish HF. 1989. A glucose transport protein expressed predominantly in insulin-responsive tissues. Proc Natl Acad Sci USA 86: 2535-2539.

Chipkin SR, Van Bueren A, Bercel E, Garrison CR, McCall AL. 1998. Effects of dexamethasone in vivo and in vitro on hexose transport in brain microvasculature. Neurochem Res 23: 645-652.

Choeiri C, Staines W, Messier C. 2002. Immunohistochemical localization and quantification of glucose transporters in the mouse brain. Neuroscience 111: 19-34.

Choeiri C, Hewitt K, Durkin J, Simard CJ, Renaud JM, et al. 2005a. Longitudinal evaluation of memory performance and peripheral neuropathy in the Ins2C96Y Akita mice. Behav Brain Res 157: 31-38.

Choeiri C, Staines W, Miki T, Seino S, Messier C. 2005b. Glucose transporter plasticity during memory processing. Neuroscience 130: 591-600.

Conrad CD, Lupien SJ, Thanasoulis LC, McEwen BS. 1997. The effects of Type I and Type II corticosteroid receptor agonists on exploratory behavior and spatial memory in the Y-maze. Brain Res 759: 76-83.

De Santi S, de Leon MJ, Rusinek H, Convit A, Tarshish CY, et al. 2001. Hippocampal formation glucose metabolism and volume losses in MCI and AD. Neurobiol Aging 22: 529-539.

De Vivo DC, Trifiletti RR, Jacobson RI, Ronen GM, Behmand RA, et al. 1991. Defective glucose transport across the blood-brain barrier as a cause of persistent hypoglycorrhachia, seizures, and developmental delay. N Engl J Med 325: 703-709.

Dick AP, Harik SI, Klip A, Walker DM. 1984. Identification and characterization of the glucose transporter of the blood-brain barrier by cytochalasin B binding and immunological reactivity. Proc Natl Acad Sci USA 81: 7233-7237.

Doege H, Schürmann A, Bahrenberg G, Brauers A, Joost HG. 2000. GLUT8, a novel member of the sugar transport facilitator family with glucose transport activity. J Biol Chem 275: 16275-16280.

Doré S, Kar S, Rowe W, Quirion R. 1997. Distribution and levels of $[^{125}I]$IGF-I, $[^{125}I]$IGF-II and $[^{125}I]$Insulin receptor binding sites in the hippocampus of aged memory-unimpaired and -impaired rats. Neuroscience 80: 1033-1040.

Duara R, Grady C, Haxby J, Sundaram M, Cutler NR, et al. 1986. Positron emission tomography in Alzheimer's disease. Neurology 36: 879-887.

Duelli R, Kuschinsky W. 2001. Brain glucose transporters; relationship to local energy demand. News Physiol Sci 16: 71-76.

Duelli R, Staudt R, Duembgen L, Kuschinsky W. 1999. Increase in glucose transporter densities of Glut3 and decrease of glucose utilization in rat brain after one week of hypoglycemia. Brain Res 831: 254-262.

Farrell CR, Pardridge WM. 1991. Blood-brain barrier glucose transporter is assymmetrically distributed on brain capillary endothelial lumenal and ablumenal membranes: An electron microscopic immunogold study. Proc Natl Acad Sci USA 88: 5779-5783.

Farrell CR, Yang J, Pardridge WM. 1992. GLUT-1 glucose transporter is present within the apical and basolateral membranes of brain epithelial interfaces and in microvascular endothelia with and without tight junctions. J Histochem Cytochem 40: 193-199.

Friedland RP, Jagust WJ, Heusman RH, Koss E, Knittel B, et al. 1989. Regional cerebral glucose transport and utilization in Alzheimer's disease. Neurology 39: 1427-1434.

Garcia ML, Millan C, Balmaceda-Aguilera C, Castro T, Pastor P, et al. 2003. Hypothalamic ependymal-glial cells express the glucose transporter GLUT2, a protein involved in glucose sensing. J Neurochem 86: 709-724.

Garvey WT, Hardin D, Juhaszova M, Dominguez JH. 1993. Effects of diabetes on myocardial glucose transport system in rats: Implications for diabetic cardiomyopathy. Am J Physiol 264: H837-H844.

Gerhart DZ, Le Vasseur RJ, Broderius MA, Drewes LR. 1989. Glucose transporter localization in brain using light and electron immunocytochemistry. J Neurosci Res 22: 464-472.

Gerhart DZ, Leino RL, Borson ND, Taylor WE, Gronlund KM, et al. 1995. Localization of glucose transporter GLUT 3 in brain: Comparison of rodent and dog using species-specific carboxyl-terminal antisera. Neuroscience 66: 237-246.

Giaume C, Tabernero A, Medina JM. 1997. Metabolic trafficking through astrocytic gap junctions. Glia 21: 114-123.

Gispen WH, Biessels G-J. 2000. Cognition and synaptic plasticity in diabetes mellitus. Trends Neurosci 23: 542-549.

Gould E, Cameron HA, Daniels DC, Woolley CS, McEwen BS. 1992. Adrenal hormones suppress cell division in the adult rat dentate gyrus. J Neurosci 12: 3642-3650.

Gould E, McEwen BS, Tanapat P, Galea LA, Fuchs E. 1997. Neurogenesis in the dentate gyrus of the adult tree shrew is regulated by psychosocial stress and NMDA receptor activation. J Neurosci 17: 2492-2498.

Grillo CA, Piroli GG, Wood GE, Reznikov LR, McEwen BS, Reagan LP. 2005. Immunocytochemical analysis of synaptic proteins provides new insights into diabetes mediated plasticity in the rat hippocampus. Neuroscience 136: 477-486.

Haber RS, Weinstein SP, O'Boyle E, Morgello S. 1993. Tissue distribution of the human GLUT3 glucose transporter. Endocrinology 132: 2538-2543.

Harr SD, Simonian NA, Hyman BT. 1995. Functional alterations in Alzheimer's disease: Decreased glucose transporter 3 immunoreactivity in the perforant pathway terminal zone. J Neuropathol Exp Neurol 54: 38-41.

Heilig C, Brosius F, Siu B, Concepcion L, Mortensen R, et al. 2003. Implications of glucose transporter protein type 1 (GLUT1)-haplodeficiency in embryonic stem cells for their survival in response to hypoxic stress. Am J Pathol 163: 1873-1885.

Ibberson M, Uldry M, Thorens B. 2000. GLUTx1, a novel mammalian glucose transporter expressed in the central nervous system and insulin-sensitive tissues. J Biol Chem 275: 4607-4612.

Ibberson M, Riederer BM, Uldry M, Guhl B, Roth J, et al. 2002. Immunolocalization of GLUTX1 in the testis and to specific brain areas and vasopressin containing neurons. Endocrinology 143: 276-284.

Joost HG, Bell GI, Best JD, Birnbaum MJ, Charron MJ, et al. 2002. Nomenclature of the GLUT/SLC2A family of sugar/polyol transport facilitators. Am J Physiol Endocrinol Metab 282: E974-E976.

Kahn BB, Flier JS. 1990. Regulation of glucose-transporter gene expression in vitro and in vivo. Diabetes Care 13: 548-564.

Kainulainen H, Breiner M, Schurmann A, Marttinen A, Virjo A, et al. 1994. In vivo glucose uptake and glucose transporter proteins GLUT1 and GLUT4 in heart and various types of skeletal muscle from streptozotocin-diabetic rats. Biochim Biophys Acta 1225: 275-282.

Kalaria RN, Harik SI. 1989. Reduced glucose transporter at the blood-brain barrier and in cerebral cortex in Alzheimer disease. J Neurochem 53: 1083-1088.

Kang L, Routh VH, Kuzhikandathil EV, Gaspers LD, Levin BE. 2004. Physiological and molecular characteristics of rat hypothalamic ventromedial nucleus glucosensing neurons. Diabetes 53: 549-559.

Kasanicki MA, Cairns MT, Davies A, Gardiner RM. 1987. Identification and characterization of the glucose-transport protein of the bovine blood-brain barrier. Biochem J 247: 101-108.

Kasanicki MA, Jessen KR, Baldwin SA, Boyle JM, Davies A, et al. 1989. Immunocytochemical localization of the glucose-transport protein in mammalian brain capillaries. Histochem J 21: 47-51.

Katz EB, Stenbit AE, Hatton K, Depinho R, Charron MJ. 1995. Cardiac and adipose tissue abnormalities but not diabetes in mice deficient in GLUT4. Nature 377: 151-155.

Kayano T, Fukumoto H, Eddy RL, Fan Y-S, Byers MG, et al. 1988. Evidence for a family of human glucose transporter-like proteins. J Biol Chem 263: 15245-15248.

Kayano T, Burant CF, Fukumoto H, Gould GW, Fan YS, et al. 1990. Human facilitative glucose transporters. Isolation, functional characterization, and gene localization of cDNAs encoding an isoform (GLUT5) expressed in small intestine, kidney, muscle, and adipose tissue and an unusual glucose transporter pseudogene-like sequence (GLUT6). J Biol Chem 265: 13276-13282.

Klepper J, Diefenbach S, Kohlschutter A, Voit T. 2004. Effects of the ketogenic diet in the glucose transporter 1 deficiency syndrome. Prostaglandins Leukot Essent Fatty Acids 70: 321-327.

Kobayashi M, Nikami H, Morimatsu M, Saito M. 1996. Expression and localization of insulin-regulatable glucose transporter (GLUT4) in rat brain. Neurosci Lett 213: 103-106.

Kumagai AK, Kang YS, Boado RJ, Pardridge WM. 1995. Upregulation of blood-brain barrier GLUT1 glucose transporter protein and mRNA in experimental chronic hypoglycemia. Diabetes 44: 1399-1404.

Leino RL, Gerhart DZ, Bueren Van AM, McCall AL, Drewes LR. 1997. Ultrastructural localization of GLUT1 and GLUT3 glucose transporters in rat brain. J Neurosci Res 49: 617-626.

Le Loup C, Arluison M, Lepetit N, Cartier N, Marfaing-Jallat P, et al. 1994. Glucose transporter 2 (GLUT 2): Expression in specific brain nuclei. Brain Res 638: 221-226.

Le Loup C, Arluison M, Kassis N, Lepetit N, Cartier N, et al. 1996. Discrete brain areas express the insulin-responsive glucose transporter GLUT4. Mol Brain Res 38: 45-53.

Le Loup C, Orosco M, Serradas P, Nicolaidis S, Penicaud L. 1998. Specific inhibition of GLUT2 in arcuate nucleus by antisense oligonucleotides suppresses nervous control of insulin secretion. Brain Res Mol Brain Res 57: 275-280.

Levin BE, Dunn-Meynell AA, Routh VH. 2001. Brain glucosensing and the K_{ATP} channel. Nat Neurosci 4: 459-460.

Levin BE, Routh VH, Kang L, Sanders NM, Dunn-Meynell AA. 2004. Neuronal glucosensing: What do we know after 50 years? Diabetes 53: 2521-2528.

Li SH, McNeill JH. 2001. In vivo effects of vanadium on GLUT4 translocation in cardiac tissue of STZ-diabetic rats. Mol Cell Biochem 217: 121-129.

Li B, Xi X, Roane DS, Ryan DH, Martin RJ. 2003. Brain Res Mol Brain Res 113: 139-142.

Lisinski I, Schurmann A, Joost HG, Cushman SW, Al-Hasani H. 2001. Targeting of GLUT6 (formerly GLUT9) and GLUT8 in rat adipose cells. Biochem J 358: 517-522.

Lund-Anderen H. 1979. Transport of glucose from blood to brain. Physiol Rev 59: 305-310.

Magistretti PJ, Pellerin L, Rothman DL, Shulman RG. 1999. Energy on demand. Science 283: 496-497.

Maher F, Vannucci S, Takeda J, Simpson IA. 1992. Expression of mouse-GLUT3 and human-GLUT3 glucose transporter proteins in brain. Biochem Biophys Res Commun 182: 703-711.

Maher F, Vannucci SJ, Simpson IA. 1994. Glucose transporter proteins in brain. FASEB J 8: 1003-1011.

Marcus RG, England R, Nguyen K, Charron MJ, Briggs JP, et al. 1994. Altered renal expression of the insulin-responsive glucose transporter GLUT4 in experimental diabetes mellitus. Am J Physiol 267: F816-F824.

Marger MD, Saier MH Jr. 1993. A major superfamily of transmembrane facilitators that catalyse uniport, symport and antiport. Trends Biochem Sci 18: 13-20.

Marks JL, Porte D Jr, Stahl WL, Baskin DG. 1991. Localization of insulin receptor mRNA in rat brain by in situ hybridization. Endocrinology 127: 3234-3236.

McCall AL. 1992. The impact of diabetes on the CNS. Diabetes 41: 557-570.

McCall AL, Van Bueren AM, Moholt-Siebert M, Cherry NJ, Woodward WR. 1994. Immunohistochemical localization of the neuron-specific glucose transporter (GLUT3) to neuropil in adult rat brain. Brain Res 659: 292-297.

McEwen BS. 1998. Protective and damaging effects of stress mediators. N Engl J Med 338: 171-179.

McEwen BS. 1999. Stress and hippocampal plasticity. Annu Rev Neurosci 22: 105-122.

McEwen BS. 2003. Mood disorders and allostatic load. Biol Psychiatry 54: 200-207.

McEwen BS, Reagan LP. 2004. Glucose transporter expression in the central nervous system: Relationship to synaptic function. Eur J Pharmacol 490: 13-24.

Messari SE, LeLoup C, Quignon M, Brisorgueil M-J, Penicaud L, et al. 1998. Immunocytochemical localization of the insulin-responsive glucose transporter 4 (Glut4) in the rat central nervous system. J Comp Neurol 399: 492-512.

Messier C. 2004. Glucose improvement of memory: A review. Eur J Pharmacol 490: 33-57.

Mooradian AD, Chung HC, Shah GN. 1997. GLUT-1 expression in the cerebra of patients with Alzheimer's disease. Neurobiol Aging 18: 469-474.

Morgello S, Uson RR, Schwartz EJ, Haber RS. 1995. The human blood-brain barrier glucose transporter (GLUT1) is a glucose transporter of gray matter astrocytes. Glia 14: 43-54.

Nagamatsu S, Kornhauser JM, Burant CF, Seino S, Mayo KE, et al. 1992. Glucose transporter expression in brain. J Biol Chem 267: 467-472.

Nagamatsu S, Sawa H, Kamada K, Nakamichi Y, Yoshimoto K, et al. 1993. Neuron-specific glucose transporter (NSGT): CNS distribution of GLUT3 rat glucose transporter (RGT3) in rat central neurons. FEBS Lett 334: 289-295.

Ngarmukos C, Baur EL, Kumagai AK. 2001. Co-localization of GLUT1 and GLUT4 in the blood-brain barrier of the rat ventromedial hypothalamus. Brain Res 900: 1-8.

Pardridge WM. 1983. Brain metabolism: A perspective from the blood-brain barrier. Physiol Rev 63: 1481-1535.

Pardridge WM, Boado RJ, Farrell CR. 1990. Brain-type glucose transporter (GLUT-1) is selectively localized to the blood-brain barrier. J Biol Chem 265: 18035-18040.

Park CR. 2001. Cognitive effects of insulin in the central nervous system. Neurosci Biobehav Rev 25: 311-323.

Pascual JM, Wang D, Lecumberri B, Yang H, Mao X, et al. 2004. GLUT1 deficiency and other glucose transporter diseases. Eur J Endocrinol 150: 627-633.

Pavlides C, Watanabe Y, McEwen BS. 1993. Effects of glucocorticoids on hippocampal long-term potentiation. Hippocampus 3: 183-192.

Payne J, Maher F, Simpson I, Mattice L, Davies P. 1997. Glucose transporter Glut 5 expression in microglial cells. Glia 21: 327-331.

Pellerin L, Magistretti PJ. 2004. Neuroenergetics: Calling upon astrocytes to satisfy hungry neurons. Neuroscientist 10: 53-62.

Pessin JE, Thurmond DC, Elmendorf JS, Coker KJ, Okada S. 1999. Molecular basis of insulin-stimulated GLUT4 vesicle trafficking. J Biol Chem 274: 2593-2596.

Pierre K, Pellerin L, Debernardi R, Riederer BM, Magistretti PJ. 2000. Cell-specific localization of monocarboxylate transporters, MCT1 and MCT2, in the adult mouse brain revealed by double immunohistochemical labeling and confocal microscopy. Neuroscience 100: 617-627.

Piert M, Koeppe RA, Giordani B, Berent S, Kuhl DE. 1996. Diminished glucose transport and phosphorylation in Alzheimer's disease determined by dynamic FDG-PET. J Nucl Med 37: 201-208.

Piroli GG, Grillo CA, Hoskin EK, Znamensky V, Katz EB, et al. 2002. Peripheral glucose administration stimulates the translocation of GLUT8 glucose transporter to the endoplasmic reticulum in the rat hippocampus. J Comp Neurol 452: 103-114.

Piroli GG, Grillo CA, Charron MJ, McEwen BS, Reagan LP. 2004. Biphasic effects of stress upon GLUT8 glucose transporter expression and trafficking in the diabetic rat hippocampus. Brain Res 1006: 28-35.

Rand EB, Depaoli AM, Davidson NO, Bell GI, Burant CF. 1993. Sequence, tissue distribution, and functional characterization of the rat fructose transporter GLUT5. Am J Physiol 264: G1169-G1176.

Rayner DV, Thomas MEA, Trayhurn P. 1994. Glucose transporters (GLUTs 1–4) and their mRNAs in regions of the rat brain: Insulin-sensitive transporter expression in the cerebellum. Can J Physiol Pharmacol 72: 476-479.

Reagan LP. 2002. Glucose, stress and hippocampal neuronal vulnerability. Int Rev Neurobiol 51: 289-324.

Reagan LP, Ye X, Mir R, DePalo LP, Fluharty SJ. 1990. Upregulation of angiotensin II receptors by in vitro differentiation of murine N1E-115 neuroblastoma cells. Mol Pharm 38: 878-886.

Reagan LP, Magariños AM, Lucas LR, Van Bueren A, McCall AL. 1999. Regulation of GLUT3 glucose transporter in the hippocampus of diabetic rats subjected to stress. Am J Physiol 276: E879-E886.

Reagan LP, Gorovits N, Hoskin EK, Alves SE, Katz EB, et al. 2001. Localization and regulation of GLUTx1 glucose transporter in the hippocampus of streptozotocin diabetic rats. Proc Natl Acad Sci USA 98: 2820-2825.

Reagan LP, Rosell DR, Alves SE, Hoskin EK, McCall AL, et al. 2002. GLUT8 glucose transporter is localized to excitatory and inhibitory neurons in the rat hippocampus. Brain Res 932: 129-134.

Roncero I, Alvarez E, Chowen JA, Sanz C, Rabano A, Vazquez P, Blazquez E. 2004. J Neurochem 88: 1203-1210.

Rosmond R, Dallman MF, Bjorntörp P. 1998. Stress-related cortisol secretion in men: Relationships with abdominal obesity and endocrine, metabolic and hemodynamic abnormalities. J Clin Endocrinol Metab 83: 1853-1859.

Saltiel AR, Pessin JE. 2002. Insulin signaling pathways in time and space. Trends Cell Biol 12: 65-71.

Sankar R, Thamotharan S, Shin D, Moley KH, Devaskar SU. 2002. Insulin-responsive glucose transporters-GLUT8 and GLUT4 are expressed in the developing mammalian brain. Mol Brain Res 107: 157-165.

Sasaki A, Horikoshi Y, Yokoo H, Nakazato Y, Yamaguchi H. 2003. Antiserum against human glucose transporter 5 is highly specific for microglia among cells of the mononuclear phagocyte system. Neurosci Lett 338: 17-20.

Sasaki A, Yamaguchi H, Horikoshi Y, Tanaka G, Nakazato Y. 2004. Expression of glucose transporter 5 by microglia in human gliomas. Neuropathol Appl Neurobiol 30: 447-455.

Schwartz MW, Figlewicz DP, Baskin DG, Woods SC, Porte D Jr. 1992. Insulin in the brain: A hormonal regulator of energy balance. Endocr Rev 13: 387-414.

Severino C, Brizzi P, Solinas A, Secchi G, Maioli M, et al. 2002. Low-dose dexamethasone in the rat: A model to study insulin resistance. Am J Physiol Endocrinol Metab 283: E367-E373.

Sheline YI, Sanghavi M, Mintun MA, Gado MH. 1999. Depression duration but not age predicts hippocampal volume loss in medically healthy women with recurrent major depression. J Neurosci 19: 5034-5043.

Shepherd PR, Kahn BB. 1999. Glucose transporters and insulin action. Implications for insulin resistance and diabetes mellitus. N Engl J Med 341: 248-257.

Shepherd PR, Gibbs EM, Wesslau C, Gould GW, Kahn BB. 1992. Human small intestine facilitative fructose/glucose transporter (GLUT5) is also present in insulin-responsive tissues and brain. Investigation of biochemical characteristics and translocation. Diabetes 41: 1360-1365.

Shin BC, McKnight RA, Devaskar SU. 2004. Glucose transporter GLUT8 translocation in neurons is not insulin responsive. J Neurosci Res 75: 835-844.

Shulman RG, Hyder F, Rothman DL. 2001. Lactate efflux and the neuroenergetic basis of brain function. NMR Biomed 14: 389-396.

Simpson IA, Chunda KR, Davies-Hill T, Honer WG, Davies P. 1994. Decreased concentrations of GLUT1 and GLUT3 glucose transporters in the brains of patients with Alzheimer's disease. Ann Neurol 35: 546-551.

Simpson IA, Appel NM, Hokari M, Oki J, Holman GD, et al. 1999. Blood-brain barrier glucose transporter: Effects of hypo- and hyperglycemia revisited. J Neurochem 72: 238-247.

Smith U, Axelsen M, Carvalho E, Eliasson B, Jansson PA, et al. 1999. Insulin signaling and action in fat cells: Associations with insulin resistance and type 2 diabetes. Ann NY Acad Sci 892: 119-126.

Stojanovska L, Rosella G, Proietto J. 1990. Evolution of dexamethasone-induced insulin resistance in rats. Am J Physiol 258: E748-E756.

Uehara Y, Nipper V, McCall AL. 1997. Chronic insulin hypoglycemia induces GLUT-3 protein in rat brain neurons. Am J Physiol 272: E716-E719.

Vannucci S, Clark RR, Koehler-Stec E, Li K, Smith CB, et al. 1998a. Glucose transporter expression in brain: Relationship to cerebral glucose utilization. Dev Neurosci 20: 369-379.

Vannucci SJ. 1994. Developmental expression of GLUT1 and GLUT3 glucose transporters in rat brain. J Neurochem 62: 240-246.

Vannucci SJ, Simpson IA. 2003. Developmental switch in brain nutrient transporter expression in the rat. Am J Physiol Endocrinol Metab 285: E1127-E1134.

Vannucci SJ, Maher F, Simpson IA. 1997. Glucose transporter proteins in brain: Delivery of glucose to neurons and glia. Glia 21: 2-21.

Vannucci SJ, Koehler-Stec EM, Li K, Reynolds TH, Clark R, et al. 1998b. GLUT4 glucose transporter expression in rodent brain: Effects of diabetes. Brain Res 797: 1-11.

Wang D, Pascual JM, Yang H, Engelstad K, Jhung S, et al. 2005. Glut-1 deficiency syndrome: Clinical, genetic, and therapeutic aspects. Ann Neurol 57: 111-118.

Wan HZ, Hulsey MG, Martin RJ. 1998. Intracerebroventricular administration of antisense oligodeoxynucleotide against GLUT2 glucose transporter mRNA reduces food intake, body weight change and glucoprivic feeding response in rats. J Nutr 128: 287-291.

Weinstein SP, Wilson CM, Pritsker A, Cushman SW. 1998. Dexamethasone inhibits insulin-stimulated recruitment of GLUT4 to the cell surface in rat skeletal muscle. Metabolism 47: 3-6.

Woolley CS, Gould E, McEwen BS. 1990. Exposure to excess glucocorticoids alters dendritic morphology of adult hippocampal pyramidal neurons. Brain Res 531: 225-231.

Yano H, Seino Y, Inagaki N, Hinokio Y, Yamamoto T, et al. 1991. Tissue distribution and species difference of the brain type glucose transporter (GLUT3). Biochem Biophys Res Commun 31: 470-477.

Young JK, McKenzie JC. 2004. GLUT2 immunoreactivity in Gomori-positive astrocytes of the hypothalamus. J Histochem Cytochem 52: 1519-1524.

Yu S, Ding WG. 1998. The 45 kDa form of glucose transporter 1 (GLUT1) is localized in oligodendrocyte and astrocyte but not in microglia in the rat brain. Brain Res 797: 65-72.

Zeller K, Duelli R, Vogel J, Schrock H, Kuschinsky W. 1995. Autoradiographic analysis of the regional distribution of Glut3 glucose transporters in the rat brain. Brain Res 698: 175-179.

20 Peptide/Polypeptide Transport in the Central Nervous System

W. Pan · A. J. Kastin

Abstract: It has been known for three decades that certain peptides in the peripheral circulation affect various central nervous system (CNS) functions. Peptides can cross the blood–brain barrier (BBB), produce secondary mediators without entering the brain and spinal cord themselves, reach the CNS by retrograde axonal transport, or affect circumventricular organs (CVOs). The transport systems enabling direct passage of peptides from blood to the CNS or vice versa can be studied in intact animals by pharmacokinetic analyses. Because of the short half-life and relative instability of most peptides, experimental modeling is required. In vivo characterization of peptide transport across the BBB provides basal information for pharmacological design of peptides as drugs in human disorders. Illumination of intracellular trafficking and factors modulating the fate of a peptide in cerebral endothelial cells further assists our understanding of disease processes. We will discuss the transport of peptides in the CNS by categorizing them by effects such as feeding, inflammation, neurotrophism, degeneration, sleep induction, and pain modulation. Representative peptides/polypeptides discussed include leptin, urocortin, insulin-like growth factor, epidermal growth factor, basic fibroblast growth factor, transforming growth factor, platelet-derived growth factor, the interleukins, tumor necrosis factor α, leukemia inhibitory factor, some chemokines, and neurotrophins. Besides the specific transport systems, we will also discuss nonsaturable permeation of peptides across the BBB, other aspects of peptide interactions with cerebral endothelial cells composing the BBB, the efflux systems, and the special situation of CVOs that are outside the BBB. The variety of peptidergic actions of circulating peptides on the CNS indicates that they are important regulators in the neurovascular interface of the BBB.

List of Abbreviations: ACTH, corticotropin; adrenocorticotropic hormone; AgRP, agouti-regulated protein; AM, adrenomeulllin; ANP, atrial natriuretic peptide; AT, angiotensin; AVP, arginine vasopressin; BBB, blood–brain barrier; CART, cocaine-regulated and amphetamine-regulated transcript; CCK, cholecystokinin; CINC1, cytokine-induced neutrophil chemoattractant-1; CNS, central nervous system; CNTF, ciliary neurotrophic factor; CRH, corticotropin-releasing hormone; CSF, cerebrospinal fluid; CVO, circumventricular organ(s); DSIP, delta sleep-inducing peptide; EGF, epidermal growth factor; ET, endothelin; FGF, fibroblast growth factor; GALP, galanin-like peptide; GDNF, glial cell line-derived neurotrophic factor; GLP-1, glucagon-like peptide; GM-CSF, granulocyte-macrophage colony-stimulating factor; GnRH, gonadotropin-releasing hormone; HPLC, high performance liquid chromatography; IGF, insulin-like growth factor; IGFBP, IGF binding protein; IL, interleukin; K_i, unidirectional influx constant; LHRH, luteinizing hormone-releasing hormone; LIF, leukemia inhibitory factor; MCH, melanin-concentrating hormone; MIF-1, Pro-Leu-Gly-NH$_2$; MIP, macrophage inflammatory proteins; MSH, melanocyte-stimulating hormone; NPY, neuropeptide Y; PACAP, pituitary adenylate cyclase-activating polypeptide; PDGF, platelet-derived Growth factor; TGF, transforming growth factor; TNF, tumor necrosis factor; VIP, vasoactive intestinal peptide; V_i, initial volume of distribution

1   Introduction

Cerebral microvessel endothelial cells form the major constituent of the blood–brain barrier (BBB), along with pericytes, astrocytic endfeet, and extracellular matrix. This interface between central nervous system (CNS) parenchyma and its supplying capillary vessels prevents free passage of peptides and proteins, which cannot diffuse across membrane lipid bilayers. The endothelial cells are joined by tight junctions and lined with a continuous basement membrane; they have reduced pinocytotic vesicles and increased metabolic and enzymatic activities. Since the observation about four decades ago that circulating peptides can exert CNS effects, there has been much progress in the pharmacokinetics and mechanisms of direct permeation of peptides (fewer than 100 amino acids) and polypeptides (100–200 amino acids) across the BBB. This chapter will summarize developments in the field of peptide transport, most of it originating from our laboratory, and the considerable work of others in the design of peptide drugs for better delivery into the CNS. We will also assess the position of peptide/polypeptide transport systems at the BBB in the overall picture of peptide/polypeptide trafficking in the CNS.

2   Peptide Transport Across the BBB

2.1   Duration of CNS Actions Induced by Peripheral Peptides

Peptides, especially small ones, are rapidly degraded in blood. This is well known to occur when these small proteins are added to a tube of blood at room temperature. Peptides also have short half-lives when injected into the blood circulation, lasting only a few minutes in intact form, as shown for melanocyte-stimulating hormone (MSH) (Redding et al., 1978), MIF-1 (Pro-Leu-Gly-NH$_2$) (Redding et al., 1973b, 1974), and luteinizing hormone-releasing hormone (LHRH) (Redding et al., 1973a). Yet their biological effects can last much longer. This is illustrated by the persistence of electroencephalographic effects of MSH (Sandman et al., 1971; Kastin et al., 1976; Redding et al., 1978), behavioral effects of MIF-1 (Plotnikoff et al., 1971; Redding et al., 1973b, 1974; Kastin et al., 1978), and mating effects of LHRH (Pfaff, 1973) for at least an hour after peripheral administration.

2.2   The Experimental Models for In Vivo Studies

The half-life of a naturally occurring peptide in the circulation is usually short (minutes). Apart from sequestration by capillary beds and excretion by the kidney, peptides are susceptible to degradation in blood and within cells (e.g., liver) by metabolic enzymes (peptidases), and their bioavailability is also affected by the extent of protein binding and aggregation. Therefore, experimental models should consider the stability, dynamic changes of concentration, different compartments involved, and the slow rate of penetration of peptides across the BBB (as contrasted with ions, glucose, amino acids, water, and lipophilic substances).

Banks, Kastin, and colleagues coined the term multiple-time regression analysis to determine the unidirectional influx constant (K_i) and initial volume of distribution (V_i) of radioactively labeled (radiolabeled = radiotracer) peptides from blood after intravenous (i.v.) injection (Banks and Kastin, 1993). The pharmacokinetic parameters are built on a two-compartment model, modified from a series of methods previously used to study nonpeptide substances (Greenblatt and Koch-Weser, 1975; Blasberg et al., 1983; Patlak et al., 1983).

One of the prerequisites for the measurement of K_i is that the peptide remains stable during the study period, so that the radioactivity measured represents intact peptide and the amount can be calculated from the specific activity (in Ci/g). Reversed phase high-performance liquid chromatography (HPLC) is the method of choice over other chromatographic methods, gel autoradiography, and acid precipitation because of its higher sensitivity and specificity (Hoke, 1993). With gel autoradiography, for instance, it may be difficult to quantify the percent of degradation by densitometry because of the smear of degradation products. Radiotracer methods still hold many advantages over other methods in determination of the kinetics of transport in small animals. This is mainly because other methods of sample preparation, such as fluorescent tracers, ELISA, and radioimmunoassay (RIA), require further tissue treatment, at least homogenization and centrifugation, to obtain the supernatant. The recovery is incomplete and multiple controls and normalization steps are needed.

The i.v. bolus injection and multiple-time regression studies can easily incorporate a three-compartment model by use of vascular perfusion to identify the cardiovascular space and a capillary depletion procedure to differentiate the capillary fraction from the brain parenchyma. In this way, the amount of peptide in blood, tightly bound or endocytosed in the BBB and that completely transcytosed, can be identified.

Since the K_i measured after i.v. injection of radiotracer can be affected by multiple physiological variable, such as endogenous peptide concentrations (which could mask the detection of a saturable transport system), protein binding, peripheral degradation, and renal excretion, the method of in situ brain perfusion can address issues about direct interactions of peptides with the BBB. Delivery of radiotracers in perfusion buffer at a constant rate is less physiological than application of the radiolabeled peptides directly into blood. However, the in situ perfusion system is adequate to determine potential modulators for transport such as excess unlabeled peptide (a reduced K_i illustrates saturability of the transport system), inhibitors for receptor-mediated transport (such as clathrin- or caveolae-mediated pathways), inhibitors for adsorptive endocytosis, and facilitative substances that would increase the K_i.

2.3   Specific Examples of Peptide Transport in Relation to Their Function

2.3.1   Feeding-Related Peptides

Leptin   Leptin has not fulfilled its initial promise, in large part, because of "leptin resistance" whereby high concentrations of leptin in the blood do not result in the satiety induced by high concentrations in the brain. This can be explained by saturation of the blood-to-brain transport system for leptin (Banks et al., 1996). This transport system is subject to physiological signals, being decreased by food deprivation (Kastin and Akerstrom, 2000a) and increased by glucose administration (Kastin and Akerstrom, 2001a). However, we have yet to find an ingestive peptide/polypeptide that alters the transport of leptin across the BBB. The ObRa leptin receptor appears to mediate much of the transport of leptin into the brain; however, other unidentified factors must also be involved (Kastin et al., 1999). As demonstrated by Peruzoo et al. (2000), the site of action of leptin—the arcuate nucleus of the hypothalamus—lies within the BBB.

Urocortin   Urocortin, like leptin, has a saturable transport system across the BBB that is unmasked once it is activated by leptin (Kastin et al., 2000d) or pretreatment with glucose (Kastin and Akerstrom, 2001b). In vitro, its transcytosis seems to be more efficient than that of leptin. Transport of urocortin is mediated by both CRHR1 and CRHR2 receptors, and the facilitating effect of leptin on this transport involves the leptin receptors ObRa as well as ObRb (Tu et al., unpublished data).

Melanin-Concentrating Hormone   Thus far we have discussed leptin that enters by a saturable transport system and urocortin that enters after activation by leptin, perhaps related to its protein binding. Melanin-concentrating hormone (MCH) also has protein binding, but in this situation it has no influx into brain from blood (probably also explained by protein binding) and its influx is not activated by leptin. In addition to binding to blood proteins, MCH may self-aggregate (Kastin et al., 2000b).

Galanin-like Peptide   Like leptin, galanin-like peptide (GALP) decreases feeding by acting at the arcuate nucleus of the hypothalamus. Also like leptin, food deprivation decreases its saturable transport into brain, and the decrease in its rate of entry precedes the drop in blood GALP-like immunoreactivity (Kastin et al., 2001a). We found that its related peptide galanin was rapidly metabolized after i.v. injection (unpublished results).

Cocaine-Regulated and Amphetamine-Regulated Transcript   Cocaine-regulated and amphetamine-regulated transcript (CART) is another anorexic peptide regulated by leptin with actions in the arcuate nucleus. It enters brain from blood at a rapid rate but not by a saturable system (Kastin and Akerstrom, 1999a). As expected, therefore, co-injection of leptin did not influence its influx into brain.

Ghrelin   Ghrelin, produced mainly in the stomach, increases feeding. Its structure is very unusual for a peptide, being modified at its third amino acid (Ser) by posttranslational acylation with the fatty acid n-octanoic acid, a modification essential for its bioactivity. Octanoylated human, but not mouse, ghrelin has a saturable transport system both into and out of the brain. The only saturable transport system for mouse ghrelin is out of the brain. Removal of the octanoyl modification results in a peptide without a saturable transport system across the BBB (Banks et al., 2002).

Neuropeptide Y   Neuropeptide Y (NPY) is probably the most potent orexigenic substance increasing feeding. It enters the brain by passive diffusion and not by a saturable transport mechanism (Kastin and Akerstrom, 1999b). Fasting of mice for 48 h, expected to increase NPY production, failed to change NPY influx into the brain.

Orexin Another peptide increasing food consumption is orexin. Orexin B is rapidly metabolized, but orexin A enters the brain by passive diffusion, the same process used by NPY involving physicochemical properties like lipophilicity, hydrogen bonding, and conformation (Chikhale et al., 1994; Kastin and Akerstrom, 1999c).

Agouti-Related Protein Agouti-related protein (AgRP) can also result in obesity, acting mainly as an antagonist of the MC4 (and MC3) receptor. Like NPY, it mediates the effect of leptin in the arcuate nucleus of the hypothalamus. It can enter the brain, but at a very slow rate, probably explained by its self-aggregation in blood, mostly as a trimer (Kastin et al., 2000a).

Mahogany The mahogany protein, also called attractin, appears to be involved in the actions of AgRP, but relatively little attention has been given to it. Because we found it to have one of the few saturable transport systems into the brain, it deserves more investigation, at least for the suppression of diet-induced obesity (Kastin and Akerstrom, 2000b).

Glucagon-like Peptide Glucagon-like peptide (GLP-1) is a gut peptide with receptors in brain. Like CART, NPY, and AgRP, it has a high density of binding sites in the arcuate nucleus of the hypothalamus. It enters the brain nonsaturably by passive diffusion (Kastin et al., 2002a).

Exendin-4 Exendin-4 is somewhat similar in structure to GLP-1. Originally isolated from the saliva of the Gila monster, it is a potent satiety agent. It is used in clinical trials for the treatment of diabetes. It enters the brain from blood with only slight saturation, indicating that increasing doses might continue to reach the brain (Kastin and Akerstrom, 2003).

Three Peptides of the Pancreas Pancreatic polypeptide is transported by a saturable system into the brain (Banks and Kastin, 1995). Amylin enters by passive diffusion (Banks et al., 1995a), but it seems to enter faster than insulin (Banks and Kastin, 1998), which is unusual since insulin enters by a saturable transport system. The transport system for insulin is operational at physiological levels of insulin (Banks et al., 1997a, c). Mice with diabetes induced by streptozotocin or alloxin have increased transport of insulin into the brain (Banks et al., 1997b). A relatively high rate of transport of insulin was found in the olfactory bulb, which contains one of the highest brain concentrations of insulin receptors (Banks et al., 1999). Starvation may influence the retention of insulin in the brain, an event perhaps triggered by tumor necrosis factor α (TNFα) (Cashion et al., 1996).

2.3.2 Endogenous Opioid Peptides Related to Pain Modulation

When a peptide is administered peripherally and exerts a CNS effect, it is possible that the effect is indirectly mediated. The first proof that an endogenous peptide administered peripherally directly crosses the BBB to exert a biological action involved use of an analog of Met-enkephalin. This pentapeptide was shown to cause marked electroencephalographic changes, which were blocked by an opiate antagonist that crossed the BBB, but not by one that did not cross the BBB (Kastin et al., 1991). Two pioneers in the BBB field, Stanley Rapoport and Tom Davis, have used synthetic analogs of endogenous opioids to show influx from blood-to-brain (Rapoport et al., 1980; Egleton and Davis, 1997; Witt et al., 2001). However, for the endogenous opioids themselves, it seems that saturable brain-to-blood transport predominates (● *Sect. 4*).

2.3.3 Peptides Affect Learning, Attention, and Memory

α-MSH α-MSH is the first peptide shown to affect the brain unconfounded by secondary effects (Kastin et al., 1975, 1979). It was also the first to be shown to cross the BBB in intact form (Redding et al., 1978). However, it crosses by passive diffusion rather than by a saturable transport system

(Wilson, 1998), although a synthetic analog—ebiratide—enters the brain saturably (Shimura et al., 1991; Pan et al., 1997a).

Corticotropin-Releasing Hormone   Corticotropin-releasing hormone (CRH), as its name implies, is the hypothalamic peptide stimulating the release of ACTH (corticotropin) which then stimulates the adrenal gland to release cortisol in humans and corticosterone in rodents. Its saturable rate of entry into the brain is moderate, and is not shared by the urocortins (Kastin and Akerstrom, 2002). Its saturable efflux system is discussed in a later section of this chapter.

Vasopressin   Many reports have appeared on the effects of arginine vasopressin (AVP) on learning and memory. Several of them show positive effects, although it is difficult to rule out the confounding effects of this peptide on blood pressure and fluid retention. Although there were some studies not finding any entry of AVP into the CNS, by in situ brain perfusion intact AVP crosses the BBB to reach brain parenchyma (Zlokovic et al., 1992).

2.3.4   Peptides Affecting the Reproductive System

Leptin exerts a permissive action on the reproductive system, partially through the hypothalamic LHRH, also called gonadotropin-releasing hormone (GnRH), since it stimulates the release of both luteinizing hormone and follicle-stimulating hormone from the pituitary gland (Schally et al., 1973). Like human ghrelin, CRH, and PACAP 38, but no other peptide yet tested, LHRH saturably crosses the BBB in both directions (Barrera et al., 1991). It is not known for any of these peptides whether the influx transporter is the same as that responsible for efflux.

2.3.5   Peptides Affecting Sleep

Many peptides affect sleep. The absence of orexin A is responsible for narcolepsy. Delta sleep-inducing peptide (DSIP) was described as a specific sleep-inducing peptide, although it can exert a variety of other effects. Before use of the multiple-time regression analysis method for quantification of peptide influx across the BBB, we developed an RIA for DSIP that required the presence of eight of its nine constitutive amino acids. By recognizing almost the entire structure, the antibody obviated the necessity for chromatographic determination whether the peripherally administered peptide crossed in intact form. Detection of DSIP in cerebrospinal fluid (CSF) as well as brain tissue showed that the peptide crossed the BBB intact. Moreover, even before the capillary depletion method was described, identification by RIA of DSIP in samples of CSF showed that peripherally administered DSIP entered the CNS (Kastin et al., 1981; Banks et al., 1982, 1986a). Subsequent studies involving radiolabeled DSIP indicated that DSIP crosses the BBB in rats by passive diffusion (Banks et al., 1984), and this method of entry was confirmed by in vitro studies with DSIP in bovine brain microvessel endothelial cells (Raessi and Audus, 1989). Nevertheless, a study with perfused sheep choroid plexus found that DSIP crosses the blood–CSF barrier by a high-affinity, low-capacity saturable transport system (Zlokovic et al., 1988).

2.3.6   Chemokines and Cytokines

Interleukin-1α and β   Interleukin (IL)-1α and β are among the proinflammatory cytokines that have saturable influx transport systems (Banks et al., 1989, 1991, 1993c). In their studies, Banks et al. (1989, 1991) reported an influx transfer constant of 0.25–0.43 μL/g min for IL-1α and 0.47 μL/g min for IL-1β. The initial volume of distribution was 20.1 and 16.5 μL/g, respectively. The relative stability of the ILs in blood circulation and in the brain was shown by HPLC and acid precipitation. Although there is influx transport, there is no saturability of the brain-to-blood efflux transport system. This vectorial passage indicates that IL-1 is an important mediator in communications between the CNS and the periphery.

The regional difference of the rate of transport illustrates that the transport system for IL-1α is physiologically pertinent to CNS function. IL-1α enters the hypothalamus more rapidly, and there is selective uptake in the posterior division of the septum (Banks et al., 1989; Maness et al., 1995). This is probably related to the suppression of feeding and catabolic metabolism induced by IL-1α. The circumventricular organs (CVOs) account for less than 5% of the total brain uptake of IL-1α and it seems that the permeation into the CVOs is still saturable (Plotkin et al., 1996). As IL-1 is pyrogenic, reduced permeation of IL-1β in aged animals probably partially explains the diminished fever response in the elderly (McLay et al., 2000). The IL-1 receptor antagonist also competes for this transport system, in contrast to IL-2, IL-6, TNFα, or MIP-1α (Gutierrez et al., 1994).

Interleukin-2   IL-2 has binding sites in the brain where it exerts a variety of effects. It crosses the BBB from blood about ten times faster than albumin. However, this does not occur by a saturable transport system (Waguespack et al., 1994).

Interleukin-6   IL-6 also has a saturable influx transport system, shared by human and murine IL-6 and flagged murine IL-6, but not by that for IL-1 and TNFα (Banks et al., 1994). After i.v. delivery by bolus injection, intact IL-6 can be recovered from CSF at 10 min and 30 min. The lack of saturable efflux indicates that this transport system is unidirectional.

Interleukin-8   IL-8 is stable in the blood circulation and crosses the BBB only by simple diffusion. Influx into brain is limited and there is no efflux transport system (Pan and Kastin, 2004).

Interleukin-10   IL-10, a polypeptide of 160 amino acids, exerts CNS effects after peripheral administration. However, it does not enter the brain or spinal cord any faster than the vascular marker albumin (Kastin et al., 2003d).

TNFα   Although large doses of TNFα might disrupt the BBB and increase paracellular permeability of the BBB, TNFα can cross the BBB itself by a saturable influx transport system. Trace amounts of ^{125}I-TNFα are detected by HPLC in blood, brain homogenate, and CSF 30 min after i.v. delivery, without increasing the permeability of the coadministered vascular marker ^{99m}Tc-albumin (Gutierrez et al., 1993). A majority of TNFα enters brain and spinal cord parenchyma. The regional differences of the uptake are such that the spinal cord has higher permeation than the brain (Pan et al., 1997b). In the spinal cord, the cervical and lumbar segments have higher permeability reflected by a greater volume of distribution and faster influx rate. In the brain, the hypothalamus and occipital cortex appear to take up TNFα significantly faster (Banks et al., 2001). The influx of TNFα is blocked by preincubation with a soluble receptor against its p75 receptor (Banks et al., 1995b) and is absent in double TNFα receptor knockout mice (Pan and Kastin, 2002).

Leukemia Inhibitory Factor and Ciliary Neurotrophic Factor   Ciliary neurotrophic factor (CNTF) and leukemia inhibitory factor (LIF) cross the BBB by independent saturable transport systems (Pan et al., 1999b, 2000). Both have moderately fast influx rate (0.46 μL/g min for CNTF and 0.41 μL/g min for LIF). Although the two cytokines have one shared receptor subunit—gp130—there is no known cross-inhibition. The high affinity receptor gp190 is apparently involved in the transport of LIF, since a blocking antibody specifically reduced the influx transfer constant of LIF in both mouse studies and cultured brain endothelial cells (Pan W et al., unpublished observations).

Cytokine-Induced Neutrophil Chemoattractant-1   Cytokine-induced neutrophil chemoattractant-1 (CINC1) is member of the chemokine family of small, inducible, secreted proinflammatory cytokines. It also has angiogenic properties pertinent to the next section of this chapter. CINC1 has been found in brain and the cerebral vasculature after i.v. injection without evidence of a saturable system (Pan and Kastin, 2001a).

Macrophage Inflammatory Proteins 1α and 1β   Peripherally administered macrophage inflammatory proteins (MIP)-1α and -1β do not seem to enter brain tissue, being reversibly associated with the microvessels of the BBB (Banks and Kastin, 1996). Therefore, it is possible that they also could exert some effects pertinent to the following section.

2.3.7   Peptides Related to Vascular Proliferation, Cellular Adhesion, and Tumor Metastasis

Transforming Growth Factors   Transforming growth factor α (TGFα), a member of the epidermal growth factor (EGF) family, appeared to enter the brain rapidly, but most of the administered cytokine was trapped in the capillary endothelial cells composing the BBB (Pan et al., 1999d). Without substantial uptake into brain parenchyma, TGFα might possibly be involved in intracranial vascular disorders such as angiopathy. TGFβ did not enter the brain any faster than the vascular marker (Kastin et al., 2003b).

Fibroblast Growth Factor   Fibroblast growth factor (FGF) peptides (acid = 1, basic = 2) are involved in angiogenesis, cell growth, and differentiation. They also can exert neurotrophic effects as anti-apototic agents. Basic FGF(2) crosses the BBB by adsorptive endocytosis but much of it is bound to the cerebral microvessels (Deguchi et al., 2000).

Several of the neurotrophic peptides discussed below also exert actions that could fit into this section of the review.

2.3.8   Neurotrophic Peptides

Epidermal Growth Factor   Like insulin-like growth factor (IGF)-1, EGF is a trophic factor both in the periphery and CNS. EGF has a rapid, saturable transport system from blood to brain that does not seem to involve its receptor, and there is no efflux transport (Pan and Kastin, 1999). Although excess EGF as well as TGFα, which share the EGF receptor, can decrease the influx of radiolabeled EGF, a monoclonal antibody against the EGF receptor did not. A potential problem in the delivery of EGF and IGF-1 as therapeutic agents for CNS pathology is that both may promote tumor growth such as prostate cancer.

Neuregulin-1-β1   Neuregulin-1-β1 is a neurotrophic peptide representing amino acid residues 176–246 of the EGF domain of heregulin-β1, which is a product of the neuregulin family of genes. The neuregulin family binds to erbB3 and erbB4 receptors. Intact neuregulin-1-β1 enters both brain and spinal cord from blood relatively rapidly (Kastin et al., 2004). This is receptor mediated since an excess amount of neuregulin-1-β1 inhibited influx as did antibodies to erbB3 and erbB4 receptors of the EGF receptor family of tyrosine kinases. Both neuregulin-1-β1 and PDGF-AA enhance myelination of neuritis in spinal cord explants (Park et al., 2001).

Platelet-Derived Growth Factors AA and BB   Platelet-derived growth factors (PDGFs) exert neuro-modulatory and neurotrophic (see next section) effects on the CNS, but neither form of PDGF crosses the BBB any faster than the vascular marker albumin (Kastin et al., 2003a). The rapid degradation of PDGF-AA and protein binding of PDGF-BB probably play large roles in their poor permeation into the brain.

Insulin-like Growth Factor-1   The availability of IGF-1 in circulating blood to cross the BBB is significantly influenced by IGF-binding proteins (IGFBPs). To deliver sufficient amounts of IGF-1 to the CNS compartment, the binding sites of IGFBPs need to be occupied. Regardless, there is a saturable influx transport system for IGF-1 at the BBB (Pan and Kastin, 2000), which is at least partially shared with that for insulin (Yu et al., in press). The cross-inhibition of transport between IGF-1 and insulin indicates a receptor-mediated mechanism. The beneficial effects of IGF-1 include reduction of neurodegeneration and amelioration of autoimmune damage to the CNS (Raub and Audus, 1990; Liu et al., 1995; Lai et al., 1997). Thus, manipulation of the transport system and design of IGF-1 variants that can easily cross the BBB will be important goals for future research.

Glial Cell Line-Derived Neurotrophic Factor Glial cell line-derived neurotrophic factor (GDNF) has neuroprotective and neurorestorative properties that might make it an appealing thereapeutic agent. GDNF has relatively fast degradation in the blood circulation; such instability is compatible with it being produced and acting in the CNS. GDNF has no saturable transport, but diffuses across the BBB to some extent (Kastin et al., 2003c). Unlike GDNF, many other neurotrophins, such as nerve growth factor and neurotrophin-3, can be transported from blood into the CNS (Pan et al., 1998).

Ciliary Neurotrophic Factor CNTF also has neurotrophic properties. It is saturably transported across the BBB into brain, as mentioned in an earlier section of this review (Pan et al., 1999c).

Granulocyte-Macrophage Colony-Stimulating Factor Granulocyte-macrophage colony-stimulating factor (GM-CSF) has neurotrophic properties reviewed elsewhere (Franzen et al., 2004). We found that this glycoprotein enters the brain and spinal cord by a saturable transport system (McLay et al., 1997).

Pituitary Adenylate Cyclase-Activating Polypeptide Pituitary adenylate cyclase-activating polypeptide (PACAP) is related to vasoactive intestinal peptide (VIP) and exists in two forms consisting of 27 and 38 amino acids. Paradoxically, the larger 38 form enters the brain faster than the smaller form and, unlike PACAP 27, does so by a saturable transport system (Banks et al., 1993d).

2.4   Cellular Models to Study Intracellular Trafficking of Peptides

Cerebral microvessels can be isolated and used immediately for analysis of binding, endocytosis, and degradation of peptides at the BBB level. The advantages of the preparation include better characterization of binding affinity and capacity, simpler analytical procedures for endothelial-specific gene and protein expression or signal transduction, and easier in vitro treatment for modulation of peptide transport.

Growth of these isolated microvessels under optimal conditions yields primary cerebral microvessel endothelial cells. Compared with direct assays using freshly isolated microvessels, the primary culture can develop tight junctions and a monolayer of cells with high-electrical resistance that simulates the in vivo BBB. One of the major drawbacks is that the cultured cells might change their phenotype and therefore display different behavior for peptide transport than that seen in animal studies.

Generation of cerebral microvessel endothelial cell lines obviates the large amount of work involved in the isolation of microvessels from animal or human brains each time, as the primary cells, particularly those from adults, are not well suited for passage. The cerebral microvessel endothelial lines are relatively easy to maintain and have yielded many exciting results concerning peptide transport. There are two primary concerns: (1) certain transport-related molecules and machinery might have been modified or lost during the immortalization process, (2) particular questions about transcytosis cannot be directly answered without the development of a tight monolayer of cells with high-transendothelial electrical resistance. Nonetheless, a combination of endocytosis and exocytosis assays have answered many questions related to peptide transport, and the ease of fluorescent and electron microscopic trafficking studies on these cells has made it the model of choice of our cellular work (Pan et al., 2004b, 2005b).

Since endothelial cells are differentiated cells and exhibit low-transfection efficiency, we have been using other cell lines to perform overexpression studies. Other investigators also have used HEK293, CHO, and MDCK cells to overexpress potential transporting receptors for peptides such as ObRa and ObRb for leptin. In particular, MDCK epithelial cells develop tight junctions in culture and have been used for drug screening in in vitro BBB studies.

2.5   Modifications of Peptide Transport to Enhance Delivery as Prodrugs

There are two major aspects of drug design strategies: modification of the BBB, such as enhancement of the capacity of the transport system or increase of paracellular permeability, and modification of the peptides to achieve better bioavailability and greater penetration across the BBB. Upregulation of the transport system has been seen in pathological conditions such as spinal cord injury and stroke (Pan et al., 1996, 1999a, 2002, 2006; Pan and Kastin, 2001b); however, physiological modulators are yet to be determined. Methods already used for the delivery of chemotherapeutic drugs can potentially be used for peptides and include osmotic opening of the BBB by mannitol or other hyperosmotic agents and the use of vasoactive substances such as bradykinin receptor agonists (Inamura et al., 1994; Doolittle et al., 2000; Borlongan and Emerich, 2003). For the other approach, pharmaceutical design of peptide drugs includes chemical modifications, such as glycosylation and pegylation, and development of fusion proteins (Witt et al., 2001).

A different approach is to use antibodies against receptors highly expressed in the BBB, including those for transferrin and insulin. Immunoliposomes have been shown to successfully deliver neurotrophic factors and neurotrophins, which ameliorate symptoms after experimental stroke (Pardridge et al., 1994; Pardridge, 2001). Nasal delivery, which bypasses the BBB, also has been successful in reducing behavioral deficits in a rat model of stroke (Liu et al., 2001).

3   Peptides Interacting with the CNS Without Specific Transport Systems at the BBB

3.1   Vasoactive Peptides

3.1.1   Adrenomedullin

Adrenomedullin (AM) exerts its major actions on the cardiovascular system, although it can also affect feeding. In primary cultures of rat cerebral endothelial cells, there is high expression of AM (Kis et al., 1999) that can be induced by astrocyte-derived substances (Isumi et al., 1998). AM can protect rat cerebral endothelial cells against oxidative injury (Chen et al., 2005). AM reaches brain parenchyma from the circulation, but much of it is reversibly associated with the brain vasculature, suggesting that it might alter cerebral blood flow and perfusion without disruption of the BBB (Kastin et al., 2001b). AM has also been reported to increase P-glycoprotein efflux activity in rat cerebral endothelial cells (Kis et al., 2001).

3.1.2   Angiotensin

The uptake and transport of angiotensin II in bovine brain microvessel endothelial cells is mediated by the AT_1 receptor (Rose and Audus, 1999). Although fragments of angiotensin do not cross the BBB (Ganong, 1984) angiotensin in the periphery probably affects brain function only by means of AT receptors in CVOs (Unger and Scholkens, 2004).

3.1.3   Bradykinin

Circulating bradykinin can affect cerebral circulation. Since it is a potent dilator of the cerebral arteries, it can increase the permeability of the BBB. This raises the possibility that bradykinin or its analogs could be used to temporarily disrupt the BBB to facilitate the delivery of therapeutic agents (Bartus et al., 1996).

3.1.4   Substance P

Substance P is involved in the breakdown of the BBB. It mediates the enhanced permeability of the BBB resulting from IL-1β, TNF-α , and gp120 from HIV-1 (Annunziata et al., 2002). Induction of the NK-1 receptor for substance P is involved in the increased permeability of the BBB seen in stroke (Stumm et al., 2001).

3.1.5 Endothelin

Endothelin, like substance P, can increase BBB permeability and contribute to cerebral edema leading to ischemic brain injury, effects of which can be reduced by administration of an ET_A antagonist (Narushima et al., 2003). It can also decrease P-glycoprotein-mediated efflux (Hartz et al., 2004).

3.1.6 Atrial Natriuretic Peptide

Atrial natriuretic peptide (ANP) binds saturably to the BBB, as shown by in vivo and in vitro (Ermisch et al., 1991; Whitson et al., 1991), without altering its tight junctions (Nag and Pang, 1989). Blood-to-brain transport of ANP is probably negligible (Levin et al., 1987).

3.1.7 Vasoactive Intestinal Peptide

Vasoactive intestinal peptide (VIP) is a potent vasodilator, including actions in the cerebrovascular system. It can exert protective actions in inflammation, oxidative stress, and apoptosis. It crosses the BBB by passive diffusion (Dogrukol-Ak et al., 2003).

3.2 Peptides Affecting CNS Functions by Other Mediators

Cholecystokinin (CCK) reduces food intake, whereas ghrelin increases feeding. The effects of both can be mediated by vagal afferents, and there are interactions between the two ingestive peptides after peripheral administration (Date et al., 2005). Peripheral CCK-8S, as well as gastric distension, modulate neuronal cell activity in the nucleus tractus solitarius (Guevara-Guzman et al., 2005). The relay of peptidergic information, particularly, in the regulation of feeding behavior has been reviewed extensively elsewhere (Konturek et al., 2004; Guevara-Guzman et al., 2005).

3.3 Peptides Modulating Transport of Others

The classic example of this is the activation of urocortin transport by leptin. Urocortin alone does not seem to have a significant influx across the BBB; however, the presence of leptin induces a dose-related increase in the permeation of urocortin from blood to the brain which is then saturable (Kastin et al., 2000c). Later on, it was found that TNFα can also enhance the transport of urocortin (Pan et al., 2004a). The modulatory effect of leptin on facilitating urocortin transport involves urocortin receptors and signaling elements downstream to leptin receptors (Pan et al., 2004a; Tu et al., unpublished data) and shows potential modulation of food intake (Kastin et al., 2002c).

3.4 Peptides Entering the CNS by Simple Diffusion

Most of the peptides that cross the BBB by simple diffusion have been discussed previously, especially in ❯ Sect. 2.3. These include: NPY; Orexin A; MCH; CART; AgRP; AM; Amylin; GLP-1; Urocortin II; cycloHis-Pro; PACAP27; ILs 2, 6, and 8; MIP; TGF; GDNF.

3.5   Peptides Facilitating Tumor Metastasis

Several peptides/polypeptides are tumor markers and others are involved in the interactions of tumor cells with microvessel endothelial cells during the course of metastasis. Peptides that promote angiogenesis (VEGF) or serve as ligands for receptor tyrosine kinases, such as EGF and TGFα, are known to play important roles in metastasis.

4   Efflux Transport of Peptides from CSF

4.1   Tyr-MIF-1 Family of Opiate-Modulating Peptides

4.1.1   Tyr-MIF-1

Most peptides/polypeptides exit the brain at the slow rate of bulk flow and reabsorption of the CSF after intracerebroventricular (icv) injection. If one were testing the rate of entry of a substance into the brain in the usual way by measuring brain content of the injected material, then a rapid transport system out of the brain might misleadingly make it appear that entry was slow. This is what we observed for Tyr-MIF-1 (Tyr-Pro-Leu-Gly-NH$_2$) in an early study in which influx rates seemed to correlate with lipophilicity (Banks and Kastin, 1985). The saturable efflux system for the antiopiate Tyr-MIF-1 is shared with the opiate Met-enkephalin despite a lack of much structural similarity (Banks et al., 1987). However, in vitro evidence shows that the transporters for these two peptides differ from the receptors of either one (Maresh et al., 1999). For Tyr-MIF-1 itself, the structural requirements for this transport system are stringent. A change of the L-Tyr to D-Tyr results in loss of transport, as does removal of a hydroxyl group from the Tyr, resulting in Phe, as well as removal of the entire Tyr, resulting in MIF-1 (Banks et al., 1986b, 1990; Banks and Kastin, 1994).

4.1.2   Tyr-W-MIF-1

Tyr-W-MIF-1 (Tyr-Pro-Trp-Gly-NH$_2$) differs from Tyr-MIF-1 in one amino acid, Trp (W), and its opiate-modulating activity includes opiate as well as antiopiate effects (Zadina et al., 1992). It is saturably transported out of the brain by a system probably partially shared with Tyr-MIF-1 but at a slower rate (Banks et al., 1993b). It also probably shares the transport system for the endomorphins (Kastin et al., 2001c).

4.1.3   Endomorphins

Just as Tyr-MIF-1 has one amino acid different from MIF-1 and Tyr-W-MIF-1 has one amino acid different from Tyr-MIF-1, endomorphin-1 also has one amino acid different from Tyr-W-MIF-1. With exceedingly high selectivity for the μ opiate receptor, endomorphin-1 (Tyr-Pro-Phe-Gly-NH$_2$) is saturably transported out of the brain by a system that is affected by Tyr-W-MIF-1 but not by Tyr-MIF-1 (Kastin et al., 2001c). The P-glycoprotein system, keeping many therapeutic drugs out of the brain, also transports the nonselective μ opiate β-endorphin (King et al., 2001). Using P-glycoprotein knockout mice (Mdr1a), we showed that this system is not required for the saturable efflux of endomorphins, Met-enkephalin, or Tyr-MIF-1 (Kastin et al., 2002b). Moreover, using primary mouse cerebral endothelial cells, we showed that the endomorphins have a saturable, unidirectional transport system in vitro not involving the P-glycoprotein system and unrelated to μ or δ opiate receptors (Somogyvari-Vigh et al., 2004).

4.1.2   CRH

CRH has a saturable efflux system that is inhibited by verapamil, ouabain, colchicine, TNF-α, and β-endorphin and increased by corticosterone (Martins et al., 1996, 1997a, b). This is in contrast to the lack of evidence for efflux systems for leptin (Banks et al., 1996; Maness et al., 1998), NPY (Kastin and Akerstrom, 1999b), insulin (Cashion et al., 1996), AgRP (Kastin et al., 2000a), CART (Kastin and Akerstrom, 1999a), orexin A (Kastin and Akerstrom, 1999c), MCH (Kastin et al., 2000b), pancreatic polypeptide (Banks and Kastin, 1995), cyclo(His-Pro) (Banks et al., 1993a), mahogany (Kastin and Akerstrom, 2000b), GALP (Kastin et al., 2001a), GLP-1 (Kastin et al., 2002a), and AM (Kastin et al., 2001b). Even urocortin, which binds to the same CRH receptors as does CRH, does not have an efflux transport system (Kastin et al., 2000d). Central injection of less than 1 pmol ^{125}I-CRH reaches the spleen in intact form within a few minutes (Martins et al., 1997b).

4.1.3 PACAP

Although only PACAP-38 but not PACAP-27 has a saturable influx system into the brain, both are saturably transported out of the brain. Each peptide inhibits the efflux of the other, showing a shared system, but one that prefers the larger form (Banks et al., 1993d). Tyr-MIF-1, AVP, LHRH, and somatostatin are all ineffective in inhibiting PACAP efflux.

5   Actions of Peptides in Circumventricular Organs

A popular misconception is that actions of peptides in CVOs, including the choroid plexus, provide unobstructed access into the CNS. Although they do not have a classical BBB, the interstitial fluid within the CVOs is effectively isolated from the brain extracellular fluid by a layer of ependymal cell with tight junctions between them (Guillot and Audus, 1990; Johanson, 1995, 1999). Thus, the blood–CSF barrier of the CVOs (and choroid plexus) are considered part of the BBB system (Johanson, 2003).

Among the CVOs, the area postrema is the target for actions of ingestive peptides and the suprachiasmatic nucleus receives input from many peptides, such as vasopressin, VIP, NPY, nociceptin/orphanin FQ, and orexin, to name a few.

6   Conclusions

Peptides and polypeptides are universal mediators for a variety of actions on the CNS. Many of the effects exerted by peripheral peptides are direct, as there are several mechanisms used by peptides to cross the BBB. In this chapter, we mainly focused on the influx transport systems of peptides studied to date and also discussed other interactions of peptides with the BBB and CVOs. The transport of peptides/polypeptides into and out of the CNS is an important aspect of neuroendocrine and other functions. Peptide transport also can modulate plastic changes of the CNS in development and regeneration.

References

Annunziata P, Cioni C, Santonini R, Paccagnini E. 2002. Substance P antagonist blocks leakage and reduces activation of cytokine-stimulated rat brain endothelium. J Neuroimmunol 131: 41-49.

Banks WA, Kastin AJ. 1985. Peptides and the blood-brain barrier: Lipophilicity as a predictor of permeability. Brain Res Bull 15: 287-292.

Banks WA, Kastin AJ. 1993. Measurement of transport of cytokines across the blood-brain barrier. Neurobiology of

Cytokines, Part A. Conn PM, De Souza EB, editors. San Diego: Academic Press, Inc; pp. 67-77.

Banks WA, Kastin AJ. 1994. Opposite direction of transport across the blood-brain barrier for Tyr-MIF-1 and MIF-1: Comparison with morphine. Peptides 15: 23-29.

Banks WA, Kastin AJ. 1995. Regional variation in transport of pancreatic polypeptide across the blood-brain barrier. Pharmacol Biochem Behav 51: 139-147.

Banks WA, Kastin AJ. 1996. Reversible association of the cytokines MIP-1α and MIP-1β with the endothelia of the blood-brain barrier. Neurosci Lett 205: 202-206.

Banks WA, Kastin AJ. 1998. Differential permeability of the blood-brain barrier to two pancreatic peptides: Insulin and amylin. Peptides 19: 883-889.

Banks WA, Kastin AJ, Coy DH. 1982. Delta sleep inducing peptide crosses the blood-brain barrier in dogs: Some correlations with protein binding. Pharmacol Biochem Behav 17: 1009-1014.

Banks WA, Kastin AJ, Coy DH. 1984. Evidence that [^{125}I]N-Tyr-delta sleep-inducing peptide crosses the blood-brain barrier by a non-competitive mechanism. Brain Res 301: 201-207.

Banks WA, Kastin AJ, Coy DH, Angulo E. 1986a. Entry of DSIP peptides into dog CSF: Role of physicochemical and pharmacokinetic parameters. Brain Res Bull 17: 155-158.

Banks WA, Kastin AJ, Fischman AJ, Coy DH, Strauss SL. 1986b. Carrier-mediated transport of enkephalins and N-Tyr-MIF-1 across blood-brain barrier. Am J Physiol 251: E477-E482.

Banks WA, Kastin AJ, Michals EA. 1987. Tyr-MIF-1 and met-enkephalin share a saturable blood-brain barrier transport system. Peptides 8: 899-903.

Banks WA, Kastin AJ, Durham DA. 1989. Bidirectional transport of interleukin-1 alpha across the blood-brain barrier. Brain Res Bull 23: 433-437.

Banks WA, Kastin AJ, Michals EA, Barrera CM. 1990. Stereospecific transport of Tyr-MIF-1 across the blood-brain barrier by peptide transport system-1. Brain Res Bull 25: 589-592.

Banks WA, Ortiz L, Plotkin SR, Kastin AJ. 1991. Human interleukin (IL) 1α, murine IL-1α and murine IL-1β are transported from blood to brain in the mouse by a shared saturable mechanism. J Pharmacol Exp Ther 259: 988-996.

Banks WA, Kastin AJ, Akerstrom V, Jaspan JB. 1993a. Radioactively iodinated cyclo(His-Pro) crosses the blood-brain barrier and reverses ethanol-induced narcosis. Am J Physiol 267: E723-E729.

Banks WA, Kastin AJ, Ehrensing CA. 1993b. Endogenous peptide Tyr-Pro-Trp-Gly-NH$_2$ (Tyr-W-MIF-1) is transported from the brain to the blood by peptide transport system-1. J Neurosci Res 35: 690-695.

Banks WA, Kastin AJ, Gutierrez EG. 1993c. Interleukin-1α in blood has direct access to cortical brain cells. Neurosci Lett 163: 41-44.

Banks WA, Kastin AJ, Komaki G, Arimura A. 1993d. Passage of pituitary adenylate cyclase activating polypeptide$_{1-27}$ and pituitary adenylate cyclase activating polypeptide$_{1-38}$ across the blood-brain barrier. J Pharmacol Exp Ther 267: 690-696.

Banks WA, Kastin AJ, Gutierrez EG. 1994. Penetration of interleukin-6 across the murine blood-brain barrier. Neurosci Lett 179: 53-56.

Banks WA, Kastin AJ, Maness LM, Huang W, Jaspan JB. 1995a. Permeability of the blood-brain barrier to amylin. Life Sci 57: 1993-2001.

Banks WA, Plotkin SR, Kastin AJ. 1995b. Permeability of the blood-brain barrier to soluble cytokine receptors. Neuroimmunomodulation 2: 161-165.

Banks WA, Kastin AJ, Huang W, Jaspan JB, Maness LM. 1996. Leptin enters the brain by a saturable system independent of insulin. Peptides 17: 305-311.

Banks WA, Jaspan JB, Huang W, Kastin AJ. 1997a. Transport of insulin across the blood-brain barrier: Saturability at euglycemic doses of insulin. Peptides 18: 1423-1429.

Banks WA, Jaspan JB, Kastin AJ. 1997b. Effect of diabetes mellitus on the permeability of the blood-brain barrier to insulin. Peptides 18: 1577-1584.

Banks WA, Jaspan JB, Kastin AJ. 1997c. Selective, physiological transport of insulin across the blood-brain barrier: Novel demonstration by species-specific radioimmunoassays. Peptides 18: 1257-1262.

Banks WA, Kastin AJ, Pan W. 1999. Uptake and degradation of blood-borne insulin by the olfactory bulb. Peptides 20: 373-378.

Banks WA, Moinuddin A, Morley JE. 2001. Regional transport of TNF-alpha across the blood-brain barrier in young ICR and young and aged SAMP8 mice. Neurobiol Aging 22: 671-676.

Banks WA, Tschop M, Robinson SM, Heiman M. 2002. Extent and direction of ghrelin transport across the blood-brain barrier is determined by its unique primary structure. J Pharmacol Exp Ther 302: 822-8

Barrera CM, Kastin AJ, Fasold MB, Banks WA. 1991. Bidirectional saturable transport of LHRH across the blood-brain barrier. Am J Physiol 261: E312-E318.

Bartus R, Elliott P, Hayward N, Dean R, McEwen E, et al. 1996. Permeability of the blood brain barrier by the bradykinin agonist, RMP-7: Evidence for a sensitive, auto-regulated, receptor mediated system. Immunopharmacology 33: 270-278.

Blasberg RG, Fenstermacher JD, Patlak CS. 1983. Transport of α-aminoisobutyric acid across brain capillary and cellular membranes. J Cereb Blood Flow Metab 3: 8-32.

Borlongan CV, Emerich DF. 2003. Facilitation of drug entry into the CNS via transient permeation of blood brain barrier: Laboratory and preliminary clinical evidence from bradykinin receptor agonist, Cereport. Brain Res Bull 60: 297-306.

Cashion MF, Banks WA, Kastin AJ. 1996. Sequestration of centrally administered insulin by the brain: Effects of starvation, aluminum, and TNFα. Horm Behav 30: 280-286.

Chen L, Kis B, Busija D, Yamashita H, Ueta Y. 2005. Adreno-medullin protects rat cerebral endothelial cells from oxidant damage in vitro. Regul Pept 130: 27-34.

Chikhale EG, Ng KY, Burton PS, Borchardt RT. 1994. Hydrogen bonding potential as a determinant of the in vitro and in situ blood-brain barrier permeability of peptides. Pharm Res 11: 412-419.

Date Y, Toshinai K, Koda S, Miyazato M, Shimbara T, et al. 2005. Peripheral interaction of ghrelin with cholecystokinin on feeding regulation. Endocrinology 146: 3518-3525.

Deguchi Y, Naito T, Yuge T, Furukawa H, Yamada S, et al. 2000. Blood-brain barrier transport of ^{125}I-labeled basic fibroblas growth factor. Pharm Res 17: 63-69.

Dogrukol-Ak D, Banks WA, Tuncel N, Tuncel M. 2003. Passage of vasoactive intestinal peptide across the blood-brain barrier. Peptides 24: 437-444.

Doolittle ND, Miner ME, Hall WA, Siegal T, Jerome E, et al. 2000. Safety and efficacy of a multicenter study using intraarterial chemotherapy in conjunction with osmotic opening of the blood-brain barrier for the treatment of patients with malignant brain tumors. Cancer 88: 637-647.

Egleton RD, Davis TP. 1997. Bioavailability and transport of peptides and peptide drugs into the brain. Peptides 18: 1431-1439.

Ermisch A, Ruhle H, Kretzschmar R, Baethmann A. 1991. On the blood-brain barrier to peptides: Specific binding of atrial natriuretic peptide in vivo and in vitro. Brain Res 554: 209-216.

Franzen R, Bouhy D, Schoenen J. 2004. Nervous system injury: Focus on the inflammatory cytokine 'granulocyte-macrophage colony stimulating factor'. Neurosci Lett 361: 76-78.

Ganong W, 1984. The brain renin-angiotensin system. Annu Rev Physiol 46: 17-31.

Greenblatt DJ, Koch-Weser J. 1975. Clinical pharmacokinetics (second of two parts). N Engl J Med 293: 964-970.

Guevara-Guzman R, Levy F, Jean A, Nowak R. 2005. Electrophysiological responses of nucleus tractus solitarius neurons to CCK and gastric distension in newborn lambs. Cell Mol Neurobiol 25: 393-406.

Guillot FL, Audus KL. 1990. Angiotensin peptide regulation of fluid-phase endocytosis in brain microvessel endothelial cell monolayers. J Cereb Blood Flow Metab 10: 827-834.

Gutierrez EG, Banks WA, Kastin AJ. 1993. Murine tumor necrosis factor alpha is transported from blood to brain in the mouse. J Neuroimmunol 47: 169-176.

Gutierrez EG, Banks WA, Kastin AJ. 1994. Blood-borne interleukin-1 receptor antagonist crosses the blood-brain barrier. J Neuroimmunol 55: 153-160.

Hartz A, Bauer B, Fricker G, Miller D. 2004. Rapid regulation of P-glycoprotein at the blood-brain barrier by endothelin-1. Mol Pharmacol 66: 387-394.

Hoke F. 1993. Recent advances increase HPLC use in life sciences. The Scientist 7: 18-19.

Inamura T, Nomura T, Bartus RT, Black KL. 1994. Intracarotid infusion of RMP-7, a bradykinin analog: A method for selective drug delivery to brain tumors. J Neurosurg 81: 752-758.

Isumi Y, Shoji H, Sugo S, Tochimoto T, Yoshioka M, et al. 1998. Regulation of adrenomedullin production in rat endothelial cells. Endocrinology 139: 838-846.

Johanson CE. 1995. Ventricles and cerebrospinal fluid. Neuroscience in Medicine. Conn PM, editor. Philadelphia: JB Lippincott; pp. 171-196.

Johanson CE. 1999. Choroid plexus. Elsevier's Encyclopedia of Neuroscience. Adelman G, Smith BH, editors. Elsevier, Amsterdam pp. 384–387.

Johanson CE. 2003. The choroid plexus-CSF nexus. Neuroscience in Medicine. Conn PM, editor. Totowa, NJ: Humana Press, Inc; pp. 165-195.

Kastin AJ, Akerstrom V. 1999a. Entry of CART into brain is rapid but not inhibited by excess CART or leptin. Am J Physiol 277: E901-E904.

Kastin AJ, Akerstrom V. 1999b. Nonsaturable entry of neuropeptide Y into the brain. Am J Physiol 276: E479-E482.

Kastin AJ, Akerstrom V. 1999c. Orexin A but not orexin B rapidly enters brain from blood by simple diffusion. J Pharmacol Exp Ther 289: 219-223.

Kastin AJ, Akerstrom V. 2000a. Fasting, but not adrenalectomy, reduces transport of leptin into the brain. Peptides 21: 679-682.

Kastin AJ, Akerstrom V. 2000b. Mahogany (1377–1428) enters brain by a saturable transport system. J Pharmacol Exp Ther 294: 633-636.

Kastin AJ, Akerstrom V. 2001a. Glucose and insulin increase the transport of leptin through the blood-brain barrier in normal mice but not in streptozotocin-diabetic mice. Neuroendocrinology 73: 237-242.

Kastin AJ, Akerstrom V. 2001b. Pretreatment with glucose increases entry of urocortin into mouse brain. Peptides 22: 829-834.

Kastin AJ, Akerstrom V. 2002. Differential interactions of urocortin/corticotropin-releasing hormone peptides with the blood-brain barrier. Neuroendocrinology 75: 367-374.

Kastin AJ, Akerstrom V. 2003. Entry of exendin-4 into brain is rapid but may be limited at high doses. Int J Obes Relat Metab Disord 27: 313-318.

Kastin AJ, Sandman CA, Stratton LO, Schally AV, Miller LH. 1975. Behavioral and electrographic changes in rat and man after MSH. Prog Brain Res 42: 143-150.

Kastin AJ, Nissen C, Nikolics K, Medzihradszky K, Coy DH, et al. 1976. Distribution of [^{3}H]α-MSH in rat brain. Brain Res Bull 1: 19-26.

Kastin AJ, Scollan EL, Ehrensing RH, Schally AV, Coy DH. 1978. Enkephalin and other peptides reduce passiveness. Pharmacol Biochem Behav 9: 515-519.

Kastin AJ, Olson RD, Schally AV, Coy DH. 1979. CNS effects of peripherally administered brain peptides. Life Sci 25: 401-414.

Kastin AJ, Nissen C, Coy DH. 1981. Permeability of the blood-brain barrier to DSIP peptides. Pharmacol Biochem Behav 15: 955-959.

Kastin AJ, Pearson MA, Banks WA. 1991. EEG evidence that morphine and an enkephalin analog cross the blood-brain barrier. Pharmacol Biochem Behav 40: 771-774.

Kastin AJ, Pan W, Maness LM, Koletsky RJ, Ernsberger P. 1999. Decreased transport of leptin across the blood-brain barrier in rats lacking the short form of the leptin receptor. Peptides 20: 1449-1453.

Kastin AJ, Akerstrom V, Hackler L. 2000a. Agouti-related protein (83–132) aggregates and crosses the blood-brain barrier slowly. Metabolism 49: 1444-1448.

Kastin AJ, Akerstrom V, Hackler L, Zadina JE. 2000b. Phe[13], Tyr[19]-Melanin-concentrating hormone and the blood-brain barrier: Role of protein binding. J Neurochem 74: 385-391.

Kastin AJ, Akerstrom V, Pan W. 2000c. Activation of urocortin transport into brain by leptin. Peptides 21: 1811-1817.

Kastin AJ, Akerstrom V, Pan W. 2000d. Activation of urocortin transport into brain by leptin. Peptides 21: 1811-1818.

Kastin AJ, Akerstrom V, Hackler L. 2001a. Food deprivation decreases blood galanin-like peptide and its rapid entry into the brain. Neuroendocrinology 74: 423-432.

Kastin AJ, Akerstrom V, Hackler L, Pan W. 2001b. Adreno-medullin and the blood-brain barrier. Horm Metab Res 33: 19-25.

Kastin AJ, Fasold MB, Smith RR, Horner KA, Zadina JE. 2001c. Saturable brain-to-blood transport of endomorphins. Exp Brain Res 139: 70-75.

Kastin AJ, Akerstrom V, Pan W. 2002a. Interactions of glucagon-like peptide-1 (GLP-1) with the blood-brain barrier. J Mol Neurosci 18: 7-14.

Kastin AJ, Fasold MB, Zadina JE. 2002b. Endomorphins, Met-Enkephalin, Tyr-MIF-1, and the P-glycoprotein efflux system. Drug Metab Dispos 30: 231-234.

Kastin AJ, Pan WH, Akerstrom V, Hackler L, Wang CF, et al. 2002c. Novel peptide-peptide cooperation may transform feeding behavior. Peptides 23: 2189-2196.

Kastin AJ, Akerstrom V, Hackler L, Pan W. 2003a. Different mechanisms influencing permation of PDGF-AA and PDGF-BB across the blood-brain barrier. J Neurochem 87: 7-12.

Kastin AJ, Akerstrom V, Pan W. 2003b. Circulating TGF-β_1 does not cross the intact blood-brain barrier. J Mol Neurosci 21: 43-48.

Kastin AJ, Akerstrom V, Pan W. 2003c. Glial cell line-derived neurotrophic factor does not enter normal mouse brain. Neurosci Lett 340: 239-241.

Kastin AJ, Akerstrom V, Pan W. 2003d. Interleukin-10 as a CNS therapeutic: The obstacle of the blood-brain/blood-spinal cord barrier. Mol Brain Res 114: 168-171.

Kastin AJ, Akerstrom V, Pan W. 2004. Neuregulin 1-$\beta 1$ enters brain and spinal cord by receptor-mediated transport. J Neurochem 88: 965-970.

King M, Su W, Chang A, Zukerman A, Pasternak GW. 2001. Transport of opioids from the brain to the periphery by P-glycoprotein: Peripheral actions of central drugs. Nat Neurosci 4: 268-274.

Kis B, Szabo C, Pataricza J, Krizbai I, Mezei Z, et al. 1999. Vasoactive substances produced by cultured rat brain endothelial cells. Eur J Pharmacol 368: 35-42.

Kis B, Deli M, Kobayashi H, Abraham C, Yanagita T, et al. 2001. Adrenomedullin regulates blood-brain barrier functions in vitro. Neuroreport 12: 4139-4142.

Konturek SJ, Konturek JW, Pawlik T, Brzozowski T. 2004. Brain-gut axis and its role in the control of food intake. J Physiol Pharmacol 55: 137-154.

Lai EC, Felice KJ, Festoff BW, Gawel MJ, Gelinas DF, et al. 1997. Effect of recombinant human insulin-like growth factor-I on progression of ALS. A placebo-controlled study. The North America ALS/IGF-I Study Group. Neurology 49: 1621-1630.

Levin E, Frank H, Weber M, Ismail M, Mills S. 1987. Studies of the penetration of the blood brain barrier by atrial natriuretic factor. Biochem Biophys Res Commun 147: 1226-1231.

Liu X, Yao DL, Webster H. 1995. Insulin-like growth factor 1 treatment reduces clinical deficits and lesion severity in acute demyelinating experimental autoimmune encephalo-myelitis. Multiple Sclerosis 1: 2-9.

Liu XF, Fawcett JR, Thorne RG, Frey WH. 2001. Non-invasive intranasal insulin-like growth factor-I reduces infarct volume and improves neurologic function in rats following middle cerebral artery occlusion. Neurosci Lett 308: 91-94.

Maness LM, Banks WA, Zadina JE, Kastin AJ. 1995. Selective transport of blood-borne interleukin 1α into the posterior division of the septum of the mouse brain. Brain Res 700: 83-88.

Maness LM, Kastin AJ, Farrell CL, Banks WA. 1998. Fate of leptin after intracerebroventricular injection into the mouse brain. Endocrinology 139: 4556-4562.

Maresh GA, Kastin AJ, Brown TT, Zadina JE, Banks WA. 1999. Peptide transport system 1 (PTS-1) for Tyr-MIF-1 and Met-enkephalin differs from the receptors for either. Brain Res 839: 336-340.

Martins JM, Kastin AJ, Banks WA. 1996. Unidirectional specific and modulated brain to blood transport of corticotropin-releasing hormone. Neuroendocrinology 63: 338-348.

Martins JM, Banks WA, Kastin AJ. 1997a. Acute modulation of the active carrier-mediated brain-to-blood transport of corticotropin-releasing hormone. Am J Physiol 272: E312-E319.

Martins JM, Banks WA, Kastin AJ. 1997b. Transport of CRH from mouse brain directly affects peripheral production of β-endorphin by the spleen. Am J Physiol 273: E1083-E1089.

McLay RN, Kimura M, Banks WA, Kastin AJ. 1997. Granulocyte-macrophage colony-stimulating factor crosses the blood-brain and blood-spinal cord barriers. Brain 120: 2083-2091.

McLay RN, Kastin AJ, Zadina JE. 2000. Passage of interleukin-1β across the blood-brain barrier is reduced in aged mice: A possible mechanism for diminished fever in aging. Neuroimmunomodulation 8: 148-153.

Nag S, Pang S. 1989. Effect of atrial natriuretic factor on blood-brain barrier permeability. Can J Physiol Pharmacol 67: 637-640.

Narushima I, Kita T, Kubo K, Yonetani Y, Momochi C, et al. 2003. Highly enhanced permeability of blood-brain barrier induced by repeated administration of endothelin-1 in dogs and rats. Pharmacol Toxicol 92: 21-26.

Pan W, Kastin AJ. 1999. Entry of EGF into brain is rapid and saturable. Peptides 20: 1091-1098.

Pan W, Kastin AJ. 2000. Interactions of IGF-1 with the blood-brain barrier in vivo and in situ. Neuroendocrinology 72: 171-178.

Pan W, Kastin AJ. 2001a. Changing the chemokine gradient: CINC1 crosses the blood-brain barrier. J Neuroimmunol 115: 64-70.

Pan W, Kastin AJ. 2001b. Increase in TNFα transport after SCI is specific for time, region, and type of lesion. Exp Neurol 170: 357-363.

Pan W, Kastin AJ. 2001c. Upregulation of the transport system for TNFα at the blood-brain barrier. Arch Physiol Biochem 109: 350-353.

Pan W, Kastin AJ. 2002. TNFα transport across the blood-brain barrier is abolished in receptor knockout mice. Exp Neurol 174: 193-200.

Pan W, Kastin AJ. 2004. Transport of cytokines and neurotrophins across the blood-brain barrier and their regulation after spinal cord injury. Blood-spinal cord and brain barriers in health and disease. Sharma HS, Westman J, editors. San Diego, CA: Elsevier; pp. 395-407.

Pan W, Banks WA, Kennedy MK, Gutierrez EG, Kastin AJ. 1996. Differential permeability of the BBB in acute EAE: Enhanced transport of TNF-α. Am J Physiol 271: E636-E642.

Pan W, Banks WA, Kastin AJ. 1997a. Blood-brain barrier permeability to ebiratide and TNF in acute spinal cord injury. Exp Neurol 146: 367-373.

Pan W, Banks WA, Kastin AJ. 1997b. Permeability of the blood-brain and blood-spinal cord barriers to interferons. J Neuroimmunol 76: 105-111.

Pan W, Banks WA, Kastin AJ. 1998. Permeability of the blood-brain barrier to neurotrophins. Brain Res 788: 87-94.

Pan W, Kastin AJ, Bell RL, Olson RD. 1999a. Upregulation of tumor necrosis factor α transport across the blood-brain barrier after acute compressive spinal cord injury. J Neurosci 19: 3649-3655.

Pan W, Kastin AJ, Maness LM, Brennan JM. 1999b. Saturable entry of ciliary neurotrophic factor into brain. Neurosci Lett 263: 69-71.

Pan W, Kastin AJ, Maness LM, Brennan JM. 1999c. Saturable entry of ciliary neurotrophic factor into brain. Neurosci Lett 263: 69-71.

Pan W, Vallance KL, Kastin AJ. 1999d. TGF alpha and the blood-brain barrier: Accumulation in cerebral vasculature. Exp Neurol 160: 454-459.

Pan W, Kastin AJ, Brennan JM. 2000. Saturable entry of leukemia inhibitory factor from blood to the central nervous system. J Neuroimmunol 106: 172-180.

Pan W, Csernus B, Kastin AJ. 2002. Upregulation of p55 and p75 receptors mediating TNFα transport across injured blood-spinal cord barrier. J Mol Neurosci 21: 173-184.

Pan W, Akerstrom V, Zhang J, Pejovic V, Kastin AJ. 2004a. Modulation of feeding-related peptide/protein signals by the blood-brain barrier. J Neurochem 90: 455-461.

Pan W, Kastin AJ, Zankel T, van Kerkhof P, Terasaki T, et al. 2004b. Efficient transfer of receptor-associated protein (RAP) across the blood-brain barrier. J Cell Sci 117: 5071-5078.

Pan W, Ding Y, Yu Y, Ohtaki H, Nakamachi T, Kastin AJ. 2006. Stroke upregulation TNFα transport across the blood-brain barrier. Exp Neurol 103: 1581-1586.

Pan W, Yu Y, Cain CM, Nyberg F, Couraud P-O, Kastin AJ. 2005b. Permeation of growth hormone across the blood-brain barrier. Endocrinology 146: 4898-4904.

Pardridge WM. 2001. Brain drug targeting and gene technologies. Jpn J Pharmacol 87: 97-103.

Pardridge WM, Kang YS, Buciak JL. 1994. Transport of human recombinant brain-derived neurotrophic factor (BDNF) through the rat blood-brain barrier in vivo using vector-mediated peptide drug delivery. Pharmaceut Res 11: 738-746.

Park SK, Solomon D, Vartanian T. 2001. Growth factor control of CNS myelination. Dev Neurosci 23: 327-337.

Patlak CS, Blasberg RG, Fenstermacher JD. 1983. Graphical evaluation of blood-to-brain transfer constants from multiple-time uptake data. J Cereb Blood Flow Metab 3: 1-7.

Peruzzo B, Pastor FE, Blazquez JL, Schobitz K, Pelaez B, et al. 2000. A second look at the barriers of the medial basal hypothalamus. Exp Brain Res 132: 10-26.

Pfaff DW. 1973. Luteinizing hormone-releasing factor potentiates lordosis behavior in hypophysectomized ovariectomized female rats. Science 182: 1148-1149.

Plotkin SR, Banks WA, Kastin AJ. 1996. Comparison of saturable transport and extracellular pathways in the passage of interleukin-1α across the blood-brain barrier. J Neuroimmunol 67: 41-47.

Plotnikoff NP, Kastin AJ, Anderson MS, Schally AV. 1971. DOPA potentiation by a hypothalamic factor, MSH release-inhibiting hormone (MIF). Life Sci 10: 1279-1283.

Raessi S, Audus KL. 1989. In-vitro characterization of blood-brain barrier permeability to delta sleep-inducing peptide. J Pharm Pharmacol 41: 848-852.

Rapoport SI, Klee WA, Pettigrew KD, Ohno K. 1980. Entry of opioid peptides in the central nervous system. Science 207: 84-86.

Raub TJ, Audus KL. 1990. Adsorptive endocytosis and membrane recycling by cultured primary bovine brain microvessel endothelial cell monlayers. J Cell Sci 97: 127-138.

Redding TW, Kastin AJ, Gonzalez-Barcena D, Coy DH, Schalch DH, et al. 1973a. The halflife, metabolism, and excretion of tritiated luteinizing hormone releasing hormone (LHRH) in man. J Clin Endocrinol Metab 37: 626-631.

Redding TW, Kastin AJ, Nair RMG, Schally AV. 1973b. The distribution, half-life, and excretion of ^{14}C and ^{3}H-labeled L-prolyl-L-leucyl-glycinamide in the rat. Neuroendocrinology 11: 92-100.

Redding TW, Kastin AJ, Gonzalez-Barcena D, Coy DH, Hirotsu Y, et al. 1974. The disappearance, excretion, and metabolism of tritiated prolyl-leucyl-glycinamide in man. Neuroendocrinology 16: 119-126.

Redding TW, Kastin AJ, Nikolics K, Schally AV, Coy DH. 1978. Disappearance and excretion of labeled α-MSH in man. Pharmacol Biochem Behav 9: 207-212.

Rose JM, Audus KL. 1999. AT$_1$ receptors mediate angiotensin II uptake and transport by bovine brain microvessel endothelial cells in primary culture. J Cardiovasc Pharmacol 33: 30-35.

Sandman CA, Denman PM, Miller LH, Knott JR, Schally AV, Kastin AJ. 1971. Electroencephalographic measures of melanocyte stimulating hormone activity. J Comp Physiol Psychol 76: 103-109.

Schally AV, Arimura A, Kastin AJ. 1973. Hypothalamic regulating hormones. Science 179: 341-350.

Shimura T, Tabata S, Hayashi S. 1991. Brain transfer of a new neuromodulating ACTH analog, ebiratide, in rats. Peptides 12: 509-512.

Somogyvari-Vigh A, Kastin AJ, Liao J, Zadina JE, Pan W. 2004. Endomorphins exit the brain by a saturable efflux system at the basolateral surface of cerebral endothelial cells. Exp Brain Res 156: 224-230.

Stumm R, Culmsee C, Schafer M, Krieglstein J, Weihe E. 2001. Adaptive plasticity in tachykinin and tachykinin receptor expression after focal cerebral ischemia is differentially linked to gabaergic and glutamatergic cerebrocortical circuits and cerebrovenular endothelium. J Neurosci 21: 798-811.

Unger T, Scholkens B. 2004. Angiotensin vol I. and vol. II. Handbook of Experimental Pharmacology, Vol. 1. Springer-Verlag, Berlin p 163.

Waguespack PJ, Banks WA, Kastin AJ. 1994. Interleukin-2 does not cross the blood-brain barrier by a saturable transport system. Brain Res Bull 34: 103-109.

Whitson P, Huls M, Sams C. 1991. Characterization of atrial natriuretic peptide receptors in brain microvessel endothelial cells. J Cell Physiol 146: 43-51.

Wilson JF. 1998. Low permeability of the blood-brain barrier to nanomolar concentrations of immunoreactive alpha-melanotropin. Psychopharmacology (Berl) 96: 262-266.

Witt KA, Gillespie TJ, Huber JD, Egleton RD, Davis TP. 2001. Peptide drug modifications to enhance bioavailability and blood-brain barrier permeability. Peptides 22: 2329-2343.

Yu Y, Kastin AJ, Pan W. 2006. Reciprocal interactions of insulin and insulin-like growth factor 1 in receptor-mediated transport across the blood-brain barrier. Endocrinology (PMID 16497794).

Zadina JE, Kastin AJ, Kersh D, Wyatt A. 1992. Tyr-MIF-1 and hemorphin can act as opiate agonists as well as antagonists in the guinea pig ileum. Life Sci 51: 869-885.

Zlokovic BV, Segal MB, Davson H, Jankov RM. 1988. Passage of delta sleep-inducing peptide (DSIP) across the blood-cerebrospinal fluid barrier. Peptides 9: 533-538.

Zlokovic BV, Banks WA, Elkadi H, Erchegyi J, Mackic JB, et al. 1992. Transport, uptake and metabolism of blood-borne vasopressin by the blood-brain barrier. Brain Res 590: 213-218.

21 Synaptic Vesicle Recycling

E. M. Lafer

Abstract: The mechanism of synaptic vesicle recycling has been hotly debated for more than 30 years. The various mechanistic models are presented, and the evidence supporting each model is discussed. It is now well accepted that endocytosis rates span an enormous range and are highly dependent on exocytosis rates. It is also well accepted that clathrin-mediated endocytosis plays a major role in synaptic vesicle recycling. However, it remains to be determined whether endocytic pathways with dramatically different rates operate using the same or different molecular mechanisms.

List of Abbreviations: AP, action potential; AZ, active zone; CCP, clathrin-coated pit; CCV, clathrin-coated vesicle; PM, plasma membrane; PSP, postsynaptic potential; SPR, surface plasmon resonance; SV, synaptic vesicle

1   Introduction

The most fundamental way that neurons communicate with each other, and with target cells, is by the process of synaptic transmission. Calcium channels open, following depolarization of a presynaptic neuron, leading to a rise in intracellular calcium. This leads to the fusion between the synaptic vesicle (SV) membrane and the presynaptic plasma membrane and the release of neurotransmitter molecules into the synaptic cleft. The neurotransmitters diffuse across the synaptic cleft and interact with postsynaptic receptors. At the same time, the exocytosed SV membrane proteins, and excess membrane, are brought back into the nerve terminal by a process that is referred to as SV recycling.

2   General Models for Synaptic Vesicle Recycling

For more than 30 years, the mechanism which underlies SV recycling has been hotly debated (Morgan et al., 2002). This is in part due to disagreements concerning the mechanism of vesicle fusion, so before we can discuss mechanisms underlying SV recycling, we must discuss the mechanistic models for vesicle fusion (Sudhof, 2004). One model assumes that when an SV fuses with the presynaptic plasma membrane, there is a complete collapse of the vesicle into the presynaptic plasma membrane, such that the vesicle loses its unique identity. I will refer to this mode of exocytosis as "full fusion mediated." Alternatively, it has been hypothesized that the formation of a transient fusion pore is sufficient to allow neurotransmitters to diffuse into the synaptic cleft. I will refer to this mode of exocytosis as "fusion pore mediated." Note that in full fusion-mediated exocytosis, the SV loses its identity since the SV membrane proteins and lipids mix with those of the presynaptic plasma membrane following fusion. Therefore, it is expected that a sorting mechanism will be required for retrieving the SV membrane proteins and excess lipid from the plasma membrane. The sorting mechanism that was first hypothesized to be involved is clathrin-mediated endocytosis (❷ *Figure 21-1a*) (Heuser and Reese, 1973). However, in the case of fusion pore-mediated exocytosis, a sorting mechanism would not be expected to be required since the vesicle never loses its identity. Therefore, in the simplest version of this model, also referred to as "kiss and run" (Valtorta et al., 2001), exocytosis takes place by the opening of a fusion pore, while endocytosis takes place by the closing of a fusion pore (❷ *Figure 21-1b*).

Following full fusion, it is not clear to what extent the SV membrane proteins and lipids diffuse within the lipid bilayer of the presynaptic plasma membrane (❷ *Figure 21-1a*). Diffusion may be limited by the presence of unresolved SNARE complexes. Furthermore, the SV membrane proteins are believed to be able to associate with each other (Calakos et al., 1994), which would require only a subset of proteins to contain direct sorting signals. For example, synaptotagmin associates with other SV membrane proteins, including syntaxin (Chapman et al., 1995; Kee and Scheller, 1996), snap-25 (Schiavo et al., 1997) and SV2 (Schivell et al., 1996), as well as with the clathrin assembly protein AP-2 (Zhang et al., 1994; Chapman et al., 1998; Haucke et al., 2000). This would allow AP-2/AP180 complexes to initiate coated pit formation on the area

◻ **Figure 21-1**

Models for synaptic vesicle recycling. (a) Exocytosis proceeds through a full fusion mechanism, while endocytosis is mediated by clathrin and an endosomal intermediate. (b) Exocytosis proceeds by the opening of a fusion pore, while endocytosis proceeds by the closing of a fusion pore. (c) Exocytosis proceeds through a full fusion mechanism, while endocytosis is mediated by clathrin. (d) Exocytosis proceeds by the opening of a fusion pore, while endocytosis is mediated by clathrin

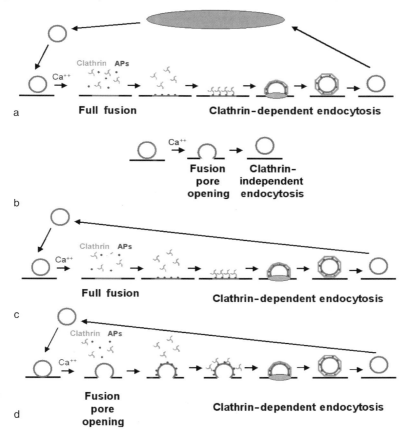

of the membrane containing the SV membrane proteins. Dynamin plays a major role in the conversion of clathrin-coated pits (CCPs) to clathrin-coated vesicles (CCVs) (Baba et al., 1995; Takei et al., 1995). The CCVs, following vesicle scission, rapidly uncoat in a reaction promoted by auxilin, Hsc70, and synaptojanin (Cremona et al., 1999; Morgan et al., 2001). The decoated vesicles are then thought to have one of two fates. They may fuse with an endosomal intermediate, and then new SVs may bud from the endosomal compartment (❯ *Figure 21-1a*). The new SVs are locally filled with neurotransmitters by neurotransmitter transporters in their membrane, and the cycle repeats. In an alternative version of this model (❯ *Figure 21-1c*), there is only a single budding step that takes place at the plasma membrane (Takei et al., 1996). Once the CCVs uncoat, they are refilled with neurotransmitter to become mature SVs. The mechanism of the second budding reaction is also controversial. While CCPs have been observed on endosomal membranes (Stoorvogel et al., 1996), work in neuroendocrine cells suggests that this step is not dependent on clathrin but is dependent on the clathrin adaptor protein AP-3 (Faundez et al., 1998).

Studies of membrane fusion in a variety of systems indicate that fusion proceeds through a number of discreet intermediates (Chernomordik and Kozlov, 2005). Indeed, fusion pore dilation is one of the intermediates on the pathway toward complete fusion. Furthermore, while the formation of SNARE complexes may inhibit the free diffusion of the SV membrane proteins and lipids, these complexes may also limit the expansion of the fusion pore. If the fusion pore does not fully expand, then it is possible that it may simply close backup after releasing neurotransmitters (❷ *Figure 21-1b*). Alternatively, the clathrin machinery may still facilitate the retrieval of SV membrane proteins even in situations where full fusion does not take place (❷ *Figure 21-1d*).

For a long time, many investigators believed that all models that are full fusion mediated are clathrin dependent, while all models that are fusion pore mediated are clathrin independent. Likewise, many investigators believed that models with slow kinetics are clathrin dependent, while models with fast kinetics are clathrin independent. However, this does not have to be the case. For example, the clathrin-dependent models that involve a single budding step (❷ *Figure 21-1c* and ❷ *21-1d*) would be much faster than the clathrin-dependent models that involve two budding steps (❷ *Figure 21-1a*). Furthermore, these models are not mutually exclusive, and multiple mechanisms may coexist. For example, if an uncoated CCV contains a full complement of active SV membrane proteins, model *c* may predominate, while if the vesicle is missing a key protein model *a* may predominate (❷ *Figure 21-1*). Likewise, if the clathrin machinery is not saturated, then model *d* may predominate, while once the components of the clathrin machinery become limited model *c* may predominate (❷ *Figure 21-1*). Therefore, let us separately consider what is known about the molecular mechanisms of SV endocytosis and what is known about the kinetics.

3   The Role of the Clathrin Pathway in Synaptic Vesicle Recycling

3.1 Morphological Studies

Let us first consider work directed at evaluating the contribution of the clathrin pathway to SV recycling. The earliest studies that were carried out were morphological. When Heuser and Reese labeled frog neuromuscular junctions with horse radish peroxidase tracer, following stimulation they were able to observe the movement of the tracer first into CCVs, then into endosomes, and lastly into new SVs (Heuser and Reese, 1973; Heuser, 1989). However, because the morphological observation of CCVs required high-frequency stimulation, some investigators felt that clathrin-mediated endocytosis only operated under high-frequency stimulation but not under lower more physiological rates of stimulation (Ceccarelli et al., 1973, 1979). Alternatively, because CCVs are known to be transient structures that rapidly uncoat, high-frequency stimulation may have been required to insure a large bolus of exocytosis and endocytosis, thereby increasing the probability that a CCV could be seen in a morphological assay. Other successful approaches at trapping CCVs included studies of the *Drosophila* mutant shibire, which has mutations in the gene encoding dynamin, the protein believed to be involved in catalyzing the scission reaction whereby CCPs become CCVs (Koenig and Ikeda, 1989). At the paralytic phenotype, one can observe an accumulation of CCPs on the plasma membrane (❷ *Figure 21-2*). Likewise, when dynamin is inhibited using GTP-γ-S in synaptosomes, one also observes an accumulation of CCPs on the plasma membrane (Takei et al., 1996). In fact, in the latter studies, the CCVs are found on deep invaginations of the plasma membrane, which looked as if the endosomes were in fact continuous with the plasma membrane, which led to the suggestion that SVs bud from the plasma membrane in a single budding reaction, not requiring an endosomal intermediate. Additional support for clathrin-dependent models comes form the finding that >90% of all CCVs isolated from brain contain SV proteins (Maycox et al., 1992).

3.2 Electrophysiological Studies

To address the role of the clathrin pathway in SV recycling under low physiological rates of stimulation, my colleagues and I carried out a series of studies at the squid giant synapse (Morgan et al., 1999, 2000, 2001, 2003; Augustine et al., 2006). In these studies, we microinjected specific inhibitors of reactions critical for

◻ Figure 21-2

The *Drosophila* mutant shibire has a phenotype consistent with a role for dynamin in vesicle scission. Typical cross-sectioned shi cervical synapses at 19°C (a) and after 8-min exposure to 29°C (b). Note depletion of synaptic vesicles in (b) and lack of compensatory increase in the perimeter of the terminal or in other membranous compartments in the cytoplasm. In (b), a number of collared pits are visible along the plasma membrane (*arrowheads*). A few larger invaginations, whose neck portions are not within the plane of section-ing, are also seen (*small arrows*). Release sites, which are characterized by pre- and postsynaptic membrane densities plus a presynaptic dense body, are designated by *large arrows*. In some instances, the dense body is out of the plane of sectioning. The *asterisk* indicates an example of one collared pit growing off another. db, presynaptic dense body; m, mitochondria; sv, synaptic vesicles. Copyright 1989, Society for Neuroscience. This is reprinted from Koenig et al. (1989) with permission from the Society for Neuroscience

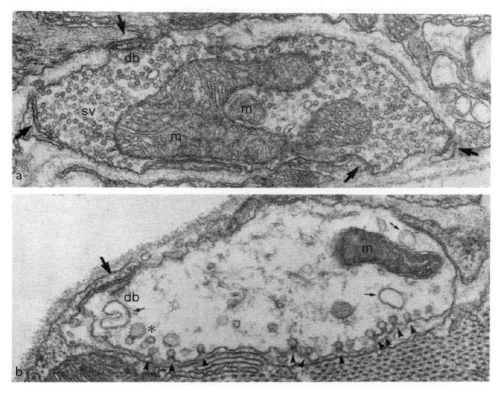

clathrin-mediated endocytosis, and then studied the effects on synaptic transmission and SV endocytosis electrophysiologically and morphologically. Examples of this approach are shown (❯ *Figures 21-3* and ❯ *21-4*) (Morgan et al., 2000, 2001). AP2 pep is a peptide synthesized from the hinge domain of the β2 subunit of AP-2, which interacts with a binding site on the N-terminal domain of the clathrin heavy chain (ter Haar et al., 2000). A control version of the peptide was also synthesized in which the DLL motif that is critical for the interaction was mutated to AAA (AP2 pep ΔDLL). We found that AP2 pep inhibited clathrin polymerization in vitro (❯ *Figure 21-3a*) and synaptic transmission in vivo (❯ *Figure 21-3b*), even at low physiological rates of stimulation (0.03 Hz). We studied other mutant versions of this peptide, and found an excellent correlation between clathrin assembly activity in vitro and inhibition of synaptic transmission in vivo (❯ *Figure 21-3c*). Terminals were fixed for electron microscopy under conditions where synaptic transmission was inhibited >90%, and morphological analyses revealed a large depletion of CCVs and SVs, with a quantitative transfer of membrane from the SV pool in the control terminals to

■ **Figure 21-3**
Clathrin assembly is essential for synaptic vesicle endocytosis. (a) AP2 pep inhibits assembly of clathrin by AP-2 in vitro. A mutant form of this peptide, AP2 pep ΔDLL, is much less effective. (b) Microinjection of AP2 pep (time indicated by the *bar*) into the squid giant presynaptic terminal reversibly inhibits neurotransmitter release. Transmitter release was assessed as the slope of PSPs evoked by presynaptic action potentials. (c) Correlation between the ability of several peptides to inhibit clathrin assembly in vitro (*abscissa*) and neurotransmitter release at the squid synapse (*ordinate*). (d) Ultrastructure of squid giant presynaptic terminals microinjected with AP2 pep (*right panel*) and the control, mutant AP2 pep ΔDLL (*left panel*). (e) The total amount of presynaptic membrane was conserved following microinjection of AP2 pep, with the decrease in membrane in SVs offset by an increase in the surface area of the presynaptic plasma membrane (PM). These changes indicate that AP2 pep inhibits endocytosis. Copyright 2000, Society for Neuroscience. This is reprinted from Morgan et al. (2000) with permission from the Society for Neuroscience

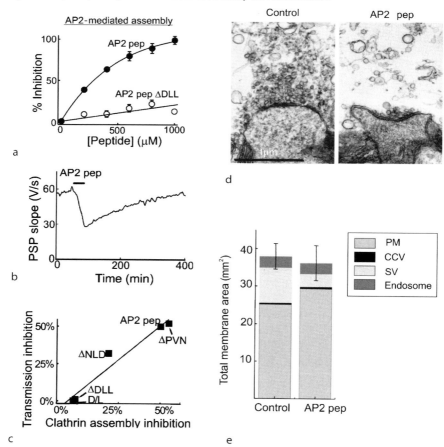

the plasma membrane in the AP2 pep injected terminals (❷ *Figure 21-3d* and ❷ *21-3e*), indicating that indeed SV recycling was inhibited at the plasma membrane step.

We also studied reagents that inhibit CCV uncoating (Morgan et al., 2001). We found that mutating the well-conserved HPD motif within auxilin to AAA (auxilin ΔHPD) eliminated its interaction with Hsc70 (❷ *Figure 21-4a*), inhibited its uncoating activity, and inhibited the ability of wild-type auxilin to uncoat (❷ *Figure 21-4b*). Microinjection of this protein into the squid giant synapse under low rates of stimulation (0.03 Hz) led to an inhibition of synaptic transmission (❯ *Figure 21-4c*) while the wild-type protein had no effect (❯ *Figure 21-4d*). Morphological analyses revealed a fivefold increase in the number of CCVs in the terminal (❯ *Figure 21-4e–g*), indicating that uncoating was inhibited in vivo. When we microinjected reagents that inhibit interactions, which regulate the efficiency of clathrin-mediated endocytosis, we found an inhibition of synaptic transmission and reductions in the numbers of CCPs and vesicles (Morgan et al., 2003). Taken together, these studies lend strong support to the idea that the clathrin pathway plays a major role in SV endocytosis, even during low physiological rates of stimulation (0.03 Hz). There is also strong support for the importance of the clathrin pathway for SV recycling based on studies carried out at the Lamprey synapse, although these studies used higher frequency stimulation (Shupliakov et al., 1997, 2002; Gad et al., 1998, 2000; Low et al., 1999; Ringstad et al., 1999; Evergren et al., 2004).

3.3 Genetic Studies

There is also strong genetic support for the importance of the clathrin pathway in SV recycling. Mutations in a large number of proteins known to be involved in clathrin-mediated endocytosis have defects in synaptic transmission and/or SV recycling. This includes loss of the clathrin assembly proteins AP180 (Zhang et al., 1998; Nonet et al., 1999) and the α-adaptin subunit of AP-2 (Gonzalez-Gaitan and Jackle, 1997), the pinchase dynamin (Kosaka and Ikeda, 1983), the clathrin accessory proteins amphiphysin (Di Paolo et al., 2002), synaptojanin (Cremona et al., 1999; Harris et al., 2000), endophilin (Guichet et al., 2002; Verstreken et al., 2002, 2003; Dickman et al., 2005), and Eps15 (Salcini et al., 2001).

4   The Kinetics of Synaptic Vesicle Recycling

A wide variety of endocytic rates have been measured in nerve terminals and neurosecretory cells, ranging from milliseconds (Sun et al., 2002), to seconds (Klingauf et al., 1998; Kavalali et al., 1999; Pyle et al., 2000; Richards et al., 2000; Sankaranarayanan and Ryan, 2000), to tens of seconds (Betz et al., 1992; Ryan et al., 1993, 1996; Wu and Betz, 1996). Moreover, endocytic rates, even within the same preparation, have been found to vary as a function of stimulation. This has now been seen in multiple preparations (von Gersdorff and Matthews, 1994; Wu and Betz, 1996; Sankaranarayanan and Ryan, 2000; Sun et al., 2002). This is well illustrated in the seminal work from Ling-Gang Wu's lab (Sun et al., 2002) (❯ *Figure 21-5*). These experiments were conducted at the Calyx of Held, a central synapse. In these studies, the investigators were able to resolve the fusion and retrieval of single as well as multiple vesicles through the use of capacitance measurements following mild, physiological stimuli. They found that the time constant for endocytosis

■ **Figure 21-4**
Interactions between Hsc70 and auxilin are essential for coated vesicle uncoating. (a) Time course of binding of Hsc70 to auxilin as monitored by SPR. Traces illustrate the SPR response as a function of time. During the time indicated by the bars, Hsc70 was passed over surfaces to which either wild-type auxilin or auxilin ΔHPD had been covalently coupled. (b) Uncoating of clathrin cages occurs in vitro when Hsc70 and wild-type auxilin (0.1 μM) are present. Auxilin ΔHPD produces a concentration-dependent inhibition of uncoating. (c) Time course of inhibition of neurotransmitter release by auxilin ΔHPD in vivo. Mutant protein was injected during the time indicated by the bar. (d) In contrast, wild-type auxilin has little effect on transmitter release. (e and f) Electron microscope images of terminals injected with auxilin ΔHPD (e) or auxilin (f). Terminals injected with auxilin ΔHPD exhibited an increase in the number of CCVs (*circles*) and a decrease in SVs. (g) Quantification of the number of CCVs in terminals injected with these two reagents. Data represent the mean values and standard error of 167 AZs analyzed from two auxilin-injected terminals and 264 AZs analyzed from two terminals injected with auxilin ΔHPD. Auxilin ΔHPD caused a fivefold increase in CCVs. Copyright 2001, Elsevier. This is reprinted from Morgan et al. (2001) with permission from Elsevier

■ Figure 21-4 (continued)

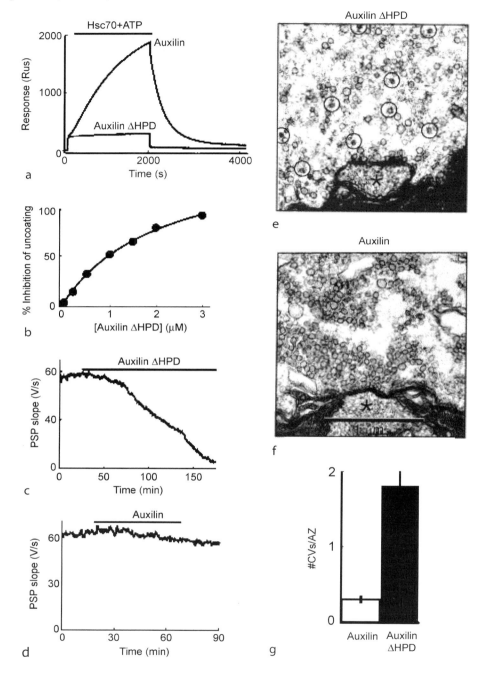

a

b

c

d

e

f

g

□ Figure 21-5

Frequency-dependent inhibition of endocytosis at the Calyx of Held. (a) In the presynaptic cell-attached configuration, a current injection (I_{stim}, 3 ms, 400 pA) induced an action potential (prespike, *arrow*) and thus an EPSC. For calculation of the evoked vesicle number, a mean mEPSC was obtained from 47 mEPSCs. (b) In the presynaptic whole-cell configuration, an AP-e (V_{stim}: 1-ms step from −80 to 7 mV) induced a presynaptic Ca^{2+} current (I_{Ca}) and an EPSC. A mean mEPSC was obtained from 58 mEPSCs. (c) The C_m, G_m, and G_s induced by the AP-e shown in (b). The decay of C_m was fitted with a single exponential function (gray) with $\tau = 115$ ms. Application of cadmium (200 μM) blocked δC_m (*dotted*), I_{Ca}, and the EPSC (b, *dotted*). Data in (a-c) were from the same synapse. Capacitance traces were low-pass-filtered at 100 Hz. (d) Sampled I_{Ca} and C_m induced by paired AP-e at 2 (*upper*), 20 (*middle*), and 333 (*lower*) Hz. Gray curves are single exponential fits with τ labeled (applies to f). G_m and G_s (*lower*) were shown only for 333 Hz (applies to f). (e) The endocytic after paired AP-e plotted versus the frequency. (f) Sampled I_{Ca} and C_m (labels as in d) induced by ten AP-e at 2 (*upper*), 20 (*middle*), and 333 (*lower*) Hz. The scale for I_{Ca} applies to other traces. (g) The endocytic after a train of AP-e at 2 (*squares*), 20 (*triangles*), and 333 (*circles*) Hz plotted versus the number of AP-e. Copyright 2002, Macmillan Publishers Ltd. This is reprinted from Sun et al. (2002) with permission from Macmillan Publishers Ltd.

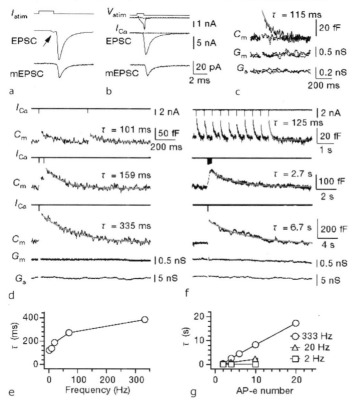

following the fusion of a single SV is 56 ms. As the frequency and number of action potentials are increased, the time constant for endocytosis increases to tens of seconds.

While investigators now agree that endocytosis rates can span a 1,000-fold range (Wu, 2004), and that endocytosis rates are highly dependent on exocytosis rates (Sankaranarayanan and Ryan, 2000; Sun et al., 2002), the molecular mechanisms which underlie these different endocytic rates are not understood. While some investigators have attributed the fast rates to kiss and run and the slow rates to a clathrin pathway, it is possible that they share a common molecular mechanism that becomes limited as a function of the amount of exocytosis. One approach is to ask whether reagents that block the action of specific molecules inhibit the faster versus the slower components of endocytosis. However, one must be cautious in interpreting these kinds of studies since the rate at which the inhibitor is capable of acting slower than the process that one is trying to inhibit. For example, it was found that the rapid capacitance changes shown by the "rapid endocytosis" of dense core vesicles in PC12 cells can be inhibited by antibodies to dynamin but not clathrin (Artalejo et al., 1995). One interpretation of this experiment is that "rapid" endocytosis is dynamin dependent but clathrin independent. An alternative interpretation is that indeed it is clathrin dependent since it is inhibited by a reagent that inhibits a key reaction in the clathrin pathway. The lack of inhibition by the clathrin antibody may be attributed to a failure of the antibody to reach its target at a fast enough rate to be effective.

5   The Endocytic Proteins That Are Key Players in Synaptic Vesicle Recycling

Excellent progress has been made in delimiting the molecular mechanisms that underlie clathrin-mediated SV recycling in nerve terminals. In this section, we will consider the proteins involved in each of the sequential steps of the coated vesicle pathway (❯ *Figure 21-6*).

◘ Figure 21-6

Molecular mechanisms of clathrin-mediated synaptic vesicle recycling. Following exocytosis, the clathrin assembly proteins AP180 and AP-2 interact with PIP₂ and synaptotagmin on the plasma membrane. This leads to the recruitment of clathrin and initiation of a CCP. Dynamin, endophilin, and amphiphysin are believed to participate in the scission reaction whereby the CCP is released from the membrane as a CCV. Auxilin then can interact with the CCV via its clathrin-binding domain, and recruit Hsc70, the uncoating ATPase, via its J domain to promote the uncoating reaction. Following uncoating, the new SV is then refilled with neurotransmitter by neurotransmitter transporters in the SV membrane and reused during a subsequent bout of exocytosis

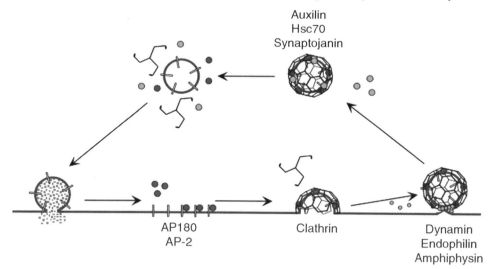

5.1 Proteins Involved in Clathrin Polymerization

Clathrin is ideally suited to serve as a coat protein since it has the property of self-assembly. In solution, or in cytosol, clathrin is found in the triskelion form (∼650 kDa). A clathrin triskelion consists of three heavy chains (180 kDa each) and three light chains (22–28 kDa each), arranged like a pinwheel. The angles made by the heavy chains as they move away from the vertex approximate the edges of a truncated icosahedron. The triskelia polymerize into basket or cagelike structures through interactions between both the proximal and distal legs of the heavy chains (Kirchhausen, 2000). If this polymerization reaction takes place on a cell membrane, it can contribute to the mechanical bending of the membrane into the shape of a CCP. Clathrin self-assembly is slow and irregular at physiological pH and ionic strength. However, clathrin assembly proteins promote the formation of homogeneously sized CCVs under physiological conditions (Ye and Lafer, 1995). The clathrin assembly proteins believed to be relevant for SV recycling are AP180 and AP-2. These proteins are major components of brain CCVs (Maycox et al., 1992). AP180 is a 92-kDa monomer (Zhou et al., 1992), while AP-2 is a ∼270-kDa heterotetramer (Keen, 1987). Each protein on its own can promote clathrin polymerization, but clathrin polymerization is more efficient by an AP180–AP-2 complex (Hao et al., 1999). Interactions between AP180 and AP-2 are regulated by protein phosphorylation (Hao et al., 1999). The accessory protein Eps15 also binds to AP180 and AP-2, and while it does not itself promote clathrin polymerization, it enhances the clathrin polymerization activities of AP180 and AP-2 (Morgan et al., 2003). Both AP180 and AP-2 also interact with inositol lipids (Gaidarov et al., 1996; Hao et al., 1997; Profit et al., 1998), helping to target clathrin polymerization to the membrane. PIP_2 is thought to be critical for this step (Ford et al., 2002). AP-2 also interacts with synaptotagmin (Zhang et al., 1994; Haucke and De Camilli, 1999), which may help to select SV membrane proteins as cargo for inclusion into nascent CCPs. Changes in inositol lipid phosphorylation and protein phosphorylation may regulate these processes.

5.2 Proteins Involved in Vesicle Scission

Dynamin is the GTPase that is thought to be involved in promoting the scission reaction as CCPs become CCVs in neurons (❷ *Figure 21-2*) (Koenig and Ikeda, 1989). Dynamin is thought to exist as a tetramer (Liu et al., 1996; Muhlberg et al., 1997), which further oligomerizes into stacks of rings (Hinshaw and Schmid, 1995; Carr and Hinshaw, 1997). If this oligomerization reaction takes place at the neck of a CCP, it will promote the scission reaction (Hinshaw and Schmid, 1995; Takei et al., 1995). Dynamin has a proline rich domain (PRD) at its C terminus, which contains numerous binding sites for SH3 domain containing proteins, including amphiphysin, endophilin, and syndapin (De Camilli et al., 2001). Interactions between dynamin and both amphiphysin and endophilin have been shown to be important for SV recycling (Shupliakov et al., 1997; Gad et al., 2000). The interaction with endophilin may also be important for the promotion of membrane scission since endophilin has been shown to promote membrane curvature (Gallop et al., 2006). It was recently shown that the interaction between dynamin and syndapin is regulated by the activity-dependent dephosporylation of dynamin by calcineurin (Anggono et al., 2006).

5.3 Proteins Involved in Vesicle Uncoating

Once a CCV is endocytosed, it is believed to be rapidly uncoated. It is thought that this happens because auxilin, which contains both a clathrin-binding domain and a J domain, is recruited to the CCVs via its clathrin-binding domain, and then in turn recruits Hsc70 and activates its ATPase activity via its J domain (Schlossman et al., 1984; Ungewickell et al., 1995; Greener et al., 2000; Pishvaee et al., 2000; Morgan et al., 2001; Newmyer and Schmid, 2001). Exactly how ATP hydrolysis by Hsc70 promotes clathrin disassembly remains to be determined. However, recent progress in this area was made by the publication of high-resolution X-ray structures of both auxilin (Jiang et al., 2003) and Hsc70 (Jiang et al., 2005), as well as cryo EM images of clathrin cages with auxilin bound (Fotin et al., 2004). Interestingly, synaptojanin knockout mice and worms both have defects in synaptic transmission characterized in part by an increase in coated vesicle number, leading to the suggestion that synaptojanin is also involved in uncoating (Cremona et al., 1999; Harris et al., 2000). Current models suggest that synaptojanin, a polyphosphoinositide phosphatase, may be destabilizing the coats by modifying the phosphorylation state of the lipids on the CCV membrane. This finding supports the idea that cycles of lipid phosphorylation may both promote clathrin polymerization onto the presynaptic plasma membrane as well as prevent clathrin from polymerizing onto mature SVs.

5.4 The Cytoskeletal Proteins

Proteins associated with the actin cytoskeleton have been implicated in endocytosis. Eps15, a protein found at the growing edges of CCPs (Tebar et al., 1996) and shown to be critical for endocytosis (Benmerah et al., 1999), binds to and activates the Arp2/3 complex which nucleates actin polymerization (Duncan et al., 2001). HIP1R, ankyrin, ACK1, and ACK2 are all clathrin-binding proteins that may be involved in rearrangements of the actin cytoskeleton (Michaely et al., 1999; Engqvist-Goldstein et al., 2001). Disruption of interactions between the actin-binding protein talin and PI4P 5-kinase type 1γ inhibits SV endocytosis at the Lamprey giant synapse (Morgan et al., 2004). All of this work is consistent with the growing picture that is emerging which suggests that there is a close relationship between actin dynamics and clathrin-mediated endocytosis (Merrifield et al., 2002, 2005; Qualmann and Kessels, 2002; Shupliakov et al., 2002). The precise role of the actin cytoskeleton during SV endocytosis is less clear. Actin has been hypothesized to be involved in a range of functions, including coated pit invagination, vesicle scission, and vesicle motility (De Camilli et al., 2001).

6   Closing Remarks

Considerable progress has been made in recent years, both in delimiting the kinetics of SV endocytosis and in elucidating underlying molecular mechanisms. It is clear that clathrin-mediated endocytosis is a major pathway for SV recycling. It is also clear that rates of SV endocytosis span an enormous range, from milliseconds to tens of seconds, and that endocytosis rates are highly dependent on exocytosis rates. However, what is not clear is whether these different endocytic rates share a common mechanism, or whether different mechanisms are operating.

Acknowledgments

I would like to thank the NIH (NS29051) and the MDA for supporting the work performed in my laboratory. I would like to thank Dr. Jennifer R. Morgan for her contributions to the artwork.

References

Anggono V, Smillie KJ, Graham ME, Valova VA, Cousin MA, et al. 2006. Syndapin I is the phosphorylation-regulated dynamin I partner in synaptic vesicle endocytosis. Nat Neurosci 9 (6): 752-760.

Artalejo CR, Henley JR, McNiven MA, Palfrey HC. 1995. Rapid endocytosis coupled to exocytosis in adrenal chromaffin cells involves Ca2+, GTP, and dynamin but not clathrin. Proc Natl Acad Sci USA 92: 8328-8332.

Augustine GJ, Morgan JR, Villalba-Galea CA, Jin S, Prasad K, et al. 2006. Clathrin and synaptic vesicle endocytosis: Studies at the squid giant synapse. Biochem Soc Trans 34: 68-72.

Baba T, Damke H, Hinshaw JE, Ikeda K, Schmid SL, et al. 1995. Role of dynamin in clathrin-coated vesicle formation. Cold Spring Harb Symp Quant Biol 60: 235-242.

Benmerah A, Bayrou M, Cerf-Bensussan N, Dautry-Varsat A. 1999. Inhibition of clathrin-coated pit assembly by an Eps15 mutant. J Cell Sci 112 (Pt. 9): 1303-1311.

Betz WJ, Mao F, Bewick GS. 1992. Activity-dependent fluorescent staining and destaining of living vertebrate motor nerve terminals. J Neurosci 12: 363-375.

Calakos N, Bennett MK, Peterson KE, Scheller RH. 1994. Protein-protein interactions contributing to the specificity of intracellular vesicular trafficking. Science 263: 1146-1149.

Carr JF, Hinshaw JE. 1997. Dynamin assembles into spirals under physiological salt conditions upon the addition of GDP and gamma-phosphate analogues. J Biol Chem 272: 28030-28035.

Ceccarelli B, Grohovaz F, Hurlbut WP. 1979. Freeze-fracture studies of frog neuromuscular junctions during intense release of neurotransmitter. II. Effects of electrical stimulation and high potassium. J Cell Biol 81: 178-192.

Ceccarelli B, Hurlbut WP, Mauro A. 1973. Turnover of transmitter and synaptic vesicles at the frog neuromuscular junction. J Cell Biol 57: 499-524.

Chapman ER, Desai RC, Davis AF, Tornehl CK. 1998. Delineation of the oligomerization, AP-2 binding, and synprint binding region of the C2B domain of synaptotagmin. J Biol Chem 273: 32966-32972.

Chapman ER, Hanson PI, An S, Jahn R. 1995. Ca2+ regulates the interaction between synaptotagmin and syntaxin 1. J Biol Chem 270: 23667-23671.

Chernomordik LV, Kozlov MM. 2005. Membrane hemifusion: Crossing a chasm in two leaps. Cell 123: 375-382.

Cremona O, Di Paolo G, Wenk MR, Luthi A, Kim WT, et al. 1999. Essential role of phosphoinositide metabolism in synaptic vesicle recycling. Cell 99: 179-188.

De Camilli P, Slepnev V, Shupliakov O, Brodin L. 2001. Synaptic vesicle endocytosis. Synapses. Cowan WM, Sudhof TC, Stevens CF, editors. Baltimore: The Johns Hopkins University Press; pp. 217-274.

Di Paolo G, Sankaranarayanan S, Wenk MR, Daniell L, Perucco E, et al. 2002. Decreased synaptic vesicle recycling efficiency and cognitive deficits in amphiphysin 1 knockout mice. Neuron 33: 789-804.

Dickman DK, Horne JA, Meinertzhagen IA, Schwarz TL. 2005. A slowed classical pathway rather than kiss-and-run mediates endocytosis at synapses lacking synaptojanin and endophilin. Cell 123: 521-533.

Duncan MC, Cope MJ, Goode BL, Wendland B, Drubin DG. 2001. Yeast Eps15–like endocytic protein, Pan1p, activates the Arp2/3 complex. Nat Cell Biol 3: 687-690.

Engqvist-Goldstein AE, Warren RA, Kessels MM, Keen JH, Heuser J, et al. 2001. The actin-binding protein Hip1R associates with clathrin during early stages of endocytosis and promotes clathrin assembly in vitro. J Cell Biol 154: 1209-1223.

Evergren E, Marcucci M, Tomilin N, Low P, Slepnev V, et al. 2004. Amphiphysin is a component of clathrin coats formed during synaptic vesicle recycling at the lamprey giant synapse. Traffic 5: 514-528.

Faundez V, Horng JT, Kelly RB. 1998. A function for the AP3 coat complex in synaptic vesicle formation from endosomes. Cell 93: 423-432.

Ford MG, Mills IG, Peter BJ, Vallis Y, Praefcke GJ, et al. 2002. Curvature of clathrin-coated pits driven by epsin. Nature 419: 361-366.

Fotin A, Cheng Y, Grigorieff N, Walz T, Harrison SC, et al. 2004. Structure of an auxilin-bound clathrin coat and its implications for the mechanism of uncoating. Nature 432: 649-653.

Gad H, Low P, Zotova E, Brodin L, Shupliakov O. 1998. Dissociation between Ca2+-triggered synaptic vesicle exocytosis and clathrin-mediated endocytosis at a central synapse. Neuron 21: 607-616.

Gad H, Ringstad N, Low P, Kjaerulff O, Gustafsson J, et al. 2000. Fission and uncoating of synaptic clathrin-coated vesicles are perturbed by disruption of interactions with the SH3 domain of endophilin. Neuron 27: 301-312.

Gaidarov I, Chen Q, Falck JR, Reddy KK, Keen JH. 1996. A functional phosphatidylinositol 3,4,5–trisphosphate/phosphoinositide binding domain in the clathrin adaptor AP-2 alpha subunit. Implications for the endocytic pathway. J Biol Chem 271: 20922-20929.

Gallop JL, Jao CC, Kent HM, Butler PJ, Evans PR, et al. 2006. Mechanism of endophilin N-BAR domain-mediated membrane curvature. EMBO J 25: 2898-2910.

Gonzalez-Gaitan M, Jackle H. 1997. Role of Drosophila alpha-adaptin in presynaptic vesicle recycling. Cell 88: 767-776.

Greener T, Zhao X, Nojima H, Eisenberg E, Greene LE. 2000. Role of cyclin G-associated kinase in uncoating clathrin-coated vesicles from non-neuronal cells. J Biol Chem 275: 1365-1370.

Guichet A, Wucherpfennig T, Dudu V, Etter S, Wilsch-Brauniger M, et al. 2002. Essential role of endophilin A in synaptic vesicle budding at the Drosophila neuromuscular junction. EMBO J 21: 1661-1672.

Hao W, Luo Z, Zheng L, Prasad K, Lafer EM. 1999. AP180 and AP-2 interact directly in a complex that cooperatively assembles clathrin. J Biol Chem 274: 22785-22794.

Hao W, Tan Z, Prasad K, Reddy KK, Chen J, et al. 1997. Regulation of AP-3 function by inosites. Identification of phosphatidylinositol 3,4,5–trisphosphate as a potent ligand. J Biol Chem 272: 6393-6398.

Harris TW, Hartwieg E, Horvitz HR, Jorgensen EM. 2000. Mutations in synaptojanin disrupt synaptic vesicle recycling. J Cell Biol 150: 589-600.

Haucke V, De Camilli P. 1999. AP-2 recruitment to synaptotagmin stimulated by tyrosine-based endocytic motifs. Science 285: 1268-1271.

Haucke V, Wenk MR, Chapman ER, Farsad K, De Camilli P. 2000. Dual interaction of synaptotagmin with mu2- and alpha-adaptin facilitates clathrin-coated pit nucleation. EMBO J 19: 6011-6019.

Heuser JE. 1989. Review of electron microscopic evidence favouring vesicle exocytosis as the structural basis for quantal release during synaptic transmission. Q J Exp Physiol 74: 1051-1069.

Heuser JE, Reese TS. 1973. Evidence for recycling of synaptic vesicle membrane during transmitter release at the frog neuromuscular junction. J Cell Biol 57: 315-344.

Hinshaw JE, Schmid SL. 1995. Dynamin self-assembles into rings suggesting a mechanism for coated vesicle budding. Nature 374: 190-192.

Jiang J, Prasad K, Lafer EM, Sousa R. 2005. Structural Basis of Interdomain Communication in the Hsc70 Chaperone. Mol Cell 20: 513-524.

Jiang J, Taylor AB, Prasad K, Ishikawa-Brush Y, Hart PJ, et al. 2003. Structure-function analysis of the auxilin J-domain reveals an extended Hsc70 interaction interface. Biochemistry 42: 5748-5753.

Kavalali ET, Klingauf J, Tsien RW. 1999. Properties of fast endocytosis at hippocampal synapses. Philos Trans R Soc Lond B Biol Sci 354: 337-346.

Kee Y, Scheller RH. 1996. Localization of synaptotagmin-binding domains on syntaxin. J Neurosci 16: 1975-1981.

Keen JH. 1987. Clathrin assembly proteins: Affinity purification and a model for coat assembly. J Cell Biol 105: 1989-1998.

Kirchhausen T. 2000. Clathrin. Annu Rev Biochem 69: 699-727.

Klingauf J, Kavalali ET, Tsien RW. 1998. Kinetics and regulation of fast endocytosis at hippocampal synapses. Nature 394: 581-585.

Koenig JH, Ikeda K. 1989. Disappearance and reformation of synaptic vesicle membrane upon transmitter release observed under reversible blockage of membrane retrieval. J Neurosci 9: 3844-3860.

Koenig JH, Kosaka T, Ikeda K. 1989. The relationship between the number of synaptic vesicles and the amount of transmitter released. J Neurosci 9: 1937-1942.

Kosaka T, Ikeda K. 1983. Reversible blockage of membrane retrieval and endocytosis in the garland cell of the temperature-sensitive mutant of Drosophila melanogaster, shibire ts1. J Cell Biol 97: 499-507.

Liu JP, Zhang QX, Baldwin G, Robinson PJ. 1996. Calcium binds dynamin I and inhibits its GTPase activity. J Neurochem 66: 2074-2081.

Low P, Norlin T, Risinger C, Larhammar D, Pieribone VA, et al. 1999. Inhibition of neurotransmitter release in the lamprey reticulospinal synapse by antibody-mediated disruption of SNAP-25 function. Eur J Cell Biol 78: 787-793.

Maycox PR, Link E, Reetz A, Morris SA, Jahn R. 1992. Clathrin-coated vesicles in nervous tissue are involved primarily in synaptic vesicle recycling. J Cell Biol 118: 1379-1388.

Merrifield CJ, Feldman ME, Wan L, Almers W. 2002. Imaging actin and dynamin recruitment during invagination of single clathrin-coated pits. Nat Cell Biol 4: 691-698.

Merrifield CJ, Perrais D, Zenisek D. 2005. Coupling between clathrin-coated-pit invagination, cortactin recruitment, and membrane scission observed in live cells. Cell 121: 593-606.

Michaely P, Kamal A, Anderson RG, Bennett V. 1999. A requirement for ankyrin binding to clathrin during coated pit budding. J Biol Chem 274: 35908-35913.

Morgan JR, Augustine GJ, Lafer EM. 2002. Synaptic vesicle endocytosis: The races, places, and molecular faces. Neuromolecular Med 2: 101-114.

Morgan JR, Di Paolo G, Werner H, Shchedrina VA, Pypaert M, et al. 2004. A role for talin in presynaptic function. J Cell Biol 167: 43-50.

Morgan JR, Prasad K, Hao W, Augustine GJ, Lafer EM. 2000. A conserved clathrin assembly motif essential for synaptic vesicle endocytosis. J Neurosci 20: 8667-8676.

Morgan JR, Prasad K, Jin S, Augustine GJ, Lafer EM. 2001. Uncoating of clathrin-coated vesicles in presynaptic terminals: Roles for Hsc70 and auxilin. Neuron 32: 289-300.

Morgan JR, Prasad K, Jin S, Augustine GJ, Lafer EM. 2003. Eps15 homology domain–NPF motif interactions regulate clathrin coat assembly during synaptic vesicle recycling. J Biol Chem 278: 33583-33592.

Morgan JR, Zhao X, Womack M, Prasad K, Augustine GJ, et al. 1999. A role for the clathrin assembly domain of AP180 in synaptic vesicle endocytosis. J Neurosci 19: 10201-10212.

Muhlberg AB, Warnock DE, Schmid SL. 1997. Domain structure and intramolecular regulation of dynamin GTPase. EMBO J 16: 6676-6683.

Newmyer SL, Schmid SL. 2001. Dominant-interfering Hsc70 mutants disrupt multiple stages of the clathrin-coated vesicle cycle in vivo. J Cell Biol 152: 607-620.

Nonet ML, Holgado AM, Brewer F, Serpe CJ, Norbeck BA, et al. 1999. UNC-11, a Caenorhabditis elegans AP180 homologue, regulates the size and protein composition of synaptic vesicles. Mol Biol Cell 10: 2343-2360.

Pishvaee B, Costaguta G, Yeung BG, Ryazantsev S, Greener T, et al. 2000. A yeast DNA J protein required for uncoating of clathrin-coated vesicles in vivo. Nat Cell Biol 2: 958-963.

Profit AA, Chen J, Gu QM, Chaudhary A, Prasad K, et al. 1998. Probing the phosphoinositide binding site of the clathrin assembly protein AP-2 with photoaffinity labels. Arch Biochem Biophys 357: 85-94.

Pyle JL, Kavalali ET, Piedras-Renteria ES, Tsien RW. 2000. Rapid reuse of readily releasable pool vesicles at hippocampal synapses. Neuron 28: 221-231.

Qualmann B, Kessels MM. 2002. Endocytosis and the cytoskeleton. Int Rev Cytol 220: 93-144.

Richards DA, Guatimosim C, Betz WJ. 2000. Two endocytic recycling routes selectively fill two vesicle pools in frog motor nerve terminals. Neuron 27: 551-559.

Ringstad N, Gad H, Low P, Di Paolo G, Brodin L, et al. 1999. Endophilin/SH3p4 is required for the transition from early to late stages in clathrin-mediated synaptic vesicle endocytosis. Neuron 24: 143-154.

Ryan TA, Reuter H, Wendland B, Schweizer FE, Tsien RW, et al. 1993. The kinetics of synaptic vesicle recycling measured at single presynaptic boutons. Neuron 11: 713-724.

Ryan TA, Smith SJ, Reuter H. 1996. The timing of synaptic vesicle endocytosis. Proc Natl Acad Sci USA 93: 5567-5571.

Salcini AE, Hilliard MA, Croce A, Arbucci S, Luzzi P, et al. 2001. The Eps15 C. elegans homologue EHS-1 is implicated in synaptic vesicle recycling. Nat Cell Biol 3: 755-760.

Sankaranarayanan S, Ryan TA. 2000. Real-time measurements of vesicle-SNARE recycling in synapses of the central nervous system. Nat Cell Biol 2: 197-204.

Schiavo G, Stenbeck G, Rothman JE, Sollner TH. 1997. Binding of the synaptic vesicle v-SNARE, synaptotagmin, to the plasma membrane t-SNARE, SNAP-25, can explain docked vesicles at neurotoxin-treated synapses. Proc Natl Acad Sci USA 94: 997-1001.

Schivell AE, Batchelor RH, Bajjalieh SM. 1996. Isoform-specific, calcium-regulated interaction of the synaptic vesicle proteins SV2 and synaptotagmin. J Biol Chem 271: 27770-27775.

Schlossman DM, Schmid SL, Braell WA, Rothman JE. 1984. An enzyme that removes clathrin coats: Purification of an uncoating ATPase. J Cell Biol 99: 723-733.

Shupliakov O, Bloom O, Gustafsson JS, Kjaerulff O, Low P, et al. 2002. Impaired recycling of synaptic vesicles after acute perturbation of the presynaptic actin cytoskeleton. Proc Natl Acad Sci USA 99: 14476-14481.

Shupliakov O, Low P, Grabs D, Gad H, Chen H, et al. 1997. Synaptic vesicle endocytosis impaired by disruption of dynamin-SH3 domain interactions. Science 276: 259-263.

Stoorvogel W, Oorschot V, Geuze HJ. 1996. A novel class of clathrin-coated vesicles budding from endosomes. J Cell Biol 132: 21-33.

Sudhof TC. 2004. The synaptic vesicle cycle. Annu Rev Neurosci 27: 509-547.

Sun JY, Wu XS, Wu LG. 2002. Single and multiple vesicle fusion induce different rates of endocytosis at a central synapse. Nature 417: 555-559.

Takei K, McPherson PS, Schmid SL, De Camilli P. 1995. Tubular membrane invaginations coated by dynamin rings are induced by GTP-gamma S in nerve terminals. Nature 374: 186-190.

Takei K, Mundigl O, Daniell L, De Camilli P. 1996. The synaptic vesicle cycle: A single vesicle budding step involving clathrin and dynamin. J Cell Biol 133: 1237-1250.

Tebar F, Sorkina T, Sorkin A, Ericsson M, Kirchhausen T. 1996. Eps15 is a component of clathrin-coated pits and vesicles and is located at the rim of coated pits. J Biol Chem 271: 28727-28730.

ter Haar E, Harrison SC, Kirchhausen T. 2000. Peptide-in-groove interactions link target proteins to the beta-propeller of clathrin. Proc Natl Acad Sci USA 97: 1096-1100.

Ungewickell E, Ungewickell H, Holstein SE, Lindner R, Prasad K, et al. 1995. Role of auxilin in uncoating clathrin-coated vesicles. Nature 378: 632-635.

Valtorta F, Meldolesi J, Fesce R. 2001. Synaptic vesicles: Is kissing a matter of competence? Trends Cell Biol 11: 324-328.

Verstreken P, Kjaerulff O, Lloyd TE, Atkinson R, Zhou Y, et al. 2002. Endophilin mutations block clathrin-mediated endocytosis but not neurotransmitter release. Cell 109: 101-112.

Verstreken P, Koh TW, Schulze KL, Zhai RG, Hiesinger PR, et al. 2003. Synaptojanin is recruited by endophilin to promote synaptic vesicle uncoating. Neuron 40: 733-748.

von Gersdorff H, Matthews G. 1994. Dynamics of synaptic vesicle fusion and membrane retrieval in synaptic terminals. Nature 367: 735-739.

Wu LG. 2004. Kinetic regulation of vesicle endocytosis at synapses. Trends Neurosci 27: 548-554.

Wu LG, Betz WJ. 1996. Nerve activity but not intracellular calcium determines the time course of endocytosis at the frog neuromuscular junction. Neuron 17: 769-779.

Ye W, Lafer EM. 1995. Bacterially expressed F1-20/AP-3 assembles clathrin into cages with a narrow size distribution: Implications for the regulation of quantal size during neurotransmission. J Neurosci Res 41: 15-26.

Zhang B, Koh YH, Beckstead RB, Budnik V, Ganetzky B, et al. 1998. Synaptic vesicle size and number are regulated by a clathrin adaptor protein required for endocytosis. Neuron 21: 1465-1475.

Zhang JZ, Davletov BA, Sudhof TC, Anderson RG. 1994. Synaptotagmin I is a high affinity receptor for clathrin AP-2: implications for membrane recycling. Cell 78: 751-760.

Zhou S, Sousa R, Tannery NH, Lafer EM. 1992. Characterization of a novel synapse-specific protein. II. cDNA cloning and sequence analysis of the F1-20 protein. J Neurosci 12: 2144-2155.

22 Lysosomal Membrane Transport in the Central Nervous System

P. Morin · C. Sagné · B. Gasnier

Abstract: The lysosome represents a major intracellular site for the degradation of macromolecules and the sole mechanism for the degradation of organelles through the processes of endocytosis and autophagy. After hydrolysis, the resulting catabolites are exported to the cytosol by secondary active transporters driven by the lysosomal H^+-ATPase. Most of these transporters are still unknown at the molecular level, but the study of lysosomal storage diseases defective for a membrane protein and the design of a whole-cell transport assay based on the inhibition of lysosomal protein sorting have recently shed light on a few proteins involved in these processes. After an overview of this topic of cell biology, we review in more detail the type 1 lysosomal amino acid transporter (LYAAT1) and its endosomal paralogue PAT2, as well as transporters or putative transporters defective in rare neurological diseases: sialin, the Batten disease protein CLN3, and the Niemann–Pick type C disease protein 1 (NPC1). Whereas LYAAT1 and sialin may have specialized roles in neurons aside from their housekeeping function in lysosomal catabolite recycling, elucidating the molecular activity of CLN3 and NPC1 should clarify the role of lysosomes and autophagy in neuronal survival.

List of Abbreviations: ABC, ATP-binding cassette; DMT1, divalent metal transporter type-1; γ interferon-inducible lysosomal thioreductase; ISSD, infantile sialic acid storage disorder; LYAAT1, lysosomal amino acid transporter type 1; MAG, myelin-associated glycoprotein; MHCI, major histocompatibility complex class I; NPC1, Niemann–Pick type C disease protein 1; NCL, neuronal ceroid lipofuscinoses; RND, resistance–nodulation–division; SLC36, solute carrier family 36; SSDs, sterol-sensing domains; SCAP, sterol-regulatory element binding protein cleavage-activating protein; SREBP, sterol-regulatory element binding protein; TOR, target of rapamycin; PPT1, palmitoyl protein thioesterase 1; TPP1, tripeptidyl peptidase 1; TMDs, transmembrane domains

1   Introduction

Lysosomes are intracellular organelles characterized by low internal pH and the presence of multiple hydrolases able to degrade proteins, carbohydrates, lipids, and nucleic acids. Diverse pathways, including receptor-mediated endocytosis, pinocytosis, phagocytosis, chaperone-mediated autophagy, microautophagy, and macroautophagy deliver macromolecules from the extracellular medium, the plasma membrane, and the cytoplasm to the lysosomal lumen. The last process represents the sole mechanism for the turnover of damaged organelles. After these macromolecules are degraded, their elementary constituents are exported from the lysosome by membrane transporters and channels to allow recycling in novel rounds of macromolecule synthesis. This chapter focuses on these lysosomal transport proteins. It begins with a general overview of this neglected field of cell biology and proceeds to mammalian transporters relevant to the physiology and pathophysiology of the central nervous system.

2   An Overview of Lysosomal Metabolite Transport

2.1 Approaches Used to Characterize These Processes

The first studies on lysosomal permeability were based on the capacity of impermeant compounds to accumulate into and enlarge lysosomes in vivo or to protect them from osmotic lysis in vitro. For example, in contrast to D-glucose, sucrose induces vacuoles when present at millimolar concentrations in the culture medium (Cohn and Ehrenreich, 1969) and its use as a major osmolyte (250 mM) prevents the release of lysosomal enzymes from purified subcellular fractions (Lloyd, 1969) because it does not significantly permeate the lysosomal membrane. Both assays were used to characterize the permeability of diverse small molecules. However, with the exception of a few later studies showing stereoselectivity (Docherty et al., 1979; Bird and Lloyd, 1990), the picture that emerged from these experiments was that of a membrane acting as a passive molecular sieve governed by the molecular mass or, in a revisited version, the hydrogen-bonding capacity of permeant species (Iveson et al., 1989).

This failure to reveal the existence of transport proteins probably reflects the fact that both techniques necessitate cytosolic (in vitro assay) or luminal (in vivo assay) concentrations of substrate in the 10–100 mM range, which largely exceeds the K_M of the transport processes. These indirect experiments were thus dominated by the nonspecific permeability of the lipid bilayer of the organelle.

The picture changed in 1982 when the study of an inherited disease, cystinosis, and the use of radiotracer flux techniques revealed the existence of a cystine transporter in the lysosomal membrane (Gahl et al., 1982; Jonas et al., 1982). Lysosomal cystine efflux was found to be abolished in cystinotic lysosomes and slowed to a half-normal value in those of heterozygous individuals. Interestingly, these experiments benefited from an elegant biochemical technique that allowed loading lysosomes with any amino acid by incubating them with a methyl ester derivative at micromolar concentrations: when the neutral, protonated ester passively enters the organelle, it is cleaved by lysosomal esterases and trapped inside as a free amino acid (Goldman and Kaplan, 1973; Reeves, 1979). This technique allows to perform counter-transport experiments in which the presence of substrate in the *trans* (luminal) compartment stimulates translocation of a *cis* (cytosolic) compound, with two critical advantages over previous techniques: (1) the phenomenon of *trans*-stimulation is a hallmark of transporter-mediated processes; (2) since esters are cleaved only in lysosomes, contaminating organelles do not contribute to the measured uptake. Therefore, in contrast with less sophisticated radiotracer flux protocols, controversies on the level of purity of the lysosomal fraction could be avoided.

This breakthrough opened the way for a series of biochemical studies that showed the existence of several lysosomal transporters for amino acids, sugars, and other small molecules (see upper part of ❷ *Table 22-1*). Two other groups of lysosomal disease associated with impaired solute transport were also identified: on one hand, Salla disease and its allelic, lethal form infantile sialic acid storage disorder (ISSD) and, on the other hand, cobalamin F disease, which are defective in sialic acid and vitamin B_{12} efflux, respectively (Rosenblatt et al., 1985; Renlund et al., 1986; Tietze et al., 1989; Mancini et al., 1991).

The molecular era of this field began with the positional cloning of the genes underlying cystinosis and sialic acid storage disorders (Town et al., 1998; Verheijen et al., 1999). However, the activity of the corresponding proteins, cystinosin and sialin, remained uncharacterized until the identification of the type 1 lysosomal amino acid transporter (LYAAT1) serendipitously revealed a novel, easier approach to study these transporters. Indeed, despite its predominant lysosomal localization, the molecular function of LYAAT1 was identified in whole transfected cells owing to the presence of a small amount of protein at the plasma membrane (Sagné et al., 2001). The advantage of this whole-cell assay is to provide the equivalent of an "inside-out lysosome" in which the poorly accessible, outward organelle transport is replaced by a classical cellular uptake (❷ *Figure 22-1*). Lysosomal transporters can thus be characterized using small amounts of transiently transfected cells, without the time- and cell-consuming steps of lysosome purification: culture wells are merely incubated with the labeled substrate at acidic extracellular pH.

This strategy was then rationally applied to cystinosin by mutating its tyrosine-based lysosomal-sorting signal to redirect massively the protein to the plasma membrane (Kalatzis et al., 2001). It has now been successfully applied to sialin, the nucleoside transporter ENT3, as well as pathogenic mutants of cystinosin and sialin (Kalatzis et al., 2004; Morin et al., 2004; Baldwin et al., 2005; Wreden et al., 2005). It may prove useful in the future for other candidate transporters revealed by the study of lysosomal diseases (see below) or by proteomic analysis of the lysosomal membrane (Bagshaw et al., 2005; Boonen et al., 2006).

2.2 Current State of Knowledge

The activities and proteins identified thus far are listed in ❷ *Table 22-1*. For clarity, they will be presented here according to the biological function they fulfil in the cell.

Export of lysosomal proteolysis products. The digestion of polypeptides in lysosomes results in a mixture of amino acids and small peptides. These products are exported by at least 12 different systems and, except for Asn and Gln, at least one system has been assigned for each amino acid. Three amino acid transporters have been identified and characterized at molecular level: the cystine transporter cystinosin (Town et al., 1998; Kalatzis et al., 2001), the small neutral amino acid transporter LYAAT1 (Sagné et al., 2001) and the

Table 22-1

Transport processes and proteins of the lysosomal and late-endosomal membranes. Amino acids are indicated by their three-letter code

Known activity by unknown protein (substrates using a common pathway)	References
Arg, Lys (system c)	Pisoni et al. (1985, 1987b)
Asp, Glu (system d)	Collarini et al. (1989)
Ala, Ser, Thr (system e)	Pisoni et al. (1987a)
Cysteine[a]	Pisoni et al. (1990)
Leu, Ile, Phe, Trp, Tyr, iodo-tyrosine (system h)	Bernar et al. (1986)
Leu, Ile, Val, Met, Phe (system l)	Stewart et al. (1989)
Phe, Trp, Tyr (system t)	Stewart et al. (1989)
Pro, Ala, Ser, Thr (system f)	Pisoni et al. (1987a)
Pro (system p)	Pisoni et al. (1987a)
Di- and tripeptides	Thamotharan et al. (1997)
N-acetyl-D-glucosamine, N-acetyl-D-galactosamine	Jonas et al. (1989)
Polymannoses[a]	Saint-Pol et al. (1997, 1999)
Folylpolyglutamates[a]	Barrueco et al. (1992); Barrueco and Sirotnak (1991)
Vitamin B_{12}	Idriss and Jonas (1991)
PO_4^-	Pisoni (1991)
SO_4^-	Jonas and Jobe (1990)
Ca^{2+}	Lemons and Thoene (1991)
Heavy metals $(Ag^{2+}, Cu^{2+}, Cd^{2+})$[a]	Havelaar (1998a)
Acetyl moieties[a] (through acetyl-CoA/α-glucosaminide-N-acetyltransferase activity)	Bame and Rome (1985); Klein et al. (1978)

Known activity and protein			
Substrates	Protein	Mechanism	
H^+[a]	V-ATPase	ATP-dependent uptake	Nishi and Forgac (2002); Sun-Wada et al. (2004)
Cystine	Cystinosin	H^+ symport	Kalatzis et al. (2001); Town et al. (1998)
Pro, Ala, Gly	LYAAT1	H^+ symport	Sagné et al. (2001)
His, dipeptides	PHT2	H^+ symport	Sakata et al. (2001)
D-Glucose	GLUT8	Uniport or H^+ symport	Augustin et al. (2005); Doege et al. (2000); Ibberson et al. (2000)
Sialic acids, acidic hexoses	Sialin	H^+ symport	Morin et al. (2004); Verheijen et al. (1999)
Nucleosides	ENT3	Uniport or H^+ symport	Baldwin et al. (2005)
Fe^{2+} and other divalent metals	DMT1 (IRE^+ isoform)	H^+ symport	Gunshin et al. (1997); Tabuchi et al. (2002)
Cl^-[a]	CLC-7	H^+ antiport?	Jentsch et al. (2005)
Monovalent cations; Ca^{2+}?	Mucolipin-1	Channel	Bach (2005)
≥6-mer peptides[a]	ABCB9	ATP-dependent uptake	Wolters et al. (2005)

[a] Substrates that are imported into the lysosome under physiological conditions. See the text for more details

□ **Figure 22-1**

A novel approach for the study of lysosomal transporters. In vivo, lysosomal transporters export lysosomal hydrolysis products to the cytosol by an active process driven by the H⁺-ATPase of these organelles (*panel a*). In recent studies, because the lysosomal lumen is poorly accessible, transporters have been relocalized to the plasma membrane by mutating their lysosomal-sorting motif. Intact cells expressing these mutated constructs (*panel b*) actively take up substrates from the extracellular medium at acidic pH (*shaded area*) by a process equivalent to lysosomal efflux. See Kalatzis et al. (2001) for more details

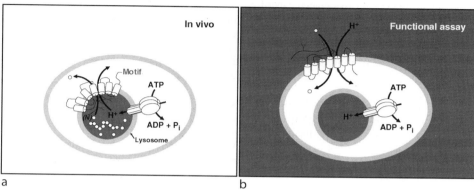

a   b

histidine and dipeptide transporter PHT2 (Sakata et al., 2001). These proteins operate as H⁺ symporters, implying that they actively export their substrates to the cytosol under physiological conditions. A recent study has suggested that the Batten disease protein CLN3 is involved in the transport of arginine across the lysosomal membrane (Ramirez-Montealegre and Pearce, 2005). However, as discussed later, the molecular function of CLN3 is still unclear.

Most amino acid transporters identified in premolecular biology times remain unknown. This includes systems *c* and *d*, which export cationic (Arg, His, and Lys) and anionic (Asp and Glu) amino acids, respectively (Pisoni et al., 1985; Collarini et al., 1989). The first one is of medical interest since it is able to transport the mixed disulfide cysteine–cysteamine, which resembles lysine (Pisoni et al., 1987b). This feature is important for the treatment of cystinosis, because it allows cysteamine to deplete cystine from patients' lysosomes through an alternative efflux pathway (Thoene et al., 1976; Pisoni et al., 1985).

Small neutral amino acids are exported by three distinct routes. Proline is recognized by two different systems with low and high affinities (*p* and *f*, respectively) in addition to LYAAT1, whereas system *e* translocates alanine, serine, and threonine, but not proline (Pisoni et al., 1987a). Despite their similarity, system *f* and LYAAT1 differ in their capacity to recognize D-proline (Sagné et al., 2001). Three transporters have been described for large, neutral amino acids. System *t* translocates aromatic amino acids, whereas system *l* prefers branched aliphatic compounds (Stewart et al., 1989). Although its selectivity overlaps those of systems *t* and *l*, system *h* probably represents a distinct transporter responsible for the salvage of iodine in thyroid cells (Bernar et al., 1986; Andersson et al., 1990).

Finally, another biochemical study described with some detail the transport of di- and tripeptides across the lysosomal membrane (Thamotharan et al., 1997). Further characterization of PHT2 (Sakata et al., 2001) is needed to determine whether one or several proteins are involved in this process.

Export of sugar and nucleic acid catabolites. Lysosomal metabolism also generates monosaccharides from polysaccharides, glycoproteins, and glycolipids. The majority of these products are hexoses, including neutral (D-glucose, D-galactose, D-mannose, L-fucose, N-acetylglucosamine, and N-acetylgalactosamine) and anionic compounds (D-glucuronic acid, L-iduronic acid), along with the nine-carbon sialic acids found at the terminal position of cell-surface sugar chains. Acidic sugars are exported by sialin, the protein defective in sialic acid storage disorders (Verheijen et al., 1999; Morin et al., 2004) (see below), whereas neutral monosaccharides exit lysosomes through two different systems: one specific for acetylhexosamines

(Jonas et al., 1989) and another for other neutral monosaccharides (Jonas et al., 1990; Mancini et al., 1990). The latter probably corresponds to the protein GLUT8, a member of the glucose transporter family that has been recently located to late endosomes and lysosomes (Doege et al., 2000; Ibberson et al., 2000; Augustin et al., 2005). D-Glucosamine is not recognized by the neutral sugar transporters, but its conversion to N-acetylglucosamine by an acetyltransferase that uses acetyl groups translocated from the cytosolic compartment (Bame and Rome, 1985) prevents its accumulation in the lysosomal lumen. This acetyltransferase is deficient in mucopolysaccharidosis type IIIC (Klein et al., 1978; Bame and Rome, 1986), but its molecular identity remains unknown (Ausseil et al., 2006).

It should be noted that D-ribose and D-deoxyribose are not produced in lysosomes because the degradation of nucleic acids does not proceed beyond the nucleoside level. These compounds leave lysosomes through a member of the equilibrative nucleoside transporter family, ENT3, activated at acidic luminal pH (Pisoni and Thoene, 1989; Baldwin et al., 2005). Phosphate (Pisoni, 1991) and sulfate ions (Jonas and Jobe, 1990) resulting from the degradation of nucleic acids and sugars are exported through distinct, unknown transporters.

Lipids. Lipid catabolites are also produced in the lysosomal lumen and must then be exported. Triglycerides are hydrolyzed into glycerol and fatty acids. Glycerol seems to be able to cross the lysosomal membrane by passive diffusion. In principle, fatty acids and cholesterol should also diffuse freely since their transbilayer movement (flip–flop) across protein-free membranes occurs on a millisecond timescale (Hamilton, 2003). However, the lysosomal accumulation of free cholesterol and other lipids in Niemann–Pick disease type C indicate that they are protein mediated, although the exact molecular function of the underlying NPC1 protein remains elusive (see below). The lysosomal ABC transporter ABCA2 (Zhou et al., 2001) may also transport lipids.

Lysosomal transporters also fulfil three other functions besides recycling lysosomal catabolites.

Cellular nutrition. Some nutriments enter eukaryotic cells by endocytosis and subsequent endolysosomal export rather than by permeating the plasma membrane. Such a role of the lysosomal membrane in cellular nutrition is illustrated by the presence of an unidentified transporter for vitamin B_{12}, which is defective in cobalamin F disease (Rosenblatt et al., 1985; Idriss and Jonas, 1991).

Iron represents another well-known example of such a two-step cell entry process. After internalization of iron-loaded transferrin by endocytosis, ferric iron is released in the acidic endosomal lumen, reduced to ferrous iron by an unknown enzyme, and exported to the cytosol by the type-1 divalent metal transporter, DMT1 (Fleming et al., 1997; Gunshin et al., 1997; Mackenzie and Hediger, 2004). This process has been well documented at the level of recycling endosomes. However, recent studies have shown that a splicing variant of DMT1 resides in late endosomes and lysosomes, and thus may play a similar role in these organelles (Tabuchi et al., 2002; Abouhamed et al., 2006). This isoform might be important in epithelial cells to rescue iron delivered to the lysosome by cubilin-mediated endocytosis of transferrin (Kozyraki et al., 2001).

Lysosomal import of oligomeric metabolites. Another function of lysosomal transporters is to feed hydrolytic enzymes with specific substrates rather than to export their products. Indeed, although most transporters operate in the efflux direction, some metabolites are imported into the lumen under physiological conditions. For instance, lysosomes import free polymannose oligosaccharides through an unknown process, which depends on ATP hydrolysis but not the H^+-ATPase, suggesting that it is operated by an ATP-binding cassette (ABC) transporter (Saint-Pol et al., 1997, 1999). Its presumed role is to allow lysosomal degradation of oligosaccharides derived from dolichol precursors or from misfolded, ER-retro-translocated glycoproteins. Folylpolyglutamates and other γ-glutamyl conjugates are also imported by an unknown H^+-driven transporter for subsequent degradation by lysosomal γ-glutamyl hydrolase (Barrueco and Sirotnak, 1991; Barrueco et al., 1992). This process also recognizes short peptides with a C-terminal glutamate.

The half-type ABC transporter ABCB9 (Yamaguchi et al., 1999), which shares homology with those involved in antigen presentation by class I major histocompatibility complex (MHCI) molecules (Koch and Tampé, 2006), provides another example. ABCB9 uses ATP hydrolysis to translocate peptides from six up to at least sixty residues across membranes (Wolters et al., 2005), and it has been reported to localize on lysosomes (Zhang et al., 2000; but see Kobayashi et al., 2004). ABCB9 thus appears to import peptides into the lysosomal lumen. This activity might fulfil diverse biological functions. A general function might be to complete the degradation of peptides escaping from the proteasome. Since the upper limit of ABCB9 substrates is unknown, it might also import unfolded proteins through a pathway parallel to (or related to) chaperone-mediated autophagy (Majeski and Dice, 2004). Finally, in some cells, it might be involved in the presentation of autoantigens by MHCII molecules (Dani et al., 2004).

Control of the lysosomal pH and other parameters. A third "additional" function of lysosomal transporters is to control the physicochemical state of the lumen. The major player for the acidification of the lysosome is obviously the V-type H^+-ATPase (Nishi and Forgac, 2002; Sun-Wada et al., 2004). However, other transport proteins are needed to prevent the development of a positive electric potential, which would rapidly block the ATPase after a few protons are translocated. Intracellular members of the CLC chloride channel family are believed to sustain and regulate H^+ pumping by providing an electric shunt through a chloride channel or H^+/chloride antiport mechanism (Jentsch et al., 2005b). Although the molecular activity of the lysosomal isoform CLC-7 has not yet been characterized, it is probably a H^+ antiporter since it possesses a glutamate residue which acts as a cytosolic H^+ transfer site and is specific of the transporter subclass (Accardi et al., 2005; Miller, 2006). The Batten disease protein CLN3 (see below) and mucolipin-1 (Soyombo et al., 2006) may also regulate the lysosomal pH.

Another physicochemical parameter which is probably controlled by secondary transporters is the redox state of the lysosome. Indeed, an unknown H^+-driven transporter actively imports cysteine in this organelle (Pisoni et al., 1990) and, on the other hand, the oxidized form of this amino acid (cystine) is exported by cystinosin and reduced in the cytosol by glutathione. The two proteins may thus act in concert to create a cysteine/cystine shuttle, which imports reducing equivalents into the lumen. This reducing environment would protect the active site of lysosomal serine proteases and facilitate the unfolding of proteins destined for degradation by disrupting their disulfide bonds (Lloyd, 1986; Pisoni et al., 1990). Although few data are available on the redox state of the lysosome, the hypothesis of a reducing environment is supported by the existence of a γ interferon-inducible lysosomal thioreductase (GILT), which uses cysteine as electron donor and is necessary for the MHCII-restricted presentation of epitopes constrained by disulfide bonds (Arunachalam et al., 2000; Maric et al., 2001).

Lysosomes also take up heavy metals with a micromolar affinity by an unknown protein (Havelaar et al., 1998a). The Wilson disease protein ATP7B, a P-type ATPase involved in biliary copper excretion (Bull et al., 1993; Tanzi et al., 1993) and recently reported to reside in late endosomes (Harada et al., 2005), represented a likely candidate. However, the uptake is still observed in ATP7B-deficient lysosomes (Havelaar et al., 1998a). The biological significance of this activity is unclear. A low-affinity Ca^{2+} uptake has also been described in an earlier study (Lemons and Thoene, 1991).

We now review lysosomal transporters believed to play a specific function in the nervous system or associated with neurological conditions. Recent reviews are available for transport proteins that are not addressed here, such as cystinosin (Gahl et al., 2002; Kalatzis and Antignac, 2003), DMT1 (Mackenzie and Hediger, 2004), CLC-7 (Jentsch et al., 2005a; Jentsch et al., 2005b), ABCA2 (Schmitz and Kaminski, 2002), and mucolipin-1 (Bach, 2005).

3   LYAAT1 and Other Members of the SLC36 Family

3.1 Discovery of LYAAT1

LYAAT1 was identified as a distant paralogue of the synaptic vesicle transporter for inhibitory amino acids (McIntire et al., 1997; Sagné et al., 1997, 2001). In our first experiments, it appeared as a plasmalemmal GABA transporter activated at acidic pH. However, its biological function was unclear because the distribution of its transcript was not selective for GABAergic neurons and more efficient plasmalemmal GABA transporters were already described (Kanner, 1994). Since the pH dependence suggested a H^+ symport mechanism, we reasoned that the protein might be involved in the export of substrates from acidic organelles. We thus hypothesized a lysosomal localization and a transport activity tailored to proteinogenic amino acids. Both hypotheses proved true and LYAAT1 was thus identified as a H^+ symporter involved in the export of proline, alanine, and glycine from lysosomes (Sagné et al., 2001).

However, as mentioned above, its activity is distinct from that of system f (Pisoni et al., 1987a) since LYAAT1 recognizes D-proline.

Subsequent studies revealed that, in addition to its lysosomal function in many cell types, LYAAT1 is also responsible for the apical uptake of GABA and proline in the intestinal epithelial cell line Caco-2 (Boll et al., 2002; Chen et al., 2003a), in agreement with the H^+-driven transport described in this cell line (Thwaites et al., 1993, 2000). It is also present at the intestinal brush-border membrane (Anderson et al., 2004). Because the Na^+/H^+ exchanger NHE3 creates an acidic microenvironment outside the brush border, LYAAT1 may be involved in the intestinal absorption of dietary amino acids.

This transporter thus has a dual role and cellular localization, depending on the cell type (Boll et al., 2004). A similar duality in endosomal export and intestinal absorption has been previously described for the iron transporter DMT1 (Mackenzie and Hediger, 2004). In the latter case, the subcellular localization is regulated by alternative splicing because of the presence of distinct targeting motifs in the protein isoforms (Tabuchi et al., 2002; Lam-Yuk-Tseung and Gros, 2006). However, in the case of LYAAT1, identical mRNAs are expressed in Caco-2 and nonepithelial cells and the mechanism by which the cellular environment controls the intracellular localization is still unknown.

3.2 Phylogeny and Functional Properties of the SLC36 Transporters

LYAAT1 belongs to a superfamily of eukaryotic amino acid transporters found in plants, yeasts, and animals (Young et al., 1999; Wipf et al., 2002). The LYAAT1 family, known as the solute carrier family 36 (SLC36) in the Human Genome Organization nomenclature, comprises four members. The *SLC36A4* gene has been mapped to human chromosome 11 whereas the three others are clustered in the 5q33.1 region (Bermingham and Pennington, 2004; Boll et al., 2003b, 2004). LYAAT1 is encoded by *SLC36A1*. SLC36 proteins have ~500 amino acid and 9 or 11 transmembrane domains (TMDs) depending on the topology predictions. An even number of TMDs is not possible for LYAAT1 since its N terminus is present in the cytosol (Agulhon et al., 2003), in contrast to its C terminus (C. Sagné and B. Gasnier, unpublished data).

Only two members of the family, LYAAT1 (also known as PAT1) and PAT2 (*SLC36A2* gene), have been functionally characterized (Sagné et al., 2001; Boll et al., 2002; Chen et al., 2003a, b; Wreden et al., 2003; Foltz et al., 2004; Rubio-Aliaga et al., 2004). They both cotransport small neutral L-α-amino acids (glycine, L-alanine, L-proline) and protons with 1:1 stoichiometry. However, their activities differ in some aspects. In contrast to LYAAT1, PAT2 is fully activated at neutral pH (Foltz et al., 2004; Rubio-Aliaga et al., 2004; but see Chen et al., 2003b). On the other hand, LYAAT1 has lower affinity and broader substrate selectivity, as it recognizes amino acids with longer aliphatic chain (GABA), methyl substitutions of the amino group (sarcosine, betaine), and D-enantiomers (Boll et al., 2003a; Metzner et al., 2005). Because of its broad selectivity and its presence at the intestinal brush border, LYAAT1 may serve as an oral delivery route for pharmaceutically active compounds, including the neuromodulatory agents D-serine and D-cycloserine (Thwaites et al., 1995; Boll et al., 2003a) and the GABA analogues vigabatrin and homotaurine (Metzner et al., 2005; Abbot et al., 2006).

3.3 Physiological Roles of LYAAT1 and PAT2 in the Nervous System

Despite its presumed housekeeping role in the lysosome, LYAAT1 exhibits a specific distribution in the central nervous system. It is widely expressed throughout the rodent brain and spinal cord where it is present in neurons, choroid plexus, and ependymal epithelial cells, but absent from glial cells (Sagné et al., 2001; Agulhon et al., 2003; Wreden et al., 2003). Light, confocal, and electron microscopies showed that LYAAT1 is massively present in lysosomes and late endosomes of the perikarya and proximal dendrites, but seems absent from axons and terminal boutons (Agulhon et al., 2003). Interestingly, the level of expression varies among neuronal populations, independently of the neurotransmitter used. LYAAT1 mRNA and protein are at highest levels in mitral cells of the olfactory bulb, pyramidal cells of the hippocampus, Purkinje cells of the cerebellum, and in diverse neurons of the tenia tecta, indusium griseum, thalamus, and brainstem. On the contrary, they are absent or weakly detected in the caudate putamen and hypothalamus, as well as in some neurons scattered in many brain regions (Agulhon et al., 2003).

This cell-specific expression pattern raises two questions: first, which protein ensures the lysosomal export of proline, alanine, and glycine in glial and other LYAAT1-negative cells? Second, why do some neurons require a high level of LYAAT1? The unidentified system f transporter (Pisoni et al., 1987a) or other members of the SLC36 family (Boll et al., 2004) may provide an answer to the first question. On the other hand, two hypotheses could explain the requirement for a high level of LYAAT1 in, for instance, hippocampal pyramidal neurons. This feature may simply reflect the existence of an intense lysosomal proteolysis in these cells and, therefore, of the necessity to avoid an engorgement of lysosomes with amino acids. In support of this hypothesis, LYAAT1-positive neurons contain high levels of the lysosomal aspartyl proteinase cathepsin-D (although some cathepsin-D-positive neurons are devoid of LYAAT1), and the two proteins colocalize strongly at subcellular level (Agulhon et al., 2003). The importance of lysosomal proteolysis in neuronal function is also highlighted by the neurodegenerative symptoms induced by cathepsin-D deficiency (Koike et al., 2000; Tyynela et al., 2000; Myllykangas et al., 2005; Siintola et al., 2006; Steinfeld et al., 2006).

Alternatively, the expression pattern of LYAAT1 may reflect a specific role in neuronal subpopulations, besides its housekeeping function. Consistent with this idea, LYAAT1 has been shown to localize to extralysosomal sites in primary cultures of hippocampal neurons (Wreden et al., 2003). In addition to the somatodendritic lysosomes, it is found in this cellular model at the plasma membrane and in axons, where it colocalizes with a component of the exocyst complex, sec6. As the role of the exocyst is to determine the sites of exocytosis at the target membrane, LYAAT1 may define a novel class of secretory lysosomes in neurons (Blott and Griffiths, 2002; Wreden et al., 2003).

The second transporter, PAT2, is widely found throughout the CNS with prominent expression in cerebellum, olfactory bulb, cerebral cortex, hippocampus, hypothalamus, and brainstem (Rubio-Aliaga et al., 2004). Like LYAAT1, it is expressed in neurons independently of the neurotransmitter phenotype; it seems absent from glial cells and cells with a strong PAT2 immunoreactivity include mitral cells of the olfactory bulb, hippocampal pyramidal cells, cerebellar Purkinje cells, and spinal motoneurons. However, the two paralogues differ in their subcellular localization since PAT2 is found in the endoplasmic reticulum and rab4-positive recycling endosomes but is excluded from late endosomes and lysosomes (Rubio-Aliaga et al., 2004). PAT2 has also been described at the paranodes and Schmidt–Lanterman incisures of myelinating Schwann cells in the peripheral nervous system (Bermingham et al., 2002).

Rubio-Aliaga and coworkers (2004) propose three hypotheses for the physiological function of PAT2 in the CNS. First, PAT2 could export amino acids from recycling endosomes. Although these organelles are not viewed as a place of high proteolytic activity, the higher affinity of PAT2 for amino acids as compared with LYAAT1 (Boll et al., 2002; Foltz et al., 2004) and the fact that it shows maximal transport rate at moderately acidic pH (Rubio-Aliaga et al., 2004) are consistent with this proposal. Second, the authors speculate that PAT2 might traffic from the endosome to the plasma membrane and participate to the homeostasis of extracellular glycine. At high glycine concentration, it could provide a low-affinity uptake pathway to assist the high-affinity transporters GLYT1 and GLYT2 in the clearance of glycine. In our opinion, this hypothesis is unlikely since a marginal presence at the plasma membrane would not be sufficient to provide a high transport capacity. A third related hypothesis proposed that the putative plasmalemmal pool of PAT2 might locally release glycine and activate NMDA receptors because its Na^+ independence prompts it to operate in the efflux mode at the plasma membrane (Rubio-Aliaga et al., 2004). However, actual measurements in neurons are needed to substantiate this hypothesis.

To conclude this section, it should be mentioned that genetic studies in *Drosophila* have suggested that some members of the SLC36 family have an amino-sensing function distinct from their transport activity. This proposal is based on the fact that two SLC36-related proteins of the fly, each of which genetically interacts with the nutrient- and growth factor-regulated intracellular kinase TOR (target of rapamycin), differ more than 400-fold in their amino acid uptake capacity (Goberdhan et al., 2005). A similar metabolite-sensing function of secondary active transporters has been previously reported in the yeast *Saccharomyces cerevisiae* (Van Belle and Andre, 2001). If this proposal holds true for LYAAT1 or PAT2 in mammalian brains, it will be interesting to examine whether they intervene in the regulation of neuronal growth by amino acids.

4   Sialin: The Sialic Acid Transporter

4.1   An Acidic Monosaccharide Transporter Defective in Sialic Acid Storage Diseases

Sialin is the product of a gene mutated in two allelic diseases characterized by defective lysosomal export of sialic acids. The first disease, infantile sialic acid storage disorder (ISSD), (MIM 269920) is a very rare autosomal recessive disease that presents with facial dysmorphism, hepatosplenomegaly, severe motor retardation, failure to thrive, and early death (<2 years) (Aula and Gahl, 2001). About 35 cases have been reported worldwide in the literature (Froissart et al., 2005). Salla disease (MIM 604369), which prevails in Finland, is a milder, progressive form in which patients exhibit an almost normal lifespan. Neurological symptoms such as hypotonia, ataxia, and delayed motor development, as well as impaired speech development and mental retardation predominate over somatic signs in this disease (Aula and Gahl, 2001). In both diseases, magnetic resonance imaging of the brain show cerebellar atrophy and central hypomyelination with a marked thinning of the corpus callosum (Haataja et al., 1994; Sonninen et al., 1999; Parazzini et al., 2003). Peripheral dysmyelination has also been reported in older Salla patients (Varho et al., 2000).

The underlying gene, *SLC17A5*, which maps to chromosome arm 6q14-q15, encodes a 495-amino acid protein, which shares homology with the type 1 phosphate transporter and the vesicular glutamate transporters (Verheijen et al., 1999; Reimer and Edwards, 2004). In nonneuronal cells, human and rat sialin localize to lysosomes and late endosomes owing to the presence of a dileucine-based lysosomal-sorting motif near their N-terminal ends (Aula et al., 2002; Morin et al., 2004; Wreden et al., 2005). By mutating this sorting motif, these proteins were mislocalized to the plasma membrane and their transport activity was characterized using the whole-cell assay described in ❷ *Figure 22-1*. Both studies (Morin et al., 2004; Wreden et al., 2005) show that mammalian sialin is a H^+-driven transporter that recognizes acidic, but not neutral, monosaccharides in the millimolar range, in agreement with previous biochemical studies on human and rat lysosomes (Mancini et al., 1989, 1991). In particular, it exports glucuronic, gluconic, and iduronic acids from the lysosome in addition to the sialic acids. It also recognizes aliphatic monocarboxylates (Havelaar et al., 1998b; Morin et al., 2004), but the biological significance of this feature is unclear.

4.2   Localization of Sialin in the Nervous System

Two studies have examined the distribution of sialin in the mouse brain (Aula et al., 2004; Yarovaya et al., 2005). The distribution pattern and immunoblotting analysis of primary cultures showed that the protein is more abundant in neurons than in glial cells (Aula et al., 2004). The expression starts early in development (E13–E15), and in the adult brain predominates in the cerebral and cerebellar cortices, the hippocampus, the striatum, and some nuclei of the midbrain. Both studies reported a clear immunolabeling of neuronal cell bodies such as those of hippocampal pyramidal cells, cerebellar Purkinje cells, and mitral cells of the olfactory bulb. However, they differed for the distribution of sialin in other neuronal compartments since one study reported a predominant labeling of the neuropil in many brain regions without significant immunoreactivity of the white matter (Yarovaya et al., 2005) whereas a strong labeling of axonal tracts was observed in another study (Aula et al., 2004). This discrepancy may originate from the use of distinct antibodies or from the fact that older brains were analyzed in the second study (up to 6 months versus 1 month). This issue deserves further investigation.

The subcellular distribution has been analyzed in more detail in neuronal cultures (Aula et al., 2004). Endogenous and transfected sialin was found not only in vesicular structures present in the soma but also along the axon as well as in the growth cone. In cell bodies, the sialin puncta appeared distinct from those immunopositive for the lysosomal/late-endosomal marker LAMP-1, in contrast to what occurs in non-neuronal cells (Aula et al., 2002; Aula et al., 2004; Morin et al., 2004). It was thus concluded that sialin is exclusively nonlysosomal in neurons (Aula et al., 2004). However, we do observe a colocalization of human sialin with LAMP1 in transfected neurons (P. Morin, C. Sagné, and B.Gasnier, unpublished data).

The authors also reported the presence of sialin at the plasma membrane based on its detection in nonpermeabilized neurons. However, this observation is in contradiction with the presumed cytosolic localization of the epitope used in this study (Aula et al., 2004).

4.3 Genotype–Phenotype Relationship and Potential Pathogenic Mechanisms

Salla disease is characterized by a missense mutation of a conserved arginine, R39C, in the sialin sequence (Verheijen et al., 1999; Aula et al., 2000). Most patients are homozygous for this mutation, but compound heterozygotes with the R39C mutation on one allele and another mutation common to ISSD on the other allele are also observed and often display increased severity. ISSD patients present diverse mutations such as large deletions, premature stops, a small in-frame deletion (ΔSSLRN), and some missense mutations (H183R, P334R, G371V), but the Scandinavian founder mutation R39C is never observed (Aula et al., 2000).

To examine how these missense mutations and the small in-frame deletion affect the transport activity, we introduced them into a human construct devoid of its dileucine-based sorting motif and analyzed the ability of whole transfected cells to take up neuraminic acid at low pH (Morin et al., 2004). Interestingly, we found that whereas ISSD mutations abolished the transport activity, the R39C mutation slowed down, but did not block the transporter, thus suggesting that the lesser severity of Salla disease and, in particular, the absence of somatic signs are due to a residual lysosomal efflux of sialic acids. Another study introduced the human mutations into the rat protein and found similar effects (Wreden et al., 2005). The correlation between residual transport and the lack of somatic signs was confirmed by the fact that a mutation (K136E) previously found as the second allele of a Salla compound heterozygote, which induces a molecular phenotype similar to that of R39C (Morin et al., 2004; Wreden et al., 2005), was later found in the homozygous state in a patient with a severe form of Salla disease (Biancheri et al., 2005).

It should be noted that previous biochemical studies failed to detect residual sialic acid transport in lysosomal membranes derived from Salla patients (Renlund et al., 1986; Mancini et al., 1991). However, this is not in contradiction with the 10% (Wreden et al., 2005) to 30% (Morin et al., 2004) residual activity measured in the whole-cell assay since the R39C and K136E mutations also induce a partial mislocalization of the protein (Aula et al., 2002; Morin et al., 2004; but see Wreden et al., 2005 for a divergent observation). The actual level of sialin activity in Salla lysosomes is thus probably much lower than 10%.

To determine whether the reduced sialin activity impacts exclusively on the lysosome or, more broadly, on the whole sialic acid metabolism in the cell, we performed saturation kinetics of the R39C and K136E mutants and found a reduced maximal velocity (Morin et al., 2004). Therefore, the accumulation of sialic acid in Salla lysosomes cannot compensate for the decreased activity, and the cytosolic availability of these sugars will rest essentially on de novo biosynthesis. Since a reduced biosynthesis induces a reduced sialylation of glycoconjugates, we predicted a similar hyposialylation in Salla disease and ISSD, particularly at the level of brain gangliosides which represent the most abundant sialoglycoconjugates. If this hyposialylation is confirmed, it should affect the axoglial interaction between gangliosides and the myelin-associated glycoprotein (MAG), thus explaining the central dysmyelination observed in these diseases (Morin et al., 2004).

5   The Batten Disease Protein CLN3

5.1 A Brief Overview of Neuronal Ceroid Lipofuscinoses

CLN3 has been identified as the product of a gene defective in an inherited, childhood-onset neurodegenerative disease known as juvenile ceroid lipofuscinosis or Batten disease (MIM 204200) (Consortium, 1995). Neuronal ceroid lipofuscinoses (NCL) constitute a subgroup of lysosomal disorders characterized by the lysosomal accumulation of fluorescent lipofuscin-like material in many tissues, including neurons, and similar neurodegenerative pathologies (Hofmann and Peltonen, 2001; Mole et al., 2005). They represent the most common cause of neurodegeneration in childhood with a worldwide incidence of 1 in 20,000 live births. Symptoms include progressive blindness, epileptic seizures, psychomotor deterioration, and premature death with an age of onset ranging from infancy to adulthood depending on the genetic defect. Brain resonance magnetic imaging shows cerebellar and cortical atrophy. The clinical forms also differ in the ultrastructural profile of the storage material, which appears as granular, curvilinear, or fingerprint like. A common biochemical feature, the lysosomal accumulation of mitochondrial ATP synthase subunit c, has been described in several types of NCL (Palmer et al., 1992), but this may represent a nonspecific phenomenon indicative of increased or impaired autophagy in lysosomal diseases (Elleder et al., 1997; Tanaka et al., 2000; Ko et al., 2005; Koike et al., 2005; Cao et al., 2006).

At least nine genetically distinct forms of NCLs have been identified, most of them inherited in an autosomal recessive manner, and seven human genes have been identified (Hofmann and Peltonen, 2001; Mole et al., 2005). Four genes encode soluble proteins of the lysosomal lumen: palmitoyl protein thioesterase 1 (PPT1, also named CLN1), an enzyme which removes fatty acids from cysteine residues in proteins; tripeptidyl peptidase 1 (TPP1 or CLN2), an exopeptidase which cleaves tripeptides sequentially from protein amino termini; the endoprotease cathepsin-D; and CLN5, a vertebrate-specific protein of unknown function. Three genes encode membrane proteins of unknown function present in lysosomes and late endosomes (CLN3) and in the endoplasmic reticulum (CLN6, CLN8).

Defective CLN3 is associated to a juvenile clinical phenotype, with visual loss at 6–7 years of age (Hofmann and Peltonen, 2001; Mole et al., 2005). Progressive mental and motor deterioration eventually occurs with epilepsy, leading to death in the second or third decade of life. Diagnostic criteria include retinal degeneration, the presence of intracellular vacuoles, and the accumulation of autofluorescent lipopigments in lymphocytes, dermal cells, or other available cell types, with a characteristic fingerprint profile of the storage material under electron microscopy. Treatment is largely supportive (anticonvulsants) because there is no specific therapy.

5.2 The CLN3 Protein

Human CLN3 comprises 438 amino acids and 6–11 predicted TMDs. Current experimental data support a six-TMD topological model (reviewed in Phillips et al., 2005), but in the absence of a systematic study using, for instance, glycosylation- or cysteine-scanning methods, the existence of additional TMDs cannot be excluded. Although early studies led to conflicting results, it is now clearly established that CLN3 resides on lysosomes and late endosomes in nonneuronal cells (Jarvela et al., 1998; Kida et al., 1999; Haskell et al., 2000; Kyttala et al., 2004; Storch et al., 2004). Two sorting signals are responsible for this localization: a nonclassical dileucine-type motif present in the loop connecting TMDs 4 and 5 an unconventional signal with critical methionine and glycine residues (M-(X)9-G) in the C-terminal tail (Kyttala et al., 2004; Storch et al., 2004). Although the first motif is necessary for intracellular sorting by the AP-1 and AP-3 adaptors, the unconventional motif is sufficient to target CLN3 to the lysosome, and mutation of both signals is necessary to retain the protein at the plasma membrane (Kyttala et al., 2004, 2005; Storch et al., 2004).

Interestingly, in neurons, CLN3 localizes to vesicular structures of the axon and presynaptic terminals in addition to the lysosomes of the cell soma and dendrites (Luiro et al., 2001). These axonal structures, which differ from synaptic vesicles, have been recently identified as early endosomes (Luiro et al., 2004). Disruption of the two targeting signals impair lysosomal/late-endosomal, but not early-endosomal, localization in neurons (Kyttala et al., 2004).

Diverse mutations of the *cln3* gene have been observed in Batten patients. The most frequent mutation is a 1.02-kb deletion, which results in a truncated protein comprising the first 153 residues of CLN3 followed by 28 novel amino acids, but other mutations including seven missense mutations have been reported (Munroe et al., 1997; see also http://www.ucl.ac.uk/ncl/index.html). Three of these missense mutations (L101P, L170P, E295K) have been associated with an atypical phenotype displaying retinopathy without CNS dysfunction (Munroe et al., 1997). Interestingly, five missense mutations, including the three latter ones, have no effect on the lysosomal localization, and should therefore impair the molecular activity of the protein (Jarvela et al., 1999; Haskell et al., 2000).

5.3 Putative Transport Function of CLN3

The molecular and cellular functions of CLN3 remain unclear. Several proposals have been made including the transport of arginine (Kim et al., 2003; Ramirez-Montealegre and Pearce, 2005), regulation of lysosomal pH (Pearce et al., 1999a, b; Holopainen et al., 2001; Gachet et al., 2005; Ramirez-Montealegre and Pearce, 2005); membrane trafficking (Chattopadhyay et al., 2003; Luiro et al., 2004), and control of apoptosis (Puranam et al., 1999; Persaud-Sawin et al., 2002). We discuss here the evidence for the first hypothesis.

In addition to the distant homology of CLN3 to members of the major facilitator superfamily (Baldwin et al., 2004), the transporter hypothesis is supported by genetic and biochemical studies of the *S. cerevisiae* homologue Btn1p. This protein shares 39% identity and 59% similarity to human CLN3 and it localizes to the vacuole (Pearce and Sherman, 1998; Pearce et al., 1999b), the yeast equivalent of mammalian lysosomes. Deletion of Btn1p results in a tenfold decrease in the level of vacuolar arginine and lysine, associated with a decreased uptake of these amino acids into the organelle. Transport was restored by expression of Btn1p or human CLN3, thus leading to the proposal that these proteins represent basic amino acid transporters (Kim et al., 2003). More recently, the same laboratory extended and slightly modified this conclusion by reporting that lysosomes derived from the lymphoblasts of patients with Batten disease differ from those of normal controls by their incapacity to import arginine, but not lysine (Ramirez-Montealegre and Pearce, 2005).

This last result is in contrast with previous description of a transport system common to both amino acids in human lysosomes (Pisoni et al., 1985, 1987b). Another puzzling fact is that, whereas previous experiments showed that ATP inhibits influx and stimulates efflux of cationic amino acids (Pisoni et al., 1985, 1987b), ATP was reported to stimulate arginine influx in the Batten lysosome study, thus leading to the conclusion that the CLN3-dependent system should import arginine under physiological conditions (Ramirez-Montealegre and Pearce, 2005), in contrast to system *c*. Further studies are needed to clarify these apparent discrepancies and, if the existence of distinct arginine transporters working in opposite direction is confirmed, the biological significance of the novel import system and how cells avoid the creation of a futile arginine cycle across the lysosomal membrane should be investigated.

6 The Niemann–Pick Type C Disease Protein 1 (NPC1)

Niemann–Pick type C (NPC) (MIM 257220) disease is a rare autosomal recessive disease characterized by hepatosplenomegaly and progressive neurodegeneration leading to death before adulthood (Patterson et al., 2001). Its prevalence is about 1 in 150,000. A biochemical hallmark is the accumulation of exogenously added cholesterol as a free (unesterified) species in the endolysosomal compartment. Staining of intracellular cholesterol with the fluorescent antibiotic filipin in dermal fibroblasts is used for diagnosis. Neuropathological findings include the accumulation of swollen vacuoles in neuronal perikarya, formation of ectopic dendrites and axonal swellings, neurofibrillary tangles, and progressive neuronal loss, particularly in the cerebellum (Walkley and Suzuki, 2004).

6.1 The NPC1 and NPC2 Proteins

Two underlying genes *NPC1* (Carstea et al., 1997) and *NPC2* (Naureckiene et al., 2000) have been identified, with mutations in *NPC1* accounting for 95% of NPC cases. The two genetic subtypes are clinically and biochemically indistinguishable, and the phenotype of a mouse model disrupted in both genes is similar to that of single mutants (Sleat et al., 2004), thus strongly suggesting that the NPC1 and NPC2 proteins act sequentially in a common pathway.

NPC1 primarily resides in late endosomes at steady state but is also transiently associated to lysosomes and the trans-Golgi network (Higgins et al., 1999; Ikonen and Holtta-Vuori, 2004). It possesses 1278 amino acids presumably organized in 13 TMDs, a large N-terminal domain, two large hydrophilic loops protruding in the endosomal lumen and a short, cytosolic C-terminal tail. TMDs 3–7 are homologous to the sterol-sensing domains (SSDs) of key components of cholesterol homeostasis, the sterol-regulatory element binding protein (SREBP) cleavage-activating protein (SCAP) and 3-hydroxy-3-methyl-glutaryl coenzyme A (HMG-CoA) reductase, the rate-limiting enzyme in cholesterol synthesis (Carstea et al., 1997). An SSD is also found in the morphogen receptor Patched. Sterols or sterol-conjugated proteins directly interact with SSDs and trigger a conformational change, which alters the interaction of the membrane protein with its partners (Sever et al., 2003). Whether the SSD domain of NPC1 works in a similar way is unknown, but its does bind cholesterol, as shown by photoaffinity labeling (Ohgami et al., 2004), and its functional importance is highlighted by the fact that most natural mutations affecting this region are associated with a severe clinical phenotype. NPC2 is a small soluble protein (132 amino acids) present in the lysosomal lumen, which binds cholesterol with nanomolar affinity (Ko et al., 2003).

NPC1 and NPC2 are widely expressed in the mammalian brain (Patel et al., 1999; Hu et al., 2000; Ong et al., 2004). They display the same regional distribution, with predominant expression in the cerebral cortex, septum, amygdala, striatum, inferior olivary nucleus, cerebellar cortex, and deep cerebellar nuclei and weaker levels in the thalamus, hypothalamus, subthalamic nucleus, and brainstem. This regional codistribution supports the hypothesis that the two proteins functionally cooperate. However, they are not expressed in the same cell types. Indeed, whereas NPC2 is found in neurons, NPC1 predominates in astrocytes (Patel et al., 1999; Ong et al., 2004). At the ultrastructural level, NPC1 is found in astrocytic processes contacting asymmetrical synapses, near the cell membrane of the soma and in lysosomes. NPC2 immunoreactivity is observed in neuronal cell bodies and dendrites (Ong et al., 2004). An attractive possibility is that they participate in a cooperative process between astrocytes and neurons. Since NPC2 can be secreted by different cell types including astrocytes (Mutka et al., 2004) and recaptured by adjacent cells via the mannose-6-phosphate receptor pathway, it could shuttle between neurons and astrocytes and transfer cholesterol from one cell type to another. Interestingly, an independent line of investigation showed that cholesterol secreted from astrocytes regulates the formation and maintenance of synapses (Mauch et al., 2001; Slezak and Pfrieger, 2003).

6.2 Molecular Function of NPC1

The exact function of NPC1 is unknown. Its weak homology to the resistance–nodulation–division (RND) family of prokaryotic permeases suggested a role in membrane transport (Davies et al., 2000). Since NPC is a cholesterol storage disease, it has been initially proposed that NPC1 catalyzes the efflux of cholesterol from late endosomes. The recent demonstration that NPC1L1, a paralogue of NPC1, plays an essential role in the ezetimibe-sensitive absorption of dietary cholesterol reinforces this hypothesis (Davis et al., 2004).

On the other hand, several lines of evidence argue against this conclusion. First, some data suggest that cholesterol accumulation is not the primary defect in NPC disease. Other lipids, such as sphingomyelin, glucosylceramide, the GM2 and GM3 gangliosides, and lysobisphosphatidic acid accumulate and, in neurons, ganglioside accumulation precedes that of cholesterol (Zervas et al., 2001). Genetic disruption of the ability to synthesize GM2 and GD2 gangliosides in NPC mice prevents cholesterol accumulation (Gondre-Lewis et al., 2003). Moreover, a dominant mutation in the SSD of the yeast orthologue NCR1, which shares 35% identity with human NPC1, alters sphingolipid, but not sterol, distribution in S. cerevisiae—curiously, however, no phenotype was associated with the null mutant (Malathi et al., 2004). NPC1 might thus export gangliosides as well. However, since cholesterol and sphingolipids associate in lipid microdomains ("rafts"), it is difficult to dissect out one process from the other and the proposal that NPC may be a primary sphingolipidosis is still a matter of debate.

A second line of evidence challenging the cholesterol transport hypothesis is that heterologous expression of NPC1 in bacteria resulted in transport of lipophilic dyes and fatty acids, but not cholesterol, across their plasma membranes (Davies et al., 2000). However again, a study of fatty acid distribution and metabolism in NPC1 fibroblasts found no evidence for defective lysosomal and late-endosomal efflux (Passeggio and Liscum, 2005).

In conclusion, the identity of NPC1 substrates remains elusive, and it is still unclear whether its primary function is transmembrane transport, intracellular trafficking, or even signalling. A potential drawback of the transport experiments performed until now is that they may not have addressed the relevant process.

Indeed, as mentioned earlier in this chapter, biophysical studies have shown that fatty acids and cholesterol diffuse very rapidly from one membrane leaflet to another (millisecond timescale). By contrast, their desorption from the membrane to the water phase is much slower, with half-lives in the range of seconds (long-chain fatty acids) and even hours (cholesterol) (Hamilton, 2003). Accordingly, the current emerging view of established cholesterol flippases, such as ABCA1, is that they are not genuine lipid translocators, but rather membrane adaptors able to "project" cholesterol molecules out of the membrane to facilitate their transfer to soluble lipid-binding proteins (Hamilton, 2003; Devaux et al., 2006). Future experiments on the putative transport function of NPC1 should thus concentrate on this desorption process.

Acknowledgments

Our research is supported by the Centre National de la Recherche Scientifique, the Fonds National de la Science (Action Concertée Incitative "Biologie cellulaire, moléculaire, et structurale"), the Institut National de la Santé et de la Recherche Médicale, the charity Vaincre les Maladies Lysosomales, and the Agence Nationale de la Recherche (programme Maladies Rares).

References

Abbot EL, Grenade DS, Kennedy DJ, Gatfield KM, Thwaites DT. 2006. Vigabatrin transport across the human intestinal epithelial (Caco-2) brush-border membrane is via the H⁺-coupled amino-acid transporter hPAT1. Br J Pharmacol 147: 298-306.

Abouhamed M, Gburek J, Liu W, Torchalski B, Wilhelm A, et al., 2006. Divalent metal transporter 1 in the kidney proximal tubule is expressed in late endosomes/lysosomal membranes: Implications for renal handling of protein-metal complexes. Am J Physiol Renal Physiol. 290: F1525-F1533.

Accardi A, Walden M, Nguitragool W, Jayaram H, Williams C, et al. 2005. Separate ion pathways in a Cl⁻/H⁺ exchanger. J Gen Physiol 126: 563-570.

Agulhon C, Rostaing P, Ravassard P, Sagné C, Triller A, et al. 2003. Lysosomal amino acid transporter LYAAT-1 in the rat central nervous system: An in situ hybridization and immunohistochemical study. J Comp Neurol 462: 71-89.

Anderson CM, Grenade DS, Boll M, Foltz M, Wake KA, et al. 2004. H⁺/amino acid transporter 1 (PAT1) is the imino acid carrier: An intestinal nutrient/drug transporter in human and rat. Gastroenterology 127: 1410-1422.

Andersson HC, Kohn LD, Bernardini I, Blom HJ, Tietze F, et al. 1990. Characterization of lysosomal monoiodotyrosine transport in rat thyroid cells. Evidence for transport by system h. J Biol Chem 265: 10950-10954.

Arunachalam B, Phan UT, Geuze HJ, Cresswell P. 2000. Enzymatic reduction of disulfide bonds in lysosomes: Characterization of a γ-interferon-inducible lysosomal thiol reductase (GILT). Proc Natl Acad Sci USA 97: 745-750.

Augustin R, Riley J, Moley KH. 2005. GLUT8 contains a [DE] XXXL[LI] sorting motif and localizes to a late endosomal/lysosomal compartment. Traffic 6: 1196-1212.

Aula N, Jalanko A, Aula P, Peltonen L. 2002. Unraveling the molecular pathogenesis of free sialic acid storage disorders: Altered targeting of mutant sialin. Mol Genet Metab 77: 99-107.

Aula N, Kopra O, Jalanko A, Peltonen L. 2004. Sialin expression in the CNS implicates extralysosomal function in neurons. Neurobiol Dis 15: 251-261.

Aula N, Salomaki P, Timonen R, Verheijen F, Mancini G, et al. 2000. The spectrum of SLC17A5-gene mutations resulting in free sialic acid-storage diseases indicates some genotype–phenotype correlation. Am J Hum Genet 67: 832-840.

Aula P, Gahl WA. 2001. Disorders of free sialic acid storage. The metabolic and molecular bases of inherited disease. Scriver CR, Beaudet AL, Sly WS, Valle D, editors. New York: McGraw-Hill; pp. 5109-5120.

Ausseil J, Landry K, Seyrantepe V, Trudel S, Mazur A, et al. 2006. An acetylated 120-kDa lysosomal transmembrane protein is absent from mucopolysaccharidosis IIIC fibroblasts: A candidate molecule for MPS IIIC. Mol Genet Metab 87: 22-31.

Bach G. 2005. Mucolipin 1: Endocytosis and cation channel–a review. Pflugers Arch 451: 313-317.

Bagshaw RD, Mahuran DJ, Callahan JW. 2005. A proteomic analysis of lysosomal integral membrane proteins reveals the diverse composition of the organelle. Mol Cell Proteomics 4: 133-143.

Baldwin SA, Beal PR, Yao SY, King AE, Cass CE, et al. 2004. The equilibrative nucleoside transporter family, SLC29. Pflugers Arch 447: 735-743.

Baldwin SA, Yao SY, Hyde RJ, Ng AM, Foppolo S, et al. 2005. Functional characterization of novel human and mouse equilibrative nucleoside transporters (hENT3 and mENT3) located in intracellular membranes. J Biol Chem 280: 15880-15887.

Bame KJ, Rome LH. 1985. Acetyl coenzyme A: α-glucosaminide N-acetyltransferase. Evidence for a transmembrane acetylation mechanism. J Biol Chem 260: 11293-11299.

Bame KJ, Rome LH. 1986. Genetic evidence for transmembrane acetylation by lysosomes. Science 233: 1087-1089.

Barrueco JR, O'Leary DF, Sirotnak FM. 1992. Facilitated transport of methotrexate polyglutamates into lysosomes derived from S180 cells. Further characterization and evidence for a simple mobile carrier system with broad specificity for homo- or heteropeptides bearing a C-terminal glutamyl moiety. J Biol Chem 267: 19986-19991.

Barrueco JR, Sirotnak FM. 1991. Evidence for the facilitated transport of methotrexate polyglutamates into lysosomes derived from S180 cells. Basic properties and specificity for polyglutamate chain length. J Biol Chem 266: 11732-11737.

Bermingham JR Jr, Pennington J. 2004. Organization and expression of the SLC36 cluster of amino acid transporter genes. Mamm Genome 15: 114-125.

Bermingham JR Jr, Shumas S, Whisenhunt T, Sirkowski EE, O'Connell S, et al. 2002. Identification of genes that are downregulated in the absence of the POU domain transcription factor pou3f1 (Oct-6, Tst-1, SCIP) in sciatic nerve. J Neurosci 22: 10217-10231.

Bernar J, Tietze F, Kohn LD, Bernardini I, Harper GS, et al. 1986. Characteristics of a lysosomal membrane transport system for tyrosine and other neutral amino acids in rat thyroid cells. J Biol Chem 261: 17107-17112.

Biancheri R, Rossi A, Verbeek HA, Schot R, Corsolini F, et al. 2005. Homozygosity for the p.K136E mutation in the SLC17A5 gene as cause of an Italian severe Salla disease. Neurogenetics 6: 195-199.

Bird SJ, Lloyd JB. 1990. Evidence for a dipeptide porter in the lysosome membrane. Biochim Biophys Acta 1024: 267-270.

Blott EJ, Griffiths GM. 2002. Secretory lysosomes. Nat Rev Mol Cell Biol 3: 122-131.

Boll M, Daniel H, Gasnier B. 2004. The SLC36 family: Proton-coupled transporters for the absorption of selected amino acids from extracellular and intracellular proteolysis. Pflugers Arch 447: 776-779.

Boll M, Foltz M, Anderson CM, Oechsler C, Kottra G, et al. 2003a. Substrate recognition by the mammalian proton-dependent amino acid transporter PAT1. Mol Membr Biol 20: 261-269.

Boll M, Foltz M, Rubio-Aliaga I, Daniel H. 2003b. A cluster of proton/amino acid transporter genes in the human and mouse genomes. Genomics 82: 47-56.

Boll M, Foltz M, Rubio-Aliaga I, Kottra G, Daniel H. 2002. Functional characterization of two novel mammalian electrogenic proton-dependent amino acid cotransporters. J Biol Chem 277: 22966-22973.

Boonen M, Hamer I, Boussac M, Delsaute AF, Flamion B, et al. 2006. Intracellular localization of p40, a protein identified in a preparation of lysosomal membranes. Biochem J 395: 39-47.

Bull PC, Thomas GR, Rommens JM, Forbes JR, Cox DW. 1993. The Wilson disease gene is a putative copper transporting P-type ATPase similar to the Menkes gene. Nat Genet 5: 327-337.

Cao Y, Espinola JA, Fossale E, Massey AC, Cuervo AM, 2006. Autophagy is disrupted in a knock-in mouse model of juvenile neuronal ceroid lipofuscinosis. J Biol Chem.

Carstea ED, Morris JA, Coleman KG, Loftus SK, Zhang D, et al. 1997. Niemann–Pick C1 disease gene: Homology to mediators of cholesterol homeostasis. Science 277: 228-231.

Chattopadhyay S, Roberts PM, Pearce DA. 2003. The yeast model for Batten disease: A role for Btn2p in the trafficking of the Golgi-associated vesicular targeting protein, Yif1p. Biochem Biophys Res Commun 302: 534-538.

Chen Z, Fei YJ, Anderson CM, Wake KA, Miyauchi S, et al. 2003a. Structure, function and immunolocalization of a proton-coupled amino acid transporter (hPAT1) in the human intestinal cell line Caco-2. J Physiol 546: 349-361.

Chen Z, Kennedy DJ, Wake KA, Zhuang L, Ganapathy V, et al. 2003b. Structure, tissue expression pattern, and function of the amino acid transporter rat PAT2. Biochem Biophys Res Commun 304: 747-754.

Cohn ZA, Ehrenreich BA. 1969. The uptake, storage, and intracellular hydrolysis of carbohydrates by macrophages. J Exp Med 129: 201-225.

Collarini EJ, Pisoni RL, Christensen HN. 1989. Characterization of a transport system for anionic amino acids in human fibroblast lysosomes. Biochim Biophys Acta 987: 139-144.

Consortium 1995. Isolation of a novel gene underlying Batten disease, CLN3. The International Batten Disease Consortium. Cell 82: 949–957.

Dani A, Chaudhry A, Mukherjee P, Rajagopal D, Bhatia S, et al. 2004. The pathway for MHCII-mediated presentation of endogenous proteins involves peptide transport to the endo-lysosomal compartment. J Cell Sci 117: 4219-4230.

Davies JP, Chen FW, Ioannou YA. 2000. Transmembrane molecular pump activity of Niemann–Pick C1 protein. Science 290: 2295-2298.

Davis HR Jr., Zhu LJ, Hoos LM, Tetzloff G, Maguire M, et al. 2004. Niemann–Pick C1 Like 1 (NPC1L1) is the intestinal phytosterol and cholesterol transporter and a key modulator of whole-body cholesterol homeostasis. J Biol Chem 279: 33586-33592.

Devaux PF, Lopez-Montero I, Bryde S. 2006. Proteins involved in lipid translocation in eukaryotic cells. Chem Phys Lipids 141: 119-132.

Docherty K, Brenchley GV, Hales CN. 1979. The permeability of rat liver lysosomes to sugars. Evidence for carrier-mediated facilitated diffusion. Biochem J 178: 361-366.

Doege H, Schurmann A, Bahrenberg G, Brauers A, Joost HG. 2000. GLUT8, a novel member of the sugar transport facilitator family with glucose transport activity. J Biol Chem 275: 16275-16280.

Elleder M, Sokolova J, Hrebicek M. 1997. Follow-up study of subunit c of mitochondrial ATP synthase (SCMAS) in Batten disease and in unrelated lysosomal disorders. Acta Neuropathol (Berl) 93: 379-390.

Fleming MD, Trenor CC 3rd, Su MA, Foernzler D, Beier DR, et al. 1997. Microcytic anaemia mice have a mutation in Nramp2, a candidate iron transporter gene. Nat Genet 16: 383-386.

Foltz M, Oechsler C, Boll M, Kottra G, Daniel H. 2004. Substrate specificity and transport mode of the proton-dependent amino acid transporter mPAT2. Eur J Biochem 271: 3340-3347.

Froissart R, Cheillan D, Bouvier R, Tourret S, Bonnet V, et al. 2005. Clinical, morphological and molecular aspects of sialic acid storage disease manifesting in utero. J Med Genet. 42: 829-836.

Gachet Y, Codlin S, Hyams JS, Mole SE. 2005. btn1, the Schizosaccharomyces pombe homologue of the human Batten disease gene CLN3, regulates vacuole homeostasis. J Cell Sci 118: 5525-5536.

Gahl WA, Bashan N, Tietze F, Bernardini I, Schulman JD. 1982. Cystine transport is defective in isolated leukocyte lysosomes from patients with cystinosis. Science 217: 1263-1265.

Gahl WA, Thoene JG, Schneider JA. 2002. Cystinosis. N Engl J Med 347: 111-121.

Goberdhan DC, Meredith D, Boyd CA, Wilson C. 2005. PAT-related amino acid transporters regulate growth via a novel mechanism that does not require bulk transport of amino acids. Development 132: 2365-2375.

Goldman R, Kaplan A. 1973. Rupture of rat liver lysosomes mediated by L-amino acid esters. Biochim Biophys Acta 318: 205-216.

Gondre-Lewis MC, McGlynn R, Walkley SU. 2003. Cholesterol accumulation in NPC1-deficient neurons is ganglioside dependent. Curr Biol 13: 1324-1329.

Gunshin H, Mackenzie B, Berger UV, Gunshin Y, Romero MF, et al. 1997. Cloning and characterization of a mammalian proton-coupled metal-ion transporter. Nature 388: 482-488.

Haataja L, Parkkola R, Sonninen P, Vanhanen SL, Schleutker J, et al. 1994. Phenotypic variation and magnetic resonance imaging (MRI) in Salla disease, a free sialic acid storage disorder. Neuropediatrics 25: 238-244.

Hamilton JA. 2003. Fast flip-flop of cholesterol and fatty acids in membranes: Implications for membrane transport proteins. Curr Opin Lipidol 14: 263-271.

Harada M, Kawaguchi T, Kumemura H, Terada K, Ninomiya H, et al. 2005. The Wilson disease protein ATP7B resides in the late endosomes with Rab7 and the Niemann–Pick C1 protein. Am J Pathol 166: 499-510.

Haskell RE, Carr CJ, Pearce DA, Bennett MJ, Davidson BL. 2000. Batten disease: Evaluation of CLN3 mutations on protein localization and function. Hum Mol Genet 9: 735-744.

Havelaar AC, de Gast IL, Snijders S, Beerens CE, Mancini GM, et al. 1998a. Characterization of a heavy metal ion transporter in the lysosomal membrane. FEBS Lett 436: 223-227.

Havelaar AC, Mancini GM, Beerens CE, Souren RM, Verheijen FW. 1998b. Purification of the lysosomal sialic acid transporter. Functional characteristics of a monocarboxylate transporter. J Biol Chem 273: 34568-34574.

Higgins ME, Davies JP, Chen FW, Ioannou YA. 1999. Niemann–Pick C1 is a late endosome-resident protein that transiently associates with lysosomes and the trans-Golgi network. Mol Genet Metab 68: 1-13.

Hofmann SL, Peltonen L. 2001. The neuronal ceroid lipofuscinoses. The metabolic and molecular bases of inherited disease. Scriver, CR, Beaudet AL, Sly WS, Valle D, editors. New York: McGraw-Hill; pp. 3877-3894.

Holopainen JM, Saarikoski J, Kinnunen PK, Jarvela I. 2001. Elevated lysosomal pH in neuronal ceroid lipofuscinoses (NCLs). Eur J Biochem 268: 5851-5856.

Hu CY, Ong WY, Patel SC. 2000. Regional distribution of NPC1 protein in monkey brain. J Neurocytol 29: 765-773.

Ibberson M, Uldry M, Thorens B. 2000. GLUTX1, a novel mammalian glucose transporter expressed in the central nervous system and insulin-sensitive tissues. J Biol Chem 275: 4607-4612.

Idriss JM, Jonas AJ. 1991. Vitamin B_{12} transport by rat liver lysosomal membrane vesicles. J Biol Chem 266: 9438-9441.

Ikonen E, Holtta-Vuori M. 2004. Cellular pathology of Niemann–Pick type C disease. Semin Cell Dev Biol 15: 445-454.

Iveson GP, Bird SJ, Lloyd JB. 1989. Passive diffusion of non-electrolytes across the lysosome membrane. Biochem J 261: 451-456.

Jarvela I, Lehtovirta M, Tikkanen R, Kyttala A, Jalanko A. 1999. Defective intracellular transport of CLN3 is the molecular basis of Batten disease (JNCL). Hum Mol Genet 8: 1091-1098.

Jarvela I, Sainio M, Rantamaki T, Olkkonen VM, Carpen O, et al. 1998. Biosynthesis and intracellular targeting of the CLN3 protein defective in Batten disease. Hum Mol Genet 7: 85-90.

Jentsch TJ, Neagoe I, Scheel O. 2005a. CLC chloride channels and transporters. Curr Opin Neurobiol 15: 319-325.

Jentsch TJ, Poet M, Fuhrmann JC, Zdebik AA. 2005b. Physiological functions of CLC Cl^{-1} channels gleaned from human genetic disease and mouse models. Annu Rev Physiol 67: 779-807.

Jonas AJ, Jobe H. 1990. Sulfate transport by rat liver lysosomes. J Biol Chem 265: 17545-17549.

Jonas AJ, Conrad P, Jobe H. 1990. Neutral-sugar transport by rat liver lysosomes. Biochem J 272: 323-326.

Jonas AJ, Smith ML, Schneider JA. 1982. ATP-dependent lysosomal cystine efflux is defective in cystinosis. J Biol Chem 257: 13185-13188.

Jonas AJ, Speller RJ, Conrad PB, Dubinsky WP. 1989. Transport of N-acetyl-D-glucosamine and N-acetyl-D-galactosamine by rat liver lysosomes. J Biol Chem 264: 4953-4956.

Kalatzis V, Antignac C. 2003. New aspects of the pathogenesis of cystinosis. Pediatr Nephrol 18: 207-215.

Kalatzis V, Cherqui S, Antignac C, Gasnier B. 2001. Cystinosin, the protein defective in cystinosis, is a H$^+$-driven lysosomal cystine transporter. EMBO J 20: 5940-5949.

Kalatzis V, Nevo N, Cherqui S, Gasnier B, Antignac C. 2004. Molecular pathogenesis of cystinosis: Effect of CTNS mutations on the transport activity and subcellular localization of cystinosin. Hum Mol Genet 13: 1361-1371.

Kanner BI. 1994. Sodium-coupled neurotransmitter transport: Structure, function and regulation. J Exp Biol 196: 237-249.

Kida E, Kaczmarski W, Golabek AA, Kaczmarski A, Michalewski M, et al. 1999. Analysis of intracellular distribution and trafficking of the CLN3 protein in fusion with the green fluorescent protein in vitro. Mol Genet Metab 66: 265-271.

Kim Y, Ramirez-Montealegre D, Pearce DA. 2003. A role in vacuolar arginine transport for yeast Btn1p and for human CLN3, the protein defective in Batten disease. Proc Natl Acad Sci USA 100: 15458-15462.

Klein U, Kresse H, von Figura K. 1978. Sanfilippo syndrome type C: Deficiency of acetyl-CoA: α-glucosaminide N-acetyltransferase in skin fibroblasts. Proc Natl Acad Sci USA 75: 5185-5189.

Ko DC, Binkley J, Sidow A, Scott MP. 2003. The integrity of a cholesterol-binding pocket in Niemann–Pick C2 protein is necessary to control lysosome cholesterol levels. Proc Natl Acad Sci USA 100: 2518-2525.

Ko DC, Milenkovic L, Beier SM, Manuel H, Buchanan J, et al. 2005. Cell-autonomous death of cerebellar Purkinje neurons with autophagy in Niemann–Pick type C disease. PLoS Genet 1: 81-95.

Kobayashi A, Maeda T, Maeda M. 2004. Membrane localization of transporter associated with antigen processing (TAP)-like (ABCB9) visualized in vivo with a fluorescence protein-fusion technique. Biol Pharm Bull 27: 1916-1922.

Koch J, Tampé R. 2006. The macromolecular peptide-loading complex in MHC class I-dependent antigen presentation. Cell Mol Life Sci 63: 653-662.

Koike M, Nakanishi H, Saftig P, Ezaki J, Isahara K, et al. 2000. Cathepsin D deficiency induces lysosomal storage with ceroid lipofuscin in mouse CNS neurons. J Neurosci 20: 6898-6906.

Koike M, Shibata M, Waguri S, Yoshimura K, Tanida I, et al. 2005. Participation of autophagy in storage of lysosomes in neurons from mouse models of neuronal ceroid-lipofuscinoses (Batten disease). Am J Pathol 167: 1713-1728.

Kozyraki R, Fyfe J, Verroust PJ, Jacobsen C, Dautry-Varsat A, et al. 2001. Megalin-dependent cubilin-mediated endocytosis is a major pathway for the apical uptake of transferrin in polarized epithelia. Proc Natl Acad Sci USA 98: 12491-12496.

Kyttala A, Ihrke G, Vesa J, Schell MJ, Luzio JP. 2004. Two motifs target Batten disease protein CLN3 to lysosomes in transfected nonneuronal and neuronal cells. Mol Biol Cell 15: 1313-1323.

Kyttala A, Yliannala K, Schu P, Jalanko A, Luzio JP. 2005. AP-1 and AP-3 facilitate lysosomal targeting of Batten disease protein CLN3 via its dileucine motif. J Biol Chem 280: 10277-10283.

Lam-Yuk-Tseung S, Gros P. 2006. Distinct targeting and recycling properties of two isoforms of the iron transporter DMT1 (NRAMP2, Slc11A2). Biochemistry 45: 2294-2301.

Lemons RM, Thoene JG. 1991. Mediated calcium transport by isolated human fibroblast lysosomes. J Biol Chem 266: 14378-14382.

Lloyd JB. 1969. Studies on the permeability of rat liver lysosomes to carbohydrates. Biochem J 115: 703-707.

Lloyd JB. 1986. Disulphide reduction in lysosomes. The role of cysteine. Biochem J 237: 271-272.

Luiro K, Kopra O, Lehtovirta M, Jalanko A. 2001. CLN3 protein is targeted to neuronal synapses but excluded from synaptic vesicles: New clues to Batten disease. Hum Mol Genet 10: 2123-2131.

Luiro K, Yliannala K, Ahtiainen L, Maunu H, Jarvela I, et al. 2004. Interconnections of CLN3, Hook1 and Rab proteins link Batten disease to defects in the endocytic pathway. Hum Mol Genet 13: 3017-3027.

Mackenzie B, Hediger MA. 2004. SLC11 family of H$^+$-coupled metal-ion transporters NRAMP1 and DMT1. Pflugers Arch 447: 571-579.

Majeski AE, Dice JF. 2004. Mechanisms of chaperone-mediated autophagy. Int J Biochem Cell Biol 36: 2435-2444.

Malathi K, Higaki K, Tinkelenberg AH, Balderes DA, Almanzar-Paramio D, et al. 2004. Mutagenesis of the putative sterol-sensing domain of yeast Niemann–Pick C-related protein reveals a primordial role in subcellular sphingolipid distribution. J Cell Biol 164: 547-556.

Mancini GM, Beerens CE, Aula PP, Verheijen FW. 1991. Sialic acid storage diseases. A multiple lysosomal transport defect for acidic monosaccharides. J Clin Invest 87: 1329-1335.

Mancini GM, Beerens CE, Verheijen FW. 1990. Glucose transport in lysosomal membrane vesicles. Kinetic demonstration of a carrier for neutral hexoses. J Biol Chem 265: 12380-12387.

Mancini GM, de Jonge HR, Galjaard H, Verheijen FW. 1989. Characterization of a proton-driven carrier for sialic acid in the lysosomal membrane. Evidence for a group-specific transport system for acidic monosaccharides. J Biol Chem 264: 15247-15254.

Maric M, Arunachalam B, Phan UT, Dong C, Garrett WS, et al. 2001. Defective antigen processing in GILT-free mice. Science 294: 1361-1365.

Mauch DH, Nagler K, Schumacher S, Goritz C, Muller EC, et al. 2001. CNS synaptogenesis promoted by glia-derived cholesterol. Science 294: 1354-1357.

McIntire SL, Reimer RJ, Schuske K, Edwards RH, Jorgensen EM. 1997. Identification and characterization of the vesicular GABA transporter. Nature 389: 870-876.

Metzner L, Kottra G, Neubert K, Daniel H, Brandsch M. 2005. Serotonin, L-tryptophan, and tryptamine are effective inhibitors of the amino acid transport system PAT1. FASEB J 19: 1468-1473.

Miller C. 2006. ClC chloride channels viewed through a transporter lens. Nature 440: 484-489.

Mole SE, Williams RE, Goebel HH. 2005. Correlations between genotype, ultrastructural morphology and clinical phenotype in the neuronal ceroid lipofuscinoses. Neurogenetics 6: 107-126.

Morin P, Sagné C, Gasnier B. 2004. Functional characterization of wild-type and mutant human sialin. EMBO J 23: 4560-4570.

Munroe PB, Mitchison HM, O'Rawe AM, Anderson JW, Boustany RM, et al. 1997. Spectrum of mutations in the Batten disease gene, CLN3. Am J Hum Genet 61: 310-316.

Mutka AL, Lusa S, Linder MD, Jokitalo E, Kopra O, et al. 2004. Secretion of sterols and the NPC2 protein from primary astrocytes. J Biol Chem 279: 48654-48662.

Myllykangas L, Tyynela J, Page-McCaw A, Rubin GM, Haltia MJ, et al. 2005. Cathepsin D-deficient Drosophila recapitulate the key features of neuronal ceroid lipofuscinoses. Neurobiol Dis 19: 194-199.

Naureckiene S, Sleat DE, Lackland H, Fensom A, Vanier MT, et al. 2000. Identification of HE1 as the second gene of Niemann–Pick C disease. Science 290: 2298-2301.

Nishi T, Forgac M. 2002. The vacuolar H^+-ATPases–nature's most versatile proton pumps. Nat Rev Mol Cell Biol 3: 94-103.

Ohgami N, Ko DC, Thomas M, Scott MP, Chang CC, et al. 2004. Binding between the Niemann–Pick C1 protein and a photoactivatable cholesterol analog requires a functional sterol-sensing domain. Proc Natl Acad Sci USA 101: 12473-12478.

Ong WY, Sundaram RK, Huang E, Ghoshal S, Kumar U, et al. 2004. Neuronal localization and association of Niemann–Pick C2 protein (HE1/NPC2) with the postsynaptic density. Neuroscience 128: 561-570.

Palmer DN, Fearnley IM, Walker JE, Hall NA, Lake BD, et al. 1992. Mitochondrial ATP synthase subunit c storage in the ceroid-lipofuscinoses (Batten disease). Am J Med Genet 42: 561-567.

Parazzini C, Arena S, Marchetti L, Menni F, Filocamo M, et al. 2003. Infantile sialic acid storage disease: Serial ultrasound and magnetic resonance imaging features. AJNR Am J Neuroradiol 24: 398-400.

Passeggio J, Liscum L. 2005. Flux of fatty acids through NPC1 lysosomes. J Biol Chem 280: 10333-10339.

Patel SC, Suresh S, Kumar U, Hu CY, Cooney A, et al. 1999. Localization of Niemann–Pick C1 protein in astrocytes: Implications for neuronal degeneration in Niemann–Pick type C disease. Proc Natl Acad Sci USA 96: 1657-1662.

Patterson MC, Vanier MT, Suzuki K, Morris JA, Carstea ED, et al. 2001. Niemann–Pick disease C: A lipid trafficking disorder. The Metabolic and Molecular Bases of Inherited Disease. Scriver CR, Beaudet AL, Sly WS, Valle D, editors. New York: McGraw-Hill; pp. 2625-2639.

Pearce DA, Sherman F. 1998. A yeast model for the study of Batten disease. Proc Natl Acad Sci USA 95: 6915-6918.

Pearce DA, Carr CJ, Das B, Sherman F. 1999a. Phenotypic reversal of the btn1 defects in yeast by chloroquine: A yeast model for Batten disease. Proc Natl Acad Sci USA 96: 11341-11345.

Pearce DA, Ferea T, Nosel SA, Das B, Sherman F. 1999b. Action of BTN1, the yeast orthologue of the gene mutated in Batten disease. Nat Genet 22: 55-58.

Persaud-Sawin DA, Van Dongen A, Boustany RM. 2002. Motifs within the CLN3 protein: Modulation of cell growth rates and apoptosis. Hum Mol Genet 11: 2129-2142.

Phillips SN, Benedict JW, Weimer JM, Pearce DA. 2005. CLN3, the protein associated with batten disease: Structure, function and localization. J Neurosci Res 79: 573-583.

Pisoni RL. 1991. Characterization of a phosphate transport system in human fibroblast lysosomes. J Biol Chem 266: 979-985.

Pisoni RL, Thoene JG. 1989. Detection and characterization of a nucleoside transport system in human fibroblast lysosomes. J Biol Chem 264: 4850-4856.

Pisoni RL, Acker TL, Lisowski KM, Lemons RM, Thoene JG. 1990. A cysteine-specific lysosomal transport system provides a major route for the delivery of thiol to human fibroblast lysosomes: Possible role in supporting lysosomal proteolysis. J Cell Biol 110: 327-335.

Pisoni RL, Flickinger KS, Thoene JG, Christensen HN. 1987a. Characterization of carrier-mediated transport systems for small neutral amino acids in human fibroblast lysosomes. J Biol Chem 262: 6010-6017.

Pisoni RL, Thoene JG, Lemons RM, Christensen HN. 1987b. Important differences in cationic amino acid transport by lysosomal system c and system y+ of the human fibroblast. J Biol Chem 262: 15011-15018.

Pisoni RL, Thoene JG, Christensen HN. 1985. Detection and characterization of carrier-mediated cationic amino acid transport in lysosomes of normal and cystinotic human fibroblasts. Role in therapeutic cystine removal? J Biol Chem 260: 4791-4798.

Puranam KL, Guo WX, Qian WH, Nikbakht K, Boustany RM. 1999. CLN3 defines a novel antiapoptotic pathway operative in neurodegeneration and mediated by ceramide. Mol Genet Metab 66: 294-308.

Ramirez-Montealegre D, Pearce DA. 2005. Defective lysosomal arginine transport in juvenile Batten disease. Hum Mol Genet 14: 3759-3773.

Reeves JP. 1979. Accumulation of amino acids by lysosomes incubated with amino acid methyl esters. J Biol Chem 254: 8914-8921.

Reimer RJ, Edwards RH. 2004. Organic anion transport is the primary function of the SLC17/type I phosphate transporter family. Pflugers Arch 447: 629-635.

Renlund M, Tietze F, Gahl WA. 1986. Defective sialic acid egress from isolated fibroblast lysosomes of patients with Salla disease. Science 232: 759-762.

Rosenblatt DS, Hosack A, Matiaszuk NV, Cooper BA, Laframboise R. 1985. Defect in vitamin B_{12} release from lysosomes: Newly described inborn error of vitamin B_{12} metabolism. Science 228: 1319-1321.

Rubio-Aliaga I, Boll M, Vogt Weisenhorn DM, Foltz M, Kottra G, et al. 2004. The proton/amino acid cotransporter PAT2 is expressed in neurons with a different subcellular localization than its paralog PAT1. J Biol Chem 279: 2754-2760.

Sagné C, Agulhon C, Ravassard P, Darmon M, Hamon M, et al. 2001. Identification and characterization of a lysosomal transporter for small neutral amino acids. Proc Natl Acad Sci USA 98: 7206-7211.

Sagné C, El Mestikawy S, Isambert MF, Hamon M, Henry JP, et al. 1997. Cloning of a functional vesicular GABA and glycine transporter by screening of genome databases. FEBS Lett 417: 177-183.

Saint-Pol A, Bauvy C, Codogno P, Moore SE. 1997. Transfer of free polymannose-type oligosaccharides from the cytosol to lysosomes in cultured human hepatocellular carcinoma HepG2 cells. J Cell Biol 136: 45-59.

Saint-Pol A, Codogno P, Moore SE. 1999. Cytosol-to-lysosome transport of free polymannose-type oligosaccharides. Kinetic and specificity studies using rat liver lysosomes. J Biol Chem 274: 13547-13555.

Sakata K, Yamashita T, Maeda M, Moriyama Y, Shimada S, et al. 2001. Cloning of a lymphatic peptide/histidine transporter. Biochem J 356: 53-60.

Schmitz G, Kaminski WE. 2002. ABCA2: A candidate regulator of neural transmembrane lipid transport. Cell Mol Life Sci 59: 1285-1295.

Sever N, Yang T, Brown MS, Goldstein JL, DeBose-Boyd RA. 2003. Accelerated degradation of HMG CoA reductase mediated by binding of insig-1 to its sterol-sensing domain. Mol Cell 11: 25-33.

Siintola E, Partanen S, Stromme P, Haapanen A, Haltia M, et al. 2006. Cathepsin D deficiency underlies congenital human neuronal ceroid-lipofuscinosis. Brain 129: 1438-1445.

Sleat DE, Wiseman JA, El-Banna M, Price SM, Verot L, et al. 2004. Genetic evidence for nonredundant functional cooperativity between NPC1 and NPC2 in lipid transport. Proc Natl Acad Sci USA 101: 5886-5891.

Slezak M, Pfrieger FW. 2003. New roles for astrocytes: Regulation of CNS synaptogenesis. Trends Neurosci 26: 531-535.

Sonninen P, Autti T, Varho T, Hamalainen M, Raininko R. 1999. Brain involvement in Salla disease. AJNR Am J Neuroradiol 20: 433-443.

Soyombo AA, Tjon-Kon-Sang S, Rbaibi Y, Bashllari E, Bisceglia J, et al. 2006. TRP-ML1 regulates lysosomal pH and acidic lysosomal lipid hydrolytic activity. J Biol Chem 281: 7294-7301.

Steinfeld R, Reinhardt K, Schreiber K, Hillebrand M, Kraetzner R, et al. 2006. Cathepsin-D deficiency is associated with a human neurodegenerative disorder. Am J Hum Genet 78: 988-998.

Stewart BH, Collarini EJ, Pisoni RL, Christensen HN. 1989. Separate and shared lysosomal transport of branched and aromatic dipolar amino acids. Biochim Biophys Acta 987: 145-153.

Storch S, Pohl S, Braulke T. 2004. A dileucine motif and a cluster of acidic amino acids in the second cytoplasmic domain of the Batten disease-related CLN3 protein are required for efficient lysosomal targeting. J Biol Chem 279: 53625-53634.

Sun-Wada GH, Wada Y, Futai M. 2004. Diverse and essential roles of mammalian vacuolar-type proton pump ATPase: Toward the physiological understanding of inside acidic compartments. Biochim Biophys Acta 1658: 106-114.

Tabuchi M, Tanaka N, Nishida-Kitayama J, Ohno H, Kishi F. 2002. Alternative splicing regulates the subcellular localization of divalent metal transporter 1 isoforms. Mol Biol Cell 13: 4371-4387.

Tanaka Y, Guhde G, Suter A, Eskelinen EL, Hartmann D, et al. 2000. Accumulation of autophagic vacuoles and cardiomyopathy in LAMP-2-deficient mice. Nature 406: 902-906.

Tanzi RE, Petrukhin K, Chernov I, Pellequer JL, Wasco W, et al. 1993. The Wilson disease gene is a copper transporting ATPase with homology to the Menkes disease gene. Nat Genet 5: 344-350.

Thamotharan M, Lombardo YB, Bawani SZ, Adibi SA. 1997. An active mechanism for completion of the final stage of protein degradation in the liver, lysosomal transport of dipeptides. J Biol Chem 272: 11786-11790.

Thoene JG, Oshima RG, Crawhall JC, Olson DL, Schneider JA. 1976. Cystinosis. Intracellular cystine depletion by aminothiols in vitro and in vivo. J Clin Invest 58: 180-189.

Thwaites DT, Armstrong G, Hirst BH, Simmons NL. 1995. D-cycloserine transport in human intestinal epithelial (Caco-2) cells: Mediation by a H^+-coupled amino acid transporter. Br J Pharmacol 115: 761-766.

Thwaites DT, Basterfield L, McCleave PM, Carter SM, Simmons NL. 2000. γ-Aminobutyric acid (GABA) transport across human intestinal epithelial (Caco-2) cell monolayers. Br J Pharmacol 129: 457-464.

Thwaites DT, McEwan GT, Cook MJ, Hirst BH, Simmons NL. 1993. H^+-coupled (Na^+-independent) proline transport in human intestinal (Caco-2) epithelial cell monolayers. FEBS Lett 333: 78-82.

Tietze F, Seppala R, Renlund M, Hopwood JJ, Harper GS, et al. 1989. Defective lysosomal egress of free sialic acid (N-acetylneuraminic acid) in fibroblasts of patients with infantile free sialic acid storage disease. J Biol Chem 264: 15316-15322.

Town M, Jean G, Cherqui S, Attard M, Forestier L, et al. 1998. A novel gene encoding an integral membrane protein is mutated in nephropathic cystinosis. Nat Genet 18: 319-324.

Tyynela J, Sohar I, Sleat DE, Gin RM, Donnelly RJ, et al. 2000. A mutation in the ovine cathepsin D gene causes a congenital lysosomal storage disease with profound neurodegeneration. EMBO J 19: 2786-2792.

Van Belle D, Andre B. 2001. A genomic view of yeast membrane transporters. Curr Opin Cell Biol 13: 389-398.

Varho T, Jaaskelainen S, Tolonen U, Sonninen P, Vainionpaa L, et al. 2000. Central and peripheral nervous system dysfunction in the clinical variation of Salla disease. Neurology 55: 99-104.

Verheijen FW, Verbeek E, Aula N, Beerens CE, Havelaar AC, et al. 1999. A new gene, encoding an anion transporter, is mutated in sialic acid storage diseases. Nat Genet 23: 462-465.

Walkley SU, Suzuki K. 2004. Consequences of NPC1 and NPC2 loss of function in mammalian neurons. Biochim Biophys Acta 1685: 48-62.

Wipf D, Ludewig U, Tegeder M, Rentsch D, Koch W, et al. 2002. Conservation of amino acid transporters in fungi, plants and animals. Trends Biochem Sci 27: 139-147.

Wolters JC, Abele R, Tampé R. 2005. Selective and ATP-dependent translocation of peptides by the homodimeric ATP binding cassette transporter TAP-like (ABCB9). J Biol Chem 280: 23631-23636.

Wreden CC, Johnson J, Tran C, Seal RP, Copenhagen DR, et al. 2003. The H^+-coupled electrogenic lysosomal amino acid transporter LYAAT1 localizes to the axon and plasma membrane of hippocampal neurons. J Neurosci 23: 1265-1275.

Wreden CC, Wlizla M, Reimer RJ. 2005. Varied mechanisms underlie the free sialic acid storage disorders. J Biol Chem 280: 1408-1416.

Yamaguchi Y, Kasano M, Terada T, Sato R, Maeda M. 1999. An ABC transporter homologous to TAP proteins. FEBS Lett 457: 231-236.

Yarovaya N, Schot R, Fodero L, McMahon M, Mahoney A, et al. 2005. Sialin, an anion transporter defective in sialic acid storage diseases, shows highly variable expression in adult mouse brain, and is developmentally regulated. Neurobiol Dis 19: 351-365.

Young G, Jack D, Smith D, Saier MJ. 1999. The amino acid/auxin:proton symport permease family. Biochim Biophys Acta 1415: 306-322.

Zervas M, Somers KL, Thrall MA, Walkley SU. 2001. Critical role for glycosphingolipids in Niemann–Pick disease type C. Curr Biol 11: 1283-1287.

Zhang F, Zhang W, Liu L, Fisher CL, Hui D, et al. 2000. Characterization of ABCB9, an ATP binding cassette protein associated with lysosomes. J Biol Chem 275: 23287-23294.

Zhou C, Zhao L, Inagaki N, Guan J, Nakajo S, et al. 2001. ATP-binding cassette transporter ABC2/ABCA2 in the rat brain: A novel mammalian lysosome-associated membrane protein and a specific marker for oligodendrocytes but not for myelin sheaths. J Neurosci 21: 849-857.

23 Efflux Transporters in the Brain

H. Potschka · W. Löscher

Abstract: Efflux transporters in the brain can limit brain penetration as well as the intra- and extracellular distribution of a variety of endogenous and exogenous compounds. Thereby, efflux transporters critically contribute to homeostasis of endogenous substrates, but also protect the brain tissue from potentially harmful xenobiotics. During the last decade, the role of efflux transporters in the treatment of central nervous system (CNS) diseases has been recognized. Effective extrusion from the brain by transporters is a frequent cause for the pharmaceutical industry to exclude novel compounds from further development of CNS therapeutics. Moreover, high transporter expression levels that are present in individual patients, or may be generally associated with the pathophysiology, seem to be a major cause of therapeutic failure in a variety of CNS diseases including brain tumors, epilepsy, brain HIV infection, and psychiatric disorders. On the basis of the impact of brain efflux transporters on pathophysiology and therapy of CNS diseases, knowledge about the structure, function, distribution, and regulation of expression of efflux transporters in the brain is of critical interest.

List of Abbreviaitons: ABC, ATP-binding cassette; BBB, blood–brain barrier; BCSFB, blood–cerebrospinal fluid barrier; CNS, central nervous system; HPA, hypothalamic–pituitary–adrenal gland axis; LTC4, Leukotriene C4; MRPs, multidrug resistance proteins; MVP, major vault protein; OAT-family, organic anion transporter-family; OATP-family, organic anion transporting–polypeptide family; PXR, pregnane X receptor; Pgp, P-glycoprotein; SNP, Single nucleotide polymorphisms; SXR, steroid and xenobiotic receptor; TNF, tumor necrosis factor

1   Introduction

The selective permeability of cell membranes is a critical presupposition to maintain a chemical composition in the cytoplasm, which is different from the external environment. In addition, the limited membrane permeability of cells that are constituents of blood–tissue barriers critically contributes to a protection of tissues from putatively harmful xenobiotics.

Membrane-bound proteins determine these selective permeability properties, which are a critical aspect of life. It has been estimated that around 10% of all genes encode proteins that have a role in membrane permeability (Higgins and Linton, 2003). These genes encode ion channels that promote the passive movement across membranes down its electrochemical gradient. However, the shift of molecules against a concentration gradient requires energy-dependent active transport. ATP-binding cassette (ABC) transporters form the largest and most physiologically diverse of these active transport families (Higgins and Linton, 2003).

Efflux transporters in the brain and especially at the blood–brain barrier (BBB) and blood–cerebrospinal fluid barrier (BCSFB) protect the central nervous system (CNS) tissue against changes in the environment by restricting penetration into and facilitating extrusion from brain tissue (Leslie et al., 2005). Because the transporter molecules do no distinguish between harmful xenobiotics and xenobiotics, which are used as drugs to treat CNS diseases, the brain efflux transporters can also mediate undesirable effects in limiting brain access of drugs that are administered to act in the CNS (Löscher and Potschka, 2005a). Actually, several brain efflux transporters like P-glycoprotein (Pgp, ABCB1) have been linked to limited brain penetrations of CNS-active drugs, which restricts drug effectiveness or may even result in mere drug resistance.

On the basis of physiological function and also the contribution to therapeutic failure in different CNS diseases, the structure and function of brain efflux transporters are of particular interest.

2   Efflux Transporters in the Blood–Brain Barrier

The BBB is a physical and metabolic barrier that controls the passage of compounds from the blood to the CNS. A monolayer of brain capillary endothelial cells is a major component of the BBB. The restriction of brain uptake arises by the presence of tight junctions (zonula occludens) between adjacent endothelial cells, and the relative paucity of fenestrae and pinocytotic vesicles. A basal membrane, pericytes, and astrocyte foot processes surround the brain capillary endothelial cells. Due to the BBB, circulating compounds can gain access to the brain only via lipid-mediated transport of small nonpolar molecules through the BBB by free (passive) diffusion or by catalyzed transport (Pardridge, 1999). Numerous membrane transporters are present in brain capillary endothelial cells that are involved in the influx or efflux of various essential substrates including electrolytes, nucleosides, amino acids, and glucose (Lee et al., 2001). More than a decade ago, Pgp was the first drug efflux transporter to be identified in the BBB (Cordon-Cardo et al., 1989; Thiebaut et al., 1989). Data accumulated since then indicate a critical role of different BBB efflux transporters in limiting the brain uptake of a variety of therapeutic agents (Löscher and Potschka, 2005a).

The most important efflux transporters that were so far identified at the blood–brain barrier belong to the class of ABC transporters (❯ *Figure 23-1*). ABC transporters characteristically comprise two transmembrane domains and two nucleotide-binding domains (Higgins and Linton, 2003). The domains may also be

❏ Figure 23-1

Different localizations of BBB transporters that are in an appropriate position to enhance efflux from the brain. (A) Transporters in the apical membrane of brain capillary endothelial cells can directly shuttle drugs into the capillary lumen. Efflux transporters described in this localization include Pgp, MPR1, MRP2, MRP4, MRP5, and BCRP. Rodent Oatp2 and Oatp3 have also been identified in the apical membrane of endothelial cells. On the basis of available data, it is highly likely that these Oatps are capable of bidirectional transport. (B) Transporters that mediate intracellular uptake in the basolateral membrane may act in concert with efflux transporters at the apical membrane, thereby enhancing extrusion of their substrates from the brain. Transporters described in this localization include OAT3 and rodent Oatp2. Again Oatp2 is likely to mediate bidirectional transport. (C) Transporters in astrocytic endfeet may shuttle drugs in the direction of capillary endothelial cells and may act in concert with efflux transporter systems of the endothelial cells, thereby promoting extrusion from the brain. Transporters described in this localization include Pgp, MRP1, MRP3, MRP4, and MRP5. It needs to be emphasized that the localizations of some of these transporters have not been verified in an unquestionable manner. In some cases, data are based on ex vivo or in vitro preparations with which transporter expression rates may change in a considerable manner as compared to the in vivo situation. Furthermore, the localization of a specific transporter may differ between species. Thus, this figure and the list of transporters must be considered as a simplified scheme of the current view of BBB efflux transporter distribution

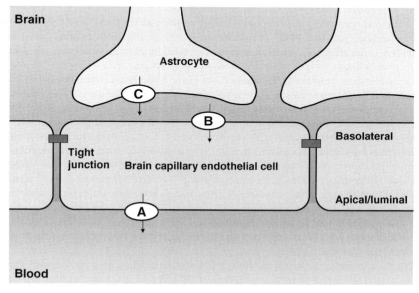

encoded by two separate polypeptides. The transmembrane domains generally determine the substrate specificity (Higgins and Linton, 2003). For several ABC transporters, for example Pgp, there is more than one substrate-binding site per transporter, allowing for a broad substrate spectrum. The nucleotide-binding domains consist of a core of about 215 amino acids, the conserved ABC domain by which these transporters are defined (Higgins et al., 1986). This core domain includes the Walker A and B and so called "ABC signature" motifs. Transport by ABC transporters involves major conformational changes (Martin et al., 2001). The transport cycle is initiated by the interaction of a substrate with specific binding sites. Substrate binding then induces a conformation change, which is transmitted to the nucleotide binding domains to initiate ATP binding. ATP binding seems to induce the major conformational change, which is associated with alterations in affinity and orientation of the substrate binding sites such that the substrate is released at the extracellular face of the membrane (Martin et al., 2001). Subsequently, hydrolysis of ATP resets the transporter for the next cycle (Senior et al., 1995).

Based on structural features of the encoded transporters, ABC genes are divided into a number of families (*ABCA, ABCB, ABCC, ABCD, ABCE, ABCF,* and *ABCG*). Due to the fact that the old nomenclature is used in the majority of the publications cited in this review, this will be used throughout the chapter. The new nomenclature is given at least once with the first mention of the respective transporter.

Efflux transporters discussed in this chapter include members of the ABCB, ABCC, and ABCG family: Pgp (ABCB1), members of the multidrug-resistance associated protein family (MRP/ABCC family), and breast cancer-related protein (BCRP/ABCG2).

2.1 P-Glycoprotein

Discovered in the late 1970s as a prototypic transporter involved in multidrug resistance of cancer cells (Juliano and Ling, 1976), Pgp (ABCB1) was also the first ABC transporter that was detected in endothelial cells of the human BBB in 1989 (Cordon-Cardo et al., 1989; Thiebaut et al., 1989). Pgp is a "full" transporter that comprises two transmembrane domains and two attached nucleotide-binding domains in one molecule. In humans, there are two types of Pgp: type I encoded by the *MDR1* gene, which confers the drug resistance phenotype and mediates BBB efflux, and type II encoded by the *MDR2* gene present in the canalicular membrane of hepatocytes and functioning as a phosphatidylcholine translocase (Demeule et al., 2002). In rodents, the multidrug resistance type I transporter protein is encoded by two genes, *mdr1a* and *mdr1b*. Distribution of the Pgp isoform encoded by *mdr1a* and *mdr1b* in rodents as well as their functional features suggest that *mdr1a* and *mdr1b* together perform the same set of functions in rodents as MDR1 Pgp in humans (Schinkel, 1999). In rodents, the *mdr1a* encoded isoform proved to be predominant in brain capillary endothelial cells, whereas *mdr1b* is expressed in brain parenchymal cells (Demeule et al., 2002; Regina et al., 1998).

With its predominant presence in the luminal site of the BBB endothelium, Pgp is in the appropriate localization as a BBB efflux transporter (Cordon-Cardo et al., 1989) (❷ *Figure 23-1*), a function that has been intensely studied and repeatedly substantiated. Identification of Pgp in brain capillary endothelial cells of several species including humans and other primates, rodents, cattle, and pigs suggested that Pgp may serve as a general defense mechanism in the mammalian BBB, which limits the penetration of harmful lipophilic compounds into the CNS (Schinkel, 1999). At the subcellular level, the majority of available data point to a principal expression of Pgp at the luminal (apical) membrane of brain capillary endothelial cells. In this localization Pgp may readily shuttle drugs, which just entered the endothelial cell membrane, back into the blood (Demeule et al., 2002). In addition, active transport by Pgp at the apical membrane decreases intracellular endothelial drug concentrations and thus increases the concentration gradient between endothelial cell cytoplasm and brain extracellular space. As a consequence, extrusion of the drug from the brain extracellular space will be enhanced, and the drug can then be shuttled into the blood by Pgp in the apical membrane (Pardridge, 2003).

Regarding the localization of Pgp at the BBB, controversial data have been published by Pardridge et al. (1997), who suggested a predominant localization of BBB Pgp in astrocytic endfeet, which are closely attached to brain capillary endothelial cells. The data let Pardridge and colleagues conclude a revised model of Pgp function in multidrug resistance. These conclusions have been criticized based on the fact that only one antibody was used in the study (Schinkel et al., 1999; Abbott et al., 2002). It needs to be considered that epitopes can be shielded in specific cell types, and that preparation and fixation procedures have a major impact on immunohistological detection of membrane proteins such as Pgp (O'Brien and Cordon-Cardo, 1996; Schinkel, 1999; Volk et al., 2005). Based on these methodological issues, immunolocalizations of membrane transporters can only be considered reliable when consistent results are obtained with at least two, but preferably three or more, different antibodies (Schinkel, 1999; Scheffer and Scheper, 2002). In a recent study, using another antibody and fixation procedure, Schlachetzki and Pardridge (2003) demonstrated a dual expression of Pgp at both astrocytes and endothelium of the normal primate brain, thereby resolving previous conflicting results. However, most other groups still did not detect Pgp in astrocytes of normal tissue, indicating that fixation and staining variables may be critical.

In brain capillary endothelial cells, the intracellular localization of Pgp may vary. Although the largest proportion of Pgp is localized in the cell membrane, Pgp may generally also be expressed in intracellular compartments (Shapiro et al., 1998; Bendayan et al., 2002; Rajagopal and Simon, 2003). In cytoplasmic vesicles, Pgp may concentrate drugs in the interior of the vesicles and may thus sequester drugs away from their subcellular targets (Shapiro et al., 1998; Rajagopal and Simon, 2003). Within the cell membrane, a large fraction of Pgp seems to be localized in caveolae (Jodoin et al., 2003), i.e., flask shaped plasma membrane invaginations involved in many cellular events, including transport of macromolecules across cells by transcytosis (Demeule et al., 2000; Jodoin et al., 2003; Schlachetzki and Pardridge, 2003). These differences in subcellular localization of Pgp are likely to have an impact on Pgp activity, and due to influences on epitope presentation, also on immunohistochemical detection of Pgp.

2.2 Multidrug Resistance Proteins

The ABCC family currently has 12 members (including MRP1–9) that act as organic anion transporters but can also transport neutral organic drugs (Borst et al., 2000). Like Pgp, multidrug resistance proteins (MRPs) are located in excretory organs and a variety of blood–tissue barriers including the BBB (Borst et al., 2000). Some MRPs, like MRP2 and MRP4, are located in apical cell membranes of tissues, which in the BBB is the appropriate position for a cytoprotective role by an efflux transporter (❷ *Figure 23-1*). In contrast, other MRPs, such as MRP1, MRP3, and MRP5, are located basolaterally in most cell types studied in this regard (Borst et al., 1999; Schinkel and Jonker, 2003). Expression of MRPs in brain microvessel endothelial cells that form the BBB has been reported for several species, including humans (Begley, 2004). Using primary cultured bovine brain microvessel endothelial cells and the capillary-enriched fraction from bovine brain homogenates, RT-PCR analysis demonstrated the presence of mRNAs coding for MRP1, MRP4, MRP5, and MRP6 as well as low levels of MRP3 mRNA, whereas MRP2 mRNA was absent (Zhang et al., 2000). However, using immunostaining of PGP and MRP2 in isolated capillaries from rat and pig brain, both multidrug transporters were localized to the luminal surface of the capillary endothelium (Miller et al., 2000). Using cDNA arrays to determine MRP expression in brain capillary endothelial cells isolated from humans, high expression levels of mRNAs coding for MRP1 and low expression levels of mRNAs coding for MRP2, MRP3, and MRP5 were reported by Dombrowski et al. (2001). Thus, taken together, at least six MRPs are expressed at the BBB of different species. However, the exact subcellular localization (apical vs. basolateral) of most of these MRPs in brain capillary endothelial cells remains to be determined, particularly because of the lack of selective antibodies. Only those MRPs which are located at the luminal plasma membrane of brain capillary endothelial cells can be considered to be major contributors to BBB function.

The functional role of MRPs in BBB permeability has been demonstrated by experiments in which inhibitors of MRPs, such as probenecid or MK-571, were shown to enhance drug penetration into the brain or to inhibit drug efflux from isolated brain endothelial cells (Gutmann et al., 1999; Potschka and Löscher, 2001; Potschka et al., 2001). The recent generation of *mrp* gene knockout mice is providing more specific information on the physiological functions of MRPs in these different localizations. The brain penetration of the MRP1 substrate fluorescein is not altered in *mrp1* knockout mice (Sun et al., 2001), indicating that MRP1 function in the BBB is limited. Investigations in an *mrp2*-deficient rat mutant (TR$^-$)

(Koopen et al., 1998) further elucidated the role of MRP2 in BBB permeability. Brain extracellular levels of the antiepileptic drug phenytoin are significantly enhanced compared to normal rats (whereas plasma drug levels are the same), indicating that MRP2 expression at the BBB restricts brain entry of this compound (Potschka et al., 2003). Interestingly, a recent study demonstrated a tremendous upregulation of Pgp in brain capillary endothelial cells of mrp2-deficient rats (Hoffmann and Loscher, 2006). These data give indirect evidence for an overlap between MRP2 and Pgp function at the BBB, so that upregulation of Pgp expression can at least partly compensate for loss of MRP2.

2.3 Breast Cancer-Related Protein

The breast cancer-related protein BRCP/ABCG2 is a so called half transporter with two proteins assembling to a functional homodimer. As a characteristic of all members of the ABCG subfamily, the nucleotide-binding domain is located at the N terminus. BCRP received its name based on its first description in a chemotherapy resistant breast cancer cell line (Schinkel and Jonker, 2003). However, its expression and function proved to be not restricted to breast cancer cells. Comparative studies of tissue distribution demonstrated an extensive overlap of BCRP expression with Pgp expression (Schinkel and Jonker, 2003). BCRP has been detected in capillary endothelial cells of humans (Cooray et al., 2002), pigs (Eisenblatter et al., 2003), and mice (Cisternino et al., 2004). Its main expression at the luminal surface suggested a contribution to BBB efflux (❷ *Figure 23-1*). The role of BCRP in limiting brain penetration has also been demonstrated on a functional level for prazosin and mitoxantrone (Cisternino et al., 2004). Interestingly, *mdr1a* knockout mice had about three times more BCRP in the brain microvessels than normal mice, indicating that an upregulation of BCRP can at least partly compensate for the lack of Pgp in the BBB (Cisternino et al., 2004).

2.4 Other Efflux Transporters

Apart from ABC transporters, several members of the organic anion transporting–polypeptide family (OATP-family) and the organic anion transporter-family (OAT-family) are expressed in the brain. A series of transport studies indicate that these transporters may also play a significant role in drug efflux at the BBB (Gao and Meier, 2001; Lee et al., 2001; Kim, 2003; Sun et al., 2003; Hagenbuch and Meier, 2003). In contrast to ABC efflux transporters such as Pgp, OATs and OATPs are not primary hydrolyzers of ATP and cannot transport against the concentration gradient or from a low energy situation to a higher one. OATs and OATPs generally function as exchangers, which exchange one molecule for another molecule and which are driven by a concentration gradient. The exact localization of most OATPs and OATs in the brain is not clear so far (Lee et al., 2001; Sun et al., 2003; Fricker and Miller, 2004). Rat Oatp2, a bidirectional transport protein that is involved in drug transport, proved to be expressed in the apical and basolateral membrane of brain capillary endothelial cells (Fricker and Miller, 2004) (❷ *Figure 23-1*). With a predominantly ablumi-nal localization, OAT3 may mediate abluminal drug uptake, thereby supplying substrates to efflux transporters in the lumenal membrane (Fricker and Miller, 2004) (❷ *Figure 23-1*). In addition, the human OATP-A has been identified by immunostaining in brain capillaries (Gao et al., 2000). Transport data indicated that OATs and OATPs have an overlapping transport spectrum with some of the MRPs, indicating that the efflux transport of certain organic anions across the BBB may involve a concerted action of multiple transport systems (Sun et al., 2003).

Another molecule that has been suggested to function as a BBB transporter is the major vault protein (MVP). Expression of MVP in normal brain tissue and in epileptic brain tissue has been demonstrated with a cellular localization not only in blood vessels but also in astrocytes and neurons (Sisodiya et al., 2003; Aronica et al., 2004). However, it has not yet been demonstrated that MVP can transport xenobiotics.

In addition, RLIP76/RalBP1 may contribute to BBB function. Awasthi et al. (2005) reported that this molecule is expressed in brain capillary endothelial cells of epileptic patients and that it extrudes the antiepileptic drug phenytoin from these cells. Based on these data, the authors suggested that the human isoform RalBP1 may function as a mechanism of drug resistance in epileptic patients (Awashti et al., 2005). However, additional studies are necessary in order to define the role of RLIP76/RalBP1 as a BBB efflux transporter more precisely.

3   Efflux Transporters in the Blood–CSF Barrier

The blood–CSF barrier is formed by ependymal epithelial cells, which are linked by tight junctions. In contrast to the BBB capillaries, the choroid plexus capillaries do not contribute to the barrier function since they are fenestrated and have no tight junctions. Another component of the blood–CSF barrier is the arachnoid membrane, which envelops the brain. Transport of drugs mainly involves the solute carrier and transporter of the ABC transporter superfamily (Lee et al., 2001; Sun et al., 2003; de Lange, 2004). Rao et al. (1999) first described the expression of Pgp and MRP (later shown to be MRP1) in the epithelia of the choroid plexus and their contribution in a bipolar permeation barrier for selected drugs. Pgp was described to be localized subapically at the choroid plexus epithelium, putatively conferring transport in the direction of the CSF (Rao et al., 1999). However, based on the subapical localization, its functional contribution to drug transport is controversially discussed. In contrast to Pgp, MRP1 is localized basolaterally, conferring transport to the blood side of the epithelial cells (Rao et al., 1999). The role of MRP1 in inhibiting drug penetration into the CSF was further supported by functional studies in knockout mice (Wijnholds et al., 2000). Rao et al. (1999) suggested that Pgp and MRP1 together might coordinate secretion and reabsorption of several compounds into and out of the CNS. Surprisingly, the association of Pgp with the apical membrane would rather promote an increase of concentrations in the CSF, which would be in apparent contrast to Pgp function at the BBB (de Lange, 2004). However, further research is necessary to better understand the role of Pgp at the choroid plexus (Sun et al., 2003).

Although MRP2 and MRP3 are only expressed at very low levels at the blood–CSF barrier (Choudhuri et al., 2003; Lee et al., 2004), MRP4 and MRP5 exhibit high expression levels in choroidal epithelial cells. Lee et al. (2004) suggested that both MRPs may contribute to the efflux of organic anions from the CSF. Several members of the OATP/OAT families, including Oatp1, Oatp2, Oatp3, and Oat3, have also been identified in the choroid plexus (Hagenbuch and Meier, 2004; de Lange, 2004). So far, the role of these and other drug transporters in blood–CSF barrier function is only incompletely understood and more studies need to be done to fully elucidate the contribution of these transporters to drug efflux at the choroid plexus (Sun et al., 2003; de Lange, 2004).

4   Efflux Transporters in Brain Parenchymal Cells

Although Pgp is expressed at high levels in brain capillary endothelial cells, only weak expression can be detected in perivascular and parenchymal astroglia (Löscher and Potschka, 2005a). In both human patients and rodents, astroglial expression may be enhanced with certain brain diseases like epilepsy (Löscher and Potschka, 2005a). In addition to astroglia, Pgp is also expressed and is functional in microglia (Lee et al., 2001). Furthermore, following seizures, Pgp expression has been determined in neurons of the rat hippocampus (Volk et al., 2004). In support of these data, neuronal Pgp expression was also observed in epileptogenic brain tissue of patients with drug refractory epilepsy (Sisodiya et al., 2002; Aronica et al., 2003).

With respect to the MRP family, MRP1 is present in higher levels in astrocytes than in brain capillary endothelial cells when this transporter is studied in rat brain cell culture or in rat brain tissue (Decleves et al., 2000; Mercier et al., 2004). Studies in primary rat brain cell cultures enriched for neurons, astrocytes, oligodendrocytes, and microglia gave evidence that MRP1 and MRP5 mRNA show higher abundance in all four cell culture types than mRNAs of other MRP transporters. mRNAs coding for MRP3 and MRP4 were found at significant levels in cultured astrocytes and microglial cells, whereas cultures of neurons and oligodendrocytes contained only marginal quantities of these mRNAs (Hirrlinger et al., 2002). In primary cell cultures from bovine brain, mRNAs for MRP1, MRP4, MRP5, and MRP6 were detected in glia cells, whereas Pgp, MRP2, MRP3, and MRP7 mRNAs were below detection level (Berezowski et al., 2004). It is important to note that such semiquantitative comparisons of transporter mRNA expression in different cell lines have to be interpreted with caution, because drug efflux transporter expression levels are sensitive to the preparation procedure as well as to in vitro cell culturing. In human brain tissue, MRP4 and MPR5 were detected in astrocytes (Nies et al., 2004). Furthermore, MRP5 was also identified in pyramidal neurons (Nies et al., 2004).

Although efflux transporters in perivascular glia may contribute to BBB function (❯ *Figure 23-1*), the functional role of such transporters in parenchymal astroglia and other parenchymal cells is only incompletely understood. Especially in pathological conditions, with increased expression of Pgp in astrocytes, astrocytic Pgp activity may influence drug compartmentalization. In line with this possibility, Marchi et al. (2004) recently reported that Pgp-overexpressing astrocytes from epileptogenic brain tissue exhibit a reduced uptake of ^{14}C-phenytoin compared to control astrocytes. This reduction in uptake could be counteracted by the Pgp inhibitor tariquidar (Marchi et al., 2004). Furthermore, evidence exists that parenchymal expression of efflux transporters may protect from cellular damage. Unconjugated bilirubin proved to induce upregulation of MRP1 in astrocytes, which then confers protection of the astrocytes from cell damage by bilirubin (Gennuso et al., 2004).

5   Brain-to-Blood Efflux of Endogenous Substrates

Transporters in BBB endothelial cells seem to play a critical role in limiting the brain level of different endogenous substrates produced either in the brain or in peripheral organs. Besides specific efflux transporters for different neurotransmitters, broad spectrum efflux transporters in brain capillary endothelial cells also contribute to brain-to-blood efflux of endogenous compounds (❯ *Table 23-1*).

■ Table 23-1

Endogenous substrates of BBB efflux transporters

Type of substrate	Examples	Transporters
Neuroactive steroids	Dehydroepiandrosterone, progesterone	Pgp, MRPs, OATPs, OATs
Glucocorticoids	Corticosterone, cortisol	Pgp
Macromolecules	β-amyloid peptide	Pgp
	Opioid peptides	Pgp, MRPs
Uremic toxins	3-carboxy-4-methyl-5-propyl-2-furapropionate, hippurate, indole acetate, indoxyl sulfate	Oat3, Oatp2
Cytokines and inflammatory mediators	Leukotriene C$_4$	MRPs and Oatp1
	Leukotriene D4 and E4	MRP1
	Prostaglandin E2	Oatp2
	Interleukin-2, interleukin-4, interferon-γ, tumor necrosis factor-α	Pgp
Degradation product of hemoglobin	Unconjugated bilirubin	Pgp

Neuroactive steroids can reach the brain following synthesis in peripheral endocrine glands but can also be synthesized in the CNS. The regulation of their brain concentration is of specific interest because neuroactive steroids including dehydroepiandrosterone and progesterone can modulate synaptic plasticity and can mediate neuroprotection in different pathological conditions (Wojtal et al., 2006). Brain concentrations of steroids regardless of the site of synthesis are limited by different efflux transporters including

Pgp, MRP transporters, OATs, and OATPs (Terasaki and Ohtsuki, 2005). Transport efficacy, which can change with different CNS pathologies, may critically contribute to factors that determine the outcome following a brain insult.

Access of the glucocorticoids corticosterone and cortisol to the brain proved to be regulated by Pgp. Malfunctions of a glucocorticoid-mediated negative feedback on the hypothalamic–pituitary–adrenal gland (HPA) axis have been reported to be pathophysiological mechanisms in the development of depression (e.g., Plotsky et al., 1998). Due to the fact that several antidepressants have been substantiated as Pgp substrates (Uhr et al., 2003), these may competitively inhibit Pgp, thereby promoting brain penetration rates of endogenous glucocorticoids and restoring the glucocorticoid-mediated negative feedback mechanism (Pariante et al., 2004).

An increase in the brain β-amyloid (Aβ) burden is generally considered to contribute to the pathophysiology of Alzheimer's disease. Pgp has been identified as an Aβ efflux pump (Lam et al., 2001). Several studies indicated that Pgp expression and efflux function in BBB endothelial cells is inversely correlated with the Aβ disposition (Vogelgesang et al., 2002, 2004; Cirrito et al., 2005; Thomas, 2005). Thus, it has been hypothesized that Pgp is a critical factor for Aβ clearance from the brain, and that low levels of Pgp activity are associated with an increased risk for Alzheimer's disease. The fact that brain Pgp activity decreases with aging (Toornvliet et al., 2006) may thereby promote Aβ disposition and disease progression in the elderly.

Renal failure can result in uremic encephalopathy as a consequence of brain penetration of uremic toxins. Rat Oat3 and Oatp2 proved to function as a CNS detoxification system that limits brain access of the uremic toxins 3-carboxy-4-methyl-5-propyl-2-furanpropionate, hippurate, indole acetate, and indoxyl sulfate (Terasaki and Ohtsuki, 2005; Deguchi et al., 2006).

Pgp has been implicated in BBB efflux of unconjugated bilirubin (Hanko et al., 2003). Inhibitors of Pgp proved to increase distribution of bilirubin to the brain. Thus, it has been speculated that drugs known to inhibit Pgp may worsen bilirubin encephalopathy in hyperbilirubinemic infants. However, in view of the limited knowledge about Pgp activity in the newborn, it is currently difficult to define the role of Pgp in CNS pathology associated with hyperbilirubinemia.

BBB transport of endogenous opioid peptides plays a critical role in the regulation of opioid pharmacokinetics and of pain modulation. Both, Pgp and MRP transporters seem to be involved in brain-to-blood efflux of different endogenous opioid peptides (Kastin et al., 2001; Ganapathy and Miyauchi, 2005).

Leukotriene C4 (LTC4) has been identified as a substrate of different MRP transporters and of rat Oatp1 (Kusuhara et al., 1998). These transporters seem to be responsible for a unidirectional efflux of LTC4 from the brain into the circulating blood (Kusuhara et al., 1998). Other prostanoids may also be subject to active brain-to-blood efflux. Leukotriene D4 and E4 are substrates of MRP1, whereas prostaglandin E2 seems to be a substrate of rat Oatp2 (Löscher and Potschka, 2005a). In addition, modulation of inflammatory and immunological reactions may also occur via Pgp-mediated efflux of cytokines, including interleukin-2, interleukin-4, interferon-γ, and tumor necrosis factor α from the brain.

6 Xenobiotics as Substrates of Efflux Transporters

Efflux transporters at the BBB and the blood–CSF barrier play a pivotal role in limiting brain uptake and in extrusion of xenobiotics (❯ Table 23-2). With a localization at the apical membrane of BBB endothelial cells, these transporters can mediate an active extrusion of their substrates back into the capillary lumen (Lee et al., 2001). Efflux transporters in this apical membrane may also interact with transporters at the basolateral membrane, which shuttle drugs into the cytoplasm of the BBB endothelial cells, thereby promoting contact of the drug with the transporter in the apical membrane. Weak substrates of BBB efflux transporters generally pass the BBB to a certain extent and exert CNS effects, provided they are lipophilic enough to diffuse through the BBB. However, their effectiveness may be critically influenced by expression rates and the functional state of the relevant efflux transporter. In contrast, strong substrates of BBB efflux transporters do not pass the BBB to a relevant extent, and their pharmacodynamic effects are restricted to the periphery.

■ Table 23-2
Important xenobiotic substrates of BBB efflux transporters

Type of substrate	Examples	Transporters
Anticancer drugs	Doxorubicin, daunorubicin, vinblastine, vincristine, paclitaxel, etoposide, topotecan	Pgp, MRPs, BCRP,
Immunosuppressants	Cyclosporine A, tacrolimus	Pgp
Corticoids	Dexamethasone, prednisolone	Pgp
Analgesics	Morphine, methadone, fentanyl	Pgp
HIV protease inhibitors	Amprenavir, indinavir, saquinavir	Pgp, MRPs
Antidiarrheal agents	Loperamide	Pgp
Anthelmintic agents	Ivermectin, abamectin	Pgp
Antipsychotic agents	Olanzapine, amisulpride	Pgp
Histamine H_1-receptor antagonists	Fexofenadine, terfenadine	Pgp, Oatp1
Histamine H_2-receptor antagonists	Cimetidine	Pgp
β-Adrenoceptor antagonists	Bunitrolol, carvedilol, celiprolol	Pgp
Calcium channel blocker	Verapamil, nifedipine, diltiazem	Pgp
Antiepileptic drugs	Phenytoin, carbamazepine, lamotrigine, phenobarbital	Pgp, MRPs
Antiemetics	Domperidone, ondansetron	Pgp
Cardiac glycosides	Digoxin, digitoxin, ouabain	Pgp, Oatp1, Oatp2
Antidepressants	Amitriptyline, nortriptiline, venlafaxine, paroxetine	Pgp
Antibiotics	Erythromycin, tetracyclines, fluoroquinolones, cephalosporins	Pgp, OAT3
Lipid-lowering agents	Lovastatin, cerivastatin, atorvastatin	Pgp
Angiotensin-converting enzyme inhibitors	Enalapril, temocaprilat	Oatp1

For comprehensive listing of known substrates also see Löscher and Potschka (2005a). Please note that the transporters listed do not necessarily transport all compounds given, but in some cases only transport single compounds of the pharmacological group

For the pharmaceutical industry, the question whether a developmental compound is a transporter substrate is of particular interest. On one hand, low affinity to BBB efflux transporters is advantageous for the development of CNS therapeutics that need to reach high concentrations in the brain. On the other hand, high affinity to BBB efflux transporters is advantageous for the development of drugs, which should act in the periphery in order to avoid CNS side effects. Although strong efforts have been made to define the criteria that allow a prediction whether a specific compound is an efflux transporter substrate (Seelig and Landwojtowicz, 2000; Crivori et al., 2006), reliable predictions are still not possible yet. The structure of Pgp substrates often includes hydrophobic regions and planar aromatic domains as well as tertiary amino groups or positive charges at physiological pH (Seelig and Landwojtowicz, 2000). MRPs preferably transport anions, but transport of cations and neutral compounds is also possible and is known to be facilitated by the binding of glutathione to the transporter molecule (Borst et al., 2000).

Efflux transporters are capable of transporting a vast and chemically diverse array of toxically relevant compounds including dietary and environmental carcinogens, pesticides, metals, and lipid peroxidation products (Leslie et al., 2005). A link between brain pathology, efflux transporters, and pesticide exposure has recently been reported for Parkinsons's disease. Parkinson's disease results from the oxidative-stress-induced death of neurons in the substantia nigra region of the brain. Several pesticides, which are Pgp substrates, are capable of inducing oxidative stress and have been implicated in the pathophysiology of Parkinson's disease in a subpopulation of patients (Lai et al., 2002; Kamel and Hoppin, 2004). Interestingly,

Pgp genotypes proved to be correlated with sensitivity to pesticide exposure and the resulting increased incidence of Parkinson's disease (Furuno et al., 2002; Drozdzik et al., 2003). Thus, Pgp may be a relevant protection mechanism against Parkinson's disease.

As already outlined, transport of pharmaceutical compounds by brain efflux transporters can critically influence drug efficacy and tolerability. Based on up-to-date knowledge, ABC transporters are the major contributors to active drug efflux in the brain. A large variety of pharmacological compounds proved to be transported by ABC transporters at the BBB.

Anticancer agents were among the first drugs that were identified to be substrates of Pgp as well as MRPs and BCRP. Efflux of anticancer agents from the brain remains to be a major research focus due to its potential to limit the therapeutic efficacy of these drugs. The immunosuppressant cyclosporin A is effectively transported by Pgp and has been often used as a competitive Pgp inhibitor in experimental studies (Sakata et al., 1994; Didier and Loor, 1995).

Not only endogenous but also synthetic glucocorticoids like dexamethasone and prednisolone are subject to transport by Pgp. Synthetic glucocorticoids even proved to be more efficaciously transported than endogenous glucocorticoids (Meijer et al., 1998; Karssen et al., 2002). This observation is in line with less pronounced CNS effects of synthetic glucocorticoids as compared to endogenous glucocorticoids. Differences in the affinity to Pgp may also explain why some glucocorticoids primarily act at the anterior pituitary level to suppress ACTH release; whereas in rodents, corticosterone, which proved to be a weak Pgp substrate, primarily acts on higher levels in brain regions that have a regulatory impact on the hypothalamic–pituitary–adrenal axis.

Pgp-mediated extrusion from the brain has a tremendous impact on opiate and opioid analgesic efficacy. Modulation of Pgp function significantly affected the antinociceptive effect of morphine (Letrent et al., 1999; Thompson et al., 2000; King et al., 2001). Thus, Pgp seems to be an important issue in pain control with opioid analgesics, which may influence the onset, magnitude, and duration of the analgesic response (Dagenais et al., 2004).

Microdialysis experiments using transporter inhibitors as well as experiments in knockout mice have indicated that several antiepileptic drugs are transported by BBB Pgp, and some are also subject to transport by MRPs (Rizzi et al., 2002; Sills et al., 2002; Löscher and Potschka, 2005b). Overexpression of these transporters in epileptic tissue of drug resistant patients may thus contribute to therapeutic failure (Löscher and Potschka, 2005b).

Furthermore, Pgp seems to limit the distribution of some antibacterial drugs including fluoroquinolones and erythromycin to the brain (Schinkel, 1999; de Lange et al., 2000; Sasabe et al., 2004). Brain extrusion of these antibiotics may contribute to their limited or lack of efficacy in CNS microbial infections. On the other hand, CNS side effects have been recognized as a problem in the group of fluoroquinolones, and fluoroquinolones that enter the brain in a reduced manner due to interaction with Pgp may thus have a favorable side effect profile.

Genetic deficiency of Pgp in mice resulted in enhanced brain access of several antidepressants, indicating that these are effluxed into the blood by Pgp (Uhr et al., 2000, 2003; Uhr and Grauer, 2003; Grauer and Uhr, 2004). If this active efflux transport can contribute to therapeutic failure in depression remains to be determined.

A critical limitation of therapeutic success by efflux transporters has also been proposed for treatment of brain HIV (Potschka and Löscher, 2005b). Several HIV protease inhibitors, which have brought tremendous progress in the treatment of HIV infection, are subject to transport by Pgp and MRP2 (Kim et al., 1998a, b; Washington et al., 2000; van der Sandt et al., 2001). Therefore, efflux transport seems to critically limit HIV protease inhibitor brain access and the virus eradication by these compounds.

The antiparasitic drug ivermectin proved to be a strong Pgp substrate. Pgp deficiency in mice as well as in different herding dog breeds results in a high sensitivity to ivermectin with severe intoxications due to an increase in ivermectin brain concentrations and an associated enhancement of inhibitory neurotransmission (Mealey et al., 2001; Neff et al., 2004). Pgp-mediated efflux at the BBB also proved to be critically involved in limiting brain access of the antidiarrheal opioid receptor agonist loperamide and in restricting its action to the periphery (Schinkel et al., 1996; Sadeque et al., 2000). In contrast to first generation antihistamines, second generation antihistamines are generally nonsedating. In vitro studies in rat brain endothelial cells indicated that all second generation antihistamines are substrates of Pgp, whereas all first generation antihistamines tested showed no affinity for Pgp (Tamai et al., 2000; Chishty et al., 2001). On the basis of these data, it was postulated that Pgp-mediated efflux at the BBB explains the lack of CNS side effects of modern antihistamines.

The role of non-ABC transporters including OATs and OATPs, MVP, and RLIP76 as drug efflux transporters in the brain is less well established compared to ABC transporters such as Pgp or several of the MRPs; and for MVP it is not even established if this protein transports drugs at all (van Zon et al., 2004). Thus, these proteins are not discussed in detail here. Future investigations may further elucidate or substantiate their putative role in limiting brain uptake or brain extrusion of drugs.

To summarize, it has been demonstrated that BBB efflux transporters critically influence CNS effects of numerous therapeutically used compounds and that this influence is of clinical relevance for many of these drugs.

7   Regulation of Expression

Expression of efflux transporters is regulated in a highly dynamic manner. This regulatory process can be considered as a mechanism that allows an adaptation to changing requirements in detoxification and tissue protection. The regulation of expression has been most intensely studied for Pgp.

Recently, it has been reported that *mdr1a* mRNA, which encodes one Pgp isoform in mice, shows clear 24-h rhythmicity in the liver and intestine with a peak occurring in the second half of the light phase (Ando et al., 2005). Hitherto, it has not been investigated if such a circadian rhythmicity also occurs in the BBB. In general, circadian variation of efflux transporter expression may be involved in various chronopharmacologic phenomena.

Comparison of brain access of the Pgp substrate [^{11}C]verapamil in young and elderly volunteers gave evidence that Pgp activity declines with aging (Toornvliet et al., 2006). Consequently, the brain may be exposed to higher drug and toxin levels in elderly subjects. This increased exposure may in turn contribute to the development or progression of neurodegenerative diseases.

In general, regulation of functional efflux transporter expression in the outer membrane of cells occurs on different molecular levels including transcriptional, posttranscriptional, and posttranslational mechanisms (Shtil and Azare, 2005). Regulation of mRNA stability contributes to the control and induction of Pgp expression (Shtil and Azare, 2005). In renal proximal tubule cells, gentamicin exposure increased shuttling of MRP2/ABCC2 to the apical membrane (Notenboom et al., 2006). Comparable mechanisms may also be effective in brain capillary endothelial cells. Recently, a novel way of nongenetic transfer of Pgp by direct intercellular transfer of the protein has been demonstrated in tumor cells (Ambudkar et al., 2005). Further research is necessary to determine if this mechanism is restricted to tumor cells or may also occur in other cells.

A variety of xenobiotics including several pharmacological compounds have been demonstrated to induce expression of multidrug transporters. In the treatment of brain cancer, induction of efflux transporter expression by chemotherapeutic drugs in tumor cells and BBB endothelial cells is a well recognized mechanism that limits drug concentrations at the target tumor cells and contributes to therapeutic failure (Lee and Bendayan, 2004; Löscher and Potschka, 2005b). Orphan nuclear receptors have been recognized as master regulators of drug-induced changes in expression of metabolizing enzymes and of members of the multidrug transporter families (Masuyama et al., 2005). The orphan nuclear receptor PXR/SXR (termed pregnane X receptor (PXR) in rodents and steroid and xenobiotic receptor (SXR) in humans) proved to be expressed in rat brain capillaries (Bauer et al., 2004). Its functional relevance for regulation of efflux transporters in the BBB was indicated by the observation that the PXR ligand dexamethasone increased Pgp expression and Pgp-specific transport (Bauer et al., 2004). Thus, PXR/SXR may be a key xenobiotic sensor in brain capillary endothelial cells, which mediates induction of Pgp. However, using intestinal and lung carcinoma cell lines, it was demonstrated that induction of efflux drug transporter by xenobiotics and especially chemotherapeutics does not necessarily depend on PXR (Huang et al., 2006). On the basis of the fact that the group also demonstrated that the modes of regulation can be cell specific, it is currently not clear if these data can be extrapolated to brain capillary endothelial cells. Baker et al. (2005) reported that epigenetic changes in the MDR1 promoter occur in response to chemotherapeutic drugs which then enhance the MDR phenotype. Dramatic changes in the temporal and spatial pattern of histone modifications occurred within the 5′-hypomethylated region of MDR1, which directly correlated with MDR1 upregulation (Baker et al., 2005).

Apart from involved receptors or changes in the promotor region, a variety of mechanisms that contribute in cellular stress responses, including phospholipase C, protein kinase C, mitogen-activated protein kinase cascades, mobilization of intracellular Ca^{2+}, cytokines, nuclear factor-κB, and heat shock factor 1, regulate multidrug transporter genes such as MDR1 (McRae et al., 2003; Shtil and Azare, 2005; Ho and Piquette-Miller, 2006; Tchenio et al., 2006). Using primary cultured rat brain endothelial cells to examine the effect of oxidative stress on expression of transporters, Felix and Barrand (2002) found a stress-induced increase in Pgp expression and function, whereas no such alterations were observed for MRP1.

Hartz et al. (2004, 2006) defined a signaling pathway as part of the innate immune response through which Pgp activity is rapidly modulated. Their findings suggested that the inflammatory cytokine tumor necrosis factor (TNF)-α reduces Pgp activity via, TNF-R1 receptor activation, endothelin-1 release, and endothelin-B receptor signaling.

Knowledge about the regulation of BBB efflux transporter activity is of particular interest because it may prepare the ground for the development of strategies to specifically manipulate BBB function in order to improve pharmacotherapy of CNS diseases. This underlines the specific importance of further research focusing on the different mechanisms of regulation and their interaction.

8 CNS Diseases and Efflux Transporter Expression and Function

8.1 Genetic Variants of Efflux Transporters and Disease

Single-nucleotide polymorphisms (SNPs) in efflux transporter genes have been associated with interindividual differences in transport activity (Sakaeda et al., 2004). Concerning the effects of genetic polymorphisms on pharmacotherapy, the best characterized transporter is the multidrug resistant transporter Pgp, the gene product of MDR1. Pharmacogenetics of Pgp have been suggested to critically influence the individual response to pharmacotherapy (Sakaeda et al., 2004; Kerb, 2006). More than 50 SNPs have been identified in the human MDR1 gene. A SNP in exon 26 of MDR1 seems to have an impact on Pgp expression and activity. This SNP has been linked to the therapeutic response in epilepsy, depression, schizophrenia, and brain HIV (Fellay et al., 2002; Roberts et al., 2002; Siddiqui et al., 2003; Soranzo et al., 2004; Zimprich et al., 2004; Yasui-Furukori et al., 2006). Other studies in epileptic patients failed to demonstrate a correlation between this polymorphism, associated haplotypes, and drug response (Tan et al., 2004; Sills et al., 2006; Kim et al., 2006). These controversial data may be due to differences in inclusion criteria, in the definition of therapeutic success or failure, and in the ethnic composition of the patient population.

Genetic variants of ABCB1 may not only be critical for therapeutic success in the treatment of CNS diseases but may also influence the individual risk to develop specific diseases like Parkinson's disease (Lee and Bendayan, 2004; Tan et al., 2004). Genotypes associated with low expression levels of Pgp proved to be more frequent in patients with early onset of Parkinson's disease and Parkinson's disease patients with prior pesticide exposure (Furuno et al., 2002; Drozdzik et al., 2003). This result is of particular interest, because epidemiological studies suggested an association between pesticides that are substrates of Pgp and Parkinson's disease (Lai et al., 2002; Kamel and Hoppin, 2004).

8.2 Impact of CNS Pathologies on Efflux Transporter Activity

Several CNS pathologies have been associated with changes in efflux transporter expression or function. Epilepsy, which is characterized by recurrent spontaneous seizures, is one of the most common neurological disorders. In animal models of epilepsy, a transient increase in Pgp and MRP2 expression was observed in brain capillary endothelial cells, astroglia, and neurons after seizures, which indicates that seizures themselves can induce overexpression of drug transporters (Sisodiya, 2003; Löscher and Potschka, 2005b). This seizure-induced overexpression proved to be restricted to brain regions involved in seizure initiation and spread. These data are in line with investigations in human epileptogenic tissue dissected from pharmacoresistant patients during epilepsy surgery, which also indicated high expression rates of efflux transporters (Sisodiya, 2003; Löscher and Potschka, 2005b). However, definite conclusions from these studies are hampered by the lack of adequate control tissue, because patients who are treated successfully do not generally undergo surgical resection of epileptogenic foci. The cellular mechanisms involved in seizure-induced overexpression of efflux transporters still need to be elucidated. With respect to the excessive glutamate release associated with seizures, it is of particular interest that glutamate proved to upregulate Pgp expression via an NMDA receptor mechanism (Zhu and Liu, 2004). Thus, glutamate is likely to be involved in seizure-mediated induction of Pgp expression.

Inflammation in the CNS proved to produce dynamic changes in Pgp expression and activity. Intraventricular administration of *Escherichia coli* lipopolysaccharide in rodents induced a local inflammatory reaction that was associated with a loss of *mdr1a* mRNA and increased brain access and retention of the Pgp substrates digoxin and (99m)Tc-sestamibi (Goralski et al., 2003; Wang et al., 2005). Reduced expression and activity of Pgp may thus be one mechanism that contributes to changes in drug distribution as a consequence of brain inflammation.

Infection of the CNS by HIV is a frequent event in the course of AIDS. It can produce neurological symptoms, and can also lead to the establishment of a lifelong latent viral reservoir in the brain. In cases of HIV encephalitis, an altered Pgp expression has been described in brain tissue with intense staining of glial cells (Langford et al., 2004). Among the different factors that can contribute to CNS alterations associated with HIV infection, the HIV-Tat protein is considered to play a critical role (Hayashi et al., 2005). Treatment of brain microvascular endothelial cells with the Tat-protein induced Pgp expression both at mRNA and protein levels.

8.3 Treatment-Induced Changes in Efflux Transporter Activity

As already discussed, a variety of pharmacological compounds including several CNS therapeutics can induce transporter expression (Lee and Bendayan, 2004; Löscher and Potschka, 2005b). Probably due to their pronounced toxic effects on cells and to the induction of a cellular stress response, anticancer chemotherapeutic drugs are very potent inducers of efflux transporters. Overexpression of efflux transporters in tumor cells and the BBB is considered to be a major contributor to therapeutic failure (Regina et al., 2001; Thomas and Coley, 2003; Kemper et al., 2004). Efflux transporter expression in brain tumor cells can be intrinsic, i.e., present before exposure to chemotherapeutic drugs, but can also be acquired as a consequence of chemotherapy.

Chemotherapy-induced transporter overexpression can cause multidrug resistance, which develops during the treatment following an initial treatment response (Thomas and Coley, 2003). Induction may also occur at the BBB, thereby limiting overall brain penetration rates (Kemper et al., 2004).

8.4 Transporter Overexpression as a Cause of Drug Resistance

The effectiveness of pharmacological therapies for many CNS diseases including brain cancer, epilepsy, depression, schizophrenia, and HIV-associated encephalopathy is limited by poor response or complete resistance to drug treatment. Besides a variety of mechanisms, alterations in drug uptake into the brain or into brain parenchymal target cells are considered an important reason for therapeutic failure (Löscher and Potschka, 2005b; Thuerauf and Fromm, 2006). Disease-associated or therapy-induced changes in efflux transporter expression are thought to critically affect brain pharmacokinetics of a variety of important CNS-active drugs.

The poor efficacy of systemically administered anticancer chemotherapeutic drugs is at least partly due to the activity of BBB efflux transporters (Bart et al., 2000; Kemper et al., 2004) and not only a result of expression of multidrug transporters by the brain tumor cells themselves. The impact of BBB Pgp has been impressively demonstrated in a mouse glioblastoma model (Fellner et al., 2002). Brain penetration and efficacy of systemically administered paclitaxel could be enhanced significantly by coadministration of the Pgp inhibitor valspodar (Fellner et al., 2002).

In view of the fact that several antiepileptic drugs seem to be transported by efflux transporters at the BBB, seizure-induced overexpression of efflux transporters renders a feasible explanation for multidrug resistance of epilepsy based on limited access of antiepileptic drugs to their target sites. Important support for this concept came from experiments in two different models of drug-resistant epilepsy. Pgp expression in drug-resistant rats significantly exceeded those in drug-responsive rats (Potschka et al., 2004; Volk and Löscher, 2005). Recent experimental studies, in which it was demonstrated that drug resistance of seizures can be overcome by transporter inhibitors, rendered further proof for the multidrug transporter hypothesis of drug resistant epilepsy (Clinckers et al., 2005; Brandt et al., 2006). The first clinical case reports with coadministration of verapamil to the individual antiepileptic drug regimen resulted in improved seizure control (Summers et al., 2004). This improvement may be due to a modulatory effect of verapamil, which is known to competitively inhibit Pgp. This modulation of Pgp transport function may have also contributed to the impressing effect of verapamil coadministration in a patient with a refractory status epilepticus at day 37 of ongoing electrographic seizures (Iannetti et al., 2005). Clinical studies in larger cohorts of patients will be necessary to render final proof-of-principle. Furthermore it must be taken into consideration that drug resistance of epilepsy must be considered as a multifactorial problem, and thus, the relative importance of efflux transporter overexpression needs to be elucidated.

A role of BBB efflux transporters in drug resistance of mood disorders or schizophrenia is generally conceivable based on the fact that some antidepressants and antipsychotic drugs are substrates of Pgp (Uhr et al., 2000; Boulton et al., 2002; Uhr and Grauer, 2003; Ejsing and Linnet, 2005). However, due to the lack of models for treatment-resistant psychiatric disorders, it is difficult to test the validity of the hypothesis, which therefore still remains rather speculative. Recently, first indirect support for the hypothesis came from a genetic analysis in schizophrenic patients treated with bromperidol. The MDR1 genotype showed some correlation with the therapeutic response to bromperidol (Yasui-Furukori et al., 2006).

In the treatment of HIV infection, the development of HIV protease inhibitors has promoted considerable progress. However, a major limitation in their efficacy is the restricted access to the brain, which leaves the brain viral reservoir unaffected. Pgp-mediated efflux has been hypothesized to contribute to the limited brain penetration rates of HIV protease inhibitors like saquinavir, amprenavir, nelfinavir, and indinavir (Kim et al., 1998a; Washington et al., 2000; Edwards et al., 2002). Pgp upregulation at the BBB by the HIV-Tat protein (Hayashi et al., 2005) may further reduce penetration and efficacy of the HIV protease inhibitors. In addition to Pgp, MRP1, MRP2, and MRP4 also accept HIV protease inhibitors as substrates and might therefore be involved in the limitation of their brain access. Because HIV primarily targets microglia and astrocytes, enhanced glial Pgp expression as reported for cases of HIV encephalopathy (Langford et al., 2004) may further limit access of the HIV protease inhibitors to their targets.

9   Efflux Transporters as Drug Targets

Increasing awareness of the impact of efflux transporters on success in the pharmacotherapy of CNS diseases promotes efforts to develop strategies to modulate transporter activity (Löscher and Potschka, 2005b; Thuerauf and Fromm, 2006). Because Pgp is known to transport a large number of commonly prescribed drugs, efforts so far especially concentrate on this transporter. Mechanisms by which Pgp activity in the BBB can be modulated include direct inhibition by specific inhibitors, functional modulation, and transcriptional modulation (Bauer et al., 2005). First and second generation Pgp inhibitors were hampered by additional pharmacodynamic effects or by additional effects on drug metabolism (Thomas and Coley, 2003). The development of third generation Pgp inhibitors rendered selective and potent modulators, such as tariquidar, laniquidar, zosuquidar, and elacridar (Bates et al., 2002; Thomas and Coley, 2003). In view of the complexity of efflux transport, an aim that suggests itself is to develop dual or multipotent inhibitors. Jekerle et al. (2006) recently reported the development of the novel inhibitor, WK-X-34, which modulates both Pgp and BCRP in experimental models. In the clinical setting, coadministration of Pgp inhibitors together with chemotherapeutic drugs in oncology has shown some efficacy (Breedveld et al., 2006), although not all studies yielded promising data. Therefore, the continued development of these agents must be awaited in order to establish the true potential of Pgp-mediated reversal of multidrug resistance in the treatment of brain cancer and other CNS diseases. In this context, it is of particular interest that a recent study reported a differential sensitivity of Pgp located in different cells and blood–tissue barriers (Choo et al., 2006). Thereby, Pgp localized in the BBB proved to be more resistant to inhibition than at other tissue sites (Choo et al., 2006). This resistance can be overcome by a sufficiently high dose of an inhibitor. However, whether this is safely attainable in the clinical situation remains to be determined.

In general, any modulation of transporter function has to consider the potential hazards of such a modulation. First, complications with a combination of a Pgp inhibitor or modulator with a CNS-active therapeutic drug may be related to the intended aim. An influence on pharmacokinetics of the therapeutic drug will not only affect the target tissue or target brain region. Enhanced drug concentrations in other brain regions and also in peripheral tissues may promote side effect potentiation. Second, multidrug transporters such as Pgp serve a variety of physiological functions including the protection from xenobiotics. Other xenobiotics taken up by the body may be more harmful in the presence of efflux transporter inhibitors due to the influence on their distribution. Furthermore Pgp and MRPs may protect brain parenchymal cells from apoptosis (Pallis et al., 2003; Gennuso et al., 2004), and transporter inhibition may thus promote cell death. Nevertheless, transient inhibition of efflux transporters by short-term administration of inhibitors may be a tolerable strategy to reverse or prevent drug resistance due to overexpression of transporters in brain tumor cells or at the BBB.

An alternative approach which avoids compromise of the protective function of efflux transporters is to bypass transporter molecules. Different strategies are followed in this regard, including peptide conjugation (Mazel et al., 2001) or nanoparticle encapsulation (Huwyler et al., 1996; Kreuter, 2001; Fricker and Miller, 2004) of transporter substrates. Furthermore, as pointed out above, increasing knowledge about the regulation of transporter expression may help to develop strategies to interfere with the induction of transporter expression.

The development of imaging techniques based on positron emission tomography renders the opportunity to noninvasively study Pgp mediated transport and its modulation in vivo (Hendrikse and Vaalburg, 2002; Elsinga et al., 2004; Lee et al., 2006). This opens possibilities for selection of patients who may benefit from coadministration of efflux transporter inhibitors in order to enhance brain penetration and efficacy of the CNS-active drugs that they receive.

10   Conclusions

In recent years, awareness of the impact of brain efflux transporters on protection of brain tissue and on treatment of CNS diseases has increased progressively. Cumulative knowledge about the structure, function, localization, and substrate specificities of brain efflux transporters helps to develop and validate strategies to deal with the activity of these transporters in a clinical setting. Special interest arose in the regulation of transporter expression or function in pathophysiological conditions, which may contribute to disease development or progression but may also influence the pharmacotherapeutic outcome. The contribution of efflux transporter to therapeutic failure in CNS diseases has led to the recognition of brain efflux transporters as targets to modulate brain penetration rates.

Future research focusing on both the physiological and pathophysiological functions of brain efflux transporters and their regulation should help to further elucidate the role of such transporters. Gain in knowledge may allow optimization of strategies for modulation of transporter function taking their spectrum of protective functions into consideration.

References

Abbott NJ, Khan EU, Rollinson CMS, Reichel A, Janigro D, et al. 2002. Drug resistance in epilepsy: The role of the blood-brain barrier. Mechanisms of Drug Resistance in Epilepsy. Lessons from Oncology. Ling V, editor. Chichester: Wiley; pp. 38-47.

Ambudkar SV, Sauna ZE, Gottesman MM, Szakacs G. 2005. Trends Pharmacol Sci 26: 385-387.

Ando H, Yanagihara H, Sugimoto K, Hayashi Y, Tsuruoka S, et al. 2005. Daily rhythms of P-glycoprotein expression in mice. Chronobiol Int 22: 655-665.

Aronica E, Gorter JA, Jansen GH, van Veelen CW, van Rijen PC, et al. 2003. Expression and cellular distribution of multidrug transporter proteins in two major causes of medically intractable epilepsy: Focal cortical dysplasia and glioneuronal tumors. Neuroscience 118: 417-429.

Aronica E, Gorter JA, Ramkema M, Redeker S, Ozbas-Gercerer F, et al. 2004. Expression and cellular distribution of multidrug resistance-related proteins in the hippocampus of patients with mesial temporal lobe epilepsy. Epilepsia 45: 441-451.

Awasthi S, Hallene KL, Fazio V, Singhal SS, Cucullo L, et al. 2005. RLIP76, a non-ABC transporter, and drug resistance in epilepsy. BMC Neurosci 6: 61

Baker EK, Johnstone RW, Zalcberg JR, El-Osta A. 2005. Epigenetic changes to the MDR1 locus in response to chemotherapeutic drugs. Oncogene 24: 8061-8075.

Bart J, Groen HJ, Hendrikse NH, van der Graaf WT, Vaalburg W, et al. 2000. The blood-brain barrier and oncology: New insights into function and modulation. Cancer Treat Rev 26: 449-462.

Bates SF, Chen C, Robey R, Kang M, Figg WD, et al. 2002. Reversal of multidrug resistance: Lessons from clinical oncology. Novartis Found Symp 243: 83-96.

Bauer B, Hartz AM, Fricker G, Miller DS. 2004. Pregnane X receptor up-regulation of P-glycoprotein expression and transport function at the blood-brain barrier. Mol Pharmacol 66: 413-419.

Bauer B, Hartz AM, Fricker G, Miller DS. 2005. Modulation of P-glycoprotein transport function at the blood-brain barrier. Exp Biol Med 230: 118-127.

Begley DJ. 2004. ABC transporters and the blood-brain barrier. Curr Pharm Des 10: 1295-1312.

Bendayan R, Lee G, Bendayan M. 2002. Functional expression and localization of P-glycoprotein at the blood–brain barrier. Microsc Res Tech 57: 365-380.

Berezowski V, Landry C, Dehouck MP, Cecchelli R, Fenart L. 2004. Contribution of glial cells and pericytes to the mRNA profiles of P-glycoprotein and multidrug resistance-associated proteins in an in vitro model of the blood-brain barrier. Brain Res 1018: 1-9.

Borst P, Evers R, Kool M, Wijnholds J. 1999. The multidrug resistance protein family. Biochim Biophys Acta 1461: 347-357.

Borst P, Evers R, Kool M, Wijnholds J. 2000. A family of drug transporters: The multidrug resistance-associated proteins. J Natl Cancer Inst 92: 1295-1302.

Boulton DW, De Vane CL, Liston HL, Markowitz JS. 2002. In vitro P-glycoprotein affinity for atypical and conventional antipsychotics. Life Sci 71: 163-169.

Brandt C, Bethmann K, Gastens AM, Löscher W. 2006. The multidrug transporter hypothesis of drug resistance in epilepsy: Proof-of-principle in a rat model of temporal lobe epilepsy. Neurobiol Dis 24: 202-211.

Breedveld P, Beijnen JH, Schellens JH. 2006. Use of P-glycoprotein and BCRP inhibitors to improve oral bioavailability and CNS penetration of anticancer drugs. Trends Pharmacol Sci 27: 17-24.

Chishty M, Reichel A, Siva J, Abbott NJ, Begley DJ. 2001. Affinity for the P-glycoprotein efflux pump at the blood-brain barrier may explain the lack of CNS side-effects of modern antihistamines. J Drug Target 9: 223-228.

Choo EF, Kurnik D, Muszkat M, Ohkubo T, Shay SD, et al. 2006. Differential in vivo sensitivity to inhibition of P-glycoprotein located in lymphocytes, testes, and the blood-brain barrier. Pharmacol Exp Ther 317: 1012–1018.

Choudhuri S, Cherrington NJ, Li N, Klaassen CD. 2003. Constitutive expression of various xenobiotic and endobiotic transporter mRNAs in the choroid plexus of rats. Drug Metab Dispos 31: 1337-1345.

Cirrito JR, Deane R, Fagan AM, Spinner ML, Parsadanian M, et al. 2005. P-glycoprotein deficiency at the blood-brain barrier increases amyloid-β disposition in an Alzheimer disease mouse model. J Clin Invest 115: 3285-3290.

Cisternino S, Mercier C, Bourasset F, Roux F, Scherrmann JM. 2004. Expression, up-regulation, and transport activity of the multidrug-resistance protein Abcg2 at the mouse blood-brain barrier. Cancer Res 64: 3296-3301.

Clinckers R, Smolders I, Meurs A, Ebinger G, Michotte Y. 2005. Quantitative in vivo microdialysis study on the influence of multidrug transporters on the blood-brain barrier passage of oxcarbazepine: Concomitant use of hippocampal monoamines as pharmacodynamic markers for the anticonvulsant activity. Pharmacol Exp Ther 314: 725–731.

Cooray HC, Blackmore CG, Maskell L, Barrand MA. 2002. Localisation of breast cancer resistance protein in microvessel endothelium of human brain. Neuroreport 13: 2059-2063.

Cordon-Cardo C, O'Brien JP, Casals D, Rittman-Grauer L, Biedler JL, et al. 1989. Multidrug-resistance gene (P-glycoprotein) is expressed by endothelial cells at blood-brain barrier sites. Proc Natl Acad Sci USA 86: 695-698.

Crivori P, Reinach B, Pezzetta D, Poggesi I. 2006. Computational models for identifying potential P-glycoprotein substrates and inhibitors. Mol Pharm 3: 33-44.

Dagenais C, Graff CL, Pollack GM. 2004. Variable modulation of opioid brain uptake by P-glycoprotein in mice. Biochem Pharmacol 67: 269-276.

Decleves X, Regina A, Laplanche JL, Roux F, Boval B, et al. 2000. Functional expression of P-glycoprotein and multidrug resistance—associated protein (Mrp1) in primary cultures of rat astrocytes. J Neurosci Res 60: 594-602.

Deguchi T, Isozaki K, Yousuke K, Terasaki T, Otagiri M. 2006. Involvement of organic anion transporters in the efflux of uremic toxins across the blood-brain barrier. J Neurochem 96: 1051-1059.

de Lange EC. 2004. Potential role of ABC transporters as a detoxification system at the blood-CSF barrier. Adv Drug Deliv Rev 56: 1793-1809.

de Lange EC, Marchand S, van den Berg D, van der Sandt IC, de Boer AG, et al. 2000. In vitro and in vivo investigations on fluoroquinolones: Effects of the P-glycoprotein efflux transporter on brain distribution of sparfloxacin. Eur J Pharm Sci 12: 85-93.

Demeule M, Jodoin J, Gingras D, Beliveau R. 2000. P-glycoprotein is localized in caveolae in resistant cells and in brain capillaries. FEBS Lett 466: 219-224.

Demeule M, Regina A, Jodoin J, Laplante A, Dagenais C, et al. 2002. Drug transport to the brain: Key roles for the efflux pump P-glycoprotein in the blood-brain barrier. Vascul Pharmacol 38: 339-348.

Didier AD, Loor F. 1995. Decreased biotolerability for ivermectin and cyclosporin A in mice exposed to potent P-glycoprotein inhibitors. Int J Cancer 63: 263-267.

Dombrowski SM, Desai SY, Marroni M, Cucullo L, Goodrich K, et al. 2001. Overexpression of multiple drug resistance genes in endothelial cells from patients with refractory epilepsy. Epilepsia 42: 1501-1506.

Drozdzik M, Bialecka M, Mysliwiec K, Honczarenko K, Stankiewicz J, Sych Z. 2003. Polymorphism in the P-glycoprotein drug transporter MDR1 gene: A possible link between environmental and genetic factors in Parkinson's disease. Pharmacogenetics 13: 259-263.

Edwards JE, Brouwer KR, McNamara PJ. 2002. GF120918, a P-glycoprotein modulator, increases the concentration of unbound amprenavir in the central nervous system in rats. Antimicrob Agents Chemother 46: 2284-2286.

Eisenblatter T, Huwel S, Galla HJ. 2003. Characterisation of the brain multidrug resistance protein (BMDP/ABCG2/BCRP) expressed at the blood-brain barrier. Brain Res 971: 221-231.

Ejsing TB, Linnet K. 2005. Influence of P-glycoprotein inhibition on the distribution of the tricyclic antidepressant nortriptyline over the blood-brain barrier. Hum Psychopharmacol 20: 149-153.

Elsinga PH, Hendrikse NH, Bart J, Vaalburg W, van Waarde A. 2004. PET Studies on P-glycoprotein function in the blood-brain barrier: How it affects uptake and binding of drugs within the CNS. Curr Pharm Des 10: 1493-1503.

Felix RA, Barrand MA. 2002. P-glycoprotein expression in rat brain endothelial cells: Evidence for regulation by transient oxidative stress. J Neurochem 80: 64-72.

Fellay J, Marzolini C, Meaden ER, Back DJ, Buclin T, et al. 2002. Response to antiretroviral treatment in HIV-1-infected individuals with allelic variants of the multidrug resistance transporter 1: A pharmacogenetics study. Lancet 359: 30-36.

Fellner S, Bauer B, Miller DS, Schaffrik M, Fankhanel M, et al. 2002. Transport of paclitaxel (Taxol) across the blood-brain barrier in vitro and in vivo. J Clin Invest 110: 1309-1318.

Fricker G, Miller DS. 2004. Modulation of drug transporters at the blood-brain barrier. Pharmacology 70: 169-176.

Furuno T, Landi MT, Ceroni M, Caporaso N, Bernucci I, et al. 2002. Expression polymorphism of the blood-brain barrier component P-glycoprotein (MDR1) in relation to Parkinson's disease. Pharmacogenetics 12: 529-534.

Ganapathy V, Miyauchi S. 2005. Transport systems for opioid peptides in mammalian tissues. AAPS J 7: 852-856.

Gao B, Meier PJ. 2001. Organic anion transport across the choroid plexus. Microsc Res Tech 52: 60-64.

Gao B, Hagenbuch B, Kullak-Ublick GA, Benke D, Aguzzi A, Meier PJ. 2000. Organic anion-transporting polypeptides mediate transport of opioid peptides across blood-brain barrier. J Pharmacol Exp Ther 294: 73-79.

Gennuso F, Fernetti C, Tirolo C, Testa N, L'Episcopo F, et al. 2004. Bilirubin protects astrocytes from its own toxicity by inducing up-regulation and translocation of multidrug resistance-associated protein 1 (Mrp1). Proc Natl Acad Sci USA 101: 2470-2475.

Goralski KB, Hartmann G, Piquette-Miller M, Renton KW. 2003. Downregulation of mdr1a expression in the brain and liver during CNS inflammation alters the in vivo disposition of digoxin. Br J Pharmacol 139: 35-48.

Grauer MT, Uhr M. 2004. P-glycoprotein reduces the ability of amitriptyline metabolites to cross the blood brain barrier in mice after a 10-day administration of amitriptyline. J Psychopharmacol 18: 66-74.

Gutmann H, Torok M, Fricker G, Huwyler J, Beglinger C, et al. 1999. Modulation of multidrug resistance protein expression in porcine brain capillary endothelial cells in vitro. Drug Metab Dispos 27: 937-941.

Hagenbuch B, Meier PJ. 2003. The superfamily of organic anion transporting polypeptides. Biochim Biophys Acta 1609: 1-18.

Hanko E, Tommarello S, Watchko JF, Hansen TW. 2003. Administration of drugs known to inhibit P-glycoprotein increases brain bilirubin and alters the regional distribution of bilirubin in rat brain. Pediatr Res 54: 439-440.

Hartz AM, Bauer B, Fricker G, Miller DS. 2004. Rapid regulation of P-glycoprotein at the blood-brain barrier by endothelin-1. Mol Pharmacol 66: 387-394.

Hartz AM, Bauer B, Fricker G, Miller DS. 2006. Rapid modulation of P-glycoprotein-mediated transport at the blood-brain barrier by tumor necrosis factor-α and lipopolysaccharide. Mol Pharmacol 69: 462-470.

Hayashi K, Pu H, Tian J, Andras IE, Lee YW, et al. 2005. HIV-Tat protein induces P-glycoprotein expression in brain microvascular endothelial cells. J Neurochem 93: 1231-1241.

Hendrikse NH, Vaalburg W. 2002. Dynamics of multidrug resistance: P-glycoprotein analyses with positron emission tomography. Methods 27: 228-233.

Higgins CF, Linton KJ. 2003. ABC transporters: An introduction and overview. ABC proteins from bacteria to man. Holland IB, Cole SPC, Kuchler K, Higgins CF., editors. London: Academic Press; pp.17-23.

Higgins CF, Hiles ID, Salmond GPC, Gill DR, Downie JA, et al. 1986. A family of related ATP-binding subunits coupled to many distinct biological processes in bacteria. Nature 323: 448-450.

Hirrlinger J, Konig J, Dringen R. 2002. Expression of mRNAs of multidrug resistance proteins (MRPs) in cultured rat astrocytes, oligodendrocytes, microglial cells and neurones. J Neurochem 82: 716-719.

Ho EA, Piquette-Miller M. 2006. Regulation of multidrug resistance by pro-inflammatory cytokines. Curr Cancer Drug Targets 6: 295-311.

Hoffmann K, Löscher W. 2006. Up-regulation of brain expression of P-glycoprotein in MRP2-deficient TR- rats resembles seizure-induced up-regulation of this drug efflux transporter in normal rats. Epilepsia 69: 1-14.

Huang R, Murry DJ, Kolwankar D, Hall SD, Foster DR. 2006. Vincristine transcriptional regulation of efflux drug transporters in carcinoma cell lines. Biochem Pharmacol 71: 1695-1704.

Huwyler J, Wu D, Pardridge WM. 1996. Brain drug delivery of small molecules using immunoliposomes. Proc Natl Acad Sci USA 93: 14164-14169.

Iannetti P, Spalice A, Parisi P. 2005. Calcium-channel blocker verapamil administration in prolonged and refractory status epilepticus. Epilepsia 46: 967-969.

Jekerle V, Klinkhammer W, Scollard DA, Breitbach K, Reilly RM, et al. 2006. In vitro and in vivo evaluation of WK-X-34, a novel inhibitor of P-glycoprotein and BCRP, using radio imaging techniques. Int J Cancer 119: 414-422.

Jodoin J, Demeule M, Fenart L, Cecchelli R, Farmer S, et al. 2003. P-glycoprotein in blood-brain barrier endothelial cells: Interaction and oligomerization with caveolins. J Neurochem 87: 1010-1023.

Juliano RL, Ling V. 1976. A surface glycoprotein modulating drug permeability in Chinese hamster ovary cell mutants. Biochim Biophys Acta 455: 152-162.

Kamel F, Hoppin JA. 2004. Association of pesticide exposure with neurologic dysfunction and disease. Environ Health Perspect 112: 950-958.

Karssen AM, Meijer OC, van der Sandt IC, de Boer AG, de Lange EC, et al. 2002. The role of the efflux transporter P-glycoprotein in brain penetration of prednisolone. J Endocrinol 175: 251-260.

Kastin AJ, Fasold MB, Smith RR, Horner KA, Zadina JE. 2001. Saturable brain-to-blood transport of endomorphins. Exp Brain Res 139: 70-75.

Kemper EM, Boogerd W, Thuis I, Beijnen JH, van Tellingen O. 2004. Modulation of the blood-brain barrier in oncology: Therapeutic opportunities for the treatment of brain tumours? Cancer Treat Rev 30: 415-423.

Kerb R. 2006. Implications of genetic polymorphisms in drug transporters for pharmacotherapy. Cancer Lett 234: 4-33.

Kim AE, Dintaman JM, Waddell DS, Silverman JA. 1998a. Saquinavir, an HIV protease inhibitor, is transported by P-glycoprotein. J Pharmacol Exp Ther 286: 1439-1445.

Kim DW, Kim M, Lee SK, Kang R, Lee SY. 2006. Lack of association between C3435T nucleotide MDR1 genetic polymorphism and multidrug resistant epilepsy. Seizure 15: 344-347.

Kim RB. 2003. Organic anion-transporting polypeptide (OATP) transporter family and drug disposition. Eur J Clin Invest 33: 1-5.

Kim RB, Fromm MF, Wandel C, Leake B, Wood AJ, et al. 1998b. The drug transporter P-glycoprotein limits oral absorption and brain entry of HIV-1 protease inhibitors. J Clin Invest 101: 289-294.

King M, Su W, Chang A, Zuckerman A, Pasternak GW. 2001. Transport of opioids from the brain to the periphery by P-glycoprotein: Peripheral actions of central drugs. Nat Neurosci 4: 268-274.

Koopen NR, Wolters H, Havinga R, Vonk RJ, Jansen PL, et al. 1998. Impaired activity of the bile canalicular organic anion transporter (MRP2/cmoat) is not the main cause of ethinylestradiol-induced cholestasis in the rat. Hepatology 27: 537-545.

Kreuter J. 2001. Nanoparticulate systems for brain delivery of drugs. Adv Drug Deliv Rev 47: 65-81.

Kusuhara H, Suzuki H, Naito M, Tsuruo T, Sugiyama Y. 1998. Characterization of efflux transport of organic anions in a mouse brain capillary endothelial cell line. J Pharmacol Exp Ther 285: 1260-1265.

Lai BC, Marion SA, Teschke K, Tsui JK. 2002. Occupational and environmental risk factors for Parkinson's disease. Parkinsonism Relat Disord 8: 297-309.

Lam FC, Liu R, Lu P, Shapiro AB, Renoir JM, et al. 2001. β-Amyloid efflux mediated by P-glycoprotein. J Neurochem 76: 1121-1128.

Langford D, Grigorian A, Hurford R, Adame A, Ellis RJ, et al. 2004. Altered P-glycoprotein expression in AIDS patients with HIV encephalitis. J Neuropathol Exp Neurol 63: 1038-1047.

Lee G, Bendayan R. 2004. Functional expression and localization of P-glycoprotein in the central nervous system: Relevance to the pathogenesis and treatment of neurological disorders. Pharm Res 21: 1313-1330.

Lee G, Dallas S, Hong M, Bendayan R. 2001. Drug transporters in the central nervous system: Brain barriers and brain parenchyma considerations. Pharmacol Rev 53: 569-596.

Lee YJ, Kusuhara H, Sugiyama Y. 2004. Do multidrug resistance-associated protein-1 and -2 play any role in the elimination of estradiol-17 β-glucuronide and 2,4-dinitrophenyl-S-glutathione across the blood-cerebrospinal fluid barrier? J Pharm Sci 93: 99-107.

Lee YJ, Maeda J, Kusuhara H, Okauchi T, Inaji M, et al. 2006. In vivo evaluation of P-glycoprotein function at the blood-brain barrier in nonhuman primates using [^{11}C]verapamil. J Pharmacol Exp Ther 316: 647-653.

Leslie EM, Deeley RG, Cole SP. 2001. Toxicological relevance of the multidrug resistance protein 1 MRP1 (ABCC1) and related transporters. Toxicology 167: 3-23.

Letrent SP, Pollack GM, Brouwer KR, Brouwer KL. 1999. Effects of a potent and specific P-glycoprotein inhibitor on the blood-brain barrier distribution and antinociceptive effect of morphine in the rat. Drug Metab Dispos 27: 827-834.

Löscher W, Potschka H. 2005a. Role of drug efflux transporters in the brain for drug disposition and treatment of brain diseases. Prog Neurobiol 76: 22-76.

Löscher W, Potschka H. 2005b. Drug resistance in brain diseases and the role of drug efflux transporters. Nat Rev Neurosci 6: 591-602.

Marchi N, Hallene KL, Kight KM, Cucullo L, Moddel G, et al. 2004. Significance of MDR1 and multiple drug resistance in refractory human epileptic brain. BMC Med 2: 37.

Martin M, Higgins CF, Callaghan R. 2001. The vinblastine binding site adopts high and low affinity conformations during the transport cycle of P-glycoprotein. Biochemistry 40: 15733-15742.

Masuyama H, Suwaki N, Tateishi Y, Nakatsukasa H, Segawa T, et al. 2005. The pregnane X receptor regulates gene expression in a ligand- and promoter-selective fashion. Mol Endocrinol 19: 1170-1180.

Mazel M, Clair P, Rousselle C, Vidal P, Scherrmann JM, et al. 2001. Doxorubicin-peptide conjugates overcome multidrug resistance. Anticancer Drugs 12: 107-116.

McRae MP, Brouwer KL, Kashuba AD. 2003. Cytokine regulation of P-glycoprotein. Drug Metab Rev 35: 19-33.

Mealey KL, Bentjen SA, Gay JM, Cantor GH. 2001. Ivermectin sensitivity in collies is associated with a deletion mutation of the mdr1 gene. Pharmacogenetics 11: 727-733.

Meijer OC, de Lange EC, Breimer DD, de Boer AG, Mercier C, Masseguin C, Roux F, Gabrion J, Scherrmann JM. 2004. Expression of P-glycoprotein (ABCB1) and Mrp1 (ABCC1) in adult rat brain: Focus on astrocytes. Brain Res 1021: 32-40.

Miller DS, Nobmann SN, Gutmann H, Toeroek M, Drewe J, et al. 2000. Xenobiotic transport across isolated brain microvessels studied by confocal microscopy. Mol Pharmacol 58: 1357-1367.

Neff MW, Robertson KR, Wong AK, Safra N, Broman KW, et al. 2004. Breed distribution and history of canine mdr1–1δ, a pharmacogenetic mutation that marks the emergence of breeds from the collie lineage. Proc Natl Acad Sci USA 101: 11725-11730.

Nies AT, Jedlitschky G, Konig J, Herold-Mende C, Steiner HH, et al. 2004. Expression and immunolocalization of the multidrug resistance proteins, MRP1-MRP6 (ABCC1-ABCC6), in human brain. Neuroscience 129: 349-360.

Notenboom S, Wouterse AC, Peters B, Kuik LH, Heemskerk S, et al. 2006. Increased apical insertion of the multidrug resistance protein 2 (MRP2/ABCC2) in renal proximal tubules following gentamicin exposure. J Pharmacol Exp Ther 318: 1194-1202.

O'Brien JP, Cordon-Cardo C. 1996. P-glycoprotein expression in normal human tissues. Multidrug resistance in cancer cells. Gupta S, Tsuruo T, editors. Chichester: John Wiley & Sons; pp. 285-291.

Pallis M, Turzanski J, Grundy M, Seedhouse C, Russell N. 2003. Resistance to spontaneous apoptosis in acute myeloid leukaemia blasts is associated with P-glycoprotein expression and function, but not with the presence of FLT3 internal tandem duplications. Br J Haematol 120: 1009-1016.

Pardridge WM. 1999. Blood-brain barrier biology and methodology. J Neurovirol 5: 556-569.

Pardridge WM. 2003. Blood-brain barrier drug targeting The future of brain drug development. Mol Interv 3: 90-105.

Pardridge WM, Golden PL, Kang YS, Bickel U. 1997. Brain microvascular and astrocyte localization of P-glycoprotein. J Neurochem 68: 1278-1285.

Pariante CM, Thomas SA, Lovestone S, Makoff A, Kerwin RW. 2004. Do antidepressants regulate how cortisol affect the brain? Psychoneuroendocrinology 29: 423-447.

Plotsky PM, Owens MJ, Nemeroff CB. 1998. Psychoneuroendocrinology of depression. Hypothalamic-pituitary-adrenal axis. Psychiatr Clin North Am 21: 293-307.

Potschka H, Löscher W. 2001. Multidrug resistance-associated protein is involved in the regulation of extracellular levels of phenytoin in the brain. Neuroreport 12: 2387-2389.

Potschka H, Fedrowitz M, Löscher W. 2001. P-Glycoprotein and multidrug resistance-associated protein are involved in the regulation of extracellular levels of the major antiepileptic drug carbamazepine in the brain. Neuroreport 12: 3557-3560.

Potschka H, Fedrowitz M, Löscher W. 2003. Multidrug resistance protein MRP2 contributes to blood-brain barrier function and restricts antiepileptic drug activity. J Pharmacol Exp Ther 306: 124-131.

Potschka H, Volk HA, Löscher W. 2004. Pharmacoresistance and expression of multidrug transporter P-glycoprotein in kindled rats. Neuroreport 15: 1657-1661.

Rajagopal A, Simon SM. 2003. Subcellular localization and activity of multidrug resistance proteins. Mol Biol Cell 14: 3389-3399.

Rao VV, Dahlheimer JL, Bardgett ME, Snyder AZ, Finch RA, et al. 1999. Choroid plexus epithelial expression of MDR1 P-glycoprotein and multidrug resistance-associated protein contribute to the blood—cerebrospinal-fluid drug-permeability barrier. Proc Natl Acad Sci USA 96: 3900-3905.

Regina A, Demeule M, Laplante A, Jodoin J, Dagenais C, et al. 2001. Multidrug resistance in brain tumors: Roles of the blood-brain barrier. Cancer Metastasis Rev 20: 13-25.

Regina A, Koman A, Piciotti M, El Hafny B, Center MS, et al. 1998. Mrp1 multidrug resistance-associated protein and P-glycoprotein expression in rat brain microvessel endothelial cells. J Neurochem 71: 705-715.

Rizzi M, Caccia S, Guiso G, Richichi C, Gorter JA, et al. 2002. Limbic seizures induce P-glycoprotein in rodent brain: Functional implications for pharmacoresistance. J Neurosci 22: 5833-5839.

Roberts RL, Joyce PR, Mulder RT, Begg EJ, Kennedy MA. 2002. A common P-glycoprotein polymorphism is associated with nortriptyline-induced postural hypotension in patients treated for major depression. Pharmacogenomics 2: 191-196.

Sadeque AJ, Wandel C, He H, Shah S, Wood AJ. 2000. Increased drug delivery to the brain by P-glycoprotein inhibition. Clin Pharmacol Ther 68: 231-237.

Sakaeda T, Nakamura T, Okumura K. 2004. Pharmacogenetics of drug transporters and its impact on the pharmacotherapy. Curr Top Med Chem 4: 1385-1398.

Sakata A, Tamai I, Kawazu K, Deguchi Y, Ohnishi T, et al. 1994. In vivo evidence for ATP-dependent and P-glycoprotein-mediated transport of cyclosporin A at the blood-brain barrier. Biochem Pharmacol 48: 1989-1992.

Sasabe H, Kato Y, Suzuki T, Itose M, Miyamoto G, et al. 2004. Differential involvement of multidrug resistance-associated protein 1 and P-glycoprotein in tissue distribution and excretion of grepafloxacin in mice. J Pharmacol Exp Ther 310: 648-655.

Scheffer GL, Scheper RJ. 2002. Drug resistance molecules: Lessons from oncology. Novartis Found Symp 243: 19-31.

Schinkel AH. 1999. P-Glycoprotein, a gatekeeper in the blood-brain barrier. Adv Drug Deliv Rev 36: 179-194.

Schinkel AH, Jonker JW. 2003. Mammalian drug efflux transporters of the ATP binding cassette (ABC) family: An overview. Adv Drug Deliv Rev 55: 3-29.

Schinkel AH, Wagenaar E, Mol CA, van Deemter L. 1996. P-glycoprotein in the blood-brain barrier of mice influences the brain penetration and pharmacological activity of many drugs. J Clin Invest 97: 2517-2524.

Schlachetzki F, Pardridge WM. 2003. P-glycoprotein and caveolin-1α in endothelium and astrocytes of primate brain. Neuroreport 14: 2041-2046.

Seelig A, Landwojtowicz E. 2000. Structure-activity relationship of P-glycoprotein substrates and modifiers. Eur J Pharm Sci 12: 31-40.

Senior AE, Al-Shawi MK, Urbatsch IL. 1995. The catalytic cycle of P-glycoprotein. FEBS Lett 377: 285-289.

Shapiro AB, Fox K, Lee P, Yang YD, Ling V. 1998. Functional intracellular P-glycoprotein. Int J Cancer 76: 857-864.

Shtil AA, Azare, J. 2005. Redundancy of biological regulation as the basis of emergence of multidrug resistance. Int Rev Cytol 246: 1-29.

Siddiqui A, Kerb R, Weale ME, Brinkmann U, Smith A, et al. 2003. Association of multidrug resistance in epilepsy with a polymorphism in the drug-transporter gene ABCB1. N Engl J Med 348: 1442-1448.

Sills GJ, Kwan P, Butler E, de Lange EC, van den Berg DJ, et al. 2002. P-glycoprotein-mediated efflux of antiepileptic drugs: Preliminary studies in mdr1a knockout mice. Epilepsy Behav 3: 427-432.

Sills GJ, Mohanraj R, Butler E, Mc Crindle S, Collier L, et al. 2005. Lack of association between the C3435T polymorphism in the human multidrug resistance (MDR1) gene and response to antiepileptic drug treatment. Epilepsia 46: 643-647.

Sisodiya SM. 2003. Mechanisms of antiepileptic drug resistance. Curr Opin Neurol 16: 197-201.

Sisodiya SM, Lin WR, Harding BN, Squier MV, Thom M. 2002. Drug resistance in epilepsy: Expression of drug resistance proteins in common causes of refractory epilepsy. Brain 125: 22-31.

Sisodiya SM, Martinian L, Scheffer GL, van der Valk P, Cross JH, et al. 2003. Major vault protein, a marker of drug resistance, is upregulated in refractory epilepsy. Epilepsia 44: 1388-1396.

Soranzo N, Cavalleri GL, Weale ME, Wood NW, Depondt C, et al. 2004. Identifying candidate causal variants responsible for altered activity of the ABCB1 multidrug resistance gene. Genome Res 14: 1333-1344.

Summers MA, Moore JL, McAuley JW. 2004. Use of verapamil as a potential P-glycoprotein inhibitor in a patient with refractory epilepsy. Ann Pharmacother 38: 1631-1634.

Sun H, Dai H, Shaik N, Elmquist WF. 2003. Drug efflux transporters in the CNS. Adv Drug Deliv Rev 55: 83-105.

Sun H, Johnson DR, Finch RA, Sartorelli AC, Miller DW, Elmquist WF. 2001. Transport of fluorescein in MDCKII-MRP1 transfected cells and mrp1-knockout mice. Biochem Biophys Res Commun 248: 863-869.

Tamai I, Kido Y, Yamashita J, Sai Y, Tsuji A. 2000. Blood-brain barrier transport of H1-antagonist ebastine and its metabolite carebastine. J Drug Target 8: 383-393.

Tan NC, Heron SE, Scheffer IE, Pelekanos JT, McMahon JM, et al. 2004. Failure to confirm association of a polymorphism in ABCB1 with multidrug-resistant epilepsy. Neurology 63: 1090-1092.

Tchenio T, Havard M, Martinez LA, Dautry F. 2006. Heat shock-independent induction of multidrug resistance by heat shock factor 1. Mol Cell Biol 26: 580-591.

Terasaki T, Ohtsuki S. 2005. Brain-to-blood transporters for endogenous substrates and xenobiotics at the blood-brain barrier: An overview of biology and methodology. NeuroRX 2: 63-72.

Thiebaut F, Tsuruo T, Hamada H, Gottesman MM, Pastan I, et al. 1989. Immunohistochemical localization in normal tissues of different epitopes in the multidrug transport protein P170: Evidence for localization in brain capillaries and crossreactivity of one antibody with a muscle protein. J Histochem Cytochem 37: 159-164.

Thomas H, Coley HM. 2003. Overcoming multidrug resistance in cancer: An update on the clinical strategy of inhibiting P-glycoprotein. Cancer Control 10: 159-165.

Thomas L. 2005. Pgp deficiency increases amyloid concentrations in the brain. Lancet Neurol 4: 798-799.

Thompson SJ, Koszdin K, Bernards CM. 2000. Opiate-induced analgesia is increased and prolonged in mice lacking P-glycoprotein. Anesthesiology 92: 1392-1399.

Thuerauf N, Fromm MF. 2006. The role of the transporter P-glycoprotein for disposition and effects of centrally acting drugs and for the pathogenesis of CNS diseases. Eur Arch Psychiatry Clin Neurosci 256: 281-286.

Toornvliet R, van Berckel BN, Luurtsema G, Lubberink M, Geldof AA, et al. 2006 Effect of age on functional P-glycoprotein in the blood-brain barrier measured by use of (R)-[^{11}C]verapamil and positron emission tomography. Clin Pharmacol Ther 79: 540-548.

Uhr M, Grauer MT. 2003. abcb1ab P-glycoprotein is involved in the uptake of citalopram and trimipramine into the brain of mice. J Psychiatr Res 37: 179-185.

Uhr M, Grauer MT, Holsboer F. 2003. Differential enhancement of antidepressant penetration into the brain in mice with abcb1ab (mdr1ab) P-glycoprotein gene disruption. Biol Psychiatry 54: 840-846.

Uhr M, Steckler T, Yassouridis A, Holsboer F. 2000. Penetration of amitriptyline, but not of fluoxetine, into brain is enhanced in mice with blood-brain barrier deficiency due to mdr1a P-glycoprotein gene disruption. Neuropsychopharmacology 22: 380-387.

van der Sandt I, Vos CM, Nabulsi L, Blom-Roosemalen MC, Voorwinden HH, et al. 2001. Assessment of active transport of HIV protease inhibitors in various cell lines and the in vitro blood–brain barrier. AIDS 15: 483-491.

van Zon A, Mossink MH, Schoester M, Scheper RJ, Sonneveld P, et al. 2004. Efflux kinetics and intracellular distribution of daunorubicin are not affected by major vault protein/lung resistance-related protein (vault) expression. Cancer Res 64: 4887-4892.

Vogelgesang S, Cascorbi I, Schroeder E, Pahnke J, Kroemer HK, et al. 2002. Deposition of Alzheimer's β-amyloid is inversely correlated with P-glycoprotein expression in the brains of elderly non-demented humans. Pharmacogenetics 12: 535-541.

Vogelgesang S, Warzok RW, Cascorbi I, Kunert-Keil C, Schroeder E, et al. 2004. The role of P-glycoprotein in cerebral amyloid angiopathy: Implications for the early pathogenesis of Alzheimer's disease. Curr Alzheimer Res 1: 121-125.

Volk H, Löscher W. 2005. Multidrug resistance in epilepsy: Rats with drug-resistant seizures exhibit enhanced brain expression of P-glycoprotein compared with rats with drug-responsive seizures. Brain 128: 1358-1368.

Volk H, Potschka H, Löscher W. 2005. Immunohistochemial localization of P-glycoprotein in rat brain and detection of its increased expression by seizures are sensitive to fixation and staining variables. J Histochem Cytochem 53: 517-531.

Volk HA, Burkhardt K, Potschka H, Chen J, Becker A, et al. 2004. Neuronal expression of the drug efflux transporter P-glycoprotein in the rat hippocampus after limbic seizures. Neuroscience 123: 751-759.

Wang JH, Scollard DA, Teng S, Reilly RM, Piquette-Miller M. 2005. Detection of P-glycoprotein activity in endotoxemic rats by 99m Tc-sestamibi imaging. J Nucl Med 46: 1537-1545.

Washington CB, Wiltshire HR, Man M, Moy T, Harris SR, et al. 2000. The disposition of saquinavir in normal and P-glycoprotein deficient mice, rats, and in cultured cells. Drug Metab Dispos 28: 1058-1062.

Wijnholds J, deLange EC, Scheffer GL, van den Berg DJ, Mol CA, van der Valk M, Schinkel AH, Scheper RJ, Breimer DD, Borst P. 2000. Multidrug resistance protein 1 protects the choroid plexus epithelium and contributes to the blood-cerebrospinal fluid barrier. J Clin Invest 105: 279-285.

Wojtal K, Trojnar MK, Czuczwar SJ. 2006. Endogenous neuroprotective factors: Neurosteroids. Pharmacol Rep 58: 335-340.

Yasui-Furukori N, Saito M, Nakagami T, Kaneda A, Tateishi T, Kaneko S. 2006. Prog Neuropsychopharmacol Biol Psychiatry 30: 286-291.

Zhang Y, Han H, Elmquist WF, Miller DW. 2000. Expression of various multidrug resistance-associated protein (MRP) homologues in brain microvessel endothelial cells. Brain Res 876: 148-153.

Zhu HJ, Liu GQ. 2004. Glutamate up-regulates P-glycoprotein expression in rat brain microvessel endothelial cells by an NMDA receptor-mediated mechanism. Life Sci 75: 1313-1322.

Zimprich F, Sunder-Plassmann R, Stogmann E, Gleiss A, Dal Bianco A, et al. 2004. Association of an ABCB1 gene haplotype with pharmacoresistance in temporal lobe epilepsy. Neurology 63: 1087-1089.

24 Blood–Retina Barriers

B. Schlosshauer

Abstract: Neurons of the retina are segregated from the blood stream via two different gateways: the inner and the outer blood–retina barriers (BRBs). The inner BRB consists of endothelial cells forming retinal capillaries. The inner barrier is similar to the microvascular blood–brain barrier (BBB) within other regions of the central nervous system (CNS). The outer blood–retina barrier (oBRB) is formed by the retinal pigment epithelium (RPE), which is positioned as interface between the neural retina and the nonneural choroid. In humans, only the inner two-thirds of the 250-μm thick retina is vascularized, and thus served by the inner blood barrier. The outer one-third of the retina is devoid of any vasculature and depends on nutrient/gas exchange via the RPE. Blood components reach the RPE from fenestrated, highly permeable blood vessels of the neighboring nonneuronal choroid. Despite the fact that both the endothelial and epithelial barriers have ontogenetically different origins and very diverging cellular structures, on the molecular and functional levels many similarities are evident. These include barrier characteristics based on tight junctions, carrier features with regard to transporters including P-glycoprotein (P-gp)/multidrug resistance protein, expression patterns of biotransformation enzymes, and immunological responses.

List of Abbreviations: ABC, ATP-binding cassette; BBB, blood–brain barrier; BRB, Blood–retina barrier; oBRB, outer blood–retina barrier; CAM, chorioallantoic membrane; CMV, cytomegalovirus; EAE, experimental allergic encephalomyelitis; EAU, experimental autoimmune uveoretinitis; GABA, γ-aminobutyric acid; GFAP, glial fibrillary astrocytic protein; γGT, γ-glutamyl transpeptidase; LIF, leukemia inhibitory factor; MCP-1, monocyte chemoattractant protein-1; MMPs, matrix metalloproteinases; MRP, mdr-associated proteins; NF-κB, nuclear factor-κB; PDGF, platelet-derived growth factor; P-gp, P-glycoprotein; P-gp/mdr, P-glycoprotein/multidrug resistance-1; RANTES, regulated on activation of normal T cell expressed and released; RPE, retinal pigment epithelium; SDF-1, stromal cell-derived factor-1; VEGF, vascular endothelial cell growth factor

1 Introduction

Neurons and glial cells of the retina of many higher vertebrates interact with components of the blood stream via two different vascular systems. One system is represented by blood vessels located in the retina, whereas the other system is a tissue sheet (the retinal pigment epithelium (RPE)) positioned between the retina and the nonneuronal choroid. The multitude of blood-borne components does not have direct access to the neuronal microenvironment of the retina but is filtered through barrier structures that are different for both systems. These barriers are referred to as inner and outer blood–retina barriers (BRBs), respectively. They consist of completely different cellular structures (Kupersmith and Shakib, 1989). The inner BRB is formed by endothelial cells of blood vessels whereas the outer barrier consists of pigment epithelium, which serves as a functional interface between the systemic blood vessels of the neighboring choroid and the neural retina. Various functional aspects are similar for the inner and outer barriers, most likely because the blood composition provides identical challenges and benefits at both locations.

A major function of the blood stream is to deliver essential nutrients to the retina. In addition, many cellular and molecular components impact the regular function of retinal networks. Furthermore, the temporal variations of the blood composition owing to food uptake/starvation, stress, circadian rhythm, etc., could seriously affect neural activity. The spatiotemporally controlled ion fluxes across neural cell membranes are the basis of neural communication. As this is critically dependent on a controlled homeostasis in the tissue parenchyma, any direct or indirect blood-borne impact on the ion equilibrium could have adverse effects. Similarly, blood-borne neuropeptides and neurotransmitters could disturb ligand-gated neural transmission. Glutamate, for example, as the prevalent excitatory neurotransmitter in the central nervous system (CNS), functions at a concentration 1000-fold lower than is present in blood (Törnquist and Alm, 1986). If retinal neurons would be exposed to such a high glutamate concentration, similar neurotoxic effects as observed during penumbra formation in the course of stroke would become evident. Uncontrolled exposure to glycine or the sudden, stress-induced release of norepinephrine would also counteract regular neural transmission (Pardridge, 1995).

Beside the need to be shielded from molecular constituents, the retina might also be affected by blood-borne cells such as patrolling leucocytes. In conjunction with the lack of lymph production and drainage, restriction of cell infiltration appears to be a prerequisite for preventing autoimmune attacks and cytokine interference between neuronal and immune communication pathways (Male, 1995). Furthermore, the exclusion of infectious microorganisms and viruses by BRBs is of fundamental importance also because of the limited access of immune-competent cells to the retinal microenvironment which otherwise could counteract microbial encounter.

The major aspect discussed so far has been the restriction of entry into the retinal parenchyma from the blood side. In addition, the reverse phenomenon is also evident, as limiting the exit of selected molecules from the retina has also been reported. As an example, dopamine diffusion out of the neuronal tissue has been interpreted as a mode to support neural function by reducing the anabolic load of the synthesizing neurons, which instead recycle the transmitter by a reuptake mechanism (Dowling, 1991).

It is obvious that a simple barrier would be deleterious, simply because of the fact that cells beyond the barrier would be deprived of sufficient nutritional supply. The primary protective function of BRBs would provoke fatal consequences. Thus, it is not surprising to find various selective transport systems in the BRBs. These transport systems facilitate or actively transfer defined low-molecular weight components such as glucose for neural energy consumption, essential amino acids, proteinaceous factors such as transferrin, and others (Banks and Kastin, 1997; Murakami et al., 2000; Sugiyama et al., 2001; Abbruscato et al., 2004). Depending on the component in question transport may be uni- or bidirectional, in the direction toward the neural microenvironment or toward the blood. As a consequence, transport results in accumulation or clearance of components in and out of the retina.

Beside these barrier/carrier aspects, BRBs represent a communication interface between blood-borne immune cells and the neural parenchyma. Communication of this sort includes antigen presentation by vascular endothelial cells and could, for example, represent an antiviral defense mechanism. On the other hand it may result in pathological conditions such as multiple sclerosis (MS) in the brain and related diseases in the eye (Liversidge et al., 1988; Risau et al., 1990; Prat et al., 2002; Xu et al., 2003).

Understanding the functioning of BRBs (and blood–brain barriers (BBBs)) has become a major issue in recent days, because many neurotargeting drugs fail due to insufficient passage into the neuronal parenchyma (Duvvuri et al., 2003; Terasaki et al., 2003). The reverse is also true, that many drug candidates for nonneuronal tissues need to be abandoned because they pass aberrantly into neuronal tissue and cause severe side effects (Misra et al., 2003). This chapter summarizes some fundamental aspects of BRBs.

2 Development of Blood–Retina Barriers

2.1 Principles of Blood Barrier Formation

As the retina is part of the CNS, most regulatory mechanisms during angiogenesis and subsequent blood barrier formation in the brain are also evident in the retina. Progenitor cells from the mesoderm differentiate to become angioblasts that form blood islands from which vasculogenesis starts. Subsequently, new capillaries sprout from the preexisting vascular network—a process referred to as angiogenesis (Carmeliet and Tessier-Lavigne, 2005). In the brain, angiogenesis follows an outside–in sequence mediated by a VEGF (vascular endothelial cell growth factor) concentration gradient originating from VEGF-synthesizing cells near the ventricle (Engelhardt and Risau, 1995; Gale and Yancopoulos, 1999). Hypoxia (see below) induces a differential but synergistic expression of angiogenic ligand and receptors: a direct induction of VEGF and subsequently an indirect induction of VEGF receptor 2 (VEGFR-2) by VEGF (Kremer et al., 1997). VEGF acts as mitogen and chemoattractant for endothelial cells (Risau, 1997).

Blood barrier characteristics are not evident in early embryonic brain capillaries but are induced only later by the developing brain parenchyma. Interspecies transplantation experiments provided clues concerning the regulatory cell interactions that induce formation of BBB properties. On the basis of unique nuclear morphology of quail cells, it was feasible to identify quail cells after transplantation into the chick in order to generate quail–chick chimeras. When embryonic quail brain fragments were transplanted into the developing chick coelomic cavity, endothelial host cells without barrier characteristics vascularized the grafted brain tissue and started to display barrier features (Stewart and Wiley, 1981). Conversely, when quail somites were transplanted into brain ventricles of the chick, host endothelial cells originating from the CNS invaded the transplant and lost their barrier properties. The data suggest that the microenvironment endothelial cells encounter determines the barrier–carrier phenotype and not the cell origin.

This assumption could be verified in another transplantation paradigm. Mouse brain tissue transplanted onto the embryonic chorioallantoic membrane (CAM) of the chick egg became vascularized by extracorporal chick blood vessels which normally lack BBB features. Within the transplanted mouse CNS environment, chick endothelial cells began to express the BBB marker (Schlosshauer and Herzog, 1990; Seulberger et al., 1990). In experiments with purified cell fractions, accumulating data indicated that glial cells induce barrier characteristics in the endothelium (Goldstein, 1988; Chishty et al., 2002).

When astrocytes present in the retina of rats and humans were transplanted into the anterior chamber of the rabbit eye, astrocytic cell aggregates were vascularized by blood vessels of the iris. In the newly formed vasculature of the transplanted cell aggregates, blood–barrier formation was initiated (Janzer and Raff, 1987). Co-culture experiments substantiated the view that glia produce diffusible differentiation factors that induce barrier characteristics (Meyer et al., 1991; Tontsch and Bauer, 1991; Lobrinus et al., 1992; Nagy and Martinez, 1992; Hamm et al., 2004). These experimental data originating from the adult system are in agreement with the fact that CNS capillaries start to develop barrier properties only from that period on when astrocytes start to differentiate (Liebner and Engelhardt, 2005). Endothelial cells are not predetermined to develop a blood barrier but remain developmentally plastic for a certain period. However, endothelial cell plasticity appears to be temporally restricted in some cases, because not all adult systemic endothelial cells can be induced to acquire the BBB phenotype. Another notable aspect is that the blood barrier remains in a metastable condition and depends on a permanent inductive input. Astrocytes have been shown to be partly responsible for induction and maintenance of BBB characteristics in endothelial cells (Abbott et al., 2006; Engelhardt, 2006).

Interestingly, reverse inductive interactions take place. Endothelial cells stimulate the differentiation of astrocytes in a first step through leukemia inhibitory factor (LIF) (Mi et al., 2001) and in a second step through platelet-derived growth factor (PDGF-BB), which results in the expression of SSeCKS (human ortholog gravin) (Lee et al., 2003). As a consequence, astrocytes downregulate VEGF and upregulate the prodifferentiation factor Ang-1, stopping further angiogenesis and inducing barrier maturation. Further cross talk with interacting cells is based on pericytes that align along endothelial tubes coincidentally with accumulation of heparan sulfate proteoglycans. Concomitantly, pericytes abrogate further endothelial cell proliferation by secretion of TGF-β, and consequently, help to stabilize the microanatomical architecture (Antonelli-Orlidge et al., 1989)

2.2 The Inner Blood–Retina Barrier

During early neuroembryogenesis the retina is formed as a protrusion of the diencephalon. Angioblasts of mesenchymal origin enter the eyecup via the optic fissure and start to populate the innermost retinal layer. First, vessels form at the superficial retina layer by end-to-end apposition and subsequently invade deeper layers by virtue of a complex branching process. As in the brain, sprouting is the predominant mechanism of retinal vascularization. In mice, vascularization proceeds from the center to the periphery (❷ Figure 24-1a–c). This process takes about 10 days (Michaelson, 1948; Connolly et al., 1988). Initially, newly formed vessels lack blood barrier characteristics.

Defined cell interactions regulate the spatial formation of the retinal vascular system based partly on a double blueprint mechanism: The neuronal layout affects glial growth pattern and the emerging glial pattern determines the endothelial cell growth (❷ Figure 24-2b–d). The concentrically oriented retinal ganglion cell axons, which are extended first during retinal histogenesis, represent guiding strands for astrocytes that infiltrate the mammalian retina from the optic nerve. Glial populations spread from the center to the periphery of the tissue. Subsequently, migratory endothelial cells follow astrocytic tracks and

◻ Figure 24-1

Stereotypical timing and morphology of retinal vascularization. (a–c) In mice, retinal vessels (*grey*) arise from the optic nerve around birth (P0), then extend radially in the superficial retina over 7–10 days to reach the periphery. (d) In primates, deeper capillary networks form by endothelial sprouting (*arrowheads*) from the previously formed superficial vascular network (*blurred*, in background). (e) In primates, shortly after retinal vessels form, capillary segments adjacent to nascent arteries (*arrows*) retract, to yield a periarterial capillary-free zone. (Reprinted from Nature 438, Gariano and Gardner (2005). Retinal angiogenesis in development and disease. p. 962, copyright 2006, with permission from Nature Publishing Group.)

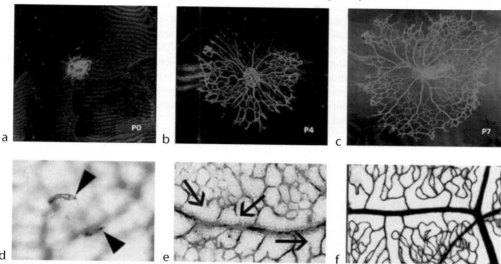

infiltrate the retina in the same direction from the optic nerve head toward the periphery. (Sandercoe et al., 1999; Gariano and Gardner, 2005). This has been shown both for the rat and cat retina (Ling and Stone, 1988; Ling et al., 1989). In the human retina, during this process a close association of both cell types and their processes has been evidenced at the ultrastructural level (Penfold et al., 1990), which is partially mediated by the cell surface adhesion molecule R-cadherin (Dorrell et al., 2002). Branching of vessels in the inner (superficial) and outer vascular plexuses is mediated by R-cadherin. Injection of antibodies directed against R-cadherin prevents the normally extensive collateralization observed during formation of the superficial network. Injection of anti-R-cadherin antibodies also dramatically affects vessels of the deep network (Dorrell et al., 2002).

Radial extension of the vascular network from the inner to outer retina layers is partly guided by Müller glia cells, which are oriented in a radial fashion through all retina layers. Astrocytes also appear to affect the formation of the collagenous matrix, which surrounds capillaries at the time of lumen formation in endothelial cells (Chan-Ling and Stone, 1992; Jiang et al., 1995). Conversely, endothelial cells direct astrocyte differentiation as demonstrated for the induction of expression of glial fibrillary acidic protein (GFAP). As indicated above, this cell–cell interaction is likely to be mediated by LIF as in the brain (Mi et al., 2001).

In the retina as well as in other tissues angiogenesis is hypoxia driven, in which an increasing demand of accumulating cells reduce the oxygen tension. This in turn stimulates the hypoxia-inducible cytokine expression of VEGF. Intracellular signaling of changing oxygen tension is mediated by the enzyme Egl9, which hydroxylates proline on the hypoxia-inducible factor HIF1α. At low oxygen levels hydroxylation fails, HIF1α dimerizes, translocates to the nucleus and binds to hypoxia-response elements of several genes, which as a whole leads to an angiogenic growth (Ohh et al., 2000; Jaakkola et al., 2001). With regard to directed angiogenesis, especially the matrix-bound isoforms VEGF164 and VEGF188 are thought to lay out

▢ Figure 24-2

Anatomy and histological organization of the retina. (a) Schematic cross-section through the human eye showing the vascularized retina lining the inner surface of the posterior two-thirds of the eye. The optic nerve (*arrow*) exits the eye at a slightly eccentric position. In primates, the central visual axis (*dotted line*) is centered on the fovea (*star*); see (f). (b–d) Similar distributions of blood vessels, neurons, and glia in a whole-mounted mouse retina. (b) Radially orientated ganglion cell axons (labeled *grey* for leptin receptor) exit the eye through the optic nerve (*arrow*). (c) Fluorescent dextran (*grey*) angiogram of adult retina; blood vessels also radiate from the optic nerve (*white arrow*) to the periphery. (d) Retinal astrocyte meshwork labeled for glial fibrillary acidic protein (*grey*) resembling that of blood vessels. (e) Human retinal cross-section showing capillaries and larger vessels (*star*) in the superficial nerve fiber layer (N). Deeper capillary networks (*arrows*) align within the ganglion cell (G) layer and along each side of the inner nuclear layer (I); the outer nuclear layer (O) is avascular, and receives blood components from choroidal vessels (*black arrow*) between the retina and the sclera (S), which is the outer white coat of the eye. Pathological angiogenesis is not confined to specific neuronal layers, and can grow into the vitreous cavity or outer retina. (f) In humans, a circular avascular zone of about 450 μm at the fovea (see *star* in (a)) improves central vision by reducing light scatter from blood vessels. (Reprinted from Nature 438, Gariano and Gardner (2005). Retinal angiogenesis in development and disease. p. 961, copyright 2006, with permission from Nature Publishing Group.)

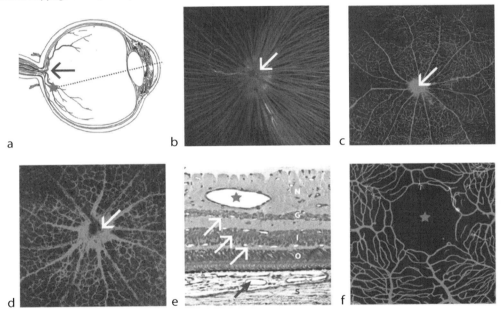

a   b   c

d   e   f

a guiding track along which growing vessels appropriately configure (Stalmans et al., 2002). Although VEGF appears to be more or less ubiquitously expressed in the retina, a variety of VEGF receptors are not (FLK1, FLK2, neuropilin-1, and -2) (Shih et al., 2003; Gariano et al., 2006). By activating corresponding receptors and different second messenger cascades, it becomes possible that a single factor sculpts the developing retinal vasculature by modifying migratory and proliferative responses selectively in closely associated endothelial cells. FLK2 activation elicits protrusion of endothelial tip cells at the leading edge of outgrowing blood vessels, whereas it stimulates mitosis in the more distal stalk cells of the same vessel (Gerhardt et al., 2003). It is noteworthy that VEGF fosters angiogenesis but would be counterproductive in barrier maturation, since it increases the leakiness of blood vessels (Ozaki et al., 1997). Therefore, after completion of angiogenesis, VEGF expression ceases in the retina (Gariano et al., 2006).

Exuberant vascular network formation and nonmixing of non-like vessels (arterial versus venous) is regulated by cell surface proteins. Repulsive ephrinB2–EphB4 signaling prevents mixing of arterial and venous endothelial cells, demarcates the boundaries between both cell populations, and secures assembly of "like" cells (Yancopoulos et al., 2000).

The overall microanatomy of the retinal vasculature resembles the cerebral circulation system and follows a similar developmental sequence. Vessels are formed initially in excess, and subsequently, the vascular network undergoes substantial remodeling during which capillary segments are pruned. In primates, shortly after retinal vessels form, capillary segments adjacent to nascent arteries retract, to yield a periarterial capillary-free zone. (❸ *Figure 24-1e*) (Hughes and Chang-Ling, 2000).

Notably, during various stages of remodeling in the retina, vascular segments lack or show reduced levels of the tight junction protein occludin (Morcos et al., 2001). Pronounced expression of occludin occurs only after vessel lumen has been formed (Russ et al., 1998). However, at most given time points, some vessels display already occludin immunoreactivity, whereas others do not or do only to a limited extent. Discontinuous occludin expression is most evident in the leading edge of vessel formation where endothelial cell migration occurs.

In summary, the development of the endothelial network and the formation of the inner BRB are characterized by a primary construction phase followed by a secondary destruction period until the adult layout is sculptured. Furthermore, the initial vascular network is leaky. The expression of barrier characteristics appears to be one of the latest steps during maturation.

2.3 The Outer Blood–Retina Barrier

The outer blood–retina barrier (oBRB) is formed by the retinal pigment epithelium (RPE). In contrast to the endothelial cell-based inner BRB barrier which is of mesodermal origin, the RPE originates from the neuroectoderm. During early embryogenesis optic vesicles arise bilaterally as dilatations of the prosencephalon. The primary optic vesicles invaginate at their lateral tips and form secondary optic vesicles (optic cups). Optic cups are bilayered in which both layers are initially separated by a ventricle-like fluid filled space. The inner layer differentiates into the neural retina and the outer layer becomes the RPE, the ultimate oBRB barrier (Mey and Thanos, 1992). Neural fate in one layer and not the other is likely to depend on the inductive action of acidic fibroblast growth factor (Guillemot and Cepko, 1992). In the future RPE, cell proliferation ceases rapidly and the potential to follow a neural fate in the native tissue environment in vivo is lost, although transdifferentiation can be still induced at later developmental stages in vitro (Zhao et al., 1997). The mature RPE is a monolayer of cubical cells underlying the neural retina.

3 Mature Blood–Retina Barriers

3.1 The Inner Blood–Retina Barrier

The vascular endothelium found in the adult retina and the brain is similar, though some differences exist, such as a higher density of interendothelial junctions and the lack of γ-glutamyl transpeptidase (γGT) in retinal endothelium (Vinores, 1995). In addition, retinal capillaries are not only invested by astrocytic processes but also by radial Müller glia cell processes, which are likely to affect maturation and maintenance of the BRB (Vinores, 1995).

Among different vertebrates specific features are evident. An inner BRB is found in humans, cats, and rats, but not in horses, rabbits, or chickens as retinas of these species are only partly or not vascularized. In the former species, the RPE provides nutritional supports only for the outer retina, in the latter species, where no retinal capillaries are present, the RPE barrier/carrier activity is essential for the complete retina (Kuwabara, 1979). In some species such as the chicken the so-called pecten is supposed to also transfer nutrients to the avascular retina. The pecten is a unique, highly vascularized structure extending into the vitreous, and consequently, not in direct contact with neuronal tissue (Wolburg et al., 1999).

For the high energy demands of the adult nervous system, oxygen and nutrients need to be delivered by a dense vascular network, with an average surface area of 100 cm^2/g tissue weight (Pardridge et al., 1990). The diffusion distance between capillaries and individual neurons does not exceed a few cell diameters in the mammalian CNS. Typically, the intercapillary distance is in the range of 50–75 μm. As outlined above, the retinal vascular system is inhomogeneous in the sense that higher vessel densities are found in the inner and outer plexuses located in the ganglion cell/optic fiber layers and the inner nuclear layer. In addition, in the outer nuclear layer capillaries are preferentially situated at the border of neighboring plexiform layers (❷ *Figure 24-2e*). Thin capillary walls (1 μm thickness) also keep diffusion distances small (Stewart and Tuor, 1994). Single endothelial cells form complete vascular tube segments. Consecutive vascular tube segments contact each other and thus form a capillary vessel.

On their abluminal surface, endothelial cells are covered by a porous basal lamina. Contractile pericytes, which are related to smooth muscle cells, are enclosed in the basal lamina sheet. Because of receptor expression for endothelin and other vasoactive amines, CNS pericytes are thought to control the luminal diameter of capillaries, and consequently blood flow. Beside that, pericytes are capable of rendering endothelial cells quiescent via transforming growth factor TGF-β. As indicated above TGF-β induces a growth arrest in endothelial cells (Orlidge and D'Amore, 1987; Kelley et al., 1988; Antonelli-Orlidge et al., 1989; Chakravarthy et al., 1992). Capillaries, including the basal lamina, pericytes, and endothelial cells, are engulfed by the endfeet of astrocytes. Though the collection of astrocytic endfeet, pericytes, and basal lamina might affect free diffusion, the inner blood barrier of the retina is exclusively related to the endothelial sheet, which displays complex arrays of tight junctions between neighboring cells (Reese and Karnovsky, 1967).

3.2 Tight Junctions at the Inner Blood–Retina Barrier

The tight junctions of nonfenestrated CNS capillaries contribute to the high transendothelial electrical resistance of some 2000 Ω cm^2 (Crone and Olesen, 1982). Tight junctions exclude even small potassium ions and water molecules, and thus abrogate paracellular diffusion via the intercellular space between neighboring endothelial cells. This is in contrast to fenestrated systemic capillaries such as those in the choroid with a very low resistance of 5–10 Ω cm^2 and fairly nonselective diffusion of substances.

Tight junctions represent the local fusion of two neighboring cell membranes that occludes the intercellular space between these cells. The continuity of the cell membranes allows diffusion of lipophilic tracers such as dipicrylamine from one cell to the other (Kachar and Reese, 1982). Tight junctions are also crucial in determining cell polarity, because tight junctions act as diffusion barriers in the plane of the cell membrane. As a consequence the surface of individual cells becomes functionally separated into an apical and a basal domain. To analyze whether the diffusion between both domains within the plane of the membrane is restricted or not, endothelial cells can be exposed to lipophilic fluorescent dyes. After photobleaching one of the surfaces and monitoring the eventual recovery of fluorescence by diffusion from the unbleached sector to the bleached one, it became evident that these tight junctions prevent free diffusion. As a result, circumscribed diffusion domains are defined by tight junctions that contribute to the asymmetric distribution of cell membrane constituents (Dragsten et al., 1981; Kachar and Reese, 1982). As depicted below, asymmetric distribution of membrane proteins participates in vectorial transport across the endothelial and epithelial barriers of the retina.

A number of proteins have been found to be associated exclusively with tight junctions. One of the first components described was the integral membrane protein occludin, which contributes both to the structure and function of tight junctions (Fujimoto, 1995; Balda et al., 1996; Wong and Gumbiner, 1997). However, occludin is found in various ocular endothelial and epithelial tissues, and consequently cannot be considered a specific marker for the BRB. Downregulation of occludin expression correlates with breakdown of the BRB in experimentally induced diabetes (Antonetti et al., 1998), aging of the rat retina (Chan-Ling et al., 1995), and with neurophil-induced BBB rupture (Bolton et al., 1998).

Other proteins of tight junctions have been identified, though they do not necessarily correlate with junctional complexity or barrier permeability. The cytoplasmic proteins ZO-1 and -2 function as intracellular linkers between occludin and cytoskeletal filaments composed of spectrin/actin (Tsukita et al., 1998). This protein–protein interaction is mediated by PDZ domains of ZO-1 and -2. Additional proteins of tight junctional complexes are members of the claudin family, which comprise more than 20 members. Only claudin-1 and claudin-5 are expressed by endothelial cells (Morita et al., 1999a, b). In the retinal context claudin-1 is primarily responsible for the formation of tight junction strands (Russ et al., 1998) (Furuse et al., 1998). Notably, claudin-1 is downregulated in human gliomas, coincidentally with an increase in microvascular permeability (Liebner et al., 2000).

Formation and possibly maintenance of tight junction complexes are critically dependent on controlled cell adhesion mediated by the calcium-dependent membrane proteins M-cadherin and E-cadherin, which are intracellularly associated with catenins (Nagafuchi and Takeichi, 1988; Reynolds et al., 1994; Tomi et al., 2004). Coincident with the decrease in tight junction resistance, β-catenin becomes phosphorylated by a junction-associated src-like tyrosine kinase. Conversely, dephosphorylation is accompanied by a return of the junctional resistance to control levels (Staddon et al., 1995). Though cadherin–catenin complexes are obviously not direct components of tight junctions, perturbation experiments with masking antibodies indicated that they are essential for the integrity of tight junctions (Gumbiner and Simons, 1986).

In summary, tight junctions are cellular structures between neighboring cells which prevent paracellular diffusion across of the inner and outer BRBs. The integrity of tight junctions depends on a number of intracellular and integral membrane proteins including ZO-1, occludin, claudins, and specific cadherins.

3.3 The Adult Outer Blood–Retina Barrier

The adult RPE is formed by a single sheet of hexagonal cells. RPE cells are interconnected at the apical side by adherence junctions, desmosomes, and tight junctions (zonula occludens), which block the free passage of water and ions (Kniesel and Wolburg, 1993; Rizzolo, 1997). Another consequence is the transepithelial resistance of 350–600 Ω cm^2 (Steinberg and Miller, 1979; Pautler and Tengerdy, 1986), which is about one-fourth of the endothelial BBB value but still more than 50 times above that of systemic capillaries (see above). In the human RPE, the cell size varies upon the concentrical position: in the central macular region of the eye the RPE cell diameter is with 10 µm considerably smaller than in the periphery where cells are 60 µm and flatter (Zinn and Benjamin-Henkind, 1979). RPE cells are polarized with an apical domain facing retinal photoreceptors and a basal domain attached to a 2-µm-thick basal lamina, called Bruch's membrane (Zinn and Benjamin-Henkind, 1979). The permeable Bruch's membrane separates the RPE from the overlying vessel-rich choroid. The apical cytoplasm of RPE cells contains a higher concentration of melanin granules (melanosomes), which function to minimize light scattering by absorbing stray light and consequently are likely to improve vision (Garcia et al., 1979). Owing to unspecific melanin binding of some drugs such as chloroquine, used to treat malaria, adverse accumulation of pharmaceutics could happen in the oBRB (Wolfensberger, 1998).

The RPE functions as a regulatory interphase between fenestrated blood vessels in the choroid and the outer neuronal retina. This function is supported by the ability of the RPE to induce sufficient fenestration of the neighboring choroidal blood vessels, which in turn facilitates the transit of blood-borne components (Burns and Hartz, 1992). On the other hand, the basal surface of RPE cells is characterized by small convoluted invaginations that increase the surface area. Thus, selective secretion and absorption involved in transport processes across the oBRB become optimized (Zinn and Benjamin-Henkind, 1979).

Beside these features that serve the (outer) retina in general, the RPE also specifically supports photoreceptor function, which has been initially only deduced from the close apposition with rods and cones. Long microvilli of RPE (❷ *Figure 24-3c, d*) envelop photoreceptor outer segments (Kuwabara, 1979). An individual RPE cell typically contacts some 45 photoreceptor cells in the human retina. Retinal adhesion to the RPE is based on the interphotoreceptor matrix, which is synthesized by the RPE (Steinberg and Wood, 1979). The viscosity and bonding properties of the matrix are critically dependent on its hydration and ionic composition, both of which are controlled by vectorial flux of water and selected ions. The net effect of several RPE pump systems is a movement of water across the RPE in the apical-to-basal i.e., retina-to-choroid direction (Zauberman, 1979). The RPE is further involved in photoreceptor outer segment

■ Figure 24-3

Retinal pigment epithelium (RPE). (a) Phase contrast—fluorescence double image of a cross-section of the porcine eye. Vitreous and sclera had been previously removed. Cell nuclei appear light blue due to fluorescent DAPI labeling. The RPE separates the neural retina from the choroid, which contains systemic blood vessels. (b) Schematic representation of different eye layers. Retina and sclera can be removed from the RPE/choroid tissue layers. (c, d) Scanning electron micrograph of (c) porcine and (d) bovine RPE. The gentle dissection procedure preserves the microvilli structures of RPE cells. Bars (a) 10 μm and (c) (also for (d)) 100 μm. (Reprinted from Brain Research Protocols 13, Steuer et al. (2004). In vitro model of the outer blood–retina barrier. pp 30–31, copyright 2006, with permission from Elsevier.)

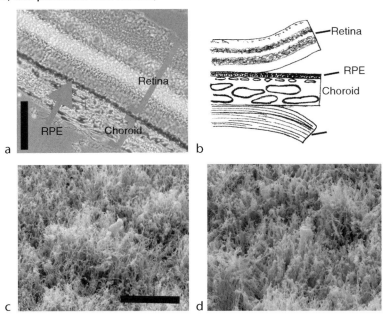

renewal. Because of continuously occurring radiation and oxidation damage to photoreceptor membranes, possibly via radical formation, each day some 100 discs of each rod photoreceptor need to be replaced. Damaged discs are phagocytosed by the RPE (Steinberg and Wood, 1979). This chapter highlights the fact that RPE functions imply blood barrier aspects as well as additional tasks that are not evident in the inner BRB.

3.4 Tapetum

In some nonhuman species, transit of blood components is affected, though not abolished by an intermediate tissue layer between the RPE and the choroid called tapetum. The tapetum, which has a species-specific composition, is a reflective layer that facilitates light capture under dim conditions (Marmor, 1998). Pigs and rabbits have a tapetum lucidum, cats and dogs have a tapetum cellulosum composed of about 20 cell layers, and some rodents and cows have a tapetum fibrosum formed by collagen fibrils. The RPE above the tapetum is always devoid of melanosomes to allow unhampered light passage. Typically, only one segment of the orbit is covered with a tapetum. Thus, many species have mixed RPE, i.e., with and without melanosomes (Kuwabara, 1979). The tapetum has not been considered part of the oBRB.

4 Retinal Barrier and Carrier Molecules

The molecular composition of the retinal vasculature and the RPE responsible for barrier properties are in many respects the same. ZO-1, occludin, cell adhesion proteins such as integrins, cadherins, and associated catenins are all expressed in the RPE as well as in the retinal endothelium (Reh and Radke, 1988). Alkaline phosphatase is expressed in the RPE at high concentrations similar to those found in CNS capillaries. Thus, in the barrier cells, a 500 times higher expression is evident as in many as systemic blood vessels (Korte et al., 1991).

4.1 Transporters

Several transport systems observed in the endothelial barrier have been also identified in the RPE. GLUT-1, the major transporter for glucose, is also expressed on apical and basolateral RPE cell surfaces as in capillary endothelial cells (Harik et al., 1990; Pardridge et al., 1990). At the apical RPE surface, the probenecid-sensitive organic anion transporter is found that mediates transport of lactate and fluorescein used for ophthalmic angiography (Koyano et al., 1993; Garcia and Burnside, 1994; Kenyon et al., 1994). Also, the membrane bound Na^+/K^+ ATPase is preferentially located at the apical (abluminal) RPE surface, similar to the polarized distribution in CNS capillaries. Identified ion transporters in both cell types include Ca^{2+} ATPase, Na^+/Ca^{2+} exchanger, $Na^+/K^+/2Cl^-$ transporter, $Na^+HCO_3^-$ transporter, and $H^+/lactate$ cotransporter (Berman, 1979; Adorante and Miller, 1990; Strauss et al., 1997). The Na^+-dependent taurine uptake mechanism is also involved in the passage of alanine and GABA (γ-aminobutyric acid). In the retina, GABA is the major inhibitory neurotransmitter (Honda et al., 1995). Other transporters found both in endothelial cells and the RPE are monocarboxylate transporter MTC1 (lactate), monocarboxylate transporter MTC3 (lactate), organic cation transporter, and GABA transporter GAT2 (Alm and Törnquist, 1985; Honda et al., 1995; Philp et al., 1998; Bergersen et al., 1999; Murakami et al., 2000; Han et al., 2001; Takanaga et al., 2001).

4.2 P-Glycoprotein/Multidrug Resistance and Multidrug Resistance-Associated Proteins

P-Glycoprotein (P-gp) is an ATP-dependent efflux pump on the luminal surface of CNS endothelial cells and the RPE (Cordon-Cordo et al., 1989). The 170-kDa protein with 12 putative transmembrane domains has an ATP-binding cassette (ABC) and an energy-dependent transporter also called traffic ATPase. Experimental evidence indicates that P-glycoprotein/multidrug resistance-1 (P-gp/mdr-1) is bifunctional, with transport and chloride-channel activities. Interconversion between functional states is mediated by conformational changes induced by different degrees of cellular tonicity (Gill et al., 1992). The pharmacological relevance of P-gp/mdr-1 stems from its ability to actively transport a variety of drugs out of cells, and thus conferring multidrug resistance by which, for example, tumor cells become insensitive to therapeutics such as actinomycin D. In the retina as well as in other parts of the CNS, P-gp/mdr-1 might act as a guardian by protecting the neuronal environment from neurotoxins (Sharom, 1997). In addition, it might control steroid hormone passage. As predicted from the protective efflux activity of P-gp/mdr-1, mice genetically engineered to lack the mdr1a gene become susceptible to otherwise nontoxic concentrations of the neurotransmitter agonist ivermectin (Schinkel et al., 1997).

The expression of P-gp/mdr-1 in the RPE has been controversial because only limited immunoreactivity has been demonstrated in the rat under control conditions (Holash and Stewart, 1993) and in humans only after pharmacological induction by daunomycin (Tervooren et al., 1998). Daunomycin is routinely used for the treatment of proliferative vitreoretinopathy. We have shown by immunocytochemistry and transport studies in vitro that P-gp/mdr-1 is expressed in porcine RPE (Steuer et al., 2005). The membrane-staining pattern elucidates the typical hexagonal cell geometry in the RPE as seen by other cytochemical techniques (Steuer et al., 2004) (❯ *Figure 24-4a*). When freshly isolated RPE tissue sheets were used as an interphase in a two chamber system, it could be shown that verapamil and rhodamine 123, two characteristic P-gp/mdr-1 substrates, are preferentially transported in a retina-to-choroid direction. In vivo this mechanism allows clearance of the retinal environment. The functional expression of P-gp/mdr-1 could further be validated when fluorescent calcein, another P-gp/mdr-1 substrate, was co-applied with verapamil. Under control conditions only small amounts of calcein accumulate in viable RPE cells, in contrast to specimens where P-gp/mdr-1 was saturated with verapamil. In the latter case RPE displayed considerably higher cell fluorescence (❯ *Figure 24-4c, e*). A similar paradigm was employed to investigate the expression of mdr-associated proteins (MRPs) in RPE. Immunocytochemistry and the application of the MRP substrate fluorescein indicated that MRP is expressed in the porcine RPE and that it is as P-gp/mdr-1 preferentially situated at the basal RPE side facing the choroid (❯ *Figure 24-4f, g*). These data are consonant with observations in other species (see above) including humans (Kennedy and Mangini, 2002).

4.3 Biotransformation Enzymes

Enzymes involved in biotransformation phase I and II show comparable distribution for both endothelial and epithelial barriers as judged from the expression of monoamino oxidase, NADPH cytochrome P450 reductase, superoxide dismutase, glutathione peroxidase, glutathione-*S*-transferase, glutathione reductase, and catalase (Schwartzman et al., 1987; Akeo et al., 1988; Singhal et al., 1999).

4.4 Receptors

Specific receptors found both on endothelial and epithelial barriers of the eye comprise the transferrin receptor, LDL receptor, vasopressin receptor, α1-adrenergic receptor, 5-HT$_{1A}$ receptor, serotonin receptor, muscarinic ACh receptor, dopamine receptors D$_1$ and D$_2$, β-adrenergic receptor, P2Y2 receptor, and the vasopressin receptor (Berman, 1979; Hayes et al., 1989; Hunt et al., 1989; Nash and Osborne, 1997; Kobayashi et al., 1998). Most interestingly, the RPE even displays the molecular addressing system of recognition molecules, MHC II induction by interferon-γ and metalloprotease activities, that appear to be integral components of leucocyte infiltration mechanisms into the brain as seen during MS (Liversidge et al., 1988; Elner et al., 1992; Padgett et al., 1997; el-Shabrawi et al., 2000) (see below).

◼ Figure 24-4

Efflux systems. (a) Immunofluorescence of the pigment epithelial whole mount showing the localization of P-glycoprotein (P-gp). (b) Vectorial transport of P-gp substrates verapamil and rhodamine 123. Application of these compounds to the retinal side of the outer blood–retina barrier (oBRB) resulted in higher permeability coefficients (P_e) than application to the choroidal side. This demonstrated a P-gp-mediated efflux from the neural tissue toward the blood ($N = 22$ and 30, respectively). (c: + verapamil; d: − verapamil) Calcein fluorescence of oBRB whole mounts in the presence or absence of competing verapamil (c: + verapamil; d: − verapamil). (e) Quantification of fluorescence intensities revealed that competing verapamil resulted in higher calcein contents inside cells, since calcein is also a P-gp substrate ($N = 12$). (f) Immunofluorescence of the pigment epithelial whole mount showing the localization of multidrug resistance-associated protein (MRP). (g) Vectorial transport of the MRP substrate fluorescein. Application of fluorescein to the retinal side of the oBRB produced a higher permeability coefficient (P_e) than application of drugs to the choroidal side. This demonstrated an MRP-mediated efflux from the neural tissue toward the blood ($N = 8$). Bars (a) 20 μm, (c) (also for (d)) 75 μm, and (f) 10 μm. (Reprinted from Investigative Ophthalmology and Visual Science 46(3), Steuer et al. (2005). Functional characterization and comparison of the outer blood–retina barrier and the blood–brain barrier. p.1051, copyright 2006, with permission from Assoc. Research in Vision and Ophthalmology.)

◘ Figure 24-4 (continued)

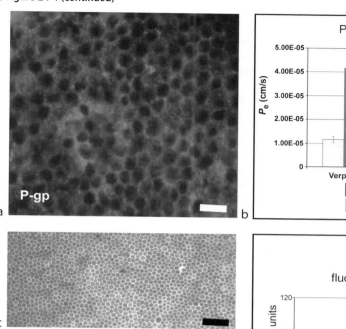

a

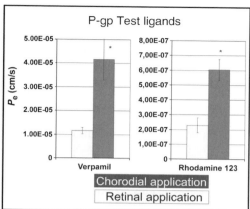

b

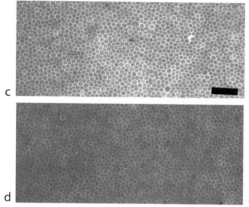

c

d

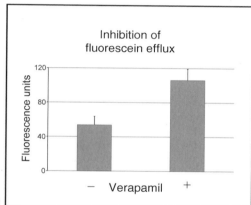

e

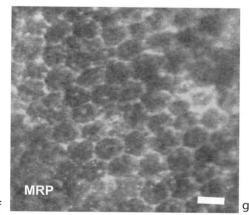

f

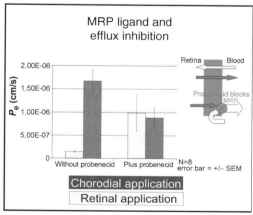

g

5   Retinal Immune Barriers

5.1 Optic Nerve

The vascular BRB and the RPE render the retina a somewhat "immune privileged" tissue (Wenkel and Streilein, 2000), though blood vessels in the retrobulbar optic nerve display some permeability for intravascular tracers, such as Evans blue (Tso et al., 1975; Chan-Ling and Stone, 1992). Under normal conditions this site harbors resident populations of MHC class II$^+$ cells. These cells are found in the lamina cribrosa region of the optic nerve and the meninges surrounding the nerve of naive rats. The MHC class II$^+$ cells with numerous cell processes are reminiscent of dendritic cells. The cell surface expression of MHC class II is indicative of the potential to present antigen during an inflammatory lesion (Lassmann et al., 1994). The inherent permeability at the optic nerve could be responsible for the susceptibility to lesion formation as observed both in MS and experimental allergic encephalomyelitis (EAE) (Guy and Rao, 1984; Hu et al., 1998). This notion is in agreement with the fact that neuronal regions that lack effective blood barriers display an early accumulation of inflammatory cells in EAE.

5.2 Retinal Endothelium as Immunological Barrier

Though the CNS including the retina has been considered to be an immune-privileged organ, it is better referred to as an immunologically specialized tissue. The CNS remains under the constant surveillance of the immune system, although retina and brain lack lymphatics and the CNS endothelium (with the exception of the circumferential organs such as the pineal gland) hinders passage of most cells. Nevertheless, small numbers of lymphocytes continuously patrol the CNS. In various pathological situations this restricted traffic increases and results in the extravasation of immune cells including T lymphocytes across capillaries. Extravasation of cells is dependent on a number of cell-surface proteins and signaling factors of both leukocytes and the vascular endothelium (Hickey, 2001).

During extravasation lymphocytes attach to the luminal vascular surface, and subsequently encounter activating factors expressed by endothelial cells, such as the chemokines MCP-1 (monocyte chemoattractant protein-1), RANTES (regulated on activation of normal T cell expressed and released), or CCL3 (Ransohoff et al., 2003). Exposure to chemokines activate integrins via Gi protein-dependent pathways in lymphocytes, resulting in integrin clustering and conformational changes that increase their avidity. Because of the concerted interaction of adhesion molecules, activated leucointegrins and endothelial receptors firm cell adhesion to the endothelial surface and flattening of lymphocytes becomes established (Greenwood et al., 2003). In a final step, lymphocytes release proteolytic matrix metalloproteinases (MMPs), which facilitate transmigration across the endothelium. During inflammatory responses, nuclear factor-κB (NF-κB) is produced and activates MMPs by binding to the NF-κB binding site (Risau et al., 1990; Lukes et al., 1999).

Activated lymphocytes that have traversed blood barriers and contact the relevant retinal tissue antigen release proinflammatory cytokines such as tumor necrosis factor-α (TNF-α), interleukin-1 (IL-1), and interferon-γ (IFN-γ) (Koizumi et al., 2003). The released cytokines activate inflammatory responses of endothelial cells, which in turn recruit more leukocytes from the blood stream with subsequent transmigration across the BBB (Franzen et al., 2003). In addition, it has been suggested that endothelial cells can be induced to express MHC class II and fulfill antigen presentation (Male et al., 1987).

The expression of chemokine receptors in the endothelium is of importance also for virus entry into the CNS. MCP-1 and the CXCR4-receptor ligand stromal cell-derived factor-1 (SDF-1) mediate transmigration of uninfected human lymphocytes as has been demonstrated in vitro. In vivo, HIV-infected blood cells enter the CNS, based on the same mechanism. In a first step, IL-1 increases the expression of CXCR4-receptor, which in turn acts as a coreceptor for HIV in order to pass through the blood barrier (Wu et al., 2000). SDF-1 and its CXCR4 receptor have also been demonstrated in the human eye (Bhutto et al., 2006).

5.3 RPE as Immunological Barrier

Despite the fact that the inner and outer BRBs are ontogenetically and structurally very different, both share many immunological features. The RPE is considered to be the first line of defense against infections in the absence of professional macrophages, owing to the fact that RPE cells express monocyte/macrophage-like features that enable the tissue to eliminate foreign antigens (Liversidge and Forrester, 1998). The RPE also expresses factors that reduce neutrophil superoxide generation during activation and protects the eye from injury (Wu and Rao, 1996). In general, the naive RPE is viewed as an immunoregulative tissue sheet that suppresses immune responses in the retina. However, inflammatory stimuli induce in the RPE the expression of MHC complexes, which allows to function as antigen-presenting cells (Liversidge et al., 1988). In vitro, RPE cells induced by IFNγ endocytose, process, and present antigens in their MHC-binding grooves to CD4$^+$ T cells.

RPE cells can produce various cytokines including MCP-1, IL-8, and RANTES, which may activate and attract lymphocytes (Holtkamp et al., 2001). Notably, after a proinflammatory stimulus with IL-1β, the changes in the chemokine production of RPE cells resemble those of retinal vascular endothelial cells (Crane et al., 2000a). The predominant chemokine receptor on RPE cells is CXCR4, whose expression can be upon TNF-α or IL-1β stimulation. This in turn leads to enhanced secretion of MCP-1 and IL-8 (Crane et al., 2000b).

Lymphocyte migration across the RPE depends on lymphocyte activation, as is true for migration across the CNS endothelium (Devine et al., 1996). Under physiological conditions, the migration of lymphocytes across unstimulated RPE cells is highly restricted. However, migration becomes reinforced after treatment with IFNγ, which results in increased levels of ICAM-1 and VCAM-1 on RPE cell surfaces. These adhesion molecules then interact with LFA-1 and VLA-4, respectively, on activated lymphocytes (Devine et al., 1996). Thus, the RPE seems to behave like brain endothelium. Similarly to the endothelium, the breakdown of the RPE barrier can be an early event in autoimmune diseases.

6 The Outer Blood–Retina Barrier in Autoimmune and Other Diseases

Various diseases of infectious or immune-mediated origin affect the visual system including the oBRB . In retinitis, the neural retina, iris, choroidea, and the ciliary body are inflamed. In uveitis, inflammation is evident in the same tissues with the exception of the retina. Uveitis/uveoretinitis with neurological complications are observed during toxoplasmosis, infection with herpes, cytomegalovirus (CMV), and HIV, lupus erythematosus, and MS. In MS patients, demyelination of the optic nerve is the predominant complication of the visual system. Inflammatory infiltration originating from the retinal vasculature has an incidence of up to 20% in MS patients (Bamford et al., 1978). During MS, lymphocytes cross probably both the inner and the outer BRBs and invade the retina. In animal models of experimental autoimmune uveoretinitis (EAU), the same cellular mechanisms become activated as in EAE. In this model the rodent immune system becomes challenged with retinal autoantigens (e.g., the calcium-binding protein S-100). Similarly, transfer of autoreactive S100β-specific T cells into rodents cause an inflammatory response in the uvea and retina (Schmidt et al., 1997). Furthermore, autoreactive antibodies against S-antigen have also been found in patients with MS (Ohguro et al., 1993).

In summary, there is a conspicuous similarity between the immunological processes at the endothelial and epithelial barriers of the eye, though several differences do exist. Both barriers actively mediate the repulsion/attraction and transmigration of lymphocytes from the blood stream into the neuronal micro-environment by similar mechanisms.

7 Conclusions

The human retina is the only part of the CNS that communicates in a "sandwich configuration" with the blood stream. Two interfaces at the inner and outer circumference of the tissue are evident. The inner BRB is to a large extent structurally identical with the endothelium-based BBB. In contrast, the oBRB is formed by the unique pigment epithelium which does not have any ontogenetic relation with the endothelial barrier and no equivalent elsewhere in the organism. Therefore, it is surprising to note that both barriers display various functional similarities. Recent, direct comparison of the RPE with two different BBB models in vitro and in vivo revealed that also permeability for a variety of pharmaceutical agents is equivalent at both sites (❯ *Figure 24-5*) (Steuer et al., 2004; Steuer et al., 2005). This provides the opportunity to employ one system for the sake of the other in order to exploit technical advantages. Thus, it has become feasible to overcome

◼ **Figure 24-5**
Comparison of in vitro/in vivo outer blood–retina barrier (oBRB)/blood–brain barrier (BBB). (a) Comparison of oBRB tissue sheets used as the interface in the perfusion system (NMI BRB) (*dark grey*) and a transfilter coculture system with purified bovine brain endothelial cells and astrocytes (BBEC-AC) (*light grey*). Permeability coefficients P_e were determined by mass spectrometry and fluorescence detection. (b) Comparison of the P_e of different compounds determined with oBRB tissue sheets used in a perfusion chamber and of the brain/plasma ratio in mice. All three systems displayed somewhat similar ranking of test agent permeabilities. (Reprinted from Investigative Ophthalmology and Visual Science 46(3), Steuer et al. (2005). Functional characterization and comparison of the outer blood–retina barrier and the blood–brain barrier. p.1051, copyright 2006, with permission from Assoc. Research in Vision and Ophthalmology.)

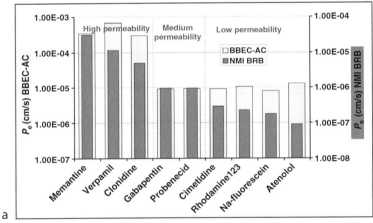

a

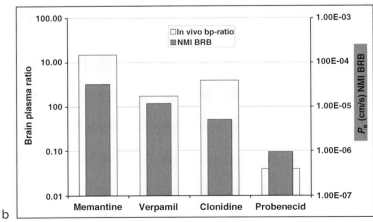

b

the notorious difficulty to gain native BBB or inner BRB preparations by using the RPE instead, which is easily dissected as intact barrier tissue (Steuer et al., 2004). By virtue of such technical progress and the expanding knowledge of molecular mechanisms involved in transport versus permeability restriction, autoimmune cell responses, and the impact of gene mutations such as in some hereditary retinitis pigmentosa forms (affecting the oBRB), the transfer of results from basic research to applied sciences will be accelerated.

Acknowledgments

I am grateful to Drs. Konrad Kohler (Tübingen, Germany) and Marteen Reith (New York, USA) for critical reading of the manuscript.

References

Abbott NJ, Ronnback L, Hansson E. 2006. Astrocyte-endothelial interactions at the blood-brain barrier. Nat Rev Neurosci 7(1): 41-53.

Abbruscato TJ, Lopez SP, Roder K, Paulson JR. 2004. Regulation of blood-brain barrier Na,K,2Cl-cotransporter through phosphorylation during in vitro stroke conditions and nicotine exposure. J Pharmacol Exp Ther 310(2): 459-468.

Adorante JS, Miller SS. 1990. Potassium-dependent volume regulation in retinal pigment epithelium is mediated by Na, K,Cl cotransport. J Gen Physiol 96: 1153-1176.

Akeo K, Curran SA, Dorey CK. 1988. Superoxide dismutase activity and growth of retinal pigment epithelial cells are suppressed by 20% oxygen in vitro. Curr Eye Res 7: 961-967.

Alm A, Törnquist P. 1985. Lactate transport through the blood-retinal and the blood-brain barrier in rats. Ophthalmic Res 17: 181-184.

Antonetti DA, Barber AJ, Khin S, Lieth E, Tarbell JM, et al. 1998. Vascular permeability in experimental diabetes is associated with reduced endothelial occludin content: Vascular endothelial growth factor decreases occludin in retinal endothelial cells. Penn State Retina Research Group. Diabetes 47(12): 1953-1959.

Antonelli-Orlidge A, Saunders KB, Smith SR, D'Amore PA. 1989. An activated form of transforming growth factor β is produced by cocultures of endothelial cells and pericytes. Proc Natl Acad Sci USA 86: 4544-4548.

Balda MS, Anderson JM, Matter K. 1996. The SH3 domain of the tight junction protein ZO-1 binds to a serine protein kinase that phosphorylates a region C-terminal to this domain. FEBS Lett 399(3): 326-332.

Bamford CR, Ganley JP, Sibley WA, Laguna JF. 1978. Uveitis, perivenous sheathing and multiple sclerosis. Neurology 28: 119-124.

Banks WA, Kastin AJ. 1997. The role of the blood-brain barrier transporter PTS-1 in regulating concentrations of methionine enkephalin in blood and brain. Alcohol 14(3): 237-245.

Bergersen I, Johannsson E, Veruki ML, Nagelhus EA, Halestrap A, et al. 1999. Cellular and subcellular expression of monocarboxylate transporters in the pigment epithelium and retina of the rat. Neuroscience 90(1): 319-331.

Berman ER. 1979. Biochemistry of the retinal pigment epithelium. The Retinal Pigment Epithelium. Marmor MF, editor. Cambridge, Massachusetts, and London, England: Harvard University Press pp. 83-102.

Bhutto IA, McLeod DS, Merges C, Hasegawa T, Lutty GA. 2006. Localisation of SDF-1 and its receptor CXCR4 in retina and choroid of aged human eyes and in eyes with age related macular degeneration. Br J Ophthalmol 90(7): 906-910.

Bolton SJ, Anthony DC, Perry VH. 1998. Loss of the tight junction proteins occludin and zonula occludens-1 from cerebral vascular endothelium during neutrophil-induced blood-brain barrier breakdown in vivo. Neuroscience 86 (4): 1245-1257.

Burns MS, Hartz MJ. 1992. The retinal pigment epithelium induces fenestration of endothelial cells in vivo. Curr Eye Res 11: 863-873.

Carmeliet P, Tessier-Lavigne M. 2005. Common mechanisms of nerve and blood vessel wiring. Nature 436(7048): 193-200.

Chakravarthy U, Gardiner TA, Anderson P, Archer DB, Trimble ER. 1992. The effect of endothelin 1 on the retinal microvascular pericyte. Microvasc Res 43: 241-254.

Chan-Ling T, Stone J. 1992. Degeneration of astrocytes in feline retinopathy of prematurity causes failure of the blood-retinal barrier. Invest Ophthalmol Vis Sci 33(7): 2148-2159.

Chan-Ling T, Gock B, Stone J. 1995. The effect of oxygen on vasoformative cell division. Evidence that "physiological hypoxia" is the stimulus for normal retinal vasculogenesis. Invest Ophthalmol Vis Sci 36(7): 1201-1214.

Chishty M, Reichel A, Begley DJ, Abbott NJ. 2002. Glial induction of blood-brain barrier-like L-system amino acid transport in the ECV304 cell line. Glia 39(2): 99-104.

Connolly SE, Hores TA, Smith LE, D'Amore PA. 1988. Characterization of vascular development in the mouse retina. Microvasc Res 36(3): 275-290.

Cordon-Cordo C, O'Brain J, Casals D, Rittman-Grauer L, Biedler JL, et al. 1989. Multidrug-resistance gene (P-glycoprotein) is expressed by endothelial cells at blood-brain barrier sites. Proc Natl Acad Sci USA 86: 695-698.

Crane IJ, Wallace CA, McKillop-Smith S, Forrester JV. 2000a. Control of chemokine production at the blood-retina barrier. Immunology 101(3): 426-433.

Crane IJ, Wallace CA, McKillop-Smith S, Forrester JV. 2000b. CXCR4 receptor expression on human retinal pigment epithelial cells from the blood-retina barrier leads to chemokine secretion and migration in response to stromal cell-derived factor 1α. J Immunol 165(8): 4372-4378.

Crone C, Olesen SP. 1982. Electrical resistance of brain microvascular endothelium. Brain Res 241: 49-55.

Devine L, Lightman S, Greenwood J. 1996. Lymphocyte migration across the anterior and posterior blood-retinal barrier in vitro. Cell Immunol 168: 267-275.

Dorrell MI, Aguilar E, Friedlander M. 2002. Retinal vascular development is mediated by endothelial filopodia, a preexisting astrocytic template and specific R-cadherin adhesion. Invest Ophthalmol Vis Sci 43(11): 3500-3510.

Dowling JE. 1991. Retinal neuromodulation: The role of dopamine. Vis Neurosci 7: 87-97.

Dragsten PR, Blumenthal R, Handler JS. 1981. Membrane asymmetry in epithelia: Is the tight junction a barrier to diffusion in the plasma membrane? Nature 294: 718-722.

Duvvuri S, Majumdar S, Mitra AK. 2003. Drug delivery to the retina: Challenges and opportunities. Expert Opin Biol Ther 3(1): 45-56.

Elner SG, Elner VM, Pavilack MA, Todd RF, Mayo-Bond L, et al. 1992. Modulation and function of intercellular adhesion molecule-1 (CD54) on human retinal pigment epithelial cells. Lab Invest 66: 200-211.

el-Shabrawi Y, Eckhardt M, Berghold A, Faulborn J, Auboeck L, et al. 2000. Synthesis pattern of matrix metalloproteinases (MMPs) and inhibitors (TIMPs) in human explant organ cultures after treatment with latanoprost and dexamethasone. Eye 2000 Jun; 14(Pt3A): 375–383, 14: 375-383.

Engelhardt B. 2006. Development of the blood-brain interface. Blood-Brain Barriers. Needergaard M, editor. Wiley-VCH. pp. 11-39.

Engelhardt B, Risau W. 1995. Development of the blood-brain barrier. New Concepts of a Blood-Brain Barrier. Segal MB, editor. New York: Plenum Press; pp. 11-31.

Franzen B, Duvefelt K, Jonsson C, Engelhardt B, Ottervald J, et al. 2003. Gene and protein expression profiling of human cerebral endothelial cells activated with tumor necrosis factor-α. Brain Res Mol Brain Res 115(2): 130-146.

Fujimoto K. 1995. Freeze-fracture replica electron microscopy combined with SDS digestion for cytochemical labeling of integral membrane proteins. Application to the immuno-gold labeling of intercellular junctional complexes. J Cell Sci 108(Pt 11): 3443-3449.

Furuse M, Fujita K, Hiiragi T, Fujimoto K, Tsukita S. 1998. Claudin-1 and -2: Novel integral membrane proteins localizing at tight junctions with no sequence similarity to occludin. J Cell Biol 141(7): 1539-1550.

Gale NW, Yancopoulos GD. 1999. Growth factors acting via endothelial cell-specific receptor tyrosine kinases: VEGFs, angiopoietins, and ephrins in vascular development. Genes Dev 13(9): 1055-1066.

Garcia DM, Burnside B. 1994. Suppression of cAMP-induced pigment granule aggregation in RPE by organic anion transport inhibitors. Invest Ophthalmol Vis Sci 35: 178-188.

Garcia RI, Szabó G, Fitzpatrick TB. 1979. Molecular and cell biology of melanin. The Retinal Pigment Epithelium. Marmor MF, editor. Cambridge, Massachusetts and London, England: Harvard University Press; pp. 124-147.

Gariano RF, Gardner TW. 2005. Retinal angiogenesis in development and disease. Nature 438(7070): 960-966.

Gariano RF, Hu D, Helms J. 2006. Expression of angiogenesis-related genes during retinal development. Gene Expr Patterns 6(2): 187-192.

Gerhardt H, Golding M, Fruttiger M, Ruhrberg C, Lundkvist A, et al. 2003. VEGF guides angiogenic sprouting utilizing endothelial tip cell filopodia. J Cell Biol 161(6): 1163-1177.

Gill DR, Hyde SC, Higgins CF, Valverde MA, Mintenig GM, et al. 1992. Separation of drug transport and chloride channel functions of the human multidrug resistance P-glycoprotein. Cell 71: 23-32.

Goldstein GW. 1988. Endothelial cell-astrocyte interactions. A cellular model of the blood-brain barrier. Ann N Y Acad Sci 529: 31-39.

Greenwood J, Amos CL, Walters CE, Couraud PO, Lyck R, et al. 2003. Intracellular domain of brain endothelial intercellular adhesion molecule-1 is essential for T lymphocyte-mediated signaling and migration. J Immunol 171(4): 2099-2108.

Guillemot F, Cepko CL. 1992. Retinal fate and ganglion cell differentiation are potentiated by acidic FGF in an in vitro assay of early retinal development. Development 114: 743-754.

Gumbiner B, Simons K. 1986. A functional assay for proteins involved in establishing an epithelial occluding barrier: Identification of an uvomorulin-like polypeptide. J Cell Biol 102: 457-468.

Guy J, Rao NA. 1984. Acute and chronic experimental optic neuritis. Alteration in the blood-optic nerve barrier. Arch Ophthalmol 102(3): 450-454.

Hamm S, Dehouck B, Kraus J, Wolburg-Buchholz K, Wolburg H, et al. 2004. Astrocyte-mediated modulation of blood-brain barrier permeability does not correlate with a loss of tight junction proteins from the cellular contacts. Cell Tissue Res 315(2): 157-166.

Han Y-H, Sweet DH, Hu D-N, Pritchard JB. 2001. Characterization of a novel cationic drug transporter in human retinal pigment epithelial cells. J Pharmacol Exp Ther 296 (2): 450-457.

Harik SI, Kalaria RN, Whitney PM, Andersson L, Lundahl P, et al. 1990. Glucose transporters are abundant in cells with "occluding" junctions at the blood-eye barriers. Proc Natl Acad Sci USA 87: 4261-4264.

Hayes KC, Lindsey S, Stephan ZF, Brecker D. 1989. Retinal pigment epithelium possesses both LDL and scavenger receptor activity. Invest Ophthalmol Vis Sci 30: 225-232.

Hickey WF. 2001. Basic principles of immunological surveillance of the normal central nervous system. Glia 36(2): 118-124.

Holash JA, Stewart PA. 1993. The relationship of astrocyte-like cells to the vessels that contribute to the blood-ocular barriers. Brain Res 629: 218-224.

Holtkamp GM, Kijlstra A, Peek R, de Vos AF. 2001. Retinal pigment epithelium-immune system interactions: Cytokine production and cytokine-induced changes. Prog Retin Eye Res 2001 Jan; 20(1): 29-48.

Honda S, Yamamoto M, Saito N. 1995. Immunocytochemical localization of three subtypes of GABA transporter in rat retina. Brain Res Mol Brain Res 33: 319-325.

Hu P, Pollard J, Hunt N, Taylor J, Chan-Ling T. 1998. Microvascular and cellular responses in the optic nerve of rats with acute experimental allergic encephalomyelitis (EAE). Brain Pathol 8(3): 475-486.

Hughes S, Chang-Ling T. 2000. Roles of endothelial cell migration and apoptosis in vascular remodeling during development of the central nervous system. Microcirculation 7(5): 317-333.

Hunt RC, Dewey A, Davis AA. 1989. Transferrin receptors on the surfaces of retinal pigment epithelial cells are associated with the cytoskeleton. J Cell Sci 92: 655-666.

Jaakkola P, Mole DR, Tian YM, Wilson MI, Gielbert J, et al. 2001. Targeting of HIF-α to the von Hippel-Lindau ubiquitylation complex by O_2-regulated prolyl hydroxylation. Science 292(5516): 468-472.

Janzer RC, Raff MC. 1987. Astrocytes induce blood-brain barrier properties in endothelial cells. Nature 325: 253-257.

Jiang B, Bezhadian MA, Caldwell RB. 1995. Astrocytes modulate retinal vasculogenesis: Effects on endothelial cell differentiation. Glia 15(1): 1-10.

Kachar B, Reese TS. 1982. Evidence for the lipidic nature of tight junction strands. Nature 296: 464-466.

Kelley C, D'Amore P, Hechtman HB, Shepro D. 1988. Vasoactive hormones and cAMP affect pericyte contraction and stress fibres in vitro. J Muscle Res Cell Motil 9: 184-194.

Kennedy BG, Mangini NJ. 2002. P-glycoprotein expression in human retinal pigment epithelium. Mol Vis 8: 422-430.

Kenyon E, Yu K, La Cour M, Miller SS. 1994. Lactate transport mechanisms at apical and basolateral membranes of bovine retinal pigment epithelium. Am J Physiol 267: C1561-C1573.

Kniesel U, Wolburg H. 1993. Tight junction complexity in the retinal epithelium of the chicken during development. Neurosci Lett 149: 71-74.

Kobayashi K, Kobayashi H, Ueda M, Honda Y. 1998. Estrogen receptor expression in bovine and rat retinas. Invest Ophthalmol Vis Sci 39: 2105-2110.

Koizumi K, Poulaki V, Doehmen S, Welsandt G, Radetzky S, et al. 2003. Contribution of TNF-α to leukocyte adhesion, vascular leakage, and apoptotic cell death in endotoxin-induced uveitis in vivo. Invest Ophthalmol Vis Sci 44(5): 2184-2191.

Korte GE, Rappa E, Andracchi S. 1991. Localization of alkaline phosphatase on basolateral plasma membrane of normal and regenerating retinal pigment epithelium. Invest Ophthalmol Vis Sci 32(13): 3187-3197.

Koyano S, Araie M, Eguchi S. 1993. Movement of fluorescein and its glucuronide across retinal pigment epithelium-choroid. Invest Ophthalmol Vis Sci 34: 531-538.

Kremer C, Breier G, Risau W, Plate KH. 1997. Up-regulation of flk-1/vascular endothelial growth factor receptor 2 by its ligand in a cerebral slice culture system. Cancer Res 57: 3852-3859.

Kupersmith MJ, Shakib M. 1989. The blood-ocular barrier. Implications of the Blood-Brain Barrier and its Manipulation. Neuwelt EA, editor. New York: Plenum Press; pp. 369-390.

Kuwabara T. 1979. Species differences in the retinal pigment epithelium. The Retinal Pigment Epithelium. Marmor MF, editor. Cambridge: Harvard University Press; pp. 58-82.

Lassmann H, Rinner W, Hickey WF. 1994. Differential role of hematogenous macrophages, resident microglia and astrocytes in antigen presentation and tissue damage during autoimmune encephalomyelitis. Neuropathol Appl Neurobiol 20(2): 195-196.

Lee SW, Kim WJ, Choi YK, Song HS, Son MJ, et al. 2003. SSeCKS regulates angiogenesis and tight junction formation in blood-brain barrier. Nat Med 9(7): 900-906.

Liebner S, Engelhardt B. 2005. Development of the blood-brain barrier. The Blood-Brain Barrier and its Microenvironment. Prat A, editor. New York: Taylor & Francis; pp. 1-26.

Liebner S, Fischmann A, Rascher G, Duffner F, Grote E-H, et al. 2000. Claudin-1 and claudin-5 expression and tight junction morphology are altered in blood vessels of human glioblastoma multiforme. Acta Neuropathol 100: 323-331.

Ling TL, Stone J. 1988. The development of astrocytes in the cat retina: Evidence of migration from the optic nerve. Brain Res Dev Brain Res 44(1): 73-85.

Ling TL, Mitrofanis J, Stone J. 1989. Origin of retinal astrocytes in the rat: Evidence of migration from the optic nerve. J Comp Neurol 286(3): 345-352.

Liversidge J, Forrester JV. 1998. Regulation of immune responses by the retinal pigment epithelium. Retinal Pigment Epithelium, Function and Disease. Wolfensberger TJ, editor. Oxford, New York: Oxford University Press; pp. 511-527.

Liversidge JM, Sewell HF, Forrester JV. 1988. Human retinal pigment epithelial cells differentially express MHC class II (HLA, DP, DR and DQ) antigens in response to in vitro stimulation with lymphokine or purified IFN-γ. Clin Exp Immunol 73: 489-494.

Lobrinus JA, Juillerat-Jeanneret L, Darekar P, Schlosshauer B, Janzer RC. 1992. Induction of the blood-brain barrier specific HT7 and neurothelin epitopes in endothelial cells of the chick chorioallantoic vessels by a soluble factor derived from astrocytes. Dev Brain Res 70: 207-211.

Lukes A, Mun-Bryce S, Lukes M, Rosenberg GA. 1999. Extracellular matrix degradation by metalloproteinases and central nervous system diseases. Mol Neurobiol 19: 267-284.

Male D. 1995. The blood-brain barrier—no barrier to a determined lymphocyte. New Concepts of a Blood-Brain Barrier. Segal MB, editor. New York: Plenum Press; pp. 311-314.

Male DK, Pryce G, Hughes CCW. 1987. Antigen presentation in brain: MHC induction on brain endothelium and astrocytes compared. Immunologie 60: 453-459.

Marmor MF. 1998. Comparative and evolutionary aspects of the retinal pigment epithelium. The Retinal Pigment Epithelium. Wolfensberger TJ, editor. New York: Oxford University Press; pp. 23-37.

Mey J, Thanos S. 1992. Development of the visual system of the chick—A review. J Hirnforsch 33: 673-702.

Meyer J, Rauh J, Galla H-J. 1991. The susceptibility of cerebral endothelial cells to astroglial induction of blood-brain barrier enzymes Depends on their proliferative state. J Neurochem 57: 1971-1977.

Mi H, Haeberle H, Barres BA. 2001. Induction of astrocyte differentiation by endothelial cells. J Neurosci 21(5): 1538-1547.

Michaelson IC. 1948. The mode of development of the vascular system of the retina, with some observations on its significance for certain diseases. Trans Ophthalmol Soc UK 68: 137-181.

Misra A, Ganesh S, Shahiwala A, Shah SP. 2003. Drug delivery to the central nervous system: A review. J Pharm Pharm Sci 6(2): 252-273.

Morcos Y, Hosie MJ, Bauer HC, Chan-Ling T. 2001. Immunolocalization of occludin and claudin-1 to tight junctions in intact CNS vessels of mammalian retina. J Neurocytol 30 (2): 107-123.

Morita K, Sasaki H, Fujimoto K, Furuse M, Tsukita S. 1999a. Claudin-11/OSP-based tight junctions of myelin sheaths in brain and Sertoli cells in testis. J Cell Biol 145(3): 579-588.

Morita K, Sasaki H, Furuse M, Tsukita S. 1999b. Endothelial claudin: Claudin-5/TMVCF constitutes tight junction strands in endothelial cells. J Cell Biol 147(1): 185-194.

Murakami H, Sawada N, Koyabu N, Ohtani H, Sawada Y. 2000. Characteristics of choline transport across the blood-brain barrier in mice: Correlation with in vitro data. Pharm Res 17(12): 1526-1530.

Nagafuchi A, Takeichi M. 1988. Cell binding function of E-cadherin is regulated by the cytoplasmic domain. EMBO J 7: 3679-3684.

Nagy Z, Martinez K. 1992. Astrocytic induction of endothelial tight junction. Ann N Y Acad Sci: 394–404.

Nash MS, Osborne NN. 1997. Pharmacologic evidence for 5-HT$_{1A}$ receptors associated with human retinal pigment epithelial cells in culture. Invest Ophthalmol Vis Sci 38(2): 510-519.

Ohguro H, Chiba S, Igarashi Y, Matsumoto H, Akino T, et al. 1993. β-Arrestin and arrestin are recognized by autoantibodies in sera from multiple sclerosis patients. Proc Natl Acad Sci USA 90: 3241-3245.

Ohh M, Park CW, Ivan M, Hoffman MA, Kim TY, et al. 2000. Ubiquitination of hypoxia-inducible factor requires direct binding to the β-domain of the von Hippel-Lindau protein. Nat Cell Biol 2(7): 423-427.

Orlidge A, D'Amore PA. 1987. Inhibition of capillary endothelial cell growth by pericytes and smooth muscle cells. J Cell Biol 105: 1455-1462.

Ozaki H, Hayashi H, Vinores SA, Moromizato Y, Campochiaro PA, et al. 1997. Intravitreal sustained release of VEGF causes retinal neovascularization in rabbits and breakdown of the blood-retinal barrier in rabbits and primates. Exp Eye Res 64: 505-517.

Padgett LC, Lui GM, Werb Z, La Vail MM. 1997. Matrix metalloproteinase-2 and tissue inhibitor of metalloproteinase-1 in the retinal pigment epithelium and interphotoreceptor matrix: Vectorial secretion and regulation. Exp Eye Res 64: 927-938.

Pardridge WM. 1995. Transport of small molecules through the blood-brain barrier: Biology and methodology. Adv Drug Deliv Rev 15: 5-36.

Pardridge WM, Triguero D, Yang J, Cancilla PA. 1990. Comparison of in vitro and in vivo models of drug transcytosis through the blood-brain barrier. J Pharmacol Exp Ther 253 (2): 884-891.

Pautler EL, Tengerdy C. 1986. Transport of acidic amino acids by the bovine pigment epithelium. Exp Eye Res 43: 207-214.

Penfold PL, Provis JM, Madigan MC, van Driel D, Billson FA. 1990. Angiogenesis in normal human retinal development: The involvement of astrocytes and macrophages. Graefes Arch Clin Exp Ophthalmol 228(3): 255-263.

Philp NJ, Yoon H, Grollman EF. 1998. Monocarboxylate transporter MCT1 is located in the apical membrane and MCT3 in the basal membrane of rat RPE—Rapid Communication. Am J Physiol Regul Integr Comp Physiol 43(6): R1824-R1828.

Prat A, Biernacki K, Lavoie JF, Poirier J, Duquette P, et al. 2002. Migration of multiple sclerosis lymphocytes through brain endothelium. Arch Neurol 59(3): 391-397.

Ransohoff RM, Kivisakk P, Kidd G. 2003. Three or more routes for leukocyte migration into the central nervous system. Nat Rev Immunol 3(7): 569-581.

Reese TS, Karnovsky MJ. 1967. Fine structural localization of a blood-brain barrier to exogenous peroxidase. J Cell Biol 34: 207-217.

Reh TA, Radke K. 1988. A role for the extracellular matrix in retinal neurogenesis in vitro. Dev Biol 129: 283-293.

Reynolds AB, Daniel J, McCrea PD, Wheelock MJ, Wu J, et al. 1994. Identification of a new catenin: The tyrosine kinase substrate p120cas associates with E-cadherin complexes. Mol Cell Biol 14: 8333-8342.

Risau W. 1997. Mechanisms of angiogenesis. Nature 386: 671-674.

Risau W, Engelhardt B, Wekerle H. 1990. Immune function of the blood-brain barrier: Incomplete presentation of protein (auto-)antigens by rat brain microvascular endothelium in vitro. J Cell Biol 110: 1757-1766.

Rizzolo LJ. 1997. Polarity and the development of the outer blood-retinal barrier. Histol Histopath 12: 1057-1067.

Russ PK, Davidson MK, Hoffman LH, Haselton FR. 1998. Partial characterization of the human retinal endothelial cell tight and adherens junction complexes. Invest Ophthalmol Vis Sci 39(12): 2479-2485.

Sandercoe TM, Madigan MC, Billson FA, Penfold PL, Provis JM. 1999. Astrocyte proliferation during development of the human retinal vasculature. Exp Eye Res 69(5): 511-523.

Schinkel AH, Mayer U, Wagenaar E, Mol CA, van Deemter L, et al. 1997. Normal viability and altered pharmacokinetics in mice lacking mdr1-type (drug-transporting) P-glycoproteins. Proc Natl Acad Sci USA 94: 4028-4033.

Schlosshauer B, Herzog K-H. 1990. Neurothelin: An inducible cell surface glycoprotein of blood-brain barrier-specific endothelial cells and distinct neurons. J Cell Biol 110: 1261-1274.

Schmidt S, Linington C, Zipp F, Sotgiu S, de Waal Malefyt R, et al. 1997. Multiple sclerosis: Comparison of the human T-cell response to S100 β and myelin basic protein reveals parallels to rat experimental autoimmune panencephalitis. Brain 120: 1437-1445.

Schwartzman ML, Masferrer J, Dunn MW, McGiff JC, Abraham NG. 1987. Cytochrome P450, drug metabolizing enzymes and arachidonic acid metabolism in bovine ocular tissues. Curr Eye Res 6: 623-630.

Seulberger H, Lottspeich F, Risau W. 1990. The inducible blood-brain barrier specific molecule HT7 is a novel immunoglobulin-like cell surface glycoprotein. EMBO J 9: 2151-2158.

Sharom FJ. 1997. The p-glycoprotein efflux pump: How does it transport drugs? J Membr Biol 160: 161-175.

Shih SC, Ju M, Liu N, Smith LE. 2003. Selective stimulation of VEGFR-1 prevents oxygen-induced retinal vascular degeneration in retinopathy of prematurity. J Clin Invest 112(1): 50-57.

Singhal SS, Godley BF, Chandra A, Pandya U, Jin GF, et al. 1999. Induction of glutathione S-transferase hGST 5.8 is an early response to oxidative stress in RPE cells. Invest Ophthalmol Vis Sci 40: 2652-2659.

Staddon JM, Herrenknecht K, Smales C, Rubin LL. 1995. Evidence that tyrosine phosphorylation may increase tight junction permeability. J Cell Sci 108: 609-619.

Stalmans I, Ng YS, Rohan R, Fruttiger M, Bouche A, et al. 2002. Arteriolar and venular patterning in retinas of mice selectively expressing VEGF isoforms. J Clin Invest 109(3): 327-336.

Steinberg RH, Miller SS. 1979. Transport and membrane properties of the retinal pigment epithelium. The Retinal Pigment Epithelium. Marmor MF, editor. Cambridge, Massachusetts and London, England: Harvard University Press; pp. 205-225.

Steinberg RH, Wood I. 1979. The relationship of the retinal pigment epithelium to photoreceptor outer segments in human retina. The Retinal Pigment Epithelium. Marmor MF, editor. Cambridge, Massachusetts and London, England: Harvard University Press; pp. 32-44.

Steuer H, Jaworski A, Elger B, Kaussmann M, Keldenich J, et al. 2005. Functional characterization and comparison of the outer blood-retina barrier and the blood-brain barrier. Invest Ophthalmol Vis Sci 46(3): 1047-1053.

Steuer H, Jaworski A, Stoll D, Schlosshauer B. 2004. In vitro model of the outer blood-retina barrier. Brain Res Brain Res Protoc 13(1): 26-36.

Stewart PA, Tuor UI. 1994. Blood-eye barriers in the rat—Correlation of ultrastructure with function. J Comp Neurol 340: 566-576.

Stewart PA, Wiley MJ. 1981. Developing nervous tissue induces formation of blood-brain barrier characteristics in invading endothelial cells: A study using quail-chick transplantation chimeras. Dev Biol 84: 183-192.

Strauss O, Mergler S, Wiederholt M. 1997. Regulation of L-type calcium channels by protein tyrosine kinase and protein kinase C in cultured rat and human retinal pigment epithelial cells. FASEB J 11: 859-867.

Sugiyama D, Kusuhara H, Shitara Y, Abe T, Meier PJ, et al. 2001. Characterization of the efflux transport of 17β-estradiol-D-17β-glucuronide from the brain across the blood-brain barrier. J Pharmacol Exp Ther 298(1): 316-322.

Takanaga H, Ohtsuki S, Hosoya K, Terasaki T. 2001. GAT2/BGT-1 as a system responsible for the transport of γ-aminobutyric acid at the mouse blood-brain barrier. J Cereb Blood Flow Metab 21: 1232-1239.

Terasaki T, Ohtsuki S, Hori S, Takanaga H, Nakashima E, et al. 2003. New approaches to in vitro models of blood-brain barrier drug transport. Drug Discov Today 8(20): 944-954.

Tervooren D, Heimann K, Bartz-Schmidt KU, Walter P, Weller M. 1998. Intravitreal daunomycin induces multidrug resistance in proliferative vitreoretinopathy. Invest Ophthalmol Vis Sci 39(1): 164-170.

Tomi M, Abukawa H, Nagai Y, Hata T, Takanaga H, et al. 2004. Retinal selectivity of gene expression in rat retinal versus brain capillary endothelial cell lines by differential display analysis. Mol Vis 10: 537-543.

Tontsch U, Bauer H-C. 1991. Glial cells and neurons induce blood-brain barrier related enzymes in cultured cerebral endothelial cells. Brain Res 539: 247-253.

Törnquist P, Alm A. 1986. Carrier-mediated transport of amino acids through the blood-retinal and the blood-brain barriers. Graefe's Arch Clin Exp Ophthalmol 224: 21-25.

Tso MO, Shih CY, McLean IW. 1975. Is there a blood-brain barrier at the optic nerve head? Arch Ophthalmol 93(9): 815-825.

Tsukita S, Furuse M, Itoh M. 1998. Molecular dissection of tight junctions: Occludin and ZO-1. Introduction to the Blood-Brain Barrier. Pardridge WM, editor. Cambridge: Cambridge University Press.

Vinores SA. 1995. Assessment of blood-retinal barrier integrity. Histol Histopath 10: 141-154.

Wenkel H, Streilein JW. 2000. Evidence that retinal pigment epithelium functions as an immune-privileged tissue. Invest Ophthalmol Vis Sci 2000 Oct 41(11): 3467–3473, 41: 3467-3473.

Wolburg H, Liebner S, Reichenbach A, Gerhardt H. 1999. The pecten oculi of the chicken: A model system for vascular differentiation and barrier maturation. Int Rev Cytol 187: 111-159.

Wolfensberger TJ. 1998. Toxicology of the retinal pigment epithelium. The Retinal Pigment Epithelium. Wolfensberger TJ, editor. Oxford: Oxford University Press; pp. 621-647.

Wong V, Gumbiner BM. 1997. A synthetic peptide corresponding to the extracellular domain of occludin perturbs the tight junction permeability barrier. J Cell Biol 136 (2): 399-409.

Wu DT, Woodman SE, Weiss JM, McManus CM, D'Aversa TG, et al. 2000. Mechanisms of leukocyte trafficking into the CNS. J Neurovirol 6 (Suppl. 1): S82-S85.

Wu GS, Rao NA. 1996. A novel retinal pigment epithelial protein suppresses neutrophil superoxide generation. I. Characterization of the suppressive factor. Exp Eye Res 63: 713-725.

Xu H, Forrester JV, Liversidge J, Crane IJ. 2003. Leukocyte trafficking in experimental autoimmune uveitis: Breakdown of blood-retinal barrier and upregulation of cellular adhesion molecules. Invest Ophthalmol Vis Sci 44(1): 226-234.

Yancopoulos GD, Davis S, Gale NW, Rudge JS, Wiegand SJ, et al. 2000. Vascular-specific growth factors and blood vessel formation. Nature 407(6801): 242-248.

Zauberman H. 1979. Adhesive forces between the retinal pigment epithelium and sensory retina. The Retinal Pigment Epithelium. Marmor MF, editor. Cambridge, Massachusetts and London, England: Harvard University Press; pp. 192-204.

Zhao S, Rizzolo LJ, Barnstable CJ. 1997. Differentiation and transdifferentiation of the retinal pigment epithelium. Int Rev Cytol 171: 225-266.

Zinn KM, Benjamin-Henkind JV. 1979. Anatomy of the human retinal pigment epithelium. The Retinal Pigment Epithelium. Marmor MF, editor. Cambridge, Massachusetts and London, England: Harvard University Press; pp. 3-31.

Index

Printing: Krips bv, Meppel
Binding: Stürtz, Würzburg